PLUMER'S
PRINCIPLES & PRACTICE OF
INFUSION THERAPY

TH EDITION

PLUMER'S
PRINCIPLES & PRACTICE OF
INFUSION THERAPY

NINTH EDITION

Sharon M. Weinstein, MS, RN, CRNI®, FACW, FAAN

President, Core Consulting Group
Buffalo Grove, Illinois
President, Global Education Development Institute
Adjunct Clinical Assistant Professor
The University of Illinois, Chicago College of Nursing
Advisory Board, Kaplan University School of Nursing
Chicago, Illinois

Infusion Nursing Consultant
Editorial Board, Journal of Infusion Nursing
Former Chair and Director Member
Board of Directors–Infusion Nurses Certification Corporation
Past President
Infusion Nurses Society, Inc.
Norwood, Massachusetts

Leader, Intravenous Therapy Delegations to People's Republic of China,
    Austria, Germany, Commonwealth of Independent States, and Egypt

Mary E. Hagle, PhD, RN, FAAN

Nurse Scientist, Department of Nursing Education and Research
Clement J. Zablocki VA Medical Center
Adjunct Clinical Assistant Professor
University of Wisconsin–Milwaukee
Milwaukee, Wisconsin

Member
Infusion Nurses Society Standards of Practice Committee
Former Director Member
Board of Directors–Infusion Nurses Certification Corporation
Norwood, Massachusetts

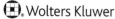 Wolters Kluwer

Health

Philadelphia · Baltimore · New York · London
Buenos Aires · Hong Kong · Sydney · Tokyo

Acquisitions Editor: Shannon Magee
Product Development Editor: Ashley Fischer
Production Project Manager: David Saltzberg
Senior Manufacturing Manager: Kathleen Brown
Marketing Manager: Mark Wiragh
Design Coordinator: Stephen Druding
Production Service: SPi Global

Library of Congress Cataloging-in-Publication Data
Weinstein, Sharon, author.
  Plumer's principles & practice of infusion therapy / Sharon M. Weinstein, Mary E. Hagle. — Ninth edition.
       p. ; cm.
  Plumer's principles and practice of infusion therapy
  Principles and practice of infusion therapy
  Preceded by Plumer's principles & practice of intravenous therapy / Sharon M. Weinstein. 8th ed. c2007.
  Includes bibliographical references and index.
  ISBN 978-1-4511-8885-1
  I. Hagle, Mary E., author. II. Title. III. Title: Plumer's principles and practice of infusion therapy.
IV. Title: Principles and practice of infusion therapy.
    [DNLM: 1. Infusions, Intravenous—methods. 2. Infusions, Intravenous—nursing. 3. Evidence-Based Medicine.
 4. Fluid Therapy—methods. 5. Nurse's Role. 6. Parenteral Nutrition—methods. WB 354]
  RM170
  615'.6—dc23
                                                                                              2013041203

Care has been taken to confirm the accuracy of the information presented and to describe generally accepted practices. However, the authors, editors, and publisher are not responsible for errors or omissions or for any consequences from application of the information in this book and make no warranty, expressed or implied, with respect to the currency, completeness, or accuracy of the contents of the publication. Application of the information in a particular situation remains the professional responsibility of the practitioner.

The authors, editors, and publisher have exerted every effort to ensure that drug selection and dosage set forth in this text are in accordance with current recommendations and practice at the time of publication. However, in view of ongoing research, changes in government regulations, and the constant flow of information relating to drug therapy and drug reactions, the reader is urged to check the package insert for each drug for any change in indications and dosage and for added warnings and precautions. This is particularly important when the recommended agent is a new or infrequently employed drug.

Some drugs and medical devices presented in the publication have Food and Drug Administration (FDA) clearance for limited use in restricted research settings. It is the responsibility of the health care provider to ascertain the FDA status of each drug or device planned for use in their clinical practice.

To purchase additional copies of this book, call our customer service department at (800) 638-3030 or fax orders to (301) 223-2320. International customers should call (301) 223-2300.

net: at LWW.com. Lippincott Williams & Wilkins customer service

RRS1401

10 9 8 7 6 5 4 3 2 1

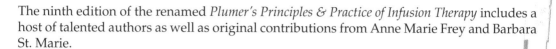

The ninth edition of the renamed *Plumer's Principles & Practice of Infusion Therapy* includes a host of talented authors as well as original contributions from Anne Marie Frey and Barbara St. Marie.

About Anne Marie Frey, BSN, RN, CRNI®, VA-BC

Anne Marie Frey is a Clinician Nurse Level Four, Vascular Access Service/I.V. Team at the Children's Hospital of Philadelphia (CHOP). Nationally certified by the Infusion Nurses Society (INS) since 1985, Anne Marie has served on national committees and has contributed to the nursing literature. She is a frequent presenter at professional society meetings. She was honored to receive the IV Nurse of the Year award from INS in 2008. She has contributed the Pediatrics Chapter to the Plumer book since the fifth edition; she is also the author of Infusion Therapy in Children in *Infusion Nursing: An Evidence-Based Approach*. With over 30 years in infusion therapy practice, Anne Marie is a renowned knowledge and practice expert.

About Barbara St. Marie, PhD, ANP, GNP

Barbara St. Marie is a nurse practitioner–supervisor in Pain and Palliative Care within the Fairview Health System. She is board certified as an Adult Nurse Practitioner, Gerontology Nurse Practitioner, and Pain Management Certified. She received her doctoral degree at the University of Wisconsin–Milwaukee and completed her postdoctoral research at the University of Iowa under Professor Keela Herr. Dr. St. Marie is editor of the Core Curriculum for Pain Management Nursing and original author of the Pain Management section of Plumer.

Acknowledgments

The authors acknowledge the expertise of **Emily Dix, RD, CNSC, CD**, dietitian for the cardiac intensive care unit at Children's Hospital of Wisconsin, in the development of Chapter 21, Pediatric Infusion Therapy. The contributions of Ms. Dix added greatly to this chapter. We also thank **Lynn Czaplewski, MS, RN, ACNS-BC, CRNI®, AOCNS**, Clinical Nurse Specialist at Froedert Hospital, Milwaukee, for her contribution to Chapter 16, Parenteral Nutrition. Several professionals associated with the Clement J. Zablocki VA Medical Center contributed their expertise to this text. The content is the responsibility of the individual authors alone and does not necessarily reflect the views or policies of the Department of Veterans Affairs or the US government, nor does mention of trade names, commercial products, or organizations imply endorsement by the US government.

Contributing Authors, in Alphabetical Order

Jeanne E. Braby, MSN, RN, CCRN
Unit-Based Advanced Practice Nurse
Cardiac Intensive Care Unit
Children's Hospital of Wisconsin
Milwaukee, Wisconsin
Chapter 21

Sherry Cannizzo, BSN, RN
Case Manager—Community Living Center
Clement J. Zablocki VA Medical Center
Milwaukee, Wisconsin
Chapter 22

Linda A. Cayan, MSN, RN-BC, CPN
Nurse Educator
Clement J. Zablocki VA Medical Center
Milwaukee, Wisconsin
Chapter 5

Ann M. Cook, MSN, RN
Nursing Instructor
Waukesha County Technical College
Pewaukee, Wisconsin
Chapter 14

Jayme L. Cotter, MS, RN, AOCNS
Clinical Nurse Specialist–Inpatient Oncology
Aurora St. Luke's Medical Center
Milwaukee, Wisconsin
Chapter 19

Deborah L. Gentile, PhD, RN-BC
Senior Research Scientist
Aurora Health Care
Aurora Sinai Medical Center–Nursing
    Research
Milwaukee, Wisconsin
Chapter 20

Maureen T. Greene, PhD, RN, CNS-BC,
    ACNP-BC
Critical Care APN, Nursing Research
    Coordinator
Wheaton Franciscan–St. Joseph Hospital
Milwaukee, Wisconsin
Chapter 15

Susan Gresser, MS, GCNS-BC, APNP
Clinical Nurse Specialist—RECC
Clement J. Zablocki VA Medical Center
Milwaukee, Wisconsin
Chapter 22

Mary E. Hagle, PhD, RN, FAAN
Nurse Scientist, Department of Nursing
    Education and Research
Clement J. Zablocki VA Medical Center
Adjunct Clinical Assistant Professor
University of Wisconsin–Milwaukee
Milwaukee, Wisconsin
Chapters 7, 10, 11, 13, 14, 16

Molly Hendricks, MS, RN, CNS-BC
Clinical Nurse Specialist
Clement J. Zablocki VA Medical Center
Milwaukee, Wisconsin
Chapter 17

Valerie Kolmer, MSN, RN, ACNS-BC
Clinical Nurse Specialist
Clement J. Zablocki VA Medical Center
Milwaukee, Wisconsin
Chapter 17

Lindsey M. Ladell, PharmD, BCPS
Clinical Pharmacy Specialist, Patient Safety
    Manager
Clement J. Zablocki VA Medical Center
Milwaukee, Wisconsin
Chapter 18

Martin Mikell, BBA/BSN, RN, CEN
Staff Nurse–Emergency Department/Research
    Trainee
Clement J. Zablocki VA Medical Center
Doctoral Student
University of Wisconsin–Milwaukee
Milwaukee, Wisconsin
Chapter 13

Julie L. Millenbruch, PhD, CRRN
At the time of this writing,
Associate Chief, Nursing Education and
    Research
Clement J. Zablocki VA Medical Center
Milwaukee, Wisconsin
Currently, Lecturer, Louise Herrington School of
    Nursing
Baylor University
Dallas, Texas
Chapter 5

Abigail Ranum, MS, MLS(ASCP)^{CM}
Research Health Scientist
Clement J. Zablocki VA Medical Center
Milwaukee, Wisconsin
Chapter 7

Wendi S. Redfern, MSN, RN, CCRN
Unit-Based Advanced Practice Nurse
Children's Hospital of Wisconsin
Milwaukee, Wisconsin
Chapter 21

Tina T. Smith, MS, RN-BC
Nurse Educator
Clement J. Zablocki VA Medical Center
Milwaukee, Wisconsin
Chapter 5

Barbara St. Marie, PhD, ANP, GNP, ACHPN
Nurse Practitioner–Supervisor, Pain and
  Palliative Care
Fairview Health System
Minneapolis, Minnesota
Chapter 20

Beth Ann Taylor, DHA, RN, NEA-BC
Associate Director, Patient/Nursing Services–
  Nurse Executive
Clement J. Zablocki VA Medical Center
Milwaukee, Wisconsin
Chapter 11

Sherry A. Tennies, MSN, RN
Patient Safety Fellow
Clement J. Zablocki VA Medical Center
Doctoral Student
University of Wisconsin–Milwaukee
Milwaukee, Wisconsin
Chapter 18

Kerry A. Twite, MSN, RN, AOCNS
Clinical Nurse Specialist–Oncology
Vince Lombardi Cancer Clinics
Aurora St. Luke's Medical Center
Milwaukee, Wisconsin
Chapter 19

Sharon M. Weinstein, MS, RN, CRNI®, FACW,
  FAAN
President, Core Consulting Group
Buffalo Grove, Illinois
President, Global Education Development
  Institute
Adjunct Clinical Assistant Professor
The University of Illinois, Chicago College of
  Nursing
Advisory Board, Kaplan University School of
  Nursing
Chicago, Illinois
Chapters 1–4, 6, 8–10, 12, 23, 24

Sol A. Yoder, PharmD, RPH, BCOP
Oncology Pharmacist
Aurora St. Luke's Medical Center
Milwaukee, Wisconsin
Chapter 19

For nearly 44 years, *Plumer's Principles & Practice of Infusion Therapy* has retained its position as the most reliable, complete source of information addressing intravenous therapy for practicing clinicians, educators, and students. Completely updated and revised to meet the changing needs of our professional practice, this ninth edition, like its predecessors, provides the most current base of knowledge available to those who share the responsibility of ensuring high-quality infusion care to patients in diverse clinical settings.

The practice of infusion therapy is a multifaceted one. Infusion therapy is at the core of patient care. Our practice continually evolves as a result of changing patient care delivery systems, the impact of managed care, reengineering of the health care system, and the impact of integrated health care delivery systems. These changes have had a dramatic impact on our professional practice as we move on the continuum from care delivered in the acute care environment to care delivered in alternative sites. One thing remains unchanged, however, and that is the continuous need for an unprecedented high level of expertise for delivering infusion therapy.

Plumer's Principles & Practice of Infusion Therapy, ninth edition, has been updated and reorganized to produce a resource that clearly exceeds these needs. The addition of even more boxes, tables, safety and legal issues, step-by-step directions, nursing alerts, tables, and references to the World Wide Web and evidence-based practice create an easy-to-use format with easy-to-access references. With a focus on the Licensed Independent Practitioner (LIP), you will recognize the changes that have been implemented. An integrated approach to content results in a streamlined five-section organization. Part 1 reviews the history of infusion therapy, risk reduction and performance improvement, legal safeguards, nursing role and responsibilities, application of the Infusion Nurses Society Standards of Practice, and Nurse and Patient Education. New content addresses shared governance models, knowledge sharing, mentoring, and applications for Magnet Recognition.

Part 2 has undergone extensive change. Now addressing assessment and monitoring, this section has been expanded to encompass fluid and electrolyte balance, principles of parenteral fluid administration, relevant anatomy and physiology, laboratory data, ongoing monitoring, and complications and nursing interventions as well as evidence-based infusion practice. A new section on sentinel events and reflex sympathetic dystrophy discusses the challenging clinical outcomes that we now face.

Part 3 has been renamed Clinical Decision Making. In this section, we present current information about infusion equipment and safety; methods for assessing product and equipment needs; short peripheral lines; central vascular access; and expanded approaches to access and monitoring, which encompasses intra-arterial, reservoir, subcutaneous infusion, intraventricular and intraosseous routes. New contributing authors have created a user-friendly section that meets your continuous learning needs.

Patient-Specific Therapies are addressed in the revamped Part 4. A plethora of talented contributing authors has created the most current and complete source of information available today. Mary E. Hagle led a team of clinical experts that completely updated the section on blood and blood component therapy, including factor II and factor V Leiden disorders, consistent with the dramatic changes in practice and the revised standards. The addition of a new coauthor to the chapter on pain expanded on the solid base of information created by

Barbara St. Marie, emphasizing practical aspects of care, IV conscious sedation, and continuous local anesthesia. The chapter on pharmacology applied to infusion therapy has been updated with an emphasis on therapeutic monitoring and drug level ranges.

Part 5 addresses Special Populations. The pediatric infusion therapy chapter has new co-authors who have updated Anne Marie Frey's original work. Infusion therapy in the older adult and across the continuum of care rounds out this section. And finally, the future of infusion nursing has been renamed The Future of Infusion Nursing: A Global Approach, with a focus on the growth of the specialty worldwide. Thus, we proudly offer you an updated, state-of-the-art ninth edition.

Revised to meet the needs of the clinician responsible for delivering high-quality infusion care, regardless of the clinical setting in which care is provided, *Plumer's Principles & Practice of Infusion Therapy*, ninth edition, retains its place as the most essential tool available in infusion practice today. May you enjoy it and gain value from it.

Sharon M. Weinstein, MS, RN, CRNI®, FACW, FAAN

ACKNOWLEDGMENTS

Plumer's Principles & Practice of Infusion Therapy, ninth edition, is the result of the collaborative efforts of its original authors, Ada Lawrence Plumer and Faye Cosentino, and the contributions of veteran authors Anne Marie Frey and Barbara St. Marie, Mary E. Hagle, and myself. This edition welcomes a coauthor, Mary E. Hagle and the contributions of a team of collaborators from multiple national medical centers. We are so grateful to them for their valuable contributions to this text, and for the contributions that they have individually and collectively made to our professional practice. I would also like to thank the manufacturers of infusion products and equipment for their information and assistance, as well as the authors and publishers who permitted use of their copyrighted materials in producing this text.

A special thank you to Lisa Marshall for her encouragement, support, and technical assistance in developing a superior manuscript—one that readily supports the Plumer name.

Thanks are extended to William Eudailey, PharmD and to the late David Blaess, RPh, who served as my mentors and who taught me to apply the principles gleaned from Plumer's book to my daily practice. Men of vision, they gave me the opportunity to explore the world of infusion therapy.

There are so many professionals in the infusion specialty whose names are synonymous with quality; these individuals are seasoned professionals as well as novices. You will continue to generate passion for infusion therapy in those with whom you work for years to come. You may have been taught by one of your mentors or colleagues; you, in turn, have the responsibility to teach others. We must develop future generations of leaders in the infusion specialty practice; we must think globally with a vision for the future. Thus, once again, all proceeds from the ninth edition of Plumer will go to the Global Education Development Institute, an organization whose mission is to foster the professional and personal growth of nurse leaders in developing countries.

And so, to the countless numbers of infusion specialty nurses throughout the world who promote quality outcomes each and every day of their lives, regardless of the clinical setting in which care is delivered, this book is for you.

Finally, thanks to my husband Steve, and to my family, for delighting in and acknowledging my continuing passion for infusion therapy.   — SMW

Infusion therapy is not done in isolation, nor is advancing our practice, professional development, or creating a text that serves as a resource for nurses new to infusion therapy or experts from different areas. It has been a pleasure promoting a team of clinicians to share their expertise from all areas of practice that support infusion therapy. It is a privilege to work with Sharon again and bring a new edition to realization.

Grateful appreciation is extended to Mark and my family for their questions, humor, and limitless support to advance quality and safety in health care and infusion therapy.   —MEH

SPECIAL ACKNOWLEDGMENTS

As Plumer's reaches 44 years as the *premier* source of information in infusion therapy, it is appropriate to recognize the woman who first penned this text. The name Ada Plumer is synonymous with infusion therapy. A leader, pacesetter, and cofounder of the professional society, Plumer set the tone for our professional practice, served as a mentor to many nurses, and encouraged excellence in the delivery of intravenous nursing care. Ms. Plumer wrote, "In spite of the increasing use and importance of parenteral therapy, little training is required of the average therapist to carry it out. It is considered sufficient by some that the therapist be able to perform a venipuncture. This does not contribute to the optimal care of the patient whose prognosis depends upon intravenous therapy. The purpose of this book is to present a source of practical information essential to safe and successful therapy." Ada Plumer was a visionary; little could she know that the knowledge base would expand to such a critical level, and that infusion nurses would advance from novice to expert, continuing to educate nurses through publication of their findings, their practices, and their research.

From my first entry into this rapidly changing field to today, I have used Plumer's book as a reference, a guide, and a bible for professional practice. Plumer's retains its position today as the only complete source of information available to the practicing clinician, student, and educator. The success of the current edition is attributed to Plumer ... the growth of our practice is likewise a result of her initial efforts; we remember her with great respect. Many thanks from all of us in whom you have instilled a passion for excellence in infusion nursing practice.

CONTENTS

LIST OF TABLES

PART 1

OVERVIEW OF INFUSION THERAPY

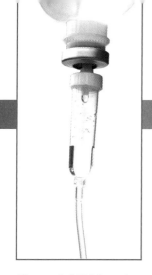

CHAPTER 1

History of Infusion Therapy

Sharon M. Weinstein

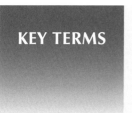

KEY TERMS	Hypotonicity	Safety
	Isotonic	Quill and Bladder
	Parenteral	Standards of Practice
	Pyrogens	

EARLY HISTORY AND METHODOLOGY

Almost 400 years have passed since the discovery of blood circulation. William Harvey's 1628 research stimulated increased experimentation, and he found that the heart is both a muscle and a pump.

Renaissance Period

In 1656, Sir Christopher Wren, the famed architect of St. Paul's Cathedral in London, injected opium intravenously into dogs. Wren, known as the father of modern intravenous (IV) therapy, used a **quill and bladder**. In 1662, Johann Majors made the first successful injection of unpurified compounds into human beings, although death resulted from infection at the injection site.

In 1665, an animal near death from loss of blood was saved by the infusion of blood from another animal. In 1667, a 15-year-old Parisian boy was the first human to receive a transfusion successfully; lamb's blood was administered directly into the boy's circulation by Jean Baptiste Denis, physician to Louis XIV (Cosnett, 1989). The enthusiasm aroused by this success led to promiscuous transfusions of blood from animals to humans with fatal results, and in 1687, by an edict of church and parliament, animal-to-human transfusions were prohibited in Europe. Nearly 150 years passed before serious attempts were again made to inject blood into people.

The 19th Century

James Blundell, an English obstetrician, revived the idea of blood transfusion. In 1834, saving the lives of many women threatened by hemorrhage during childbirth, he proved that animal blood was unfit to inject into humans and that only human blood was safe. Nevertheless, there were **safety** concerns, and complications persisted, with infections developing in donors and recipients. With the discovery of the principles of antisepsis by Pasteur and Lister, another obstacle was overcome, although reactions and deaths continued.

The first recorded attempt to prevent coagulation during transfusion was in 1821 by Jean Louis Prévost, a French physician who, with Jean B. A. Dumas, used defibrinated blood in animal transfusions (Cosnett, 1989).

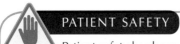

PATIENT SAFETY

Patient safety has been a concern since the 19th century.

In the middle to late 19th century, increased knowledge of bacteriology, pharmacology, and pathology led to new approaches. Ignaz Semmelweis, a Viennese obstetrician, was the first to correlate the effect of hand washing on prevention of infection. Semmelweis is credited with a 90% reduction of maternal deaths between 1846 and 1848. Meanwhile, chemist Louis Pasteur was proving that bacteria were living microorganisms, although his ideas were challenged by many researchers and practitioners.

In 1889, William Halsted of the Johns Hopkins Hospital, in cooperation with Goodyear Rubber Company, introduced the use of surgical gloves in the operating theater. Ten years later, the use of rubber gloves was widely accepted as a means of protecting patients and physicians (Sutcliff, 1992).

In 1896, the H. Wulfing Luer Company of France developed the Luer connection, allowing the head of a hypodermic needle to be easily attached and detached from a glass syringe. This connection, which is composed of tapering male and female components, is still used today to attach various pieces in an IV line. These interlocking pieces allow practitioners to change IV bags, add additional drip lines, and attach the IV tubing to the needle with minimal discomfort to the patient.

French physiologist Claude Bernard is credited with experimental injection of sugar solutions into dogs. The precursor to modern nutritional support, Bernard's experiments were followed by the subcutaneous injection of fat, milk, and camphor by Menzel and Perco in Vienna. Work in nutritional support remained at a standstill for many years.

Twentieth-Century Advances

In the 20th century, IV therapy advanced rapidly. Blood transfusions and **parenteral** fluids, which bypass the intestines, were administered, and parenteral nutrition became possible as well. Moreover, nurses became skilled in both administering and monitoring infusions.

Tʀᴀɴsfusɪᴏɴ Tʜᴇʀᴀᴘʏ

In 1900, Karl Landsteiner proved that not all human blood is alike when he identified four main classifications. In 1914, sodium citrate was found to prevent blood from clotting (Cosnett, 1989), and since then, rapid advances have been made (Table 1-1).

TABLE 1-1	TWENTIETH- AND TWENTY-FIRST-CENTURY PROGRESS IN INFUSION THERAPY
Year	Significant Advancement
1900	Karl Landsteiner discovered three of four main blood groups
1914	Sodium citrate was first used to preserve blood
	Hydrolyzed protein and fats were administered to animals
1925	Dextrose was used as an infusate
1935	Marriot and Kekwick introduced slow-drip method of transfusion
1937	Rose identified amino acids essential for growth
1940	Disposable plastic administration sets were developed
1945	Flexible intravenous (IV) cutdown catheter was introduced
1950	Rochester needle was introduced
1960	Peripherally inserted catheter lines were introduced in intensive care areas
1963–1965	First success with hyperalimentation at the University of Pennsylvania
1964	First disposable intravenous catheter introduced by Deseret
1970	Centers for Disease Control (CDC) guidelines for IV therapy were published
	First edition of *Plumer's Principles and Practice of Intravenous Therapy* was published
1972	Access with implanted ports was introduced
1972	The American Association of IV Nurses was organized by Ada Plumer, Marguerite Knight, and colleagues
1973	The professional society name was changed to reflect a more inclusive audience—National Intravenous Therapy Association (NITA)
	Broviac tunneled catheter was introduced
1976	Fat emulsions were used for nutritional support
1980	NITA Standards of Practice was published
	NITA National Office opened
	IV Nurse Day was recognized by U.S. House of Representatives
1981	CDC Guidelines were revised and published
1982	Implantable ports were used for long-term access
	First IV teaching program in People's Republic of China
1983	Home blood transfusion initiated
	Osteoport was developed
1984	Core Curriculum for Intravenous Nursing was published
1985	Intravenous Nurses Certification Corporation offered its first credentialing examination (CRNI)
1986	Use of patient-controlled analgesia increased

(Continued)

TABLE 1-1	TWENTIETH- AND TWENTY-FIRST-CENTURY PROGRESS IN INFUSION THERAPY (*Continued*)
Year	**Significant Advancement**
1987	Development by the Centers for Disease Control and Prevention (CDC) of "standard precautions"
1987	NITA changed its name to the Intravenous Nurses Society (INS)
1990	Safe Medical Device Act and Food and Drug Administration Device Reporting regulations published
	INS Revised Standards of Practice published
1992	U.S. Food and Drug Administration issued alert concerning needlestick injuries
1995	Occupational Safety and Health guidelines for handling cytotoxic drugs published
1996	LPNI examination offered to LPN/LVNs by INS
	CDC Guidelines revised and published
1998	INS celebrated its 25th Anniversary (Houston, TX)
1999	Journal of Intravenous Nursing offered CE/recertification units
2000	Core Curriculum for Intravenous Nursing, 2nd edition, published
	Revised Standards of Practice published
	INS Policies and Procedures Manual published
	CRNI Exam Preparation Guide & Practice Questions published
	First public member added to the INS board of directors
2001	The organization's name again changed to the Infusion Nurses Society reflecting the expansive role of the infusion nursing specialist
2002	Publication of the CDC *Guidelines for the Prevention of Intravascular Catheter-Related Infections* supporting the use of trained personnel
2003	Core Curriculum for Infusion Nursing, 3rd edition, published
	Infusion Nurses Society celebrates its 30th year
2004	Infusion Nurses Society Standards for Adult Patients published
2005	Revised Infusion Nurses Standards of Practice published
2006	*Plumer's Principles and Practice of Intravenous Therapy*, 8th edition, published
2006	Revised Infusion Nurses Standards of Practice published
2006	Initiation of central line bundling recommendations by the Institute for Healthcare Improvement
2011	Policies and Procedures for Infusion Nursing, 4th edition, published by the Infusion Nurses Society
2011	Revised Infusion Nurses Standards of Practice published
2012	Policies and Procedures for Infusion Nursing of the Older Adult published by the Infusion Nurses Society
2013	Infusion Nurses Society celebrates its 40th year where it began
2014	*Plumer's Principles and Practice of Infusion Therapy*, 9th edition, published with a name change to reflect current practice and a co-author

In 1911, Dr. Ottenberg of New York demonstrated the use of donor blood; his theory that safe transfusion was possible from a donor whose serum agglutinated the recipient's red blood cells was readily accepted. Dr. Ottenberg further suggested that it was unsafe to use a donor whose red blood cells were acted on by the recipient's serum. These research findings evolved into the universal donor concept still valid today.

Hugh Leslie Marriot and Alan Kekwick, English physicians, introduced the continuous slow-drip method of blood transfusion; their findings were published in 1935 (Cosnett, 1989).

The Rh factor was discovered in 1940, and the American Association of Blood Banks was formed in 1947. The invention of the first cell separator in 1951 introduced component therapy (for more information, see Chapter 19).

PARENTERAL FLUIDS

Administration of parenteral fluids by the IV route has been widely used only since the late 1950s. The difficulty in accepting this procedure resulted from the lack of safe fluids. The fluids then in use contained substances called **pyrogens**, proteins that are foreign to the body and not destroyed by sterilization. These caused chills and fever when injected into the circulation. The 1923 discovery and elimination of pyrogens led to safer and more frequent IV administration of parenteral fluids. In 1925, the most frequently used parenteral fluid was normal saline (0.9% sodium chloride). Because of its **hypotonicity**, water could not be administered IV and had to be made **isotonic**. A certain percentage of sodium chloride added to water achieved this effect (Cosnett, 1989). After 1925, dextrose was used extensively to make isotonic fluids and provide a source of calories.

By 1939, Dr. Robert Elman infused a solution of 2% casein hydrolysate and 8% dextrose without adverse effects; thus began the movement toward development of protein hydrolysates.

INFUSION NURSING

Massachusetts General Hospital is credited with many firsts in medical history. The first nurse to hold the title "IV nurse" is known to have practiced at this Boston hospital. That nurse, Ada Plumer was a cofounder of the National Intravenous Therapy Association (NITA), along with Marguerite Knight, infusion nurse at Johns Hopkins Hospital. The NITA is now known as the Infusion Nurses Society (INS). Ms. Plumer was also the original author of this text.

Early on, IV nurses were responsible for phlebotomy, transfusion therapy, venipuncture, and maintaining equipment. Emphasis was placed on the technical responsibility of maintaining the infusion and keeping the needle and tubing apparatus patent. The sole requisite for being an IV nurse was the ability to perform a venipuncture skillfully.

At the time, IV therapy was limited to use in surgery and treating dehydration. Infusates were administered through rubber administration sets and 16- to 18-gauge steel needles strategically placed in the antecubital fossa and secured with an arm board.

As knowledge of electrolyte and fluid therapy grew, more parenteral fluids became available, and additional knowledge was then needed to monitor the fluid and electrolyte status of the patient. The nurse assigned to the patient in need of IV therapy was expected to have a working knowledge of fluid and electrolyte balance and to assess the "whole" patient in terms of fluid needs. Normal saline was no longer the only electrolyte fluid. Today, more than 200 commercially prepared IV fluids are available to meet patients' needs.

PARENTERAL NUTRITION

W. C. Rose identified amino acids in 1937, leading to the development of protein hydrolysates for human infusion. A whole new approach to IV therapy and a respite to the starving patient evolved between 1963 and 1965, when members of the Harrison Department of Surgical Research at the University of Pennsylvania showed that sufficient nutrients could be given to juvenile beagles to support normal growth and development (Cosnett, 1989). This led to what is known today as *total parenteral nutrition* (TPN).

In the mid-1960s, as a result of animal TPN research, Stanley Dudrick developed the first formula for parenteral nutrition, a method by which sufficient nutrients are administered into the central vein to support life and maintain growth and development.

Fats as a calorie source were also studied, but the adverse reactions proved too severe, and the U.S. Food and Drug Administration banned the use of fats in the United States in 1964. A refined product derived from soybean and safflower oil was approved for administration in 1980.

Home TPN was introduced in 1983. Research into the use of antioxidants, the role of amino acids, and indications for medium-, short-, and long-chain triglycerides in TPN continues today (Grant, 1992).

EARLY INFUSION DEVICES AND EQUIPMENT

Until and even into the 1950s, IV sets consisted of steel reusable needles with a stylet inside to keep the lumen open. The plastic revolution evolved when Dr. David Massa, an anesthesia resident at the Mayo clinic, shortened a 16-gauge Becton Dickinson needle and inserted another steel needle as an inner stylet. A polyvinyl chloride catheter was placed over the needle and was attached to a metal hub via a crimp band. Thus, the first "over-the-needle" configuration was developed (Rivera, Strauss, vanZundert, & Mortier, 2005). After several iterations, it became the Rochester needle, a resinous catheter on the outside of a steel introducer needle. Available only as a 16-gauge, the entire unit measured 5 mm or 2 inches. On successful insertion, the catheter was slipped off the needle into the vein and the needle was removed. Desert Pharmaceutical Co. introduced the Intracath in 1958, minimizing the need for surgical cutdown; the first disposable device, the Angiocath was introduced in 1964. McGaw Laboratories introduced the first small vein set with foldable wings in 1957; this product is still known today as a winged infusion needle.

Dudrick adapted the subclavian approach for the administration of high concentrations of dextrose and proteins in 1967. Expansion of this concept led to the creation of the Broviac catheter, initially designed for use in pediatrics; a larger size (Hickman) was developed for the adult population. Since the 1980s, tunneled and nontunneled catheters have enhanced central venous access. The port soon followed, and totally implanted access devices are now used routinely. The peripherally inserted central catheter (PICC) was introduced in the last quarter of the 20th century.

The first IV fluid containers were made of glass. Plastic bags were introduced in the 1970s. Because they do not require air venting, these containers reduced the risks of air embolism and airborne contamination. Today, plastic is the primary container for IV fluids, whereas glass containers are used when fluid stability in plastic is a concern.

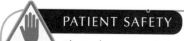

> **PATIENT SAFETY**
>
> Plastic bags were introduced in the 1970s. Because they do not require air venting, these containers reduced the risks of air embolism and airborne contamination.

In the mid-1940s, disposable plastic IV administration sets became available and eventually replaced the reusable rubber tubings. Manufacturers have continued to keep pace with demands for technologically advanced products that ensure patient safety and reliability in the delivery of infusion therapy. Polypropylene, nylon, and Dynaflex are some of the more common materials from which that IV tubing is made. As plastics, these synthetic materials can be manufactured to meet this need; they are flexible, strong, and leakproof and do not react with the chemicals transported through them. Manufacturers of IV tubing have the capacity to create tubing of various thicknesses consistent with specifications given to them.

The use of electronic infusion devices to assist in controlling flow has changed the face of infusion nursing by improving the safety and accuracy of the process and reducing adverse events. Many devices can now be connected to the institution's information system and thus enhance electronic documentation.

Progress in Clinical Practice

In the 1970s, tremendous scientific, technologic, and medical advances occurred, and IV therapy gained recognition as a highly specialized field. Nurses performed many of the functions formerly reserved for the medical staff—intra-arterial therapy, neonatal therapy, and antineoplastic therapy. Professional societies were established to provide a forum for the exchange of ideas, knowledge, and experiences, with the ultimate goal of raising standards and increasing the level of patient care.

On October 1, 1980, the United States House of Representatives recognized the profession and declared an official day of honor for IV nurses: "Resolved, that IV Nurse Day be nationally celebrated in honor of the National Intravenous Therapy Association, Inc., on January 25 of each year." The proclamation was presented by the Honorable Edward J. Mackey from the Fifth Congressional District of the Commonwealth of Massachusetts (Gardner, 1982).

Today, the infusion nurse with responsibility for PICC insertion is often involved in the reading of x-ray films to ensure placement. This has allowed timelier implementation of orders and improved patient care.

THE INFUSION NURSES SOCIETY, INC.

The INS has continued to grow worldwide. Educational offerings have expanded to include advanced studies in an effort to meet the needs of the advanced practitioner. INS is the premier resource for infusion education and knowledge sharing.

Credentialing

The Infusion Nurses Certification Corporation (INCC) has credentialed thousands of nurses across the globe. Professional IV nurses are encouraged to prepare for the credentialing process through educational programming, webinars, the INS Knowledge Center, clinical nursing forum, a revised core curriculum, the society's professional journal, clinical textbooks, and published Standards of Practice. Box 1-1 describes the vision, mission and values of the INCC.

There are nine core content areas of the examination including technology and clinical application, fluid and electrolyte therapy, pharmacology, infection control, transfusion therapy, antineoplastic and biologic therapy, parenteral nutrition, performance improvement, and pediatrics. Successful completion of the examination results in the nurse being awarded the CRNI designation. Recertification is obtained through reexamination or validation of clinical practice and documentation of 40 recertification units earned during the previous 3-year period.

Because delivery of IV therapy permeates all clinical settings, the role of the IV nurse is now well established as integral to multidisciplinary, high-quality care in all practice settings (Baranowski, 1995). The growth of this specialty practice has expanded the roles of IV nurses nationally and internationally. IV nurses are constantly striving to find new and more efficient ways to perform their services in an integrated health care environment.

BOX 1-1   INFUSION NURSES CERTIFICATION CORPORATION

Vision

Certification, by INCC, is the standard of excellence that nurses will seek in order to provide optimal infusion care that the public expects, demands, and deserves.

Mission

INCC promotes excellence in infusion nursing certification by:
- Developing and administering a comprehensive, evidence-based program
- Advocating the importance of the CRNI credential
- Supporting continuous infusion nursing education and research

Values

Integrity — We are committed to providing a psychometrically sound, legally defensible certification program.

Public Protection — We support the role certified nurses play in promoting optimal health outcomes and ensuring that our program is driven by the needs of the public.

Excellence — We are committed to providing a program of high quality and are dedicated to a process of continuous improvement.

Source: Infusion Nurses Certification Corporation. (2013). *CRNI Exam Handbook March 2013.* Retrieved from http://www.incc1.org/i4a/pages/index.cfm?pageid=1

INFUSION NURSING IN THE 21st CENTURY

Nurses continue to lead the labor sector throughout the United States, and advanced-practice nursing has grown dramatically (Kalisch & Kalisch, 1995). In the January/February 2007 issue of *Health Affairs*, Dr. David I. Auerbach and colleagues estimated that the U.S. shortage of registered nurses (RNs) will increase to 340,000 by the year 2020. The study is titled "Better Late than Never: Workforce Supply Implications of Late Entry into Nursing" (Auerbach, 2007). According to the latest projections from the U.S. Bureau of Labor Statistics (2005) published in the Monthly Labor Review, more than 1.2 million new and replacement nurses will be needed by 2014. Government analysts project that more than 703,000 new RN positions will be created through 2014, which will account for two-fifths of all new jobs in the health care sector. With new graduates producing a relatively new workforce in many institutions, there will be an increasing need for IV resource experts.

The challenge for nurses is to effect health policy through use of their knowledge and skills. Wakefield (1999) stated that the value assigned to nursing will be based on a standard that measures how the profession effects access and achieves the highest-quality care at the lowest cost. Infusion therapy has evolved from a form of treatment for the most critically ill to a highly specialized form of treatment used for 90% or more of all hospitalized patients. No longer confined to the hospital setting, infusion therapies are now delivered in alternative care sites such as the home, skilled nursing facilities, and physician offices.

Infusion nursing is now recognized as a highly specialized practice. During the last 60 years, the role of the nurse in infusion therapy has evolved tremendously. The 21st century infusion nurse is responsible for integrating the holistic principles of medicine and nursing, management, marketing, education, and performance improvement into the patient's plan of care. Clinical expertise is of utmost importance (INS, 2011).

Review Questions   *Note: Questions below may have more than one right answer.*

1. The clinical use of amino acids led to the development of which of the following?
   A. Antioxidants
   B. Home total parenteral nutrition
   C. Protein hydrolysates
   D. Triple-mix fluid

2. The initial role of the IV specialist included which of the following?
   A. Phlebotomy
   B. Crossmatching of blood
   C. Maintaining equipment
   D. Maintaining IV lines

3. Three of the four main blood groups were discovered by:
   A. Karl Landsteiner
   B. Florence Seibert
   C. William Halsted
   D. W. C. Rose

4. The first national certification examination for nurses was offered in:
   A. 1983
   B. 1985
   C. 1988
   D. 1991

5. Primary fluids in use in the mid-1950s included:

A. Lactated Ringer's injection

B. 5% Dextrose in water

C. 0.9% Sodium chloride (normal saline)

D. 0.45% Sodium chloride (half-normal saline)

References and Selected Readings　*Asterisks indicate references cited in text.*

*Auerbach, D. (2007). *Better late than never: Workforce supply implications of late entry into nursing.* http://content.healthaffairs.org/cgi/content/abstract/26/1/178

*Baranowski, L. (1995). Presidential address: Take ownership. *Journal of Intravenous Nursing, 18*(4), 163.

*Cosnett, J.E. (1989). Before our time: The origins of intravenous fluid therapy. *Lancet, 4,* 768–771.

*Gardner, C. (1982). United States House of Representatives honors the National Intravenous Therapy Association, Inc. *Journal of the National Intravenous Therapy Association, 5*(1), 14.

*Grant, J.P. (1992). *Handbook of total parenteral nutrition* (3rd ed., pp. 21–29). Philadelphia, PA: W.B. Saunders.

Griffith, J.M., Thomas, N., & Griffith, L. (1991). MDs bill for these routine nursing tasks. *American Journal of Nursing, 90*(10), 65–73.

*INS (2011). *Role of the infusion nurse in clinical practice.* http://www.ins1.org/i4a/pages/index.cfm?pageid=3563

*Kalisch, P.A., & Kalisch, B.J. (1995). *The advance of American nursing* (3rd ed.). Philadelphia, PA: J.B. Lippincott.

*Rivera, A.M., Strauss, K.W., vanZundert, A, & Mortier, E. (2005). The history of peripheral intravenous catheters: How little plastic tubes revolutionized medicine. *Acta Anaesthesiologica Belgica, 56,* 271–282, http://www.sarb.be/fr/journal/artikels_acta_2005/artikels_acta_56_3/acta_56_3_rivera.pdf

Salsberg, E., Wing, P., & Brewer, C. (1998). Projecting the future supply and demand for registered nurses. In E. O'Neil & J. Coffman (Eds.), *Strategies for the future of nursing.* San Francisco, CA: Jossey-Bass.

*Sutcliff, J. (1992). *A history of medicine.* New York: Barnes & Noble.

*Wakefield, M. (1999). Nursing's future in health care policy. In E. Sullivan (Ed.), *Creating nursing's future* (pp. 41–49). St. Louis, MO: Mosby.

*U.S. Bureau of Labor Statistics (November 2005). *Monthly Labor Review,* www.bls.gov/opub/mlr/2005/11/art5full.pdf

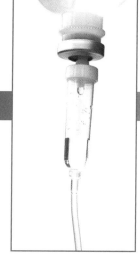

Minimizing Risk and Enhancing Performance

Sharon M. Weinstein

Benchmarking
Competence
Competency
Culture of safety
Documentation
External drivers
Licensed
   Independent
   Practitioner

Malpractice
Outcomes
Patient Safety
Performance
   Improvement
Plan of Corrective
   Action
Regulating Agencies
Sentinel Event

PROFESSIONAL NURSING PRACTICE AND LEGAL SAFEGUARDS

The goal of safe infusion care is to minimize risk and improve outcomes. The key factor in this process is ensuring **patient safety**. Each chapter in this edition addresses patient safety. This chapter focuses on a broader view and the need to create and maintain a **culture of safety**.

The law and its interpretation can lead to doubts and questions regarding the legal rights and obligations of nurses to administer infusion therapy. Legal standards are an integral component of a **performance improvement** (PI) program. As infusion practice becomes more complex and specialized, and as infusion experts gain international acceptance, nurses are becoming more involved in procedures formerly performed solely by physicians/**licensed independent practitioners** (LIPs). Because violation of the Medical Practice Act is a criminal offense, infusion nurses need to be well versed on the subject and the law, not only to protect themselves but also to ensure safe **outcomes** for their patients.

BOX 2-1 STRATEGIES FOR REDUCING RISKS RELATED TO INFUSION THERAPY

- Keep informed of laws and regulations governing practice.
- Stay up-to-date on defined standards of practice and their clinical application.
- File incident reports and record sentinel events (unforeseen outcomes resulting in a negative response to treatment) as appropriate.
- Ensure that informed consent is obtained and on file as needed.
- Participate in product evaluation processes and ensure safe use by providing internal product education.
- Maintain continued competency in your professional practice; ensure that you meet credentialing criteria.
- Monitor patients' responses and unforeseen reactions to treatment; document these events appropriately and in a timely manner.
- Ensure that safety standards are maintained; be aware of OSHA regulations; practice risk management.
- Participate in the quality improvement process in your institution.

To clarify the roles of nurses and physicians/LIPs in various aspects of health care, joint policy statements have been issued by the medical societies and nursing associations on a number of procedures, including infusion therapy (Box 2-1).

External Drivers That Influence Safety

External drivers that influence the quality of nursing care include regulation and legislation, accrediting organizations, efforts to link payment with performance, the need for interdisciplinary guidelines, the commitment of professional organizations, and the level of public engagement. **Regulating agencies** issue mandates that directly or indirectly impact the role of the health care professional, in this case, the infusion nurse. These agencies include the Food and Drug Administration (FDA), the Occupational Safety and Health Administration (OSHA), the Joint Commission (TJC), state regulatory boards, and professional organizations.

Federal Statutes

Federal statutes are laws enacted by Congress and published in the *Federal Register*. Such laws relevant to IV nursing include those addressing occupational health and safety, infection control, environmental hazards, medical device safety, control of drug abuse, federally funded insurance programs, and patient self-determination acts (Table 2-1).

Applying Law to Practice

In organizations or hospitals, as well as in states in which no written opinion relevant to IV therapy exists, nurses are legally required to perform any nursing or medical procedure they are directed to carry out by a duly licensed physician/LIP unless they have reason to

TABLE 2-1	SOURCES OF STANDARDS OF CARE RELATED TO INFUSION THERAPY	
Source	**Agency**	**Examples of Standard**
Federal statutes	OSHA	• Hazard Communication Standard Practice Guidelines for Handling Cytotoxic Drugs • Occupational Safe Exposure to Bloodborne Pathogens
	United States FDA	• Safe Medical Device Act of 1990
	Drug Enforcement Agency (DEA)	• Controlled Substances Act
State statutes	Department of Health Board of Nursing	• Licensure of health care facilities
	Board of Regents	• Nurse Practice Act
Private/ professional bodies	The Joint Commission (TJC) ANA IOM	• Accreditation manual for hospitals and health care organizations • Accreditation manual for home health care • Quality reports
	INS	Standards of Nursing Practice and position papers
	AABB	Infusion Nursing Standards of Practice
	ECRI	Technical manual
		Health devices standard nomenclature
Institutional bodies	Infusion Therapy or Nursing Department	Job descriptions; nursing policies and procedures

believe harm will result to the patient from doing so. To meet their legal responsibilities to patients, nurses must be qualified by knowledge and experience to execute the procedure; otherwise, they may properly refuse to perform it.

In cases in which the nurse finds no medical reason to question a physician/LIP's order, the nurse's failure to carry out such an order subjects him or her to liability for any consequent harm to the patient. It has been established by law that in a question of negligence, individuals are not protected because they have "carried out the physician/LIP's orders." Rather, they are held liable in relation to their knowledge, skill, and judgment or lack thereof.

Several states recommend that schools and colleges of professional nursing include an IV therapy course in the curriculum. The course should provide the student nurse with clinical instruction and experience in IV therapy. Infusion nursing specialists nationwide have been instrumental in developing the content for such programs.

CONTRACTED PERSONNEL OR FLEXIBLE STAFFING

Cyclic staff shortages create a market niche for the interim or long-term use of contracted personnel. Thus, nurses working in institutions that use contracted nurses as well as nurses whose employers are contracted agencies must be aware of their own accountability for their actions and practice in addition to their accountability to their employers, patients, and colleagues. The Institute of Medicine (IOM) report identified the need for all health care organizations to have in place mechanisms to achieve "flexible" staffing in instances when the patient census, acuity, or both demand staffing at a higher level than anticipated. The IOM recommends using internal nursing "float pools" composed of nurses employed by the health care organization. Although using floating nurses may still result in nurses being assigned to patient care units with which they are less familiar, using an organization's own float pool of employed nurses at least assures that these nurses have received the same orientation and in-house training as other nursing staff permanently assigned to specific nursing units. Float pools would also assure that, even if the floating nurses are not familiar with policies and procedures unique to individual patient care units within the organization, the nurses would be familiar with organization-wide policies and practices pertaining to patient safety, such as an organization's error reporting system, decision support systems, and information technologies (Page, 2008).

PRIVATE DUTY NURSE

A private duty nurse, who works under the direction, supervision, and control of a hospital and private physician/LIP, is subject to the rules and regulations of the hospital concerning all matters relating to nursing care. The institution's joint policy statement may note that the private duty nurse who has complied with the criteria applicable to the administration of IV therapy may give an IV infusion.

AGENCY NURSE

Nationwide, temporary staffing agencies provide valuable assistance during shortages of licensed professional personnel. When given responsibility for the administration of intravascular therapies, agency personnel must be oriented to the health care facility's policies and procedures and the functions performed by specialized department personnel. When the facility must use agency staff, every effort should be made to ensure patient safety, public protection, and viability of the IV therapy program.

ALLIED PERSONNEL

Because of downsizing, restructuring, and nursing shortages in many areas of the country, various aspects of IV therapy may be performed by allied health personnel other than by registered nurses (RNs), such as licensed practical nurses (LPNs), licensed vocational nurses (LVNs), and patient care technicians (PCTs). When performing IV care, LPNs or LVNs must have the necessary preparation and experience. In addition, they must be authorized by their employer and by the state in which they work before they perform any procedures. LPNs and LVNs are governed by the Nurse Practice Act in their state and are accountable for any procedure they accept and perform. PCTs, depending on their training and place of employment, may be trained to set up the equipment to start an IV or to monitor the IV while it is in place.

Guarding Against Malpractice

The IV nurse's risk of involvement in malpractice suits is increasing with the increasing complexity of therapy and delegation of responsibility for infusion therapy in some institutions to less qualified paraprofessionals. In many cases, the professional nurse is legally responsible for the work performed by nonlicensed assistive personnel. Therefore, many of the functions performed by the nurse have important legal consequences. An understanding of the legal principles and guidelines involved is necessary if daily professional actions are not to result in unwanted malpractice suits. Terminology related to potential litigation is presented in Box 2-2.

If the hospital/organization or involved professional person (or both) is to be charged with malpractice resulting from injury to a patient, the patient's representative should be able to demonstrate that

1. A standard of care or duty can be established.
2. The standard of care or duty was not met.
3. The patient was harmed or injured because the standard was not met.
4. It was possible to foresee that injury or harm would result from not meeting the standards (depending on state law).

Personal Liability and Protective Measures

The rule of personal liability states that "every person is liable for his (or her) own tortious conduct" (his own wrongdoing). No physician/LIP can protect a nurse from an act of negligence by bypassing this rule with verbal reassurances. The nurse cannot avoid legal liability even though another person may be sued and held liable. For example, the physician/LIP who orders placement of a peripherally inserted central catheter (PICC) cannot assume responsibility for the nurse who is negligent in implementing the action. If harm occurs as a result of the action, the nurse is held liable for this wrongdoing.

The rule of personal liability is relevant to medication errors as well. Medication errors are a common cause of malpractice claims against nurses. Negligence results from the administration of a drug to the wrong patient, at the wrong time, in an incorrect dosage, or in an improperly prescribed manner. If the physician/LIP writes an incomplete or partially illegible order and the nurse fails to clarify it before administration and harm results, the nurse is liable for negligence. The same applies to the administration of IV fluids. Nurses

---

BOX 2-2   LEGAL TERMS

- *Criminal law*—actions judged under criminal law include violation of the Nurse Practice Act, which is prosecuted by a government authority and punishable by fine or imprisonment, or both. An example of a criminal act is unlawful administration of IV therapy.
- *Civil law*—actions judged under civil law relate to conduct affecting the legal rights of the private person. According to civil law, the guilty party is responsible for damages (*compensation*).
- *Tort*—a private wrongful act (of omission or commission) for which relief may be obtained by injunction or damages. Examples of a tort include assault, battery, negligence, slander, libel, false imprisonment, and invasion of privacy. Assault includes anticipation of harm; battery is the actual infliction of harm.
- *Malpractice*—negligent conduct of professionals characterized by not acting in a prudent manner and resulting in damage to another person or property

have a legal and professional responsibility to know the purpose and effect of the IV fluids and medications they administer. They must ensure that patients receive the prescribed volume of fluid at the prescribed rate of flow.

> **PATIENT SAFETY**
>
> Nurses have a legal and professional responsibility to know the purpose and effect of the IV fluids and medications they administer.

The rule of personal liability applies to nurse administrators and to nurses under their supervision. Although administrative nurses usually are not held liable for the negligence of nurses under their supervision (because every person is liable for his or her own wrongdoing), a director is expected to know if the nurse is competent to perform assigned duties without supervision.

On the other hand, directors who are negligent in the assignment of an inexperienced nurse or a nurse who requires supervision may be held liable for the acts of the nurse. Floating nurses to units to provide direct patient care when they are not experienced at the assigned level is a good example. Some institutions float nurses only to like intensive care units.

Observe Carefully

Nursing today requires a strong knowledge base and good observation skills. The act of observation is the legal and professional responsibility of the nurse. Frequent observation is imperative for the early detection and prevention of complications. Undetected complications that are allowed to increase in severity because of failure to observe the patient constitute an act of negligence on the part of the nurse.

Establish Therapeutic Relationships

Nurse–patient relationships play a significant role in influencing patients to initiate legal liability against nurses. Nurses performing infusion therapy must be particularly aware of and attentive to the emotional needs of their patients, particularly when patients experience pain and apprehension during such procedures as catheter insertion. Clearly, specialists must foster appropriate interpersonal relationships. Nurses who are impersonal, aloof, and so busy with the technical process of starting an IV infusion that they have no time for establishing kindly relationships are the suit-prone nurses whose personalities may initiate resentment and later malpractice suits.

Patients most likely to sue may be resentful, frequently hostile, uncooperative, and dissatisfied with the level of nursing care. By demonstrating respect, care, and concern for all patients, as well as rendering skilled, efficient nursing care, nurses may avoid malpractice claims.

Review and Clarify Current Policies and Procedures

Policies and procedures should be detailed, and all nurses practicing infusion therapy should be required to know them and review them periodically. Policies and procedures should follow national guidelines established by the Centers for Disease Control and Prevention (CDC) and Standards of Practice established by the Infusion Nurses Society (INS). These guidelines provide a model for IV nurses and foster optimal care for the patient receiving IV therapy.

DOCUMENTATION

Documentation is essential as a legal record of care provided a communication tool for other health care professionals and a determinant of eligibility for reimbursement. Detailed, accurate, adequate documentation prevents reinvention of the wheel (or duplication of effort and services) by saving time, ensures that the patient masters skill sets, and protects the health care provider or the institution. Tools used to document care include nursing care plans, flow sheets, progress notes, periodic updates developed by home care providers, and discharge summaries (Rankin & Stallings, 1996).

Electronic medical records (EMR) have facilitated the process. A commercially available program involves an innovative technology that combines the safety features of an automatically programmed infusion pump with software that provides clinical visibility to real-time infusion data. The nurse validates the information, and the system begins infusing the medication to the patient as prescribed. The clinician can view the trends in real-time and in conjunction with the patient's physiologic and hemodynamic data. http://www.cerner.com/solutions/Client_Stories/Wellspan_Health/

PATIENT SAFETY

Connectivity between an infusion pump and EMR systems supports the five rights of medication administration, helping ensure that the right patient gets the right medication in the right dose at the right time through the right route of administration.

Documentation should include the intervention performed, the patient's response to the intervention, and the subsequent outcomes. Sentinel or adverse events should also be documented consistent with institutional policy. By providing an accurate record of the care delivered and by structuring that care on evidence-based nursing practice and published standards, the nurse who is responsible for providing IV care ensures safe practice. The quality of infusion therapy is evaluated by the quality of the nursing **documentation**.

Accurate and complete documentation is considered a professional standard of nursing practice. Documentation that is incomplete or not consistent with organizational policy, state regulations, or state boards of nursing can be used to support an allegation of negligent care.

PATIENT SAFETY

Integrating infusion devices into health care information technology systems will be the primary focus over the next decade. Without this integration, it will be difficult to realize additional safety and productivity gains. At the same time, integrating infusion pumps with computerized physician/LIP order entry systems, expanding bar code medication administration system to infusion pumps, directly documenting therapies from the pumps to the patient's medical record, and incorporating pump alarms into "smart" alarm systems are high priorities and will usher in a new era of infusion therapy.

Keep Credentials Current

Credentialing of IV nurses nationwide began with the first certification examination in 1985. The credentialing process consists of three components: licensure, accreditation, and certification.

Licensure represents the entry into practice level afforded to all professional nurses who successfully complete the RN examination.

Accreditation establishes that a program or service meets established guidelines. Accreditation is offered to facilities, agencies, and other health care providers by such groups as TJC, which is an accrediting body that evaluates (rates) the programs of hospitals and home care agencies.

Certification is the highest level attainable by the professional IV nurse. It is the process by which society attests to the professional and clinical **competence** of the person who successfully completes the process.

Nurse Competence

Defining and evaluating **competency** in nursing is part of the yearly assessment of professionals in all clinical settings. The IV nurse's competence in performing peripheral IV therapy should be assessed periodically. Of course, the competent IV nursing professional should be able to perform the procedure using aseptic technique. The health care environment is changing drastically to demand quality through efficiency and effectiveness in all aspects of patient care. Competency is required to attain quality and to provide the patient with optimal outcomes. Proof of infusion competency is crucial to ensure excellence in infusion care for all patients (Weinstein, 2000).

Nurse educators are challenged to implement teaching strategies that promote learners' clinical competency and critical thinking skills. Additionally, these educators are asked to base their curriculum decisions, teaching practices, and evaluation methods on current research findings. Simulation offers a unique mode for experiential learning and evaluation, but the appropriate use of the spectrum of simulation typology requires strategic planning. Although simulation provides educators with new educational opportunities, the potential use of simulation in competency testing cannot be achieved until educators and researchers acquire the knowledge and skills needed to use this education strategy, develop realistic case scenarios, and design and validate standardized and reliable testing methods (Decker, Sportsman, Puetz & Billings, 2008). Simulation laboratories in clinical environments are helpful in documenting competencies in infusion nursing.

Preserve Confidentiality

Health Insurance Portability and Accountability Act regulations have impacted confidentiality in all clinical settings. Confidentiality of patient information consists of three related components: privacy, confidentiality, and security (Conner, 1999). With current advances in communication, such as electronic mail (e-mail) and other communication systems, including fax machines, cellular or cordless telephones, phone, tablet and computer applications, answering machines, and voice mail, nurses need to be aware and vigilant in preventing the misdirection, printing, interception, rerouting, or reading of information by unintended recipients.

Technology alone cannot ensure the legal and ethical use of e-mail and other communications in the health care environment. The e-mail message, for example, accurately documents communication and, as such, is part of the medical record and a legal document.

Expert security sources recommend the use of multilevel, individual passwords for all e-mail users, as opposed to generic group sign-ons and systems that require a single pass code (Dorodny, 1998). Monitored audit trails and increased accountability of caregivers to their patients should be established (Conner, 1999). Health information has become a commodity over the Internet, and every precaution should be taken to maintain the confidentiality of electronic additions to the clinical record.

PERFORMANCE EVALUATIONS

A standard must be carefully defined for the health care institution or the nurse to evaluate adequate performance. Tools useful in guiding this process include the following:

* Standards of Practice (INS, 1998, 2000, 2006, 2011)
* State Board of Nursing regulations for RNs and licensed practical/vocational nurses
* American Nurses Association (ANA) Standards of Nursing Practice
* Policies and procedures of the employing health care institution or agency

PROFESSIONAL NURSING AND PERFORMANCE IMPROVEMENT

The complexity of infusion therapy practice today mandates a higher level of expertise and training than ever before. Do not *assume* that the nurses you hire are competent based on self-reported past experiences. Evaluate their performance of procedures with attention to proper technique, including understanding aseptic (sterile) versus clean technique in the clinical setting, adherence to infection control, hand hygiene, hub disinfection, and the use of a mask and sterile gloves during site care. Let's look at the issues associated with placement of a long-term catheter, such as the PICC.

Qualified Personnel

The placement of a PICC requires special training and demonstrated competency on the part of the professional RN. Each state sets its own practice guidelines, and not all states consider the placement of PICC catheters to be within the scope of professional nursing practice. The INS assembled a task force to standardize the usage, terminology, and adjunctive guidelines for the insertion of PICCs. Teaching programs and ongoing updates ensure the accuracy of information. Each health care facility must establish criteria that qualify nurses to insert a PICC. The criteria should be within the institution's own legal guidelines. Such a program should address

* Indications
* Care and maintenance
* Advantages
* Legal issues

- Placement technique
- Product education
- Complications

Minimal standards for successful completion of an educational program include

- Satisfactory performance during initial probationary/review period
- Successful completion of in-house IV certification course
- Clinical competency evidenced by actual practice
- Successful completion of in-house requirements for PICC insertion

Risk Reduction

Given the continued growth of infusion therapy practice and the shift to alternative care settings, the potential for associated risks is higher than ever before. The institution is responsible for the quality of care delivered by its agents. Infusion therapy itself, without complications, is complicated. Infusion nurses are required to assess, access, monitor, and maintain a variety of complex infusion devices and therapies in a diversity of practice settings. As infusion therapy continues to evolve and become more complex, it is essential that the infusion nurse maintain a level of knowledge that is current and evidence based.

Knowledge of risk–benefit analysis of all aspects of infusion therapy including those leading to **sentinel events** is critical. Sentinel events are reflective of patient safety failures. Medication errors contribute to nearly 20% of all medical injuries. Infusion errors involving the administration of high-risk medications have the greatest potential to result in patient harm. The Agency for Healthcare Research and Quality (AHRQ) focuses on the development of quality measures to increase patient safety and provide improved patient outcomes (Table 2-2).

Medical Errors

"First, do no harm" is the ethical imperative for every patient safety effort. In working to reduce the frequency of medication errors, first priority must be to prevent those errors with the greatest potential for harm. The leading cause of patient harm is medication errors, which account for a significant number of medical injuries. Twenty-eight percent of medication-related injuries (adverse drug events, ADEs) are considered preventable. Administration is the stage of the medication use process most vulnerable to error; the intravenous (IV) route of drug administration often results in the most serious outcomes of medication errors. IV infusion errors, which involve high-risk medications delivered directly into a patient's bloodstream, have been identified as having the greatest potential for patient harm.

Medical errors can result in patient harm, disability, or even death and can prolong hospital stays and raise health care costs. The IOM report has impacted awareness of safety issues. Crossing the Quality Chasm: A New Health System for the 21st Century is a follow-up report from the IOM panel of the Quality Health Care Project. Table 2-3 addresses Simple Rules for the 21st Century Health Care System. IOM-2 recommends a sweeping redesign of the American health care system. It provides overarching principles for specific direction for policymakers, health care leaders, clinicians, regulators, and purchasers. It offers

TABLE 2-2	ADVANCING PATIENT SAFETY: 14 YEARS OF ADVANCING THE EVIDENCE

1999: Healthcare Research and Quality Act of 1999; Institute of Medicine's To Err Is Human: Building a Safer Health System

2000: National Summit on Medical Errors and Patient Safety; Doing What Counts for Patient Safety: Federal Actions to Reduce Medical Errors and Their Impact

2001: AHRQ patient safety research agenda; Patient safety grants; Evidence Report No. 43: Making Health Care Safer

2002: John M. Eisenberg Patient Safety and Quality Awards

2003: Patient Safety Indicators; Patient Safety Improvement Corps; AHRQ WebM&M, Morbidity & Mortality Rounds on the Web

2004: Health information technology portfolio; National Resource Center for Health IT; "Implementing Reduced Work Hours to Improve Patient Safety"; Hospital Survey on Patient Safety Culture

2005: AHRQ PSNet, AHRQ Patient Safety Network; Advances in Patient Safety: From Research to Implementation

2006: Keystone Project; Improving Patient Safety through Simulation Research grants; TeamSTEPPS

2007: Transforming Hospitals: Designing for Safety and Quality; "Questions Are the Answer" campaign

2008: Advances in Patient Safety: New Directions and Alternative Approaches; Health care-associated infections action plan; "Project RED"; Patient Safety and Quality: An Evidence-Based Handbook for Nurses; Consumer and clinician publications on preventing blood clots

2009: Patient video and booklet on blood thinner medicines; Patient Safety Organizations and Common Formats

2009: Tenth Anniversary of the IOM Report, To Err Is Human

2010: Establishing a Global Learning Community for Incident-Reporting Systems. AHRQ 11-R018

2010: The 2010 Report. Hospital Survey on Patient Safety Culture. AHRQ 10–0026

2011: Partial Truths in the Pursuit of Patient Safety. AHRQ 11-R016

2011: From Research to Practice: Factors affecting implementation of prospective targeted injury-detection Systems. AHRQ 1-R069

2011: New Research Highlights the Role of Patient Safety Culture and Safer Care. AHRQ 11-R070

2012: Choosing a Patient Safety Organization: Tips for hospitals and health care providers. AHRQ 12–0078

2012: Variations in safety culture dimensions within and between US and Swiss Hospital Units: an exploratory study by Schwendimann and Zimmermann

2012: Alleviating "Second Victim" Syndrome: How we should handle patient harm. AHRQ 12-R030

2013: Hospital Survey on Patient Safety Culture: 2012 User Comparative Database Report prepared by Westat, Rockville, MD. AHRQ Publication No. 12–0017

Adapted and updated from AHRQ Publication No. 09(10)-0084

Current as of February 2013

- A set of performance expectations for the 21st century health care system
- A suggested organizing framework to better align the incentives inherent in payment and accountability with improvements in quality
- Key steps to promote evidence-based practice and strengthen clinical information systems
- Ten rules to guide patient–clinician relationships

TABLE 2-3	SIMPLE RULES FOR THE 21ST CENTURY HEALTH CARE SYSTEM
Current Approach	**New Rule 3**
Care is based primarily on visits	Care based on continuous healing relationships
Professional autonomy drives variability	Customization based on patient needs and values
Professionals control care	The patient as the source of control
Information is a record	Shared knowledge and free flow of information
Decision making is based on training and experience	Evidence-based decision making
Do no harm is an individual responsibility	Safety as a system property
Secrecy is necessary	The need for transparency
The system reacts to needs	Anticipation of needs
Cost reduction is sought	Continuous decrease in waste
Preference is given to professional roles over the system	Cooperation among clinicians

CARE BASED ON CONTINUOUS HEALING RELATIONSHIPS

Patients should receive care whenever they need it and, in many forms, not just face-to-face visits. This implies that the health care system should be responsive at all times (24 hours a day, every day) and that access to care should be provided over the Internet, by telephone, and by other means in addition to face-to-face visits.

CUSTOMIZATION BASED ON PATIENT NEEDS AND VALUES

The system of care should be designed to meet the most common types of needs, but have the capability to respond to individual patient choices and preferences.

THE PATIENT AS THE SOURCE OF CONTROL

Patients should be given the necessary information and the opportunity to exercise the degree of control they choose over health care decisions that affect them.

SHARED KNOWLEDGE AND THE FREE FLOW OF INFORMATION

Patients should have unfettered access to their own medical information and to clinical knowledge. Clinicians and patients should communicate effectively and share information.

EVIDENCE-BASED DECISION MAKING

Patients should receive care based on the best available scientific knowledge.

SAFETY AS A SYSTEM PROPERTY

Patients should be safe from injury caused by the care system. Reducing risk and ensuring safety require greater attention to systems that help prevent and mitigate errors.

THE NEED FOR TRANSPARENCY

The health care system should make information available to patients and their families that allow them to make informed decisions when selecting a health plan, hospital, or clinical practice, or when choosing among alternative treatments.

ANTICIPATION OF NEEDS

The health system should anticipate patient needs, rather than simply reacting to events.

TABLE 2-4	THE IOM QUALITY CHASM SERIES

To Err Is Human: Building a Safer Health System, 2000
Crossing the Quality Chasm, 2001
Leadership by Example: Coordinating Government Roles in Improving Health Care Quality, 2002
Fostering Rapid Advances in Health Care: Learning From Systems Demonstrations, 2002
Priority Areas for National Action: Transforming Health Care Quality, 2003
Health Professions Education: A Bridge to Quality, 2003
Patient Safety: Achieving a New Standard for Care, 2003
Keeping Patients Safe: Transforming the Work Environment of Nurses, 2004
Quality Through Collaboration: The Future of Rural Health Care, 2004
Preventing Medication Errors: Quality Chasm Series, 2006
Improving the Quality of Health Care for Mental and Substance-Use Conditions: Quality Chasm Series, 2006

CONTINUOUS DECREASE IN WASTE

The health system should not waste resources or patient time.

COOPERATION AMONG CLINICIANS

Clinicians and institutions should actively collaborate and communicate to ensure an appropriate exchange of information and coordination of care.

According to the IOM, 45,000 to 98,000 Americans die each year due to medical errors. Infusion nurses can effect change and safeguard patients against harm (Premier Inc., 2012) (Table 2-4).

CAUSALITY OF MEDICAL ERRORS

Cause may be attributed to technical errors, misdiagnosis, failure to prevent injury, and medication errors. From inappropriate medication to pharmacist errors, there is a growing concern related to outcomes. Many factors can lead to medication errors. The Institute for Safe Medication Practices has identified 10 key elements with the greatest influence on medication use, noting that weaknesses in these can lead to medication errors. They are

- Patient information
- Drug information
- Adequate communication
- Drug packaging, labeling, and nomenclature
- Medication storage, stock, standardization, and distribution
- Drug device acquisition, use, and monitoring
- Environmental factors
- Staff education and competency
- Patient education
- Quality processes and risk management

METHODS FOR LIMITING ERRORS

Creating a culture of safety, often referred to as a high reliability organization, is the first step in the process. Staff should be aware of, and use, the safety resources available at their facilities.

Avoiding medication errors requires vigilance and the use of appropriate technology to help ensure proper procedures are followed. Computerized physician/LIP order entry reduces errors by identifying and alerting physicians/LIPs to patient allergies or drug interactions, eliminating poorly handwritten prescriptions, and giving decision support regarding standardized dosing regimens.

The Leapfrog Group (whose mission is to trigger giant leaps forward in health care safety, quality, and affordability) supports computerized physician/LIP order entry as a way to reduce medication errors. Use of computerized physician/LIP order entry and bar codes may reduce errors by up to 50%. Human influence is also a challenge; by not circumventing the system, by adherence to policies, and by an acute awareness, we can limit errors.

REPORT PRODUCT PROBLEMS

Because risk may be increased as a result of inappropriate use of medical devices, the U.S. FDA evaluates approximately thousands of medical devices monthly. The evaluation assesses

- Good manufacturing controls
- Application for a device existing before 1976 (in current use)
- Implantable or hazardous devices

FILE UNUSUAL OCCURRENCE REPORTS

A report is required for any accident or error resulting in actual or potential injury or harm. The report should contain only factual statements regarding the incident. Each report must be immediately followed by a full investigation into all possible causes, and corrective action must be taken immediately to prevent its recurrence.

Unusual occurrence reports should be routinely filed when there is a deviation from the standards. These reports are used as an internal reporting mechanism for a facility's quality assurance program. Components of the report may be found in Box 2-3. This type of report may also be used to help identify problem patterns and institute corrective actions. Surveillance programs documented by such reports can be effective in preventing unsafe or insecure environments that can result in injuries to the patient.

BOX 2-3 COMPONENTS OF AN UNUSUAL OCCURRENCE REPORT

- Admitting diagnosis
- Date of occurrence
- Patient's room number/location
- Patient's age
- Location of occurrence
- Type of occurrence (medication error, policy and procedure)
- Factual description
- Patient's prior clinical condition
- Results/interventions

Patient Safety

Leape (Buerhaus, 1999), a health policy analyst, suggests in a study in the *Harvard Medical Practice Journal* that nearly 4% of people who are hospitalized have an adverse event. The study further states that at least two thirds of the events are preventable, meaning that approximately 1 million preventable injuries and 120,000 preventable deaths from injury occur annually. Based on the findings, Leape asserts that the cost of adverse events to health care facilities in 1998 was approximately $100 billion. Much of the increase in adverse events is attributed to a more complex health care system and to the acuity of the patient population at the turn of the century.

The National Patient Safety Foundation, established in 1997 by the American Medical Association, brought together representatives from nursing, pharmacy, medicine, and patient advocacy groups to examine ways to improve safety in health care across the health care continuum. On a hospital-wide level, organizations have continued to emphasize quality improvement processes.

Performance Improvement Process

Almost 50% of TJC standards are directly related to safety, addressing such issues as medication use, infection control, surgery and anesthesia, transfusions, restraint and seclusion, staffing and staff competence, fire safety, medical equipment, emergency management, and security. The National Patient Safety Standards related to infusion therapy are found in Table 2-5. The TJC previously mandated an ongoing program for monitoring quality-based outcomes. The trend continues to be toward process improvement, which involves pursuing opportunities to improve the quality of care and to ensure positive patient outcomes.

Starting in 1998, TJC began requiring the reporting of sentinel events. TJC updated their definition of a sentinel event in 2007 as follows:

- A sentinel event is an unexpected occurrence involving death or serious physical or psychological injury, or the risk thereof. Serious injury specifically includes loss of limb or function. The phrase "or the risk thereof" includes any process variation for which a recurrence would carry a significant chance of a serious adverse outcome.
- Such events are called "sentinel" because they signal the need for immediate investigation and response.
- The terms "sentinel event" and "medical error" are not synonymous; not all sentinel events occur because of an error, and not all errors result in sentinel events.

Reporting Sentinel Events

TJC sponsors a hotline (630-792-3700) for reporting serious events. It also provides summary information on its Web site about the occurrence and management of sentinel events. Although modifications have been made to the original policy, the critical requirement for organizations is performing a "root cause analysis" of the event to identify the true underlying cause. This highlights the understanding that most events are the result of system problems and are not cause for individual blame.

TABLE 2-5	NATIONAL PATIENT SAFETY STANDARDS RELATED TO INFUSION THERAPY	
Goal	**Description**	**Comment**
Improve accuracy of patient identification.	Use at least two patient identifiers when administering medications or blood products, venous sampling, or other treatments.	Neither identifier should be the patient's room number.
Improve communication among caregivers.	– Verbal or telephone orders, verify complete order or test result by having it read back. – Standardize a list of abbreviations, acronyms, and symbols for use within the organization. – Measure, assess, and take action to improve timeliness of reporting results and values.	IV and lab results should be read back to confirm accuracy. Use only abbreviations, acronyms, and symbols that are standardized by the facility. Report test results to the licensed caregiver as soon as possible.
Improve medication safety.	– Standardize and limit number of drug concentrations available. – Identify and annually review a list of look-alike/soundalike drugs used.	Check concentrations of medications to ensure accuracy. Check all medications at least three times.
Reduce the risk of health care–related infections.	Comply with current CDC hygiene guidelines.	Wash hands before and after each procedure. Approved antiseptic hand rubs may be used if no visible soilage is on your hands.
Accurately and completely reconcile medications across the continuum of care.	– Implement a process for obtaining and documenting a complete list of patient's current medications upon admission and with patient involvement. – A complete list is communicated to the next provider of service when the patient is referred or transferred to another setting, service, practitioner, or level of care within or outside the organization.	Ensure that all medications are recorded completely and accurately. Ensure that a complete list is provided for the patient when he or she receives service from another physician/LIP or health care facility.

Adapted from The Joint Commission. www.jcaho.org

RISK REDUCTION STRATEGIES

Risk reduction strategies that reflect reported sentinel events to date are likely to include the following:

- Restricting access to concentrated potassium chloride
- Reducing the risk of inpatient suicide
- Eliminating wrong-site surgery
- Eliminating the use of inappropriate and unsafe restraints
- Reducing the risk of infant abduction
- Reducing the risk of adverse transfusion-related events
- Minimizing operative/postoperative complications
- Reducing the risk of fatal falls
- Reducing the risk of IV infusion pump errors
- Managing "high alert" medications

IDENTIFY DEFICIENCIES OR PROBLEM AREAS

Data may be collected by interview, observation, or visual inspection. Problems and deficiencies may be readily identified through incident reports, patient complaints, employee complaints, questionnaires, patient satisfaction surveys, and suggestions from patients, visitors, or other staff. Determine the cause of the deficiency by comparing actual care with established standards. In assessing the need for further investigation, the facility should determine the character of the problem or deficiency, which in most cases involves noncompliance with standards of care. Examples of questions to ask include the following:

- Does the deficiency/problem relate to the quality of patient care?
- Does the deficiency/problem occur frequently enough to require correction?
- Can the deficiency/problem be solved?
- Do the potential benefits to patient care warrant the cost of investigation and resolution?

Methods and instruments used for evaluation may include criterion-based studies, interviews with patients and staff members, surveys, and observations. Experimental research designs can be an excellent method for assessing and collecting meaningful data about the problem, although such designs can be complex and costly. First, however, study methodology and criteria must be established before data can be collected, analyzed, and interpreted. The Standards of Practice of the INS and guidelines of the CDC, American Association of Blood Banks (AABB), and TJC may all be beneficial in developing criteria for IV practice standards by which to assess problems and measure performance (Infusion Nurses Society, 1998, 2000, 2006, 2011; AABB, 2011; CDC, 2011; TJC, 2011).

ANALYZE AND INTERPRET

In collecting, analyzing, and interpreting data related to meeting the standards of practice and care, *compliance* refers to those situations in which the criteria are met. *Noncompliance* refers to the situations in which the criteria are not met. Both compliance and noncompliance are usually expressed in percentages. The expected compliance rate should be reasonable and achievable.

In most studies, findings are compiled statistically. These statistics provide a meaningful and concise description of the deficiency or problem. The data can then be used to calculate the average result, the difference between individual results and the average, and the relationship between the average result on one part of the study and the average result on another part.

PLAN CORRECTIVE ACTION

Once the findings are compiled, analyzed, and interpreted, a **plan of corrective action** can be developed. Two major forms of deficiencies require corrective action: knowledge and performance (Alexander & Corrigan, 2004). Components of the plan may address

- Changes that the environment can best accommodate
- Potential barriers or constraints

- Areas of potential support
- Needed resources

The best method of corrective action depends on the particular problem and individual situation. Methods may include revision of policies or procedures; change of equipment such as inclusion of tamper-proof nonpermeable sharps containers in patients' rooms, at shoulder height, and emptied regularly and as needed (Alexander & Corrigan, 2004); creation of a new information system; continuous monitoring; and on-site education.

REEVALUATE

After corrective action has been implemented, a reevaluation is necessary to determine whether the applied corrective action resolves the problem. Frequently, reevaluation is performed by repeating the first evaluation and comparing preaction data with postaction data.

RESOLUTION

The final step in the process is resolution, which involves developing a plan to ensure the maintenance of the quality of care achieved with the corrective action. Periodic or continuous screening may be required.

Continuous Quality Improvement

The influence of Deming and others, who introduced the concept of total quality improvement—also called continuous quality improvement (CQI)—has had a great impact on quality in health care organizations. CQI provides a mechanism for examining the process, rather than the individual involved, and encourages participation across interdepartmental lines to improve the process itself. Quality improvement teams in an organization are appointed, and study areas are identified. Process improvement is the direct result of the CQI program (see Box 2-4 for more information).

Measurement of Outcomes and Improvement

Interest in patient outcomes and their improvement continues to escalate. One reason for this is mounting evidence of wide and perplexing variations in outcomes of care, use of resources, and costs of care.

Outcome Improvement

Outcomes are the consequences of a treatment or intervention. Indicators are valid and reliable measures related to performance. *Outcome indicators*, or measures, gauge how patients are affected by their nursing care; for example, is the rate of nosocomial infections down? Is the incidence of IV-related infections lower? *Process indicators*, such as pressure ulcers, reflect the nature and amount of care that nurses provide, for example, the frequency of assessment for peripheral IVs. Based on the INS position paper, more frequent PIV site assessments, every 4 hours, will increase dwell time (INS, 2011). *Structure indicators* assess the organization and delivery of nursing care from a standpoint of staffing. Indicators are commonly

BOX 2-4   DEMING'S 14-POINT SYSTEM FOR MANAGING QUALITY

- Create consistency of purpose for continuous product improvement.
- Adopt the new philosophy across the organization.
- Cease dependence on inspection; improve the *process*.
- Avoid awarding business on price alone.
- Constantly seek to improve.
- Provide opportunities for training and staff development.
- Institute leadership; recognize the difference between management and leadership.
- Eliminate fear; fear inhibits innovation.
- Eliminate barriers among staff.
- Eliminate slogans; involve workers in the identification of new methods.
- Eliminate numerical quotas.
- Empower workers.
- Institute a broad-based education program to engage support.
- Be proactive in achieving transformation.

Adapted from Walton, M. (1991). *Deming management at work*. New York: Putnam.

reviewed to evaluate patient status in relation to outcomes—for example, the ability to bear weight is an indicator used to evaluate ambulation.

Across the health care arena, organizations are developing national quality initiatives (Table 2-6). One such organization is ECRI (Plymouth Meeting, PA), a firm that tests medical devices and develops guidelines and test programs. Formerly known as Emergency Care and Research Institute, ECRI has developed a comprehensive guide to quality practice using

TABLE 2-6   NATIONAL QUALITY INDICATORS

Organization	Initiative	Description
TJC	ORYX	Integrates use of outcomes and performance measures
National Committee for Quality Assurance (NCQA)	Health Plan Employer Data and Information Set (HEDIS)	Targets effectiveness of care, access and availability, patient satisfaction, costs
ANA	Nursing Report Card	Provides indicators and measurement tools for evaluating quality of nursing care in acute care settings
Centers for Medicare and Medicaid Services (CMS)	OASIS (Outcome and Assessment Information Set)	Provides assessment questions used to collect clinical, financial, and administrative data in home health care
Foundation for Accountability	Foundation for Accountability	Improves information available to consumers when they are choosing health plan, provider, hospital, treatment

the principles of evidence-based disease management. Disease management is an approach to patient care that coordinates medical resources for patients across the entire health care delivery system.

In 2004, the Agency for Health Care Policy and Research (AHCPR) restructured its popular clinical practice guideline and technology assessment programs. AHCPR's Evidence-Based Practice Program now sponsors the development of technology assessments and evidence reports by 12 designated evidence-based practice centers. The new initiative includes the development of a National Guideline Clearinghouse (NGC) that will be a comprehensive database. ECRI has been chosen to create the database, abstract existing guidelines, compare guidelines on similar topics, and establish the NGC Web site.

Patient outcomes may include physiologic values (vital signs, chemical results), physical values (ability to self-administer IV therapy), mental or psychological terms (cognitive skill, affective interactions), social terms (ability to assume responsibility for self-care), and other health-related quality-of-life parameters (pain level, energy, sleep).

PROCESS IMPROVEMENT

The quality assurance technique operates on the assumption that the professional or institution is the sole cause of adverse outcomes and ignores the reality that sources of adverse outcomes are complex and include variations in policies, procedures, equipment, and techniques, as well as people (patients, professionals, support staff) and their interactions. In many cases, process improvement may be measured by developing a flowchart (*flowcharting*) to identify patterns related to the basic process, the detailed process, errors and corrective measures, and redesigns (Batalden, Nelson, & Roberts, 1994).

The flowchart begins with the basic process at admission to the institution; the flowchart continues the detailed process by highlighting areas of possible duplication, complexity, and sources of error (Batalden et al., 1994). Using the flowchart as a basic tool, many institutions have developed ways to manage the improvement process by incorporating the model known as the plan-do-check-act improvement trial. Those who use this model proceed through the following sequence: state aim, identify measures of improvement, plan and do a pilot test, check and study results, act to improve, and reflect on learning (Batalden et al., 1994):

* Aim—what are we trying to accomplish?
* Measure—how will we know that a change is an improvement?

Measurement in nursing may be traced to Florence Nightingale, who used mortality statistics as a quality-of-care measure for British soldiers during the Crimean War. The ORYX initiative of TJC integrated patient outcomes and other performance measures into the accreditation process. "Oryx" is the Latin word for gazelle. Although accreditation is still based on standards, trends in data and in an organization's response to its data are being used as part of TJC's overall assessment as the performance measures database expands (TJC, 2011). All of the National Hospital Quality Measures common to TJC and the Centers for Medicare and Medicaid Services are endorsed by the National Quality Forum and are also used for the "Hospital Quality Alliance (HWA): Improving Care through Information initiative."

The INS *Standards of Practice* were developed as a framework for establishing infusion policies and procedures in all practice settings and for defining *performance criteria* for nurses responsible for administering infusion therapy. In the 2011 INS *Standards*, the recommended frequency for site rotation of the "short" peripheral catheter (as differentiated from a midline peripheral catheter in the *Standards*) is now based on clinical indications, rather than a specific time frame. Clinical indications include assessment of the patient's condition and access site, skin and vein integrity, length and type of prescribed therapy, venue of care, and integrity and patency of the catheter.

The primary reference used to support site rotation based on clinical indications was a Cochrane systematic review of the literature. Five randomized, controlled trials that compared routine peripheral IV catheter removal with removal only when clinically indicated were included in the analysis of 3,408 trial participants that found no conclusive evidence of benefit for routine peripheral IV catheter site rotation. The impact of clinically indicated site rotation will continue to be a research priority for INS (INS, 2011).

- Possible changes—what changes can we make that we predict will lead to improvement?
- Plan—how shall we plan the pilot? Who does what? When? And with what tools and training? What baseline data need to be collected?
- Do—what are we learning as we do the pilot?
- Check—as we check and study what happened, what have we learned?
- Act—as we act to hold the gains or to abandon the pilot, what needs to be done? (Batalden et al., 1994)

A multidisciplinary quality council may be appointed within an organization to determine the best institution-wide approach to managing quality. A technique such as process management—consisting of merging comparative data analyses, operational and clinical analyses, benchmarking (comparing an institution with the best institutions nationwide), quality methods, and simulation methods—results in improvements in quality.

Some responsible and progressive hospitals and health networks have committed themselves to seeking significant improvements yearly. One goal, for example, is specific improvement in medication management by a certain year or other time frame. To achieve the overall outcome, the collaborative group may design an ideal plan for improved medication management. Some examples of the goals of the plan may be reducing medication errors within the respective facilities by 50% over a 3-year period, deploying an advanced ADE detection technique in 100% of the collaborating systems, and introducing one breakthrough technology per year.

Review Questions   *Note: Questions below may have more than one right answer.*

1. The statement "every person is liable for his own tortious conduct" is known as the rule of
   A. Negligent action
   B. Personal liability
   C. Tortious conduct
   D. Wrongdoing act

2. A nurse inserts an IV cannula against the wishes of a coherent adult patient. In this situation, the nurse could be charged with
   A. Assault
   B. Battery
   C. Assault and battery
   D. Malpractice

3. Which of the following is not a component of the credentialing process?
   A. Accreditation
   B. Certification
   C. Diploma
   D. Licensure

4. The new rules for the 21st Century Health Care System include which of the following?
   A. Customization of patient needs and values
   B. Preference to professional roles
   C. Professionals control care
   D. System reacts to patient needs

5. Data may be collected by all of the following methods **except**
   A. Interview
   B. Observation
   C. Hearsay
   D. Visual inspection

6. Researchers who have affected the quality improvement process include
   A. Conner
   B. Evanson
   C. Deming
   D. Dorodny

7. Benchmarking is the process of comparing
   A. Institution to like institutions
   B. Institution to the best institutions
   C. Practitioner to practitioner
   D. Practitioner to the best practitioner

8. Quality improvement programs examine
   A. Individuals
   B. Processes
   C. A only
   D. A and B

9. The Food and Drug Administration inspects devices on each of the following levels except
   A. Good manufacturing controls
   B. Application for a device existing before 1976 (still in common use)
   C. Implantable or hazardous device
   D. Nurse-inserted devices

10. Which of the following is **not** an external driver that influences safety?
    A. Regulation and legislation
    B. Accreditation
    C. Professional societies
    D. Hospitals

References and Selected Readings   *Asterisks indicate references cited in text.*

AHRQ/RWJF. (2012). Patient safety and quality: an evidence-based handbook for nurses. http://www.ahrq.gov/qual/nurseshdbk/

*Alexander, M., & Corrigan, A.M. (2004). *Core curriculum for infusion nursing* (pp. 428–230). Philadelphia, PA: Lippincott Williams and Wilkins.

Alspach, G. (1998). Nurse-to-nurse recognition. *Critical Care Nurse*, 18(3), 6–9.

American Association of Blood Banks. (2012). *AABB Clinical Practice Guidelines for Transfusion*. http://www.aabb.org/pressroom/pressreleases/Pages/pr120327.aspx

*American Association of Blood Banks. (2011). *Technical manual* (17th ed) . Bethesda, MD: Author.

*Batalden, P.B., Nelson, E.C., & Roberts, J.S. (1994). Linking outcomes measurement to continual improvement: The serial "V": Way of thinking about improving clinical care. *Journal on Quality Improvement*, 20(4), 168–169.

*Buerhaus, P.I. (1999). Lucian Leape on the causes and prevention of errors and adverse events in health care. Image: *Journal of Nursing Scholarship*, 31(3), 281–286.

*Centers for Disease Control and Prevention. (2011). Guidelines for prevention of intravascular catheter-related infections. http://www.cdc.gov/hicpac/pdf/guidelines/bsi-guidelines-2011.pdf

*Cohen, M.R. (2005). How to prevent errors—safety issues with patient-controlled analgesia. Part 2. ISMP medication error report analysis. *Hospital Pharmacy, 40,* 210–212.

*Conner, V.W. (1999). Patient confidentiality in the electronic age. *Journal of Infusion Nursing, 22,* 199–201.

*Decker S., Sportsman S., Puetz L., & Billings L. (2008). The evolution of simulation and its contribution to competency. *The Journal of Continuing Education in Nursing, 39*(2), 74–80.

*Dorodny, V. (1998). The highwire act of medical records security. *Advice for Health Information Executives, 2,* 24–32.

Fabian, B. (2010). Infusion therapy in the older adult. In M. Alexander, A. Corrigan, L. Gorski, J. Hankins, & R. Perucca (Eds.), *Infusion Nursing: an evidence-based approach* (3rd ed., pp. 571–582). St. Louis, MO: Saunders/Elsevier.

Ferner, R.E. (2009). The epidemiology of medication errors: the methodological difficulties. *British Journal of Clinical Pharmacology, 67*(6), 614–620.

Fields, M., & Peterman, J. (2005). IV medication safety system averts high-risk medication errors and provides actionable data. *Nursing Administration Quarterly, 29,* 77–86.

Gorski, L.A. (2007). Ethical decision making and repair of a patient's catheter. *Journal of Infusion Nursing, 30*(4), 203–204.

Hatcher I., Sullivan M., & Hutchinson J., et al. (2004). An intravenous medication safety system: Preventing high-risk medication errors at the point of care. *Journal of Nursing Administration, 34,* 437–439.

*Infusion Nurses Society. (1998). Revised infusion nursing standards of practice. *Journal of Infusion Nursing, 21*(Suppl. 1), 517, 525.

*Infusion Nurses Society. (2000). Revised standards of practice. *Journal of Infusion Nursing, 23*(Suppl. 1).

*Infusion Nurses Society. (2006). Revised Standards of practice. *Journal of Infusion Nursing, 28*(Suppl. 1).

*Infusion Nurses Society. (2011). Position Paper on Recommendations for Frequency of Assessment of the Short Peripheral Catheter Site. Available at http://www.ins1.org/i4a/pages/index.cfm?pageid=3412

*Institute of Medicine. (2006). *Preventing medication errors: Quality chasm series.* Washington, DC: National Academies Press.

Institute of Medicine of the National Academies. (1999). Report on preventing medical errors: To err is human: Building a safer health system. [On-line]. http://www.ashp.org/public/news/breaking/IOM.num.

*The Joint Commission. (2011). *Patient safety goals.* http://www.jointcommission.org/assets/1/18/2011-2012_npsg_presentation_final_8-4-11.pdf

Krahenbuhl-Melcher, A., Schlienger, R., Lampert, M., Haschke, M., Drewe, J., & Krahenbuhl, S. (2007). Drug-related problems in hospitals: A review of the recent literature. *Drug Safety, 30*(5), 379–407.

Leape L.L., Brennan T.A., Laird N., et al. (1991). The nature of adverse events in hospitalized patients. Results of the Harvard Medical Practice Study II. *New England Journal of Medicine, 324,* 377–384.

McMahon, D.D. (2002). Evaluating new technology to improve patient outcomes. *Journal of Infusion Nursing 25*(4), 250–255.

Page, A.E.K. (2008). Chapter 27 Temporary, agency, and other contingent workers. In R.G. Hughes (Ed.), *Patient safety and quality: an evidence-based handbook for nurses.* Rockville, MD: Agency for Healthcare Research and Quality (US).

*Premier, Inc. (2012). *Patient safety.* https://www.premierinc.com/safety/topics/patient_safety/index_3.jsp

Rankin, S.H., & Stallings, K.D. (1996). *Patient education issues, principle, practices* (3rd ed., pp. 122, 162–164, 183–187). Philadelphia, PA: Lippincott-Raven.

Rothschild, J.M., Landrigan, C.P., Cronin, J.W., Kaushal, R., Lockley, S.W., Burdick, E., & Bates, D.W. (2005). The Critical Care Safety Study: The incidence and nature of adverse events and serious medical errors in intensive care*. *Critical care medicine, 33*(8), 1694–1700.

Spielberg, A.R. (1998). Sociohistorical, legal and ethical implications of e-mail for the patient-physician relationship. *Journal of the American Medical Association, 280*(15), 1353–1357.

Wakefield, M.K. (2008). The quality chasm series: Implications for nursing in patient safety and quality, Chapter 4. In R.G. Hughes (Ed.), *An evidence-based handbook for nurses.* Rockville, MD: Agency for Healthcare Research and Quality (US). http://www.ncbi.nlm.nih.gov/books/NBK2677/pdf/ch4.pdf

Webster, J., Osborne, S., Rickard, C.M., & New, K. (2013). Clinically-indicated replacement versus routine replacement of peripheral venous catheters. *Cochrane Database of Systematic Reviews, 2013,*4: CD0077981.1–CD0077981.42.

*Weinstein S. (2000). Certification and credentialing to define competency-based practice. *Journal of Infusion Nursing, 23*(1), 21

Weinstein, S. (1996). Legal implications/risk management. *Journal of Infusion Nursing, 19*(3 Suppl), S16–S18.

Wilson K., & Sullivan M. (2004). Preventing medication errors with smart infusion technology. *American Journal of Health Systems Pharmacy, 61*, 177–183.

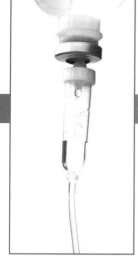

CHAPTER 3

Nursing Role and Responsibilities

Sharon M. Weinstein

KEY TERMS

Accountability
Advocate
Anesthesia
Autonomy
Blood Bank
Credentials
Infusion Nurse
   Specialist
Infusion Nursing
   Team
Innovator
Knowledge Sharer

Magnet Recognition
Magnet Team Member
Mentor
Pharmacist
Positive Practice
   Environment
Researcher
Resource Personnel
Scope of Practice
Shared Governance
Staff Nurse

ROLE DELINEATION

The practice of infusion nursing encompasses many levels of knowledge and expertise. A credentialed infusion nurse is highly qualified to provide infusion care across the patient care continuum and to participate in benchmarking efforts related to infusion nursing and patient outcomes. The role of this nursing specialist is defined in institutional policy and procedure, often based upon established Standards of Practice and consistent with the Nurse Practice Act. While the role may vary across clinical settings, the primary responsibility is to ensure quality infusion care regardless of the setting in which care is delivered. Expertise, clinical competence, credentials—these are the hallmarks of the infusion nurse.

SCOPE OF PRACTICE

The infusion nurse is a specialist and a generalist; the generalist could not be considered a specialist. One's basic nursing education prepares one to become a nursing generalist.

The infusion nurse is accountable for the defined scope of practice based on the following:

- Knowledge of anatomy and physiology
- Knowledge and understanding of the vascular system and its relationship with other body systems
- Participation in the creation of the patient's ongoing plan of care
- Possession of skills needed for the administration of infusion therapies
- Knowledge of state-of-the-art technologies associated with infusion therapies
- Knowledge of psychosocial aspects, including sensitivity to the patient's wholeness, uniqueness and significant social relationships, and knowledge, and community and economic resources (a holistic approach to care)
- Interaction and collaboration with members of the health care team and participation in the clinical decision-making process (INS, 2011)

COLLABORATIVE ROLE OF THE NURSE

Administration of safe, high-quality infusion therapy today depends on a collaborative and positive practice environment in which many members of the health care team play a key role. The nurse, in particular, plays a primary role in collaborating with other health care providers to maintain an infusion and to protect the patient from the hazards and complications associated with routine infusion (IV) therapy. Policies regarding the responsibilities of a staff nurse in relation to therapy vary significantly among health care institutions and are often influenced by the presence or absence of a full-service infusion team. In reality, many medical–surgical nurses are involved in the delivery of infusion care and have expanded their base of knowledge to prepare for the Infusion Nurses Credentialing Examination.

An essential component of the collaborative practice setting is the flexibility of the infusion nurse in adapting to changing institutional environments. Expanded roles might include mentor, knowledge sharer, Magnet team member, advocate, and researcher. The global role of the infusion nurse is addressed in this chapter.

ROLE OF INFUSION NURSING TEAMS

Research findings show that an infusion nursing team enhances the level of care that an organization provides. To ensure that the team approach provides safe IV care, the role of the team and the delineation of responsibilities must be part of the orientation program and ongoing education for all nurses. Specialized teams of infusion nurses provide clinical expertise and cost-effective care. In the ideal setting, registered nurses with clinical and theoretic expertise should be responsible for administering infusion therapy. This improves the quality of patient care because specialized nurses, freed from other responsibilities, can focus their attention on developing a high standard of performance. Such nurses, aware of the inherent risks of therapy, are vigilant and meticulous in performing and maintaining IV therapy. Their advanced skills promote trauma-free venipuncture, conserve veins for future use, and reduce routine complications. The knowledge, skills, and abilities of these specialized nurses ensure patient safety.

Benefits of an IV team include reduction in complications related to peripheral IV administration, reduction in catheter-related bloodstream infections, increased patient satisfaction, timely completion of therapies, enhanced level of clinical expertise, utilization of state-of-the-art technology, reduction in patient length of stay, potential revenue generation, and early assessment and identification of vascular access needs.

In August 2002, in a publication by the CDC entitled "Guidelines for the Prevention of Intravascular Catheter-Related Infections," where dedicated IV teams were recommended, the authors noted that specialized IV teams have shown unequivocal evidence in reducing the number of catheter-related bloodstream infections and associated complications and costs. Reports spanning decades have consistently demonstrated that risk of infection declines with standardization of aseptic care and that insertion and maintenance of central access catheters by inexperienced staff might increase the risk of catheter colonization and central line bloodstream infections.

With the majority of acute care patients receiving infusion therapy throughout the course of a hospitalization, the infusion nurse has become an integral part of the nursing process for each patient entrusted to his/her care. Once considered a technical function, the practice of infusion therapy is now recognized as a clinical specialty requiring the knowledge, skills, and abilities to offer sound assessment and interventions within the patient's plan of care.

Today's patient care models demand optimum utilization of resources, control of costs, and high quality; this is the ideal practice environment for the infusion nurse specialist who can offer comprehensive care with a high degree of safety. Even the most complex cases may be handled by the infusion specialist in an alternative care or home setting. Infusion nursing teams succeed in those institutions in which their value is recognized and appreciated. The Infusion Nurses Society published a white paper entitled Infusion Teams in Acute Care Hospitals: Call for a Business Approach (INS, 2013). Within this important document, the society emphasizes the three-tiered approach to hospital-based infusion care. No single model of service delivery works in all organizations.

PATIENT SAFETY

Patient safety is a major focus in today's clinical environment. It is critical to have highly trained and knowledgeable infusion nurses to provide care.

RESOURCE NURSE

In lieu of a full-service infusion team, the health care facility may use the services of one or more IV nurse specialists as a limited-service team or as **resource personnel**. The team may function within certain clinical units, or within given hours.

Although the coverage is not complete, it does provide for consistent, quality care by infusion nurses but leaves primary responsibility related to infusion care to staff nurses during the hours when there is no team coverage and sometimes during peak hours. In these situations, the infusion specialist may serve as educator, clinician, or team leader to a number of integrated health care organizations or home care agencies.

The role for the infusion nurse specialist is continually evolving. Changes in clinical practice and in the practice setting direct this process (Lozins Miller, 1998).

MENTOR

The infusion nurse specialist has a unique responsibility and opportunity to mentor others. This responsibility transcends the entire organization as well as members of the infusion nursing team. This is especially important when new staff is involved in the delivery of infusion care. Raising the bar and setting the standard are key responsibilities of the infusion specialist. Considerations for potential mentors may be found in Box 3-1.

BOX 3-1 MENTORING

1. Mentees need your expertise.
You have a wealth of life experience no matter what your age. You know how to listen, plan a project, make things happen, study and evaluate situations, talk to individuals and groups, influence others to take steps, bargain, write documents, parent, handle aging parents, express your feelings, and telecommute, among a multitude of other skills. Many individuals could benefit from grasping at least one thing you know.

2. Mentees need your particular slant on your expertise.
Mentees need more than just the general expertise you possess; they need your particular version of it. How do you do it differently from others? What are the unwritten rules you've learned on how to do it better, faster, more enjoyably, or with more sensitivity? No one but you knows this, and it will end with you if you don't pass it on.

3. Mentoring is less time intensive and mentor managed than it used to be.
Mentoring has changed dramatically and has evolved into a practice that truly benefits mentor and mentee.

4. Mentoring is a way to leave a legacy.
You can also leave an important legacy through the work you do, what you create, improve, and influence that makes the world and the people in it better for having you in it. Mentoring at least one person well is another powerful legacy you can leave. A part of you, your experience, and your character will be a part of that person's journey, which in turn is likely to be a part of someone else's. Mentors really can change the world one person at a time.

5. You will learn from your mentees.
An example of reverse mentoring is in the corporate world where older mentors are learning computer tips and tricks from their younger counterparts. No matter what your mentees know and can do, you'll learn something from them about their worlds and experiences.

6. It is satisfying to see someone shine.
We have the unique ability to allow others to shine, to share their successes, and to support their growth.

TABLE 3-1 BARRIERS OF KNOWLEDGE SHARING	
Knowledge-Sharing Barriers	**Possible Solutions**
Lack of trust	Establish an environment where quality of ideas is more important than status of source.
Different cultures, languages, and frames of reference	Educate people on the advantages of flexibility; employ for openness to ideas.
Lack of time and meeting places; narrow idea of productive work	Build relationships and trust through balancing between virtual and face-to-face meeting. Establish time and places for formal and informal knowledge sharing.
Status and rewards go to knowledge owners	Evaluate performance and provide rewards to those who share and reuse knowledge.
Belief that knowledge relates to specific groups	Create common ground through team work, job rotation, and other types of collaboration.
Intolerance for mistakes and lack of help	Tolerate and reward errors from creative collaboration and help a person learn from these.

Adapted from Davenport and Prusak (1998).

EDUCATOR AND KNOWLEDGE SHARER

One of the challenges of knowledge management is that of convincing people to share their knowledge. Why should people give up their hard-won knowledge when it is one of their key sources of personal advantage? In some organizations, sharing is natural. In others, the old dictum, knowledge is power, reigns. In this chapter, we explore some of the barriers and offer some pointers in overcoming them. The infusion nurse is a knowledge expert with a broad spectrum of knowledge to be shared with others.

BARRIERS

Barriers to knowledge sharing abound, and include loss of power, fear from revelation, uncertainty (especially among new nurse members), a loss of recognition or reward (because they have shared their knowledge with others), personal or institutional culture, a difference between awareness and knowledge, and conflict of motives.

OVERCOMING THE BARRIERS

The key is awareness of the organization itself—by identifying and developing complementary ways to share the knowledge management and transfer within an organization. Best practices that result in excellence include processes, methods, and strategies; identifying and sharing best practices is a critical way of incorporating the knowledge of some into the work of many (Table 3-1).

THE EVOLVING ROLE OF KNOWLEDGE SHARER

The role of the knowledge sharer involves cultural change, cooperation, and commitment (David J. Skyrme, www.skyrme.com/updates/u64_f1.htm; Accessed October 5, 2005). According to Skyrme, culture change is never easy and takes time. But cultures can be changed once the term *culture* is clearly defined. Culture is defined in many ways, such as "commonly held beliefs, attitudes, and values" and "the collective programming of the mind that distinguishes one group from another" and in many other ways that also embrace rituals, artifacts, and other trappings of the work environment. Cooperation is an essential component of knowledge sharing; we are both competitive and cooperative. In today's complex world, we need help from others with whom we compete in order to achieve our goals.

And commitment is based on culture and cooperation. Organizations need to create a commitment to culture, to change, to challenge, to compete, and to cooperate. If, as is often the case, time pressure leads to poor knowledge sharing, then there must be a commitment to allow time for it to happen. Commitment to knowledge sharing must be demonstrated throughout the organization. It is inherent in the behaviors of infusion nurse specialists who consistently share knowledge with others even if it is not formally part of their job.

THE INNOVATOR

Wilson, Whitaker, and Whitford (2012) challenge us to look at the entrepreneurial and intrapreneurial roles of nurses in the health care reform era that we currently live in. These roles vary as per employment and practice setting yet reflect the nurse as an innovator. Innovation is providing affordable health care, access to health care, collaborative practice settings, and expanding "out of the box" thinking to global partners. Nurses are the "leaders of the pack" in designing innovation in patient care.

MAGNET TEAM MEMBER

The Magnet Recognition Program recognizes health care organizations for quality patient care, nursing excellence, and innovations in professional nursing practice. Consumers rely on Magnet designation as the ultimate credential for high-quality nursing. Developed by the American Nurses Credentialing Center (ANCC), Magnet is the leading source of successful nursing practices and strategies worldwide. The program provides a vehicle for disseminating successful practices and strategies among nursing systems. To provide greater clarity and direction, as well as eliminate redundancy within the Forces of Magnetism, the latest model configures the 14 Forces of Magnetism into 5 Model Components. The simpler model reflects a greater focus on measuring outcomes and allows for more streamlined documentation, while retaining the 14 Forces as foundational to the program. Overarching the new Magnet Model Components is an acknowledgment of Global Issues in Nursing and Health Care. While not technically a Model Component, this category includes the various factors and challenges facing nursing and health care today (Box 3-2).

The Magnet Recognition Program is based on quality indicators and standards of nursing practice as defined in the American Nurses Association's *Scope and Standards for Nurse Administrators* (2003). The Magnet designation process includes the appraisal of both qualitative and quantitative factors in nursing. (See Box 3-3 for the findings of independent research on magnet-designated facilities.)

Dr. Aiken and her team surveyed more than 26,250 RNs at 567 hospitals in California, Florida, New Jersey, and Pennsylvania. Of the hospitals involved, four had achieved Magnet recognition from the ANCC. Results show that the Magnet hospitals had not only a larger number of specialty-certified nurses but also a greater proportion of nurses with a BSN

BOX 3-2   MODEL COMPONENTS

- Transformational leadership
- Structural empowerment
- Exemplary professional practice
- New knowledge, innovation, and improvements
- Empirical quality results

---

degree or higher education. In addition, the number of patients per nurse in Magnet hospitals was significantly lower than in non-Magnet hospitals. Nurses in Magnet hospitals were 18% less likely to be dissatisfied, 13% less likely to have high levels of burnout, and much less likely to report intent to leave their current position.

Three decades of evidence showing superior outcomes for Magnet hospitals place this organizational innovation in a class of its own as best practice, which deserves the attention of hospital leaders, nurses, and the public (Aiken, 2012a, 2012b) (Table 3-2).

New research from Aiken shows that surgical patients cared for in ANCC Magnet-recognized hospitals have significantly lower odds of mortality and failure-to-rescue than those cared for in non-Magnet facilities. The findings appeared in the October 2012 issue of *Medical Care*, the official journal of the Medical Care section of the American Public Health Association. Dr. Aiken and her team analyzed linked data from 564 hospitals in California, Florida, Pennsylvania, and New Jersey. Of the hospitals involved, 56 had received Magnet recognition from the ANCC. Controlling for differences in nursing, hospital, and patient characteristics, the team found that surgical patients in Magnet hospitals had 14% lower odds of inpatient death within 30 days and 12% lower odds of failure-to-rescue, compared with similar patients in non-Magnet hospitals. Although Dr. Aiken has published previous studies documenting lower mortality rates in Magnet hospitals, this was the first time she and her team directly measured the work environment with a variety of indicators, including a survey of more than 100,000 nurses. Their findings reinforced that superior practice environments for nurses are the distinguishing factor between Magnet and non-Magnet hospitals and are key to better patient outcomes. The research was funded by the National Institute of Nursing Research of the National Institutes of Health (Table 3-3).

BOX 3-3   INDEPENDENTLY SPONSORED RESEARCH CONCERNING MAGNET-DESIGNATED FACILITIES

- Consistently outperform non-Magnet organizations
- Deliver better patient outcomes
- Experience increased time spent at the bedside of patients
- Have shorter patient stays
- Have lower patient mortality rates
- Have lower incidence of needlestick injuries
- Enjoy increased nurse retention and recruitment rates

TABLE 3-2   REASSESSING THE ROLE OF THE INFUSION TEAM

Reassessment Objective	Time Frame	Accountability
Reduce IV team full-time equivalents (FTEs)	60 days	Task force
Develop and implement training plan for staff nurse generalists	30 days	IV team leader, nurse educator, IV resource clinician
Transfer 3.0 FTEs to staff nurse positions	30 days	Chair, cochair, nurse recruiter
Develop clinical practice guidelines for infusion therapy based on Infusion Nurses Society Standards of Practice	60 days	Task force
Establish advanced practice skills with 2.0 FTEs determined by caseload	60 days	IV team leader, nurse educator, medical director
Maintain level of quality	Ongoing	Task force

Adapted from Lozins Miller, P.K. (1998). Downsizing. *Journal of Infusion Nursing*, 21(2), 107.

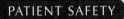 **PATIENT SAFETY**

Patient safety is recognized within this section of the Leapfrog Group survey, which scores hospitals on their commitment to staffing with highly trained nurses and putting nurses in leadership positions that afford them substantial input on patient safety issues.

Recognizing quality patient care, nursing excellence, and innovations in professional nursing practice, the Magnet Recognition Program provides consumers with the ultimate benchmark to measure the quality of care that they can expect to receive. The *U.S. News & World Report* uses Magnet designation as a primary competence indicator in its assessment of almost 5,000 hospitals in order to rank and report the best medical centers in 16 specialties. In the Leapfrog Hospital Survey, the nation's oldest survey comparing hospital performance in safety, quality, and efficiency, Magnet designation automatically earns full credit for Safe Practice No. 9: Nursing Workforce.

Magnet provides consumers with the benchmark for measuring the quality of care that they can expect to receive. As a natural outcome of this, the program elevates the reputation and standards of the nursing profession. One such standard recognizes the number of credentialed nurses in a health care organization. The Infusion Nurses Credentialing Corporation *credentials infusion nurse specialists* whose accomplishments are included in the evidence developed to support this standard.

SHARED GOVERNANCE

A cyclical nursing shortage is revitalizing shared governance. This innovative organizational model gives staff nurses control over their practice and can extend their influence into administrative areas previously controlled only by managers (Hess, 2004). Shared governance in nursing is more than a new organizational chart or committee configuration; structures can be deceiving. The key factors are those who make up the membership. The meaning of success in terms of shared governance and patient care should be the control

TABLE 3-3	THE MAGNET CHARACTERISTICS OF A PROFESSIONAL PRACTICE ENVIRONMENT FORCES OF MAGNETISM 1983 (McCLURE)

Forces of Magnetism 2005 (ANCC)	
Administration	1. Quality of nursing leadership
Quality of leadership	2. Organizational structure
Organizational structure	3. Management style
Management style	4. Personnel policies and programs
Staffing	(staffing embedded in No. 4)
Personnel policies and programs	5. Professional models of care
Professional practice	6. Quality of care
Professional practice models	7. Quality improvement
Quality of care	8. Consultation and resources
Quality assurance	9. Autonomy
Consultation and resources	10. Community and the hospital
Autonomy	11. Nurses as teachers
Community and the hospital	12. Image of nursing
Nurses as teachers	13. Interdisciplinary relationships
Image of nursing	14. Professional development (original subgroups embedded)
Nurse–physician/LIP relationships	
Professional development	
Orientation	
In-service and continuing education	
Formal education and career development	

of practice leading to better patient outcomes. Shared governance is a frequent model within Magnet facilities, and research related to Magnet-designated hospitals indicates a clear correlation between status and outcome. In nursing, shared governance models have always focused on nurses controlling their professional practice. Shared governance is an ongoing journey moving from past orientations where the few rule to an orientation where many learn to make consensual decisions. Such institutions are in a constant state of growth, renewal, and revival. The infusion nurse specialist is an important part of that process (Table 3-3).

Infusion nurses are professionally fulfilled; their work is satisfying, emotionally and professionally. **Autonomy** is a vital component of long tenure and satisfaction. Autonomy also keeps the infusion nurse highly visible within the health care organization. Nurses need to get involved in decision making, setting standards, and ensuring quality. Shared governance provides the structure for accountability for nursing practice and participation in the process.

ADVOCATE

The nurse's role as a patient *advocate* is a complex one. It encompasses informing patients of their rights, ensuring information exchange, and supporting patients in decisions they make. The Infusion Nursing Code of Ethics related to the Standards of Practice (INS, 2011) addresses patient advocacy in clinical situations related to infusion practice.

PATIENT SAFETY

The Empowered Patient Coalition is a 501(c) (3) charitable organization created by a patient advocate devoted to helping the public improve the quality and the safety of their health care. The coalition feels strongly that the first crucial steps in both patient empowerment and patient safety efforts are information and education. The public is increasingly aware that they must assume a greater role in health care issues, but they need tools, strategies, and support to assist them in becoming informed and engaged medical consumers who are able to make a positive impact on health care safety. Infusion professionals also advocate for patient safety.

http://www.empoweredpatientcoalition.org/

RESEARCHER

The infusion nurse specialist utilizes the research platform to test new ideas that will advance the practice and enhance outcomes. Contributing to the evidence base for infusion practice ensures the growth of the specialty, the dissemination of knowledge, and the clinical competencies. As the recognized practice leader, the Infusion Nurses Society (INS) recognizes the critical need for research to support the specialty practice. In partnership with Wayne State University College of Nursing, INS surveyed its members by using the Delphi approach. The qualitative responses received supported a theoretical framework on which to base an agenda. Respondents identified more problem areas in their practice than in research topics needing further exploration. Four themes, all falling under the overarching domain of patient safety, were identified (Zugcic, Davis, Gorski, & Alexander, 2010).

ROLE AS A LEADER

Traditionally, the responsibility for IV therapy has been allocated to the director of the **blood bank**, the **pharmacist**, or the **anesthesia** department. Infusion nurses fulfill several important functions. Not only do they administer blood and blood components, but they are in close alliance with the pharmacy. IV nurses administer infusions of which 50% to 80% contain additives. Moreover, they execute many of the functions performed by the anesthesiologist.

In some health care settings, IV departments may also function as self-contained cost centers within an institution's infrastructure. The infusion team has become an integral part of the nursing department, engaging in increased interaction and collaboration with nursing colleagues, especially as they seek Magnet recognition.

PATIENT SAFETY

Leaders in infusion nursing have the power to influence the quality of patient care and patient safety.

As a leader, the infusion nurse accepts responsibility for personal and professional growth. Within the Institute of Medicine report, we find a focus on full partnership with other disciplines and key players in the health care arena. In the contemporary health care environment, nurses, physicians/licensed independent practitioners (LIPs), patients, and other health professionals are increasingly interdependent. Singular solutions don't adequately address the kinds of complex problems presented to patient care decision makers. A new kind of partnership-based leadership will be necessary to improve patient outcomes, reduce errors, and impact staff engagement and satisfaction. The repeated evidence of the benefits of collaboration hasn't yet been well articulated into the activities of health professionals across the health system. Changing this culture, although not easy, will be essential to advancing quality health care (IOM, 2010).

IV DEPARTMENT CONSIDERATIONS

In organizing a department, the first consideration should be to establish a philosophy and the objectives necessary to support such a philosophy (Box 3-4). Health care facilities around the country and across the globe are establishing resource programs and outpatient infusion centers to ensure a high standard of care. The team functions must be delineated to ensure consistency, quality, and safety (Box 3-5).

Departmental Policies and Procedures

Policies and procedures play a vital role in the functioning of the department, serving as a guide to its operations, providing the nurse with adequate instruction, and ensuring the patient a high level of infusion care. They may also provide legal protection in determining

---

BOX 3-4   EXAMPLE OF MISSION AND OBJECTIVES OF AN IV DEPARTMENT

Mission

To administer safe and successful infusion therapy in the best interests of the patient, the hospital, and the nursing profession

Objectives

The objectives of an IV department are as follows:

1. To develop skills and impart knowledge that will provide a high level of safety in the practice of infusion nursing
2. To encourage further education and knowledge in the field of IV therapy
3. To assist in keeping the nursing staff educated in the maintenance of IV therapy and other nursing needs relevant to IV therapy
4. To collaborate with other personnel in the development and implementation of continuing education in infusion therapy
5. To develop nursing judgment and critical thinking in infusion therapy
6. To keep abreast of the latest scientific and medical advances and their implications in the practice of IV therapy
7. To attain and maintain certification
8. To ensure fiscal responsibility

BOX 3-5   FUNCTIONS OF AN IV DEPARTMENT

Infusion Administration

Parenteral fluids
Blood and blood components
Total parenteral nutrition
Antineoplastic therapy
Intra-arterial therapy
Pain management

IV Access and Monitoring

Peripheral lines
Pediatrics
Administration set and dressing changes
Therapeutic phlebotomy
Venous sampling
Peripherally inserted central catheters
Subcutaneous drug administration
Other alternative access devices

Patient/Family Education

Self-care
Home therapy

Preparation

Drugs in solution

Collaborative Practice

Safety committee
Quality improvement
Code team
Product evaluation
Development of policies and procedures
Magnet preparation

---

whether a person involved in negligent conduct has had adequate instruction in performing the procedure.

Policies and procedures should comply with state and federal laws, and national guidelines should be followed. The Joint Commission publishes manuals for hospital, home, ambulatory, and long-term care accreditation. The American Association of Blood Banks provides a technical manual with standards for care and administration of blood and component therapy. The Centers for Disease Control and Prevention (CDC) and the INS provide guidelines as well as Standards of Practice (CDC, 2011; INS, 2011).

Policies describing the responsibilities of the IV nurse vary significantly among facilities and practice settings and should be outlined to prevent confusion or misunderstanding. Examples of such policies are found in Box 3-6.

BOX 3-6   EXAMPLES OF POLICIES DESCRIBING INFUSION NURSE'S RESPONSIBILITIES

Administration of Parenteral Fluids

- Infusion nurses will, on written order, initiate all IVs, with the exception of those not approved for administration by the nurse.
- No more than two attempts at venipuncture will be allowed.
- Venipuncture should be avoided in the lower extremities except when the patient's condition may necessitate this use, and this location has specifically been ordered by the physician/LIP.

Preparation and Administration of IV Drugs

- Nurses will, on written order, prepare and administer only those solutions, medications, and combinations of drugs approved in writing by the pharmacy and the therapeutics committee.
- Nurses must check the patient's clinical record and question the patient regarding sensitivity to drugs that may cause anaphylaxis. They must observe the patient after initial administration of such drugs.

Nursing Care Plan

- A nursing care plan should be established within 24 hours of date/time of admission.

Peripheral Catheter Selection

- The catheter selected should be of the smallest gauge and shortest length to accommodate the prescribed therapy.

IV Nurse Qualifications

Because infusion therapy involves specialized judgment and skills, the infusion nurse must be qualified to meet the job requirements and scope of practice as defined in the Standards of Practice (CDC, 2011; INS, 2011). Any program of study for infusion nursing should be based on outcome criteria established in behavioral objectives. Both theoretical knowledge and clinical experience should be subsumed within the curriculum. The theoretical portion of the curriculum is based upon the core (Box 3-7). The success of the department depends on the selection of its personnel. Ideally, a credentialed infusion nurse specialist meets this goal.

These nurses must be not only meticulous in their actions but also accountable, conscientious, and dedicated to the specialty practice. There is no margin for error. Collaboration and teamwork are essential to the success of the department.

Mental and emotional stability are equally important to the nurse's success as an IV specialist. Manual dexterity, necessary in administering an IV, is greatly affected by the mental and emotional attitude of the nurse. Moreover, the performance of few other procedures is so easily affected by stress as a difficult venipuncture. Outstanding verbal and written communication skills are other assets necessary to the success of the nurse and the department.

BOX 3-7 NINE CORE AREAS OF A THEORETICAL CURRICULUM

- Technology and clinical application
- Pharmacology
- Neonate and pediatric patients
- Antineoplastic and biologic therapy
- Performance improvement
- Fluid and electrolytes
- Infection control
- Transfusion therapy
- Parenteral nutrition

Nursing Process Model

A study in the *Journal of Infusion Nursing* referred to the design and application of a nursing process model that illustrates infusion procedures performed in an outpatient setting. The model may be applied to other clinical settings and involves parameters for before, during, and after service. During the therapy administration phase, reconstitution of a drug or solution may occur in a hospital-based admixture service, and greet-and-escort responsibilities refer to the outpatient setting. The study further details time and motion studies associated with infusion therapy and cost justification.

Requests for Service

A system for receiving calls must be developed, with special emphasis on emergency calls. The size of the facility, number of patients, size and location of the department, and the functions to be performed must be considered when deciding which system would be most appropriate. Voice mail may be used for routine scheduling and nonemergencies. Mobile phones have transformed response time. Wireless networking has further facilitated the process, contributing to patient safety and timely documentation.

Preparation of Equipment

To maximize safety and minimize response time, the facility may choose to set up an equipment cart or designated supply cabinet on each patient care unit. Such equipment should comply with safety standards and infection control guidelines.

Before using the equipment, the professional infusion nurse ascertains the accuracy of the physician/LIP's order and then assembles the needed supplies from the cart if it is maintained on each nursing unit or from supply storage areas located elsewhere. Regardless of the method of obtaining equipment for venipuncture, the IV nurse has a crucial role in determining the accuracy of the order, assembling the appropriate equipment consistent with the therapy that has been ordered, and using the equipment in a safe manner.

During their hospital stay, patients with IVs in progress may visit ancillary hospital departments, including medical imaging, nuclear medicine, and surgery. To ensure the success and viability of an IV department or team, other departments in the institution must be oriented to the team's functions. If orders are written early in the day, it will be easier to meet all requests and ensure timely delivery of therapy to each patient under the team's care (Lozins Miller, 1998; INS, 2011).

Educational Approach

Today's methods of health care delivery demand excellence in the administration of complex infusion skills and the application of critical thinking. An adequate teaching program and criteria for evaluating the infusion nurse specialist must be established. The program curriculum and performance criteria depend on the role of the IV nurse as dictated by hospital policies. The nurse's competency must be evaluated and maintained, particularly when the infusion nurse receives on-the-job training.

The length of time involved in teaching depends on the individual and may range from 6 to 8 weeks. Content should be based on institutional policy and procedures, Standards of Practice, and the Core Curriculum for Infusion Nursing. The outline is consistent with that defined in the Core Curriculum for Infusion Nursing (Alexander & Corrigan, 2009). Principles of adult learning should be considered. Box 3-8 provides teaching strategies that are helpful for teaching IV, drug, and transfusion therapy.

Simulation models have enhanced the learning process. Virtual simulation software programs allow the learner to simulate procedures such as peripheral venipuncture via the computer. While there is no substitution for the practice needed to master a clinical skill, simulation can help the learner to gain confidence. See Table 3-4 for examples of infusion teaching models.

IMPACT OF COST CONTAINMENT ON TEAMS

In today's health care environment, it is becoming increasingly difficult for established infusion teams to justify their existence and for new teams to gain approval. The health care setting has changed dramatically; fiscal constraints are often overwhelming, forcing institutions to scrutinize methods of IV delivery for efficiency and cost-effectiveness.

BOX 3-8   TEACHING STRATEGIES

- Lecture
- Discussion
- Self-learning modules
- Simulation
- Train the trainer
- Computer-based learning
- Demonstration
- Experiential
- PowerPoint or Keynote presentation
- CD/DVD/YouTube®
- Case study

TABLE 3-4	SIMULATION TEACHING MODELS
Simulation Model	**Use**
Laerdal IV torso	External jugular insertion
Life/form Venatech IV Trainer	Peripheral placement and arterial blood gas
CentraLine Man	External jugular cannulation
Geriatric IV training arm	Peripheral IV placement
Life/form hemodialysis practice arm	Accessing fistulas
Deluxe IV training arm	Peripheral IV placement
Chester Chest	PICC, implanted port, peripheral IV, and peripheral port care
Peter PICC Line	PICC placement

Adapted from Czaplewski, L. (2011). Clinical and patient education. In M. Alexander, A. Corrigan, L. Gorski, J. Hankins, & R. Perucca (Eds.), *Infusion Nursing, an Evidence-Based Approach* (p. 71). St. Louis, MO: Saunders/Elsevier.

As a result, hospitals have downsized, restructured the workplace, and developed new patient care delivery models. Such models have had a significant impact on IV teams because ancillary services are not regarded as appropriate to the new, centralized, unit-based approach to patient care. In all practice settings, IV teams must be innovative and adaptable while maximizing capabilities and analyzing complementary practice roles and multidisciplinary care. The teams must work with their professional society to lead the way toward designing new directions for intravenous nursing practice. We now see renewed efforts at the development of infusion teams to impact safety, ensure positive outcomes, and maximize resources.

The CDC document "Guidelines for Prevention of Intravascular Device-Related Infections: An Overview" and Part 2, "Recommendations for Prevention of Intravascular Device-Related Infections," published in *Infection Control and Hospital Epidemiology* and the *American Journal of Infection Control,* suggested that eliminating infusion teams downgrades patient care by raising the risk of infection (CDC, 1998). Lozins Miller (1998) studied the use of IV clinicians to maintain high-quality venous access care in a health care system involved in downsizing its ranks. Reassigning the role of the infusion team member to an IV nurse clinician added new skill sets and an expanded role. The CDC position was updated in 2011 (CDC, 2011).

THE FUTURE OF INFUSION NURSING

This chapter addressed many expanding roles of the infusion nurse specialist; enhanced role models create a solid future for infusion practice. Team building, partnering, outreach, and collaboration—all terms of this millennium—suggest a continuing trend in health care. As the health care environments in which infusion care is delivered continue to expand, encompassing tertiary care, home care, outpatient clinics, and work sites, the need to align with strategic partners escalates. The complex process of providing infusion care requires collaboration among a diverse group of professionals with a diverse group of skills, including, but not limited to, the following: infusion nurses, infection control, oncology, pharmacy, education, quality improvement, and medicine, as well as the patients and families they serve (Weinstein, 2004).

Partnering and collaboration are the hallmark of many successful models implemented by practice and academic health care settings worldwide. Strategic partnering, within and beyond institutions, provides opportunities for personal and professional growth, outreach, and collaboration. Within the global nursing community, cross-national partnerships represent a vehicle for extending knowledge sharing, using on-site visits, teleconferencing and videoconferencing, electronic mail, and other resources. The World Wide Web has opened doors to distance learning programs that were once only a dream. The future of infusion nursing is evolving each and every day in settings around the country and across the globe.

Review Questions *Note: Questions below may have more than one right answer.*

1. Infusion specialists may provide clinical support in which of the following settings?
   A. Home care
   B. Acute care
   C. Infusion centers
   D. All of the above

2. Research about Magnet facilities demonstrates which of the following?
   A. Shorter patient stays
   B. Lower mortality rates
   C. Lower incidence of needlestick injuries
   D. All of the above

3. Policies and procedures should comply with which of the following?
   A. State and federal laws
   B. Hospital handbook
   C. County rules and regulations
   D. Local law

4. The first step in developing an infusion department is to
   A. Establish philosophy
   B. Define objectives
   C. Order supplies
   D. Create requisitions

5. A catheter selected for peripheral therapy should be
   A. Largest gauge and longest length
   B. Smallest gauge and shortest length
   C. Largest gauge and shortest length
   D. Smallest gauge and longest length

6. All of the following statements are true about mentoring *except*
   A. Mentoring is not time intensive.
   B. Mentees need your expertise.
   C. You learn from mentees.
   D. You leave a legacy.

7. The infusion nurse specialist may have an essential role in which of the following?
   A. Shared governance models
   B. Magnet recognition
   C. Mentoring programs
   D. All of the above

8. The infusion nurse specialist must have which of the following attributes?
   A. Mental and emotional stability
   B. Manual dexterity
   C. Verbal and written communication skills
   D. All of the above

9. A nursing care plan should be established within how many hours of admission?
   A. 6
   B. 12
   C. 18
   D. 24

10. The infusion specialist may serve as
    A. Resource nurse/clinician
    B. Educator
    C. A and B
    D. A only

References and Selected Readings   *Asterisks indicate references cited in text.*

*Aiken, L. (2012a). http://nursing.advanceweb.com/News/National-News/Nurse-Work-Environments-Better-at-Magnet-Hospitals-Aiken-Led-Study-Shows.aspx

*Aiken, L. (2012b). *Medical Care, Official journal of Medical Care section of the American Public Health Association.* http://www.nursecredentialing.org/Headlines/Aiken-PressRelease.pdf

*Alexander, M., & Corrigan, A.M. (Eds.). (2009). *Infusion Nurses Society core curriculum for infusion nursing* (3rd ed.). Philadelphia, PA: Lippincott Williams & Wilkins.

Alexander, M., Corrigan A., Gorski, L, Hankins, J., & Perucca R. (2008). *Infusion nursing: an evidence-based approach* (3rd ed). St Louis, MO: Saunders Elsevier.

American Nurses Credentialing Center. (2008). *Magnet recognition program: Application manual for 2005.* Silver Spring, MD: American Nurses Credentialing Center.

American Nurses Credentialing Center. (2013). Magnet Recognition Program model. http://www.nursecredentialing.org/Magnet/ProgramOverview/New-Magnet-Model

Baranowski, L. (1995). Presidential address: Take ownership. *Journal of Infusion Nursing*, *18*(4), 163.

Burggraf, V. (2012). Overview and summary: The new millennium: Evolving and emerging nursing roles. *OJIN: The Online Journal of Issues in Nursing*, *17*, 2.

*Centers for Disease Control and Prevention. (1998). Guidelines for prevention of intravascular infection. *Federal Register*, *60*(187), 49978–50006.

*Centers for Disease Control and Prevention. (2011). *Guidelines for prevention of intravascular catheter-related infections, 2011.* http://www.cdc.gov/hicpac/pdf/guidelines/bsi-guidelines-2011.pdf

*Czaplewski, L. (2011). Clinical and patient education. In M. Alexander, A. Corrigan, L. Gorski, J. Hankins, & R. Perucca (Eds.), *Infusion Nursing, an Evidence-Based Approach* (p. 71). St. Louis, MO: Saunders/Elsevier.

Davenport, T.H., & Prusak, L. (1998). *Working knowledge: how organizations manage what they know.* http://wang.ist.psu.edu/course/05/IST597/papers/Davenport_know.pdf

Fabian, B. (2010). Infusion therapy in the older adult. In M. Alexander, A. Corrigan, L. Gorski, J. Hankins, & R. Perucca., (Eds.), *Infusion nursing: An evidence-based approach* (3rd ed., pp. 571–582). St Louis, MO: Saunders/Elsevier.

Huras R. (2009). *RNs should check IVs every 4 hours to avoid malpractice.* http://news.nurse.com/apps/pbcs.dll/article?AID=2009305180015

*Hess, R. (2004). From bedside to boardroom—nursing shared governance. *Online Journal of Issues in Nursing*, *9*(1), manuscript 1. http://www.nursingworld.org/MainMenuCategories/ANAMarketplace/ANAPeriodicals/OJIN/TableofContents/Volume92004/No1Jan04/FromBedsidetoBoardroom.aspx

*Infusion Nurses Society. (2011). Infusion nursing standards of practice. *Journal of Infusion Nursing*, *34*(1S), S1–S110.

*Infusion Nurses Society. (2013). Infusion teams in acute care hospitals: Call for a business approach. www.ins1.org, accessed on November 27, 2013.

*Institute of Medicine. (2010). *The future of nursing: Leading change, advancing health* (5–2). Washington, DC: National Academies. http://www.iom.edu/Reports/2010/The-future-of-nursing-leading-change-advancing-health.aspx

Kelly, L.A., McHugh, M.D., & Aiken, L.H. (2011). Nurse outcomes in Magnet® and non-magnet hospitals. *Journal of Nursing Administration*, *41*(10), 428–433.

Kim, H., Capezuti, E., Boltz, M., & Fairchild, S. (2009). The Nursing Practice Environment and nurse-perceived quality of geriatric care in hospitals. *Western Journal of Nursing Research*, *31*(4), 480–495.

Kutney-Lee, A., McHugh, M.D., Sloane, D.M., Cimiotti, J.P., Flynn, L., & Neff D.F., et al. (2009). Nursing: A key to patient satisfaction. *Health Affairs*, *28*(4), 669–677.

Leapfrog Group. (2013). *Hospital ratings.* http://www.hospitalsafetyscore.org/about-the-score/about-the-leapfrog-group

*Lozins Miller, P.K. (1998). Downsizing. *Journal of Infusion Nursing*, *21*(2), 105–112.

Lundmark, VA. (2008). Magnet environments for professional nursing practice. In: R.G. Hughes (Ed.), *Patient safety and quality: An evidence-based handbook for nurses* (Chapter 46). Rockville, MD: Agency for Healthcare Research and Quality (US). Available from: http://www.ncbi.nlm.nih.gov/books/NBK2667/

McClure, M.L., Poulin, M.A., & Sovie, M.D., et al. (2002). Magnet hospitals: Attraction and retention of professional nurses (the original study). In M.L. McClure, & A.S. Hinshaw, (Eds.), *Magnet hospitals revisited: attraction and retention of professional nurses* (pp. 1– 24). Washington, DC: American Nurses Publishing.

McClure, M.L. (2005). Magnet hospitals: Insights and issues. *Nursing Administration Quarterly*, 29(3), 198–201.

National Electronic Library for Health. *The Knowledge Worker*. National Health Service. http://www.nelh.nhs.uk

Ostendorf, W. (2010). Intravenous and vascular access therapy. In A.G. Perry, & P. A. Potter, *Clinical nursing skills and techniques* (7th ed., pp. 740– 784). St Louis, MO: Mosby.

Shortell, S.M., & Kaluzny, A.D. (2006). *Health care management: organization design and behavior* (5th ed.). Clifton Park, NY: Thomson Delmar Learning.

Skyrme, D. (2013). *About I³ update*. www.skyrme.com/updates

*Weinstein, S.M. (2004). Strategic partnerships: Bridging the collaboration gap. *Journal of Infusion Nursing*, 27(5), 297–301.

*Wilson, A., Whitaker, N., & Whitford, D. (2012). Rising to the Challenge of Health Care Reform with entrepreneurial and intrapreneurial nursing Initiatives. *OJIN: The Online Journal of Issues in Nursing*, 17, 2, Manuscript 5.

*Zugcic, M., Davis, J.E., Gorski, L.A., & Alexander M. (2010). Establishing research priorities for the Infusion Nurses Society. *Journal of Infusion Nursing*, 33(3), 176–182.

CHAPTER 4

Standards of Practice

Sharon M. Weinstein

KEY TERMS	Beneficence	Global Authority
	Body of Evidence	Nonmaleficence
	Competencies	Practice Criteria
	Educational	Scope of Practice
	Requirements	Standards of Practice
	Fidelity	

THE STANDARDS

The Infusion Nurses Society (INS) has established the scope of practice, competencies, and educational requirements for the administration of infusion therapy and has set forth Standards of Practice. INS is recognized as the global authority in infusion nursing. As the science and research of infusion nursing expands and technology advances, the Standards are revised and updated consistent with practice. The Standards are written to be applicable to all care settings in which infusion therapy is delivered and to address all clinical patient populations. The most current edition of the Standards defines practice criteria supported by the latest available research and further ranks the strength of the body of evidence reviewed (INS, 2011).

NURSING PRACTICE

In this section, the Standards address the practice setting; patient-specific populations, including neonatal and pediatric patients and older adult patients; as well as ethics, scope of practice, competencies, quality improvement, the evidence base, and policies and procedures for clinical practice.

The Standards allow for those inside and outside the profession to judge the competency of nurses practicing infusion therapy. As a method of public protection, the Standards address the need for the nurse to be competent in the safe delivery of infusion therapy within his or her scope of practice (INS, 2011).

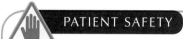

PATIENT SAFETY

Competencies are a critical element in ensuring patient safety.

Throughout this chapter, the authors highlight key standards and the relevant **practice criteria**. (*Standards are printed in italics;* practice criteria are not in italics.) How well the nurse integrates the Standards and practice criteria is one way to evaluate competence in specialty IV nursing practice. The reader is referred to the INS for a full copy of the Standards document.

Practice Setting

STANDARD

The Infusion Nursing Standards of Practice shall be applied and met in all practice settings. Administration of infusion therapy shall be established in organizational policies, procedures, and/or practice guidelines. Administration of infusion therapy shall be in accordance with rules and regulations promulgated by the state's Board of Nursing and federal and state regulatory and accrediting agencies in all practice settings.

Neonatal and Pediatric Patients

STANDARD

The nurse providing infusion therapy for neonatal and pediatric patients shall have clinical knowledge and technical expertise with regard to this population. Clinical management of neonatal and pediatric patients shall be established in organizational policy, procedures, and/or practice guidelines and in accordance with applicable standards of care. The nurse shall verify that informed consent for treatment of neonatal and pediatric patients, as well as those patients who are deemed emancipated minors of mature majors, is documented.

Ethics

STANDARD

Ethical principles shall be the foundation for decision making and patient advocacy. Guidelines and resources for ethical issues shall be outlined in organizational policies, procedures, and/or practice guidelines. The nurse shall act as a patient advocate; maintain patient confidentiality, safety, and security; and respect, promote, and preserve human anatomy, dignity, rights, and diversity. Principles of **beneficence, nonmaleficence, fidelity***, protection of patient autonomy, justice, and veracity shall dictate nursing action.*

Scope of Practice

STANDARD

The scope of practice for each type of person involved with the delivery of infusion therapy shall be organized to support patient safety and protection and shall clearly define the roles, responsibilities, tasks and range of services, and accountability for all levels of personnel involved with the delivery of infusion therapy. All licensed nursing personnel shall possess a license in standing with the state's Board of Nursing. All personal shall practice within the legal boundaries of individual license or scope of practice. The RN shall be accountable for patient safety in the delivery of infusion care. The scope continues to address communication, the role of assistive personnel, and delegation of infusion therapy tasks. The reader can clearly see that the upgraded and updated Standards reflect the specialty practice and patient safety.

PATIENT SAFETY

The scope of practice revolves around patient safety and protection.

PRACTICE CRITERIA

A. The legal scope of practice for all licensed health care professions is defined in the state statute governing each profession.
B. The method for making scope of practice decisions is different for each state's Board of Nursing and includes a decision tree model, declaratory ruling, and advisory opinions.
C. Decisions about the scope of practice for each type of personnel involved with infusion therapy should focus on nursing assistive personnel, medical assistant, licensed practical/vocational nurses, registered nurses, infusion nursing specialists (CRNI), and advanced practice nurses.

Quality Improvement

STANDARD

The nurse shall participate in quality improvement activities that advance patient care, quality, and safety.

PRACTICE CRITERIA

A. Quality improvement activities include evaluation of patient or clinical outcomes; identifying clinical indictors, benchmarks, and areas for improvement; providing best evidence; recommending and implementing changes in structures or processes; analyzing date and outcomes against benchmarks; considering the use of cost analysis; or minimizing and eliminating barriers to change and improvement.
B. The quality improvement program should create a culture that fosters the reporting and analysis of quality and safety indictor outcomes, near misses, errors, and adverse events. The program should focus on systems and processes that promote individual accountability and a just culture.

C. The knowledge gained through this process should be shared internally and externally with other health care providers and organizations.

PATIENT CARE

This section of the Standards addresses orders for the initiation and management of infusion therapy, patient education, informed consent, and the plan of care. Again, the reader is referred to the INS for the complete document.

DOCUMENTATION

Within documentation, we find evidence surrounding documentation, unusual occurrence and sentinel event reporting, product evaluation, integrity and defect reporting, as well as verification of products and medications.

INFECTION PREVENTION AND SAFETY COMPLIANCE

With a strong focus on patient safety and outcomes, this section addresses infection prevention, hand hygiene, compounding of parenteral solutions and medications, the use of scissors, safe handling and disposal of sharps, hazardous materials, hazardous waste, disinfection of durable medical equipment, transfusion-based precautions, and latex sensitivity or allergy. An example related to hand hygiene is offered.

Hand Hygiene

STANDARD

Hand hygiene shall be a routine practice established in organizational policies, procedures, and/or practice guidelines. Hand hygiene shall be performed before and after touching a patient; before handling an invasive device; before moving from a contaminated body site to another site; before donning and after removing gloves; and after contact with inanimate objects in the immediate vicinity of the patient. The nurse shall not wear artificial nails when performing infusion therapy procedures. In cases in which the nurse's hands are visibly contaminated with blood or body fluids or hands have been exposed to spore-producing pathogens, hand hygiene with either nonantiseptic or antiseptic (preferably antiseptic-containing) liquid soap and water shall be performed.

Practice Criteria

A. Alcohol-based hand rubs are preferred for routine hand hygiene.
B. Chosen hand hygiene products should be high efficiency with low potential for skin irritation. Towelettes and non–alcohol-based rubs should not be used for hand hygiene.
C. Proper hand hygiene should be taught to caregivers involved in the care of the patient.
D. Dispensers of liquid soap or antiseptic solution are recommended.
E. Single-use soap scrub packets or waterless antiseptic products should be used when clean running water is not ensured or is unavailable.

    F. The nurse shall be involved with hand hygiene evaluation.

    G. Hand hygiene is a key component of a group of evidence-based interventions to promote better outcomes for patients with intravascular catheters.

    H. Artificial nails have been associated with transmission and outbreaks of infection.

Infusion Equipment

This section of the document involves add-on devices, needleless connectors, filters, flow-control devices, blood and fluid warmers, and tourniquets. In this area, we address vascular access device selection, including short peripheral catheters, midline catheters, and central vascular access devices (nontunneled, peripherally inserted central catheter (PICC), tunneled, implanted port); arterial catheters; site selection; local anesthesia for vascular access device placement and access; vascular access site preparation and device placement; stabilization; joint stabilization: and site protection—completely updated to reflect the practice, the state of the art, safety, and outcomes.

A separate section of the document includes implanted vascular access ports, hemodialysis vascular access devices, umbilical catheters, as well as apheresis and ultrafiltration catheters.

SITE CARE AND MAINTENANCE

Here, we cover administration set changes, vascular access device removal, flushing and locking, and vascular access device site care and dressing changes.

INFUSION-RELATED COMPLICATIONS

Common complications associated with infusion therapy include phlebitis, infiltration and extravasation, infection, air embolism, catheter embolism, catheter-associated venous thrombosis, and central vascular device malposition. This is explored in great detail in the relevant chapter of this text (Table 4-1, Phlebitis Scale).

OTHER INFUSION-RELATED PROCEDURES

In this area, we address vascular access device repair, central vascular access device exchange, catheter clearance, and phlebotomy. In *nonvascular infusion devices*, we cover intraspinal access, intraosseous access, and continuing subcutaneous infusion.

INFUSION THERAPIES

PATIENT SAFETY

The health care consumer is the focus of Standards of Practice. Standards are statements of the anticipated care experience or outcome. The outcome for those receiving infusion therapies should always be focused on safety.

TABLE 4-1	PHLEBITIS SCALE
Grade	Clinical Criteria
0	No symptoms
1	Erythema at access site with or without pain
2	Pain at access site with erythema and/or edema
3	Pain at access site with erythema Streak formation Palpable venous cord
4	Pain at access site with erythema Streak formation Palpable venous cord > 1 inch in length Purulent drainage

Source: Infusion Nurses Society Standards of Practice, 2011.

The final section of the 2011 revision addresses parenteral medication and solution administration, antineoplastic therapy, biologics, patient-controlled analgesia, parenteral nutrition, transfusion therapy, moderate sedation/analgesia using intravenous infusion, and the administration of parenteral investigational drugs.

Review Questions   *Note: Questions below may have more than one right answer.*

1. The INS Standards document was most recently revised in
   A. 1995
   B. 1998
   C. 2004
   D. 2011

2. Which of the following statements is true of standards?
   A. They are written to be applicable to all care settings and to address all clinical patient populations.
   B. They provide a framework for evaluation of outcomes.
   C. They must be implemented institution wide.
   D. They should regularly be compared with existing policies.

3. Appropriate hand hygiene includes
   A. Towelettes
   B. Alcohol-based hand rubs
   C. Non–alcohol-based rubs
   D. Bar soap in lieu of other products

4. The section of the Standards labeled Infection Prevention and Safety Compliance addresses which of the following?
   A. Prevention
   B. Transmission-based precautions
   C. A and B
   D. A only

5. Which of the following is an important component of infusion practice?
   A. Umbilical catheters
   B. Apheresis and ultrafiltration catheters
   C. Flushing and locking
   D. All of the above

6. Which of the following is most important concerning infusion-related complications?
   A. They are a routine occurrence regardless of clinical setting.
   B. The assessment and treatment of infiltration or extravasation shall be established in organizational policies.
   C. Infection can be prevented.
   D. Hand hygiene plays an important role in minimizing complications.

7. Absence of symptoms, including erythema and a palpable cord, is indicative of a nonphlebitic site.
   A. True
   B. False

8. Quality improvement activities include which of the following?
   A. Evaluation of patient or clinical outcomes
   B. Identifying clinical indictors
   C. Cost analysis
   D. All of the above

9. Guidelines and resources for ethical issues shall be
   A. Defined by the hospital's board of directors
   B. Outlined in organizational policies and procedures
   C. Described in the patient's rights
   D. Identified by the infusion team

10. Decisions regarding the scope of practice should be defined for which of the following personnel?
    A. Nursing assistive personnel
    B. Registered nurses
    C. Advanced practice nurses
    D. All of the above

References and Selected Readings   *Asterisks indicate references cited in text.*

Adams, J. (2010). Utilizing evidence-based practice to support the infusion alliance. *Journal of Infusion Nursing, 33*(5), 273–277.

Ahlqvist, M., Brglund, B., Wiren, M., Klang, B., & Johansson, E. (2009). Accuracy in documentation: a study of peripheral catheters. *Journal of Clinical Nursing, 18*, 1945–1952.

American Nurses Association. (2010). *Nursing: scope and standards of practice* (2nd ed.). Silver Spring, MD: ANA.

Czaplewski, L. (2010). Clinician and patient education. In M. Alexander, A. Corrigan, L. Gorski, J. Hankins, & R.D. Perucca (Eds.), *Infusion nursing: An evidence-based approach* (3rd ed., pp. 71–94). St. Louis, MO: Saunders/Elsevier.

ECRI Institute. *Suggested guidelines for blood warmer use.* http://www.mdsr.edri.org/summary/detail.aspx?doc_id8269

Frey, A.M., & Pettit, J. (2010). Infusion therapy in children. In M. Alexander, A. Corrigan, L. Gorski, J. Hankins, & R. Perucca (Eds.), *Infusion nursing: An evidence based approach* (3rd ed., pp. 550–570), St. Louis, MO: Saunders/Elsevier.

Gorski, L., Perucca, R., & Hunter, M. (2010). Central venous access devices: Care, maintenance and potential complications. In M. Alexander, A. Corrigan, L. Gorski, J. Hankins, & R. Perucca (Eds.), *Infusion nursing: An evidence-based approach* (3rd ed., pp. 456–479). St. Louis, MO: Saunders/Elsevier.

Hadaway, L., & Richardson, D. (2010). Needleless connectors: A primer of terminology. *Journal of Infusion Nursing, 33*(1), 1–11.

Hughes R.G. (2008). Tools and strategies for quality improvement and patient safety. In R.G. Hughes (Ed.), *Patient safety and quality: An evidence-based handbook for nurses.* AHRQ publication no. 08-0043. Rockville, MD: Agency for Healthcare Research and Quality. http://www.ahrq.gov/qual/nursehdbk/docs/HughesR-QMBMP.pdf

* Infusion Nurses Society. (2011). Revised infusion nursing standards of practice. *Journal of Infusion Nursing,* *34*(1S).

Institute for Healthcare Improvement. (2013). *Implement the central line bundle.* http://www.ihi.org/IHI/ Topics/CriticalCare/IntensifeCare/Changes/ImplementtheCentralLineBundle.htm

National Quality Forum. (2009). *Safe practices for better healthcare. Update: A consensus report.* Washington, DC: NQF.

Pugliese, G., & Salahuddin, M. (1999). *Sharps injury prevention program: A step-by-step guide.* Chicago, IL: American Hospital Association.

Sims, J.M. (2008). Your role in informed consent. *Dimensions of critical care nursing, 7*(3), 118–121.

Smith, R.L., & Sheperd, M. (1995). Central venous catheter infection rates in an acute care hospital. *Journal of Infusion Nursing, 18,* 255.

U.S. Department of Health and Human Services. (2010). *Healthy people 2010: Understanding and improving health* (2nd ed.). Washington, DC: DHHS.

U.S. Food and Drug Administration. (2012). *Letter to infection control practitioners regarding positive displacement needleless connectors.* http://www.fda.gov/MedicalDevices/Safety/AlertsandNotices/ucm220459.htm

Wakefield D., & Wakefield B. (2009). Are verbal orders a threat to patient safety? *Quality and safety in health care, 18*(3), 165–168.

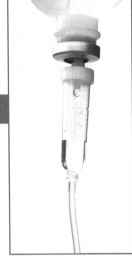

CHAPTER 5

Nurse and Patient Education

Tina T. Smith
Linda A. Cayan
Julie L. Millenbruch

KEY TERMS		
	Adult Learning Principles	Learning Needs Assessment
	Certification	Learning Style
	Competency	Low Fidelity
	Competency Assessment	Mannequin
	Competency Validation	Orientation
	Curriculum	Professional Development
	Health Literacy	Reflective Practice
	High Fidelity	SBAR
	Human Patient Simulator	Simulation
		Task Trainer

KNOWLEDGE SHARING

Approximately 80% of patients admitted to hospitals receive some form of intravenous (IV) therapy (Ozyazicioglu & Arikan, 2008), which can be high risk and also problematic. Among patients with central vascular access devices (CVADs), 5% to 26% will develop an infectious complication such as a bloodstream infection (CDC, 2011; Taylor, 2012). Furthermore, patients and families may experience stress, anxiety, and/or pain during IV therapy (Cox & Westbrook, 2005; Stafford & Emery, 2007).

Consistency in evidence-based IV insertion and site care, expert surveillance, and timely interventions by health care personnel with education and competency in infusion therapy may prevent complications (CDC, 2011) and lessen patients' emotional reactions to infusion therapy. This chapter provides content about the knowledge and skills required for nurses to be competent in infusion therapy; how infusion nurses can develop their knowledge, skills, and competence throughout their careers; and the role of the infusion nurse in teaching patients and significant others about infusion therapy.

THE INFUSION NURSE

An infusion nurse has acquired a body of knowledge that encompasses expertise in technical infusion therapy skills and clinical reasoning. The nurse focuses on patient-centered care and interpersonal communication. The individual expertly manages infusion therapy, including an awareness of the inherent risks of therapy. The infusion nurse functions in a variety of practice areas, is vigilant and meticulous in initiating and maintaining infusion therapy, and shares infusion-specific knowledge and skill to develop others, for example, nurses new to infusion therapy. Sharing knowledge and skills, and developing other nurses, helps promote competence in infusion therapy practice by all nurses when an infusion nurse may not be present on a twenty-four hour and seven-day basis.

An infusion nurse practices in all health care settings and with patients of all age groups, diagnoses, comorbidities, and severity of illness. Practice areas may include but are not limited to acute care, home health care, long-term care, outpatient clinics, surgical procedure centers, ambulatory infusion centers, and health care provider offices. Responsibilities of the infusion nurse may vary according to state nurse practice acts and organizational or departmental policies and procedures.

Promoting Effective Communication

A majority of untoward events occurring in health care settings involve miscommunication. According to The Joint Commission, patient safety is improved when communication is clear, accurate, complete, and timely; in 2008 communication was made a patient safety goal. Since that time, tools have been developed to assist health care team members in structuring focused communication. Effective communication and teamwork are critical to the delivery of quality patient care.

Communication is an essential component of all health care curricula; unfortunately, we typically focus on intradisciplinary communication. Each discipline has its own terminology, expectations, and idiosyncrasies relative to communication, all of which can impact the effectiveness of communication across disciplines. Because health care involves multiple disciplines, we need a method of standardized interdisciplinary communication to enhance quality of care and promote patient safety. SBAR, which stands for Situation-Background-Assessment-Recommendation, is one communication technique that can assist infusion nurses. SBAR is a shared model for standardized communication designed to facilitate and improve communication between and among health care personnel. It can be applied to both verbal and written communication (Haig, Sutton, & Whittington, 2006). The model has four components:

- *Situation*—statement of what is happening at the present time that has triggered the SBAR. For example, "I am calling about Mr. Jones who has a central line and the antibiotic will not infuse."
- *Background*—information that puts the situation into context and explains the circumstances that have led to the situation. Continuing the example, "The central line was inserted one week ago into the subclavian and has been used daily without difficulty. Trouble-shooting according to policy has been completed. The antibiotic is due now."
- *Assessment*—statement of the communicator's ideas about the problem. "I believe the line is occluded."
- *Recommendation*—statement of what should be done to correct the problem, by when, and by whom. "Would you want to order a thrombolytic per policy to try and open the line or should I remove the line?"

INFUSION NURSES' EDUCATION, COMPETENCY, AND PROFESSIONAL DEVELOPMENT

The American Nurses Association (ANA), in its standards (2010), identifies that registered nurses (RNs) have "the professional obligation to acquire and maintain the knowledge and competencies necessary for current nursing practice" (Kulbok, 2012, p. 123). To acquire the unique body of knowledge and skills for infusion nursing practice, the RN must pursue infusion therapy education beyond that which was learned in nursing school. Once infusion specialty knowledge and skills have been acquired and demonstrated, the infusion nurse must then maintain competence in evidence-based infusion therapy through active participation in professional development activities.

Infusion Nurses' Education

To acquire infusion therapy knowledge and skills, the RN may attend formal and/or informal classes, in-services, webinars, or complete self-learning modules on infusion therapy (Collins, Phillips, Dougherty, de Verteuil, & Morris, 2006; Roslien & Alcock, 2009). One size, or one educational approach, will not fit all. For example, an education session for a nurse with limited IV therapy knowledge and skill will include content, practice, and competency validation for IV insertion, aseptic dressing changes, pharmacology, and transfusion therapies. Education for an experienced infusion therapy nurse might focus on developing knowledge regarding IV equipment specific to the setting/patient populations or successful completion of more advanced competencies.

The nurse who desires to become expert in infusion therapy should first identify what he or she knows and does not know regarding published IV standards, guidelines, and content. The nurse then can seek out an evidence-based curriculum that incorporates these standards and guidelines and builds upon their learning needs. This planned program of study will guide learning, mastery, and competence in infusion nursing practice.

There are several resources and educational recommendations that can help the nurse gain further infusion therapy knowledge. The Infusion Nurses Society (INS) has standards

EVIDENCE FOR PRACTICE

Fakih, M. G., Jones, K., Rey, J.E., Berriel-Cass, D., Kalinicheva, T., Saravolatz, L.D. (2012). Sustained improvements in peripheral venous catheter care in non-intensive care units: A quasi-experimental controlled study of education and feedback. *Infection Control and Hospital Epidemiology, 33*(5), 449–455.

In a study of 10 non-ICU units and over 4,000 peripheral venous catheters, providing education and "real-time feedback" to nurses significantly reduced peripheral venous catheter-associated bloodstream infection. Process information provided to direct care nurses and nurse managers included dressing change documentation, dressing being intact, and correctly scrubbing the hub. Outcome information about infection rate also was provided.

of practice (2011) as well as a core curriculum (Alexander et al., 2014), which identify needed content for infusion nursing knowledge and competence. The CDC also recommends education in the following areas: (a) reasons for infusion therapy, (b) correct insertion and maintenance of IV catheters, and (c) prevention of catheter-associated infections (CDC, 2011). These and other appropriate references should inform any curriculum that prepares infusion nurses.

PATIENT SAFETY

A planned and structured orientation program for the infusion nurse using best evidence and demonstrated competency increases patient safety.

CURRICULUM DEVELOPMENT FOR INFUSION THERAPY NURSE EDUCATION

Nurses benefit from a well-conceived curriculum (Boland & Finke, 2012). A comprehensive curriculum also provides for consistency in delivery of IV content to assure that learners receive the required information. Adult teaching, learning, and assessment strategies inform the design of curricula and learning experiences so that those who attend infusion therapy education sessions are engaged, understand the learning outcomes they are to achieve, and are involved in the planning and managing of their learning (Boland & Finke, 2012). Without active and engaged learners, knowledge and skill acquisition to enhance the infusion nurse's practice may be limited.

A **curriculum**, or plan for instruction, should be developmental, based upon the learner, the learner's goals, and the learner's competency. In order for the appropriate curriculum to be created and taught, the purpose and objectives of the education should be identified after the needs of the learner are identified. An example of a curriculum plan from a needs assessment for developing RNs' knowledge and clinical skills to care for patients with peripherally inserted central catheters (PICCs) and to prevent central line–associated bloodstream infections (CLABSIs) is included in Table 5-1. This curriculum plan is one of many that could be included in evidence-based, structured, and developmental infusion therapy curricula to prepare competent infusion therapy nurses.

TABLE 5-1	CURRICULUM PLAN AND CONTENT FOR CARE OF THE PATIENT WITH A PERIPHERALLY INSERTED CENTRAL CATHETER (PICC)

Part A: Curriculum Plan

Program Purpose	Develop knowledge and clinical skills in PICC nursing care and prevention of CLABSI.
Learning Objectives	At the end of the session, the participant will be able to: • Describe a PICC. • Identify one action to prevent CLABSI in PICCs. • Perform a dressing change for a PICC. • Administer medication through a PICC.
Instructional Methods	Audience response participation system Presentation Discussion Video Simulation (task trainer)
Target Audience	Infusion Nurses
Instructional Tools for PICC Education Learning Stations	Dressing change learning station: • PICC arm with catheter • Alcohol swabs • Waterless hand sanitizer • Gloves Transparent semipermeable chlorhexidine gluconate dressing kit	Medication administration learning station: • PICC arm with catheter • Alcohol swabs • Waterless hand sanitizer • Gloves • IV tubing primary and secondary • 10 mL 0.9 NS prefilled syringes • Heparin prefilled syringe (based upon policy for PICC locking)
Instructor Resources for Planning Curriculum Content	• Alexander, M., Corrigan, A.M., Gorski, L.A., Hankins, J., & Perucca, R. (2010). *Infusion nursing: An evidence-based approach* (3rd ed.). St Louis, MO: Saunders Elsevier. • Alexander, M., Corrigan, A.M., Gorski, L.A., & Phillips, L. (2014). *Core curriculum for infusion nursing* (4th ed.). Philadelphia, PA: Lippincott Williams & Wilkins. • Bartock, L. (2010). An evidence-based systematic review of literature for the reduction of PICC line occlusions. *Journal of the Association for Vascular Access, 15*, 58–63. • Bucher, L., & Sanderson, L.V. (2011). Peripherally inserted central catheter. In D. Wiegand (Ed.), *AACN procedure manual for critical care* (6th ed., pp. 763–774). Philadelphia, PA: Saunders. • Camp-Sorrell, D. (2011). *Access device guidelines: Recommendations for nursing practice and education* (3rd ed.). Pittsburgh, PA: Oncology Nursing Society. • CDC. (2011). *Guidelines for the prevention of intravascular catheter-related infections*. http://www.cdc.gov/hicpac/pdf/guidelines/bsi-guidelines-2011.pdf • Infusion Nurses Society. (2011). Infusion nursing standards of practice. *Journal of Infusion Nursing, 34*(15), S1–S110. • Organizational policy
Preclass Learner Assignment	Instructor could assign an article for participants to review.

TABLE 5-1	CURRICULUM PLAN AND CONTENT FOR CARE OF THE PATIENT WITH A PERIPHERALLY INSERTED CENTRAL CATHETER (PICC) *(Continued)*

Kirkpatrick's Evaluation	Level 1: Class evaluation
	Level 2: Preevaluation of knowledge compared to postevaluation of knowledge using audience response system

Part B: Content

Time	Objectives	Content	Instructional Methods
15 minutes	Introduction	• Introduction of instructor • Ice breaker: name and first paying job • Review locations of restrooms and personal electronic device expectations • Review objectives • Complete preevaluation questions using audience response participation system	Audience response participation system
15 minutes	Describe a PICC	PICC suggested content: • Definition	
		• Arm anatomy for insertion sites: cephalic, basilic, median cubital, and brachial veins	Arm diagram
		• Heart anatomy: chambers, superior/inferior vena cava, circulation, tip rests in the distal superior vena cava • Rationale for use • Insertion sites, contradictions for placement, and what to avoid when a patient has a PICC	Heart diagram
		• Catheter: single or multilumen, power injectable, staggered lumen exits, various gauges and lengths, 10-mL syringe or greater for medication/blood draw/ flushing	Single- and multilumen PICC and power injectable PICC
15 minutes	Identify one action to prevent catheter-associated bloodstream infections in PICCs	Activity from audience response participation system suggested content: **Q:** Audience response: What one patient demographic increases risk for infection? **A:** Age: premature infants and patients older than 65	Audience response system slides
		Q: Audience response: Name this potential PICC complication. **A:** Phlebitis, infiltration, extravasation, infection, air embolism, catheter embolism, venous thrombosis, and malposition. Include content on why the complication occurs and prevention strategies CLABSI prevention and standard assessment-suggested content:	Pictures of complications
		• CLABSI prevention guidelines from the CDC include health care provider training, correct hand hygiene, use of maximal barrier protection, use of chlorhexidine gluconate solution for skin antisepsis, and daily review of continuation of need for access device.	
		• Standardized assessment: visual condition of site, palpation of site, patient discomfort at insertion site or arm, external catheter length, integrity of device, closed secure system, signs/symptoms of infection	Demonstrate with task trainer

(Continued)

TABLE 5-1	CURRICULUM PLAN AND CONTENT FOR CARE OF THE PATIENT WITH A PERIPHERALLY INSERTED CENTRAL CATHETER (PICC) *(Continued)*		
30 min	Perform a dressing change for a PICC	• Dressing suggested content: aseptic application, product integrity, transparent semipermeable dressing, occlusive, site label, device secure, and frequency of dressing change • Use a standardized checklist	Video demonstration and show materials
		• Learners to perform PICC dressing change with removal of dressing, placement of new dressing, and documentation based upon agency policy	Simulation: task trainer and materials
30 min	Administer medication through a PICC	• Medication administration suggested content: product integrity, add-on devices only when needed, access port integrity, aseptic technique, venous blood return and patency, flushing PICC pre- and postmedication administration, use of heparin or antireflux device based upon agency policy • Use a standardized checklist	Video Demonstration and show materials
		• Learners to perform PICC medication administration with flushing/locking of PICC line based upon agency policy	Simulation: task trainer and materials
10 min	End of class	Review objectives Complete postevaluation using audience response participation system	Audience response participation system

METHODS FOR EDUCATION

Simulation, as an instructional method for education and training and incorporated in the sample PICC curriculum plan, is not new. Simulation offers the opportunity for novice infusion nurses to practice psychomotor skills and then advance to integration of clinical decision making in the nursing process of assessment, planning, implementation, and evaluation. Simulation can be incorporated within the infusion nurse **orientation** with a combination of instructional methods including task trainers, human patient simulators, and standardized patients (Figure 5-1).

The sample PICC curriculum plan (Table 5-1) uses task trainers for learning select technical skills. A **task trainer** is a life-like model of a body part or organ; it also can be a nonanatomical device to teach a skill, such as a specialized stethoscope to learn heart sounds. A task trainer is well suited for infusion therapy instruction since it breaks down a physical activity into understandable steps. This instructional method is considered **low-fidelity** simulation as it does not place the learner in a realistic environment and the focus is on skill development.

Human patient simulators are fully automatic **mannequins** with comprehensive clinical functioning and react to the learner's actions or inactions. **High-fidelity** simulation, using a human patient simulator, addresses technical skills and integrates the dimensions of decision making and clinical judgment while incorporating teamwork in a fully interactive real work environment. High-fidelity simulation experience is as close to the live patient situation as possible and places the learner in a realistic setting and situation (Gaba, 2007; Kuehster & Hall, 2010; Taylor, 2012).

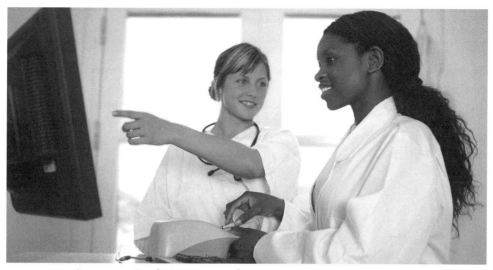

FIGURE 5-1 Computer simulation training for venipuncture. (Courtesy of Laerdal Medical.)

High-fidelity simulation allows for validation of competency of the infusion nurse as an individual, as well as within a team, and provides a setting for "learning without risk in a controlled, predictable, safe environment" (Finkelman & Kenner, 2009, p. 58). An example of a high-fidelity simulation using a human patient simulator that integrates cognitive, psychomotor, and interpersonal skills to develop practice and critical thinking for problem solving can be found in Table 5-2. Further, during and after the simulation, the learner is able to develop self-awareness and self-regulation in a nonthreatening environment through

RESEARCH ISSUE

What is the role of simulation in patient and staff education, and how will simulation impact patient safety and outcomes?

debriefing (Czaplewski, 2010). This simulation could be sequenced after the initial classroom session and patient care experiences with one-to-one preceptor support.

Simulation can be a teaching technique for education and training for infusion nurses and a validation method of competency for key aspects of knowledge, skill, and behavior (Figure 5-2). "Simulation will never replace clinical experience. It does, however, allow nurses to experience clinical situations in areas where occurrences are rare" (Kuehster & Hall, 2010, p. 127). Use of simulation as a competency validation method may be necessary when the opportunity is low volume yet high risk (e.g., chemotherapy administration with allergic reaction).

Competency

Competency as an infusion nurse is achieved as the nurse gains specialty knowledge and effective clinical reasoning and demonstrates expert technical and interpersonal skills in infusion therapy practice (INS, 2011). It is defined as "an expected and measureable level

TABLE 5-2	SIMULATION CASE WORKSHEET AND SCENARIO[a]

Part A: Simulation Case Worksheet

Scenario name	Proficiency in PICC patient assessment and medication administration
Target audience	Infusion nurse
Simulator mechanics	Simulation technical person for computer
	Facilitator: leads the session/debriefing
Patient	Human patient simulator
Standardized patient actor	Wife
Patient profile	Tom Gonzalez, admitted with infection to right foot. PICC line placed right arm basilic vein 4 d ago for long-term antibiotic administration
	Allergic to sulfa, history of atrial fibrillation, full code
	Married 44 y, lives with wife, wife has macular degeneration
	B/P 120/64, HR 72, RR 12, temp 98.9
	Orders: vancomycin 250 mg/250 mL every 12 h via PICC line

Environment and Equipment

Scenario Setting and Patient

Patient room with all equipment
Arm band, gown, sheet, pillow
Bandage to right arm
PICC line (single lumen) right basilic vein

Medications

IV fluid: 0.9 NS 1,000 mL
Vancomycin 250 mg/250 mL
10 mL 0.9 NS prefilled syringes × 4

Documentation/Charting

Patient history and physical
Lab result: CBC, BMP
PICC radiology report
Licensed independent practitioner (LIP) orders
12-lead EKG
Vital sign record

Equipment and Supplies

Infusion pump
Transparent semipermeable chlorhexidine
Gluconate dressing kit
Primary and secondary IV tubing

Gloves
Alcohol wipes

Part B: Simulation Scenario

Learner Guidelines:
1. All electronics including cell phones and pagers should be turned off
2. Learners wash hands prior to participation in the simulation and use proper PPE (personal protection equipment)
3. Sharps utilized will be disposed of using the approved red sharps containers
4. No food or drink in the simulation area
5. Mannequin's privacy should be maintained just like a real patient

Introduction to the Mannequin

Review Confidentiality

The Student Will:
1. Perform a focused PICC site assessment prior to medication administration
2. Initiate teaching to patient and family
3. Respond courteously with care and compassion to the patient/family
4. Use aseptic technique to administer IV medication through a PICC
5. Demonstrate ability to troubleshoot, and perform nursing intervention to maintain patient safety
6. Communicate to provider using SBAR

Initiation of Scenario: Mr. Gonzalez requires his 0900 antibiotic to be administered.

TABLE 5-2   SIMULATION CASE WORKSHEET AND SCENARIO[a]   *(Continued)*

State	Patient Status Monitor Settings	Learner Outcome or Actions Desired and Triggers to Next State	
Frame 0: Patient presentation/ computer setting	B/P: 120/64 RR: 16 HR: 72 Temp: 98.9 Rhythm: a-fib IV setup: 0.9 NS connected to IV tubing with sterile cap on end with secondary line not present bandage to right foot Lungs/heart/bowel: normal Vocal sounds: • Hello • Oh that hurts when you press on my arm This is my wife Caroline	**Learner Actions:** Introduces self to patient and family Performs hand hygiene Performs assessment of PICC site: • Visual inspection for signs and symptoms of infection • External length • Integrity of device • Closed system • Palpation of site Documents assessment	**Trigger:** Documents site and catheter assessment
Frame 1: Evaluation for infection	Vocal sounds: Why did that hurt when you touched my arm? Wife: Is there something wrong? You are making me nervous. The other nurse did not cause my husband pain!	**Learner Actions:** Courteously explain to patient and family/ provide reassurance Review radiology report Review lab results (infection)	**Trigger:** Reviewed chart documents and patient vital signs
Frame 2: Administration of IV antibiotcs	Vocal sounds: My wife has difficulty seeing. Wife: I thought he only had to have the antibiotic once a day? Did you wash your hands? Facilitator: Create occlusion after antibiotic infusion is started.	**Learner Actions:** Provide patient education: medication and procedure Perform hand hygiene Assemble materials Open all supply packages to be used on a sterile field Clean port with alcohol, and allow to dry Attach 0.9 NS prefilled syringe to port Obtain blood return, and flush line Luer lock the IV Infusion line to the PICC port Start the IV infusion of 0.9 NS at 25 mL/h Connect antibiotic to secondary line and back prime Program the infusion device for secondary medication administration and start administration	**Trigger:** IV infusion device alarms occlusion
Frame 3: Line occlusion and troubleshooting	Vocal sounds: How long will this medication take to give to me? I have to see the wound nurse. Facilitator: Create occlusion after learner restarts infusion pump.	**Learner Actions:** Assures all IV tubing clamps are open Assures PICC line clamp is open Visualize the site Restarts IV administration on infusion pump	**Trigger:** IV infusion device alarms occlusion

TABLE 5-2	SIMULATION CASE WORKSHEET AND SCENARIO[a] (Continued)

State	Patient Status Monitor Settings	Learner Outcome or Actions Desired and Triggers to Next State
Frame 4: Thrombosis identification/call provider using SBAR	Vocal Sounds: Why is it not working? It worked last night. Wife: Do you know what you are doing? What is wrong, why is that beeping?	**Learner Actions:** Turns off infusion device Disconnects IV infusion line from PICC Aseptically cleans the device hub Attaches 0.9 NS syringe to hub and attempts to obtain blood return—no blood return Courteously explains to patient why the PICC line is not working and intervention he/she will take Notifies LIP of potential of thrombosis using SBAR

Scenario End Point: calls LIP to report occlusion of line with request for an order for medication to obtain patency of line

Debriefing Question Examples:

- What did the initial site assessment tell you?
- What were your thoughts when Mr. Gonzalez complained of pain?
- What actions may prevent a CLABSI?
- Were there any actions that may have contributed to a CLABSI?
- How did you incorporate the patient and family into your care?
- When did you choose to notify the LIP?
- Describe the communication.
- What are two key takeaways from the learning experience

[a]Adapted from Taekman, J. (2003). *Template for simulation patient design*. Durham, NC: Duke University Medical Center.

of nursing performance that integrates knowledge, skills, abilities, and judgment, based on established scientific knowledge and expectations for nursing practice" (American Nurses Association (ANA), 2010). Competency assessment is the review and documentation of an individual's ability to achieve job expectations and performance standards (The Joint Commission, 2013). Competency validation is often used to reflect that the individual has demonstrated, in simulation or in a clinical setting, specific knowledge and skills related to a clinical practice, such as a dressing change for a CVAD. Core competencies for professional nurses in infusion therapy are based upon

- Professional standards (ANA, 2010)
- Specialty guidelines and practice standards (Camp-Sorrell, 2011; INS, 2011)

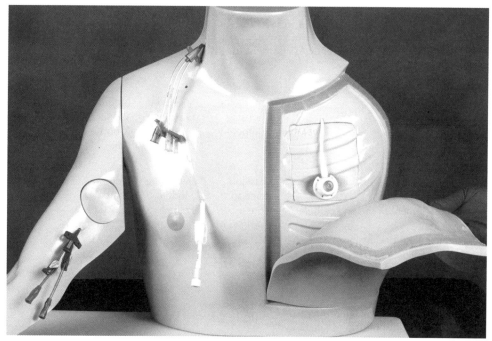

FIGURE 5-2 Low fidelity simulator chest with central vascular access devices. (Courtesy of T.T. Smith and A. Urrea; Clement J. Zablocki, VA Medical Center.)

- Key texts and core curriculum (Alexander et al., 2010; Alexander et al., 2014)
- Agency competencies

Assessment of competence in infusion therapy, whether for a beginning infusion nurse or a more experienced infusion nurse, is an important component of orientation to a new job role and/or the institution. A sample of an infusion nurse competency assessment related to PICC line care, based upon Wright's (2005) competency assessment framework, is presented in Table 5-3.

Competency of all nurses providing infusion therapy, regardless of the clinical setting in which care is delivered and/or specialty area of nursing practice (e.g., infusion nurse, medical–surgical nurse, outpatient clinic nurse), must be demonstrated and documented. Furthermore, guideline recommendations include the expectation that health care personnel performing IV therapy periodically undergo assessment of their knowledge and competency in IV therapy (CDC, 2011).

> ⚠ **PATIENT SAFETY**
>
> A high-risk and high-volume procedure, such as accessing a CVAD, requires competency validation to minimize the occurrence of CLABSIs.

TABLE 5-3	EXAMPLE OF COMPETENCY ASSESSMENT FORM[a]

Infusion Registered Nurse Competency Assessment for PICC Line Care

Name:

Department: Infusion Nurse Team

Competency Statement	Criteria for Choosing Competency	Suggested Learning	Method of Validation (Choose One)	Date Completed	Validator Signature
Role Specific					
Perform assessment and aseptic dressing change for a PICC: • Complete assessment of site and catheter for complications • Assemble materials for dressing change, maintaining sterility • Perform dressing change using standardized kit • Provide teaching • Document assessment, procedure performed, patient response, and teaching	Core job function Core Curriculum	E-learning Module Policy task trainer	Demonstrated in actual patient care or mock simulated event		
Access PICC, and administer medication using aseptic technique: • Assemble materials, maintaining sterility • Assess for complications before, during, and after procedure • Flush catheter with 10-mL 0.9 NS prior to medication administration • Perform medication administration using five rights • Flush catheter with 10-mL 0.9 NS after medication administration, and follow with heparin administration based upon policy • Document assessment, procedure performed, patient response, and teaching	Core job function Core Curriculum	Policy task trainer Preceptor	Demonstrated in actual patient care or mock simulated event		
Role-Specific Equipment					
Demonstrate technical skill and troubleshooting when programming infusion device using the safety software: • Prepare for IV medication administration • Prime administration set assuring no air in line • Load administration set • Select drug profile from library • Program infusion for medication delivery • Respond to alarms, and perform applicable nursing interventions	Core job function New piece of equipment	Equipment Manual Infusion Device Job Aid E-Learning Module	Demonstrated in actual patient care or mock simulated event		

[a]Adapted from Wright, D. (2005). Competency assessment form. In *The ultimate guide to competency assessment in health care* (3rd ed., pp. 38–39). Minneapolis MN: Creative Health Care Management.

Professional Development

Professional development for the infusion nurse is a lifelong process. As a professional, the infusion nurse strives to remain current with best practices, and obtain and/or maintain specialty certification. Wade (2009) states, "Education may be one factor that increases the effectiveness of nursing care" (p. 183). The health care environment and nursing standards are constantly changing based upon evidence. The infusion nurse must be actively engaged in continuing education, for without continuing education, positive patient outcomes and safety will be at risk.

Continuing education may include reading professional journals, attending conferences and workshops, or completing formal academic coursework. Another method to remain current with best practice is to join a professional nursing organization whose members are committed to evidence-based and professional infusion nursing practice. Two organizations, which offer resources for professional development, are the Infusion Nurses Society (INS) (www.ins1.org) and the Association for Vascular Access (AVA) (www.avainfo.org). Each organization provides journal publications, webinars, and other educational and practice resources.

The RN, as a means to further developing one's professional specialty, inclusive of knowledge, skills, and competence, is encouraged to engage in reflective practice (Johns, 2009; Johns, 2010). This is a planned and organized method of making sense of one's experiences, situations, or activities (Oelofsen, 2012). Reflective analysis and evaluation of infusion nursing experiences develop professional judgment and practice expertise.

Another method of professional development is obtaining certification. Certification is defined as "the formal recognition of the nurses' specialized knowledge, skills, and experience demonstrated by the achievement of standards identified by a nursing specialty to promote optimal health outcomes" (Joint INS/INCC Position Paper, 2009). Valente (2010) states, "Certification aims to foster continuing scholarship and enhance quality" (p. 215).

Two diverse certification exams are available, depending on one's licensure (Table 5-4). The examination offered by the Infusion Nurses Certification Corporation (INCC) certifies RNs meeting the criteria defined in Table 5-4. The credential is the standard of excellence that nurses seek in order to provide optimal infusion care. The CRNIs dual accreditations and a proven track record of more than 25 years assure patient, employers, and peers that the credential is a credible and reliable method of validating a nurse's experience in the specialty of infusion therapy.

The Vascular Access Certification Corporation (VACC) offers a multidisciplinary approach and includes a broad range of health care professionals and clinicians involved in vascular access. Acquiring certification as an infusion therapy nurse signifies to the public, patients, families, and other professionals that the infusion nurse has the requisite knowledge to perform evidence-based infusion nursing (Corrigan, 2010). While certification is a voluntary activity, it is becoming increasingly valued and, in some agencies, may be required for the infusion nurse role.

EDUCATION FOR PATIENTS RECEIVING INFUSION THERAPY

The infusion nurse plays an instrumental role in achieving positive outcomes for patients receiving infusion therapy by using evidence-based practices and age-appropriate learning principles. Providing patients with knowledge of infusion therapy increases their role in

TABLE 5-4	INFUSION NURSE CERTIFICATION AND PROVIDERS	
Certification in Infusion Nursing	Certified Registered Nurse Infusion (CRNI)	Vascular Access Board Certified (VA-BC)
Provider of Certification	Infusion Nurses Certification Corporation (INCC, 2013)	Vascular Access Certification Corporation (VACC, 2010)
Established	1985	2009
Eligibility Requirements	*Type of clinician:* Current, active, unrestricted RN license in the United States or Canada	*Type of clinician:* Licensed health care personnel actively engaged in the practice of vascular access such as nurses (RN, APN, and LPN/LVN), respiratory care professionals, LIPs, physician assistants, radiology professionals, and other clinicians actively engaged in the practice to vascular access
	Experience: 1,600 h of clinical experience in infusion therapy within the past 2 years. Nursing experience may be in the areas of nursing education, administration, research, or clinical practice within the infusion specialty.	*Experience:* Must include at least two (2) of the following activities:
	International applicants: In addition to the regular requirement of 1,600 h of clinical experience, nurses educated and practicing abroad without a US or Canadian RN license should submit documentation of their current, unrestricted RN license in the country in which they practice and a complete exam application before regular exam application deadlines.	• Assessing, planning, implementing, and evaluating the care and needs of patients and clients who require vascular access in the course of their care • Education of individuals in best practice as it pertains to vascular access • Development and revision of vascular access policies and procedures • Management of vascular access activities • Provision of consultation of vascular access activities
Exam Offered	2 months a year March and September	2 months a year June and December
Renewal Requirements	• Every 3 years • 40 CRNI recertification units: includes several activities	• Every 3 years • 30 contact hours: Activity matrix defines contact hours.
Web Site	http://www.incc1.org	www.avainfo.org

decision making, aids in ensuring the safe administration of the required therapeutics, and may reduce the risk of complications. **Adult learning principles** emphasize the importance of knowing how previous learning or experiences may facilitate new learning, the reasons behind the specific content, hands-on or problem-solving experiences, and the lesson's immediate real-world applicability (Bastable, 2008).

Educating patients and families for home therapy, in particular, is complex and commonplace as has been noted in the literature (Cox & Westbrook, 2005). Home care infusion requires intensive training that is reinforced at frequent intervals (Stafford & Emery, 2007). Patients and their families are often anxious about transitioning to home with a vascular access device. In addition, they may have anxiety and emotional responses to their diagnosis and prognosis, as exemplified by one patient's statement:

I had a PICC line inserted while hospitalized for an acute bacterial infection. My son gave me the antibiotic twice a day after I was discharged home. Whenever I was given the medicine, I was concerned about how quickly it was given and the importance of keeping everything clean and maintaining a sterile environment. I watched my son each time. It forced me, the patient, to be an integral part of the procedure every time, even when I was not feeling well. I had to really trust my family since no other alternatives were given.

The primary caregiver needs to be identified early in the discharge planning process so they can be included in all education and observe as well as participate in the care. Being a primary caregiver requires a strong commitment to learning and providing care. The following comment illustrates this, as acknowledged by the son/caregiver from the previous statement.

The only thing that concerned me was making sure everything was clean. I didn't want to do anything wrong like have air go through the tubes or giving the medicine too fast. Other than that there was nothing too hard about it. Something needed to get done, so I did it. He needed care so I took care of him. It's not like I was going to refuse to take care of him.

Challenges to learning in the hospital include patient factors such as anxiety, pain, discomfort, insomnia, and fatigue. The caregiver may also be challenged by anxiety and fatigue. The health care environment also contributes to learning barriers with interruptions from hospital staff, the number of health care providers who interact with the patient and caregiver, and inconsistency in the information provided by health care providers (Stafford & Emery, 2007). Patient education sessions are frequently scheduled around the patient's tests, procedures, and the availability of the caregiver. The stress and anxiety caused by illness often can interfere with the patient's ability to comprehend the content. Patients and caregivers may not volunteer that they do not understand the education. These challenges and time limitations are potential barriers to learning that should be considered when assessing patient and/or caregiver readiness to learn.

Assessment

Assessment is the initial step in the nursing process and is applicable prior to the infusion nurse providing patient education. The assessment of learning needs will aid in identifying gaps in knowledge, individualizing the teaching, and prioritizing needs. Actively engaging the learner in this assessment uses principles of adult learning that will foster the motivation to learn. A **learning needs assessment** should include three domains: needs of the learner, state of readiness to learn, and preferred learning style. A preferred **learning style** may use visual, auditory, or kinesthetic strategies (Bastable, 2008). Information should also be gathered about the learner's previous experience and knowledge of infusion therapy.

The learner's education level, primary language, cognitive ability, reading and comprehension skills, and health literacy also need to be assessed (INS, 2011). "**Health literacy** refers to how well an individual can read, interpret, and comprehend health information for maintaining an optimal level of wellness" (Bastable, 2008, p. 234). Health literacy is influenced by an individual's education, culture, language, and the ability of providers to effectively communicate medical information to the individual and caregivers (Institute of Medicine (IOM), 2004). In order for individuals to be able to make decisions about their health care and actively participate in caring for oneself, the individual and caregiver have to be able to grasp the content being presented by the health care provider. Any sensory

> **PATIENT SAFETY**
>
> Performing a health literacy assessment prior to providing education for the patient/caregiver ensures education is in the appropriate format and delivery method to meet the patient and caregiver's needs.

deficits and limitations in ability to care for self or others should also be identified (Billings & Halstead, 2012).

Planning

A teaching plan that includes objectives, intended audience, resources, teaching strategies, and evaluation methods guides the learning process. Table 5-5 identifies potential topics to consider when the infusion nurse develops a teaching plan for the patient and caregiver in the acute care, long-term care, or home therapy setting.

TABLE 5-5	PATIENT CARE EDUCATION CONTENT BASED ON SETTING
Acute- or long-term care setting	• Describe procedure for therapy or device insertion—what patient can expect • Describe rationale for the treatment • Therapies that will be initiated: fluids/medications including purpose, dosages or rate, and side effects • Potential complications • How to manage activities of daily living (ADLs) with catheter in place • When to notify a nurse and what to report: signs/symptoms appropriate for therapy and/or device
Home therapy setting	• Care of vascular access device • Home self-monitoring if required (i.e., blood glucose, intake and output, weight) • Infusion administration • Management of infusion pumps including response to alarms, priming of tubing, setting functions, care of battery pack • Medication/fluids: purpose, dosages or rate, side effects • Potential complications • Precautions for preventing infection and other complications including aseptic technique: hand washing, designated clean work space • Signs and symptoms of complications • When to notify provider: ER vs. nonemergency • How and who to report signs and symptoms or questions • Dressing change • Flushing of catheter: how, frequency, what to use • Problem solving • How to manage ADLs with catheter in place • Emergency procedures to follow for a break in catheter, accidental removal of cap, or catheter not secured to skin • Disposal of equipment/supplies • Where and how to obtain equipment/supplies • Storage of supplies/equipment • Maintenance of supplies • Inspection of supplies/equipment prior to use

Implementation

Structure the teaching environment so that it is supportive, unhurried, and without interruptions. A variety of teaching strategies should be used based upon the preferred learning style of the patient/caregiver. One teaching strategy would be the use of instructional videos. If possible, provide the patient and significant other with a copy for home reference. Patient education handouts that reinforce instructions should be provided. These should use clear language at a 5th grade reading level (Bastable, 2008), with easy-to-read text, simple concise illustrations, and be consistent with the information that has been taught.

"Many people read at least two to three grade levels below their reported level of formal education...For those in poverty, the gap between grade level completed and actual reading level was shown to be even greater" (Bastable, 2008). Readability assessment tools, such as the Gunning Fog Index (FOG) or the Simple Measure of Gobbledygook (SMOG), can assist in determining readability of materials (Bastable, 2008, p. 241). Developed by Robert Gunning, the FOG is one of the simplest and most effective manual tools for analyzing readability. Gunning defines hard words as those with more than two syllables. To get to a fourth grade reading level, you need to write with an average sentence length (ASL) of eight words and no more than one out of 50 words being three or more syllables. It is easy to calculate, and it is accurate within one grade level. The ideal score is 7 or 8 (Box 5-1).

Some word processing programs also provide readability statistics (e.g., reading ease and grade level in Microsoft Word). Organizations like Communication Science (CSI) specialize in preparing patient education packets specific to disease entity or procedure that facilitate learning at the suggested reading level. CSI is an innovation consultancy and product design firm. They use a design thinking process to create teaching products and processes that have the potential to be "mistake proof" (Communication Science, 2013).

Procedures that the patient and caregiver will be performing should be observed closely during return demonstrations. A procedure checklist should be used to ensure consistency among nurses providing the patient education, as well as assisting the patient to remember

---

BOX 5-1   GUNNING FOG INDEX (FOG)

Using the FOG Index to analyze writing:

- Select a 100 word sample. Count the number of sentences. Divide the total number of words in the sample by the number of sentences to get the average sentence length (ASL).
- Count the number of words with three or more syllables in the sample. Do not count (1) proper nouns, (2) hyphenated words, or (3) two-syllable verbs made into three with -es and -ed endings.
- Divide the number by the number of words in your sample. For example, 15 long words divided by 100 words give you 15 % hard words (PHW).
- Add the ASL and the PHWs, and multiply this by 0.4. The formula is as follows:

$$(ASL + PHW) \times 0.4 = \text{Grade Level.}$$

This indicates the number of years of schooling of the reader to have understood the writing sample.

the procedure steps. The learner should be given multiple opportunities for return demonstration of procedures prior to independently performing them. Teaching should be learner paced, noncondescending, and encouraging. Instructor qualities that have been identified as being helpful include competence, reassuring attitude, providing personalized support, and demonstrating understanding of the patient's situation and diagnosis (Cox & Westbrook, 2005). The following comment from a caregiver describes the feelings and experience related to learning about infusion therapy at home:

> *I had to assist my son while he was receiving IV antibiotics at home. I felt very prepared to care for the IVs. The nurses reviewed how I should care for the IV, what I should watch for and report, and how to flush the tubing. They [the nurses] watched me several times as I did this until I felt comfortable doing it myself.*

Lastly, a list of Internet resources and Web sites that include accurate information about medication safety can be provided to learners. Table 5-6 provides examples of these resources for patient and caregiver education. The infusion nurse must determine if the patient and caregiver have access to the Internet and the ability to use a computer prior to considering Web site resources as a learning method.

Evaluation

Ongoing evaluation of learning to determine effectiveness of teaching is crucial to discharge planning and outcomes for the patient and caregiver. "The results of evaluation provide practice-based evidence to support continuing an educational intervention as is or revising that intervention to enhance learning" (Bastable, 2008, p. 558). This type of evaluation allows for making adjustments in the process as soon as they are needed. The teach-back method should be used to validate that the patient and caregiver have integrated all knowledge needed to competently assume the infusion therapy prior to the health care provider attesting to their ability.

TABLE 5-6	PATIENT/CAREGIVER EDUCATION RESOURCES FOR MEDICATION	
Resource	**Web Site**	**Organization**
How to take your medication safely	www.ismp.org	Institute for Safe Medication Practices
Medication safety articles	www.consumermedsafety.org	Consumer Medication Safety
Report fact sheet: What you can do to avoid medication errors	www.IOM.edu	Institute of Medicine
Your medicine: Be smart. Be safe	www.ahrq.gov/consumer/safemeds/yourmeds.htm	Agency for Healthcare Research and Quality
Safe medication use[a]	www.fda.gov/ForConsumers/ByAudience/ForWomen/ucm116695.htm	U.S. Food and Drug Administration
Help avoid mistakes with your medicines[a]	www.jointcommission.org	The Joint Commission

[a]Available in English and Spanish versions.

			Learner Completing Competency (Insert Name)	Date Completed
TABLE 5-7	**PATIENT TEACHING EVALUATION TOOL**			
Competency	Suggested Learning	Validation Method		
Learner performs dressing change using aseptic technique.	Patient education handout: _____ Instructional video: _____ Live teaching session: *principles of aseptic technique*	Verbalizes importance of aseptic technique Demonstrates hand washing technique Assembles sterile field with equipment Performs dressing change		

Another method of evaluation might include asking the learner to repeat in his/her own words what has just been taught. Use of a patient teaching evaluation tool captures critical behaviors, learning tools, and verification methods required by the learner to assume responsibility for infusion therapy. An example of an evaluation tool that demonstrates patient and/or caregiver learning can be found in Table 5-7.

CONCLUSION

The infusion nurse in today's health care environment requires ongoing professional development in infusion practices, clinical competence, and a solid understanding of how patients learn. "Nursing education is critical for safe and effective patient care. Increasing the knowledge, confidence and psychomotor skills of RNs may impact care of patients and ultimately may improve patient outcomes" (Roslien, 2009, p. E22).

To provide high-quality, safe care, nurses need to be highly skilled, competent practitioners who can think critically and respond quickly to changing conditions. Historically, other occupations whose members needed similar skills, such as the military, aviation, and medicine, have used high-fidelity simulations (HFSs) to better prepare members to respond appropriately in diverse situations. Nursing education has long utilized simulation in some form to teach principles and skills of nursing care. Models of anatomic parts, whole body mannequins, and various computer-based learning programs have provided educators with training tools for students seeking to become professional nurses. Simulation has its roots as far back as 1911 with the introduction of "Mrs. Chase," the very first life-size mannequin (Nickerson, Morrison, & Pollard, 2011). The Institute of Medicine's report (Kohn, Corrigan, & Donaldson, 2000) recommended that nursing also increase the use of simulation to both train and ensure competency in nurses. The report (Kohn) states that "… health care organizations and teaching institutions should participate in the development and use of simulation for training novice practitioners, problem solving, and crisis management, especially when new and potentially hazardous procedures and equipment are introduced" (p. 179).

The use of human patient simulation in orientation and continuing education has the potential to meet many learning needs for the infusion nurse (Hallenbeck, 2012). Infusion nurses can practice clinical skills, critical thinking, and communication in a safe learning environment to enhance patient safety. In addition, nurses' use of adult learning principles and relevant content when teaching patients and caregivers about infusion therapy is essential to achieving the best possible outcomes.

Review Questions   *Note: Questions below may have more than one right answer.*

1. A practice area where the infusion nurse may care for patients may be all of the below except
   A. Medical oncology
   B. Long-term care
   C. Surgical procedure center
   D. Operating room

2. Which of the following methods of professional development will enhance practice?
   A. Certification
   B. Reflective practice
   C. A only
   D. A and B

3. The INS Core Curriculum for all infusion nurses is inclusive of which of the following?
   A. Fluid and electrolytes
   B. Infection control
   C. Technology and clinical application
   D. All of the above

4. Adult learning strategies should include all except
   A. Need to know the reason behind the specific learning content
   B. Hands-on experience
   C. Immediate real-world application
   D. Utilizing the same teaching strategies for all learners

5. Which of the following may be said about simulation?
   A. Controlled
   B. Predictable
   C. Low risk
   D. All of the above

6. Tina, an infusion nurse, demonstrates competency of blood administration knowledge and skill by
   A. Completion of a case study
   B. Verbalization
   C. Demonstration during patient care
   D. Completion of a posttest

7. When the infusion nurse provides education for a patient requiring education, it begins with which of the following?
   A. Implementation
   B. Assessment
   C. Planning
   D. Evaluation

8. A learning needs assessment should include
   A. State of readiness to learn, teaching strategies, and preferred learner style
   B. State of readiness to learn, preferred learner style, and evaluation
   C. Needs of the learner, state of readiness to learn, and preferred learner style
   D. Needs of the learner, state of readiness to learn, and objectives

9. Patient education materials should be written
   A. At an 8th grade reading level
   B. At a 3rd grade reading level
   C. At a 5th grade reading level
   D. At a 12th grade reading level

10. Simulation offers the opportunity for novice infusion nurses to do which of the following?
    A. Practice psychomotor skills
    B. Advance clinical decision making
    C. Create instructional methods
    D. A and B

References and Selected Readings *Asterisks indicate references cited in text.*

Alexander, M., Corrigan, A.M., Gorski, L.A., Hankins, J., & Perucca, R. (2010). *Infusion nursing: An evidence-based approach* (3rd ed.). St Louis, MO: Saunders Elsevier.

*Alexander, M., Corrigan, A.M., Gorski, L.A., & Phillips, L. (2014). *Core curriculum for infusion nursing* (4th ed.). Philadelphia, PA: Lippincott Williams & Wilkins.

*American Nurses Association. (2010). *ANA nursing scope and standards of practice* (2nd ed.). Silver Spring, MD: Nursingbooks.org

*Bastable, S. (2008). *Nurse as educator: Principles of teaching and learning for nursing practice* (3rd ed.). Sudbury, MA: Jones and Bartlett.

*Bartock, L. (2010). An evidence-based systematic review of literature for the reduction of PICC line occlusions. *Journal of the Association for Vascular Access, 15*, 58–63.

*Billings, D., & Halstead, J. (2012). *Teaching in nursing: A guide for faculty* (4th ed.). St. Louis, MO: Saunders Elsevier.

*Boland, D.L., & Finke, L.M. (2012). Curriculum designs. In D. Billings, & J. Halstead (Eds.), *Teaching in nursing: A guide for faculty* (4th ed., pp. 119–137). St. Louis, MO: Saunders Elsevier.

Bucher, L., & Sanderson, L.V. (2011). Peripherally inserted central catheter. In D. Wiegand (Ed.), *AACN Procedure Manual for Critical Care* (6th ed., pp. 763–774). Philadelphia, PA: Saunders.

*Camp-Sorrell, D. (2011). *Access device guidelines: Recommendations for nursing practice and education* (3rd ed.). Pittsburgh, PA: Oncology Nursing Society.

Cary, A.H. (2001). Certified registered nurses: Results of the study of the certified workforce. *AJN The American Journal of Nursing, 101*(1), 44–52.

*Centers for Disease Control and Prevention (CDC). (2011). *Guidelines for the prevention of intravascular catheter-related infections.* http://www.cdc.gov/hicpac/pdf/guidelines/bsi-guidelines-2011.pdf

*Collins, M., Phillips, S., Dougherty, L., de Verteuil, A., & Morris, W. (2006). A structured learning programme for venipuncture and cannulation. *Nursing Standard, 20*(26), 34–40.

Comer, S.K. (2005). Patient care simulations: role playing to enhance clinical understanding. *Nursing Education Perspectives, 26*(6), 357–361.

*Communication Science. (2013). http://www.communicationscience.com/index.html

*Corrigan, A. (2010). Infusion nursing as a specialty. In M. Alexander, A. Corrigan, L. Gorski, J. Hankins, & R. Perucca (Eds.), *Infusion Nurses Society infusion nursing: An evidence-based approach* (3rd ed., pp. 1–9), St. Louis, MO: Saunders Elsevier.

*Cox, J., & Westbrook, L. (2005). Home infusion therapy-Essential characteristics of a successful education process: A grounded theory study. *Journal of Infusion Nursing, 28*(2), 99–107.

Craven, H. (2007). Recognizing excellence: Unit-based activities to support specialty nursing certification. *Medsurg Nursing, 16*(6), 367.

*Czaplewski, L. (2010). Clinical and patient education. In M. Alexander, A. Corrigan, L. Gorski, J. Hankins, & R. Perucca (Eds.), *Infusion Nurses Society infusion nursing: An evidence-based approach* (3rd ed., pp. 71–94). St. Louis, MO: Saunders Elsevier.

Dugger, B. (1997). Intravenous nursing competency: Why is it important? *Journal of Infusion Nursing, 20*(6), 287–298.

*Fakih, M.G., Jones, K., Rey, J.E., Berriel-Cass, D., Kalinicheva, T., & Saravolatz, L.D. (2012). Sustained improvements in peripheral venous catheter care in non-intensive care units: a quasi-experimental controlled study of education and feedback. *Infection Control and Hospital Epidemiology, 33*(5), 449–455.

*Finkelman, A., & Kenner, C. (2009). *Teaching IOM: Implications of the Institute of Medicine reports for nursing education* (2nd ed.). Silver Spring, MD: American Nurses Association.

*Gaba, D. (2007). The future vision of simulation in healthcare. *Simulation Healthcare, 2*(2), 126–135.

Gentile, D.L. (2012). Applying the Novice-to-Expert model to infusion nursing. *Journal of Infusion Nursing, 35*(2), 101.

*Haig, K.M., Sutton, S., & Whittington, J. (2006). National Patient Safety Goals SBAR: A shared mental model for improving communication between clinicians. *Joint Commission Journal on Quality and Patient Safety*, *32*(3), 167–175. [PubMed].

*Hallenbeck, V. (2012). Use of high fidelity simulation for staff education/development. *Journal for Staff Development*, *28*, 260–269.

Hammer, J., & Souers, C. (2004). Infusion therapy: A multifaceted approach to teaching in nursing. *Journal of Infusion Nursing*, *27*(3), 151–156.

*Infusion Nurses Certification Corporation. (2013). *CRNI Exam Handbook March 2013*. http://www.incc1. org/i4a/pages/index.cfm?pageid=1

*Infusion Nurses Society. (2011). Infusion nursing standards of practice. *Journal of Infusion Nursing*, *34*(1S), S1–S110.

*Institute of Medicine (IOM). (2004). *Health literacy: A prescription to end confusion*. Washington, DC: The National Academies Press.

*Johns, C. (2009). *Becoming a reflective practitioner* (3rd ed.). Ames, IA: Wiley-Blackwell.

*Johns, C. (2010). *Guided reflection: A narrative approach to advancing professional practice* (2nd ed.), Ames, IA: Wiley-Blackwell.

*The Joint Commission. (2013). *Comprehensive Accreditation Manuals. Edition v4.5. Hospital: HR .01.06.01*. Oakbrook Terrace, IL: Author.

*Joint INS/INCC Position Paper. (2009). The value of certification in infusion nursing. *Journal of Infusion Nursing*, *32*, 248–250.

Katz, G.B., Peifer, K.L., & Armstrong, G. (2010). Assessment of patient simulation use in selected baccalaureate nursing programs in the United States. *Simulation in Healthcare*, *5*(1), 46.

*Kohn, L.T., Corrigan, J.M., & Donaldson, M.S., Eds. (2000). To err is human: Building a safer health system. *A report of the Committee on Quality of Health Care in America, Institute of Medicine*. Washington, DC: National Academy Press.

*Kuehster, C., & Hall, C. (2010). Simulation: Learning form mistakes while building communication and teamwork. *Journal of Staff Development*, *26*, 123–127.

*Kulbok, P.A. (2012). Chapter 11: Standard 8. Education. In K.M. White & A. O'Sullivan (Eds.), *The essential guide to nursing practice: Applying ANA's scope and standards in practice and education* (pp. 123–132). Silver Spring, MD: American Nurses Association.

Limei, Z., Chao, Q., & Junqing, W. (2010). Study for the simulation and optimization for Med-model based outpatient infusion center process. *Journal of Nurses Training*, *10*, 009.

*Nickerson, M., Morrison B., & Pollard M. (2011). Simulation in nursing staff development. *Journal for Nurses in Staff Development*, *27*(2), 81–89.

Niebuhr, B., & Biel, M. (2007). The value of specialty nursing certification. *Nursing Outlook*, *55*(4), 176.

*Oelofsen, N. (2012). Using reflective practice in frontline nursing. *Nursing Times*, *108*(24), 22–24.

*Ozyazicioglu, N., & Arikan, D. (2008). The effect of nurse training on the improvement of intravenous applications. *Nurse Education Today*, *28*, 179–185.

Parr, M.B., & Sweeney, N.M. (2006). Use of human patient simulation in an undergraduate critical care course. *Critical care nursing quarterly*, *29*(3), 188–198.

Polzien, G. (2006). Home infusion therapy-First things first: The patient and the prevention of central catheter infections. *Home Healthcare Nurse*, *24*, 681–684.

*Roslien, J., & Alcock, L. (2009). The effect of an educational intervention on the RN's peripherally inserted central catheters knowledge, confidence and psychomotor skill. *Journal for Nurses in Staff Development*, *25*(3), E19–E27.

*Stafford, J., & Emery, D. (2007). Getting the patient out of the hospital on parenteral nutrition: Catheter selection, assessment, and education. *Support Line*, *29*(3), 3–7.

Starkweather, A.R., & Kardong-Edgren, S. (2008). Diffusion of innovation: Embedding simulation into nursing curricula. *International Journal of Nursing Education Scholarship*, *5*(1).

Stromborg, M.F., Niebuhr, B., Prevost, S., Fabrey, L., Muenzen, P., Spence, C., & Valentine, W. (2005). More than a title. *Nursing Management*, *36*(5), 36.

*Taekman, J. (2003). *Template for simulation patient design.* Durham, NC: Duke University Medical Center. http://simcenter.duke.edu/support.html

*Taylor, J. (2012). Using low-fidelity simulation to maintain competency in central line care. *Journal of the Association for Vascular Access, 17*(1), 31–37.

Tilley, J.D., Gregor, F.M., & Thiessen, V. (2006). The nurse's role in patient education: Incongruent perceptions among nurses and patients. *Journal of Advanced Nursing, 12*(3), 291–301.

*Valente, S. (2010). Improving professional practice through certification. *Journal for Staff Development, 26,* 215–219.

*Vascular Access Certification Corporation. (2010). *Vascular Access Certification Candidate Handbook and Application: June 2013.* http://www.vacert.org/website/article.asp?id=280434

*Wade, C. (2009). Perceived effects of specialty nurse certification: A review of the literature. *AORN Journal, 89,* 183–192.

*Wright, D. (2005). *The ultimate guide to competency assessment in health care* (3rd ed.). Minneapolis, MN: Creative Health Care Management.

PART 2

CLINICAL ASSESSMENT AND MONITORING

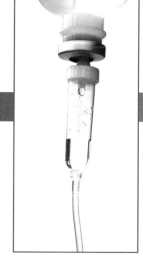

CHAPTER 6

Anatomy and Physiology Applied to Infusion Therapy

Sharon M. Weinstein

KEY TERMS		
	Aberrant Artery	Integument
	Afferent	Somatic Nervous
	Arterial Spasm	System
	Arteriovenous	Superficial Fascia
	Anastomosis	Tunica
	Autonomic Nervous	Valves
	System	Vascular System
	Clotting Cascade	Vasovagal Reaction
	Efferent	Velocity
	Extrapyramidal Side	
	Effects	

VASCULAR ANATOMY AND THERAPEUTIC GOALS

Because infusion therapy involves the administration of fluids, blood, and drugs directly into the vascular system—that is, into arteries, bone marrow, and veins—the nurse and others responsible for administering therapy need to understand the anatomy and physiology of vascular structures and related systems.

Knowing the functions of the cardiovascular system and the parts of the body that are part of it is critical in understanding the physiology of the human body. With its complex pathways of veins, arteries, and capillaries, the cardiovascular system keeps life pumping through you. The heart, blood vessels, and blood help to transport vital nutrients throughout the body as well as remove metabolic waste. They also help to protect the body and regulate body temperature.

Although the *veins*, because of their abundance and location, provide the most readily accessible route for infusion therapies, the arteries and bone marrow are also used. *Arteries* provide the route for introducing radiopaque material for diagnostic purposes, such as in arteriograms to detect cerebral disorders; blood pressure monitoring, determinations of arterial blood gas levels, and administration of chemotherapy. The dangers of **arterial spasm** and subsequent gangrene present problems that make this route of therapy hazardous for therapeutic use. The *bone marrow*, because of its venous plexus, is used for infusion therapy by the intraosseous route.

The primary goal of infusion (IV) therapy is to provide a positive outcome for the patient. Painless and effective therapy is desirable, promoting the patient's comfort, well-being, and often complete recovery from disease or trauma. An integral part of this goal is the recognition and prevention of complications. To achieve the goal and minimize the risk of complications, the IV nurse needs a solid knowledge of vascular anatomy and physiology.

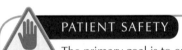

PATIENT SAFETY

The primary goal is to ensure a safe outcome for the patient.

Integration of Knowledge with Practice

By studying the superficial veins, the nurse learns to discriminate the most appropriate veins to use for infusion therapy. Factors to be considered in selecting a vein include size, location, and resilience. In addition, understanding the reaction of veins to the nervous stimulation of the vasoconstrictors and vasodilators enables the clinician to increase the size and visibility of a vein before attempting venipuncture and to relieve venous spasm and thus assist in infusion maintenance.

By studying the superficial veins of the lower extremities, the nurse becomes alert to the dangers resulting from their use. Avoiding venipuncture in veins susceptible to varicosities and sluggish circulation decreases the likelihood of complications, such as phlebitis and thrombosis, and reduces the secondary risk of pulmonary embolism.

Common Venous Complications

Phlebitis and thrombosis are by far the most common complications resulting from parenteral therapy. Although seemingly mild, phlebitis and thrombosis may have serious consequences. First, they cause moderate to severe discomfort, often taking many days or weeks to subside. Second, they limit the veins available for future therapy. Injury to the endothelial lining of the vein contributes to these local complications.

Crucial to recognizing and preventing complications is a solid knowledge of the characteristics that differentiate veins from arteries and the positions of each. Understanding this helps the nurse avoid the complications of an inadvertent arterial puncture. The knowledge also helps to reduce the risk of necrosis and gangrene and to recognize the existence of an **arteriovenous anastomosis**, a congenital or traumatic abnormality in which blood flows directly from the artery into the vein.

Failure to recognize an arteriovenous anastomosis results in repeated and unsuccessful venipunctures performed in an attempt to initiate the infusion. Repeated punctures compound the trauma to the inner lining of the vein and increase the risk of the local complications already described, any one of which limits the number of available veins, interrupts the course of therapy, and causes unnecessary pain or, possibly, dire consequences for the patient.

SYSTEMS AND ORGANS INVOLVED IN INFUSION THERAPY

Among the organs and systems closely associated with infusion therapy are the integumentary, neurologic, cardiovascular, and respiratory systems, as well as individual circulatory organs and structures.

Integument and Connective Tissue

The **integument**, or skin, is the first organ affected in IV access. It protects the body from the environment and is a natural barrier to external forces. It ranges in thickness from 1.5 to 4.0 mm, with the thickest skin appearing on the palms of the hands and plantar aspect of the feet. The skin also synthesizes vitamin D, cytokines, and other growth factors; is influenced by hormones; and assists in the control of body temperature (Standring, 2008). The skin is made up of two layers, the epidermis and the dermis. See Table 6-1: Layers of the epidermis.

Epidermis

The epidermis is the uppermost layer, which forms a protective covering for the dermis. Its thickness varies in different parts of the body and is thickest on the palms of the hands and the soles of the feet and thinnest on the inner surface of the limbs. Thickness is a variable of the aging process and medications such as prednisone. In an elderly patient, for example,

TABLE 6-1	LAYERS OF THE EPIDERMIS
Layer	Characteristics
Stratum corneum	Many layers of dead, anucleate keratinocytes completely filled with keratin The outermost layers are constantly shed.
Stratum lucidum	Two to three layers of anucleate cells This layer is found only in "thick skin" such as the palm of the hand and the sole of the foot.
Stratum granulosum	Two to four layers of cells held together by desmosomes These cells contain keratohyalin granules, which contribute to the formation of keratin in the upper layers of the epidermis.
Stratum spinosum	Eight to 10 layers of cells connected by desmosomes These cells are moderately active in mitosis.
Stratum basale	Single layer of columnar cells actively dividing by mitosis to produce cells that migrate into the upper epidermal layers and ultimately to the surface of the skin

Adapted from CliffsNotes.com. *The epidermis*. (2013). http://www.cliffsnotes.com/study_guide/The-Epidermis. topicArticleId-277792,articleId-277538.html

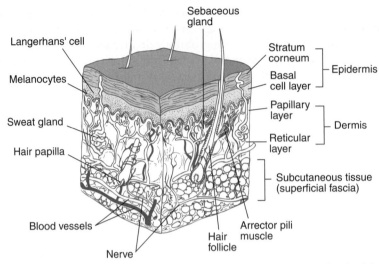

FIGURE 6-1 Layers of the skin. The epidermis protects the highly vascular dermis that lies above the superficial fascia (subcutaneous tissue).

the skin on the dorsum of the hand may be so thin that it does not adequately support the vein for venipuncture when parenteral infusions are required.

DERMIS

The dermis, or underlayer, is highly sensitive and vascular. It contains many capillaries and thousands of nerve fibers (Figure 6-1). See Table 6-2: Layers of the Dermis.

SUPERFICIAL FASCIA OR HYPODERMIS

The **superficial fascia**, or subcutaneous areolar connective tissue, lies below the two layers of skin and is, itself, another covering. The superficial veins are located in this fascia, which varies in thickness. When a catheter is inserted into this fascia, there is free movement of the skin above. Great care and meticulous aseptic technique must be observed because an infection in this loose tissue spreads easily. Such an infection is called *cellulitis* (Williams, Warwick, Dyson, & Bannister, 1995).

TABLE 6-2	LAYERS OF THE DERMIS
Layer	Characteristics
Papillary	Thin outer layer of areolar connective tissue with fingerlike projections called *dermal papillae* that protrude into the epidermis
Reticular	Thick layer of dense irregular connective tissue, which lies deep to the papillary layer and makes up most of the dermis

Adapted from CliffsNotes.com. *The dermis*. (2013). http://www.cliffsnotes.com/study_guide/The-Dermis. topicArticleId-277792,articleId-277540.html

Neurologic System

The human nervous system is an integral loop containing billions of neurons and hundreds of thousands of synaptic connections. Changes in the environment trigger a response by the main controlling organ, the brain, which coordinates and processes the information, determines a response mechanism, and then communicates that response back to the body.

Functional

Sensory Receptors

A characteristic of a living organism is its ability to respond to stimuli. The human sensory system is highly evolved and processes thousands of incoming messages simultaneously. This complexity allows you to be aware of your surroundings and take appropriate actions. They are classified by type, location, and type of stimulus detected. For example,

- Mechanoreceptors respond to physical force such as pressure (touch or blood pressure) and stretch.
- Photoreceptors respond to light.
- Thermoreceptors respond to temperature changes.
- Chemoreceptors respond to dissolved chemicals during sensations of taste and smell and to changes in internal body chemistry such as variations of O_2, CO_2, or H^+ in the blood.
- Nociceptors respond to a variety of stimuli associated with tissue damage. The brain interprets the pain (CliffsNotes, 2013).

Motor Function

Sensory information is transmitted from all areas of the nervous system into the spinal cord, brain stem, and cerebrum where it produces muscular functions transmitted to the body along efferent nerve fibers. The term **extrapyramidal side effect** is sometimes used to describe involuntary motor movements of the neck, jaw, and extremities with the administration of some types of medications (Hadaway, 2010).

Anatomical

Central Nervous System

The central nervous system (CNS) consists of the brain and spinal cord. The spinal cord extends from the medulla oblongata and occupies approximately two thirds of the length of vertebral column. The cord is enclosed within three protective layers: the pia mater, the arachnoid mater, and the dura mater, which is most distal.

Peripheral Nervous System

The peripheral nervous system (PNS) consists of nerves outside the CNS. Nerves of the PNS are classified in one of two ways: first, by how they are connected to the CNS. Cranial nerves originate from or terminate in the brain, while spinal nerves originate from or terminate at the spinal cord and then by the direction of nerve propagation. Sensory (**afferent**) neurons transmit impulses from the skin and other sensory organs or from various places within the body to the CNS. Motor (**efferent**) neurons transmit impulses from the CNS to effectors (muscles or glands). Secondly, motor neurons are further classified according to the effectors they target or function. The **somatic nervous system (SNS)** directs the contraction of skeletal muscles. The **autonomic nervous system (ANS)** controls the activities of organs, glands, and various involuntary muscles, such as cardiac and smooth muscles.

The ANS is further divided in two:

- The sympathetic nervous system is involved in the stimulation of activities that prepare the body for action, such as increasing the heart rate, increasing the release of sugar from the liver into the blood, and other activities generally considered as fight or flight responses.
- The parasympathetic nervous system activates tranquil functions, such as stimulating the secretion of saliva or digestive enzymes into the stomach and small intestine.

Both sympathetic and parasympathetic systems target the same organs but often work antagonistically. For example, the sympathetic system accelerates the heartbeat, while the parasympathetic system slows the heartbeat. Each system is stimulated as is appropriate to maintain homeostasis.

The nervous system responds to changes in the environment through sensory organs and is responsible for

- Sensory function, transmitting information from tactile, visual, and auditory receptors
- Motor functions, controlling skeletal and smooth muscle
- Autonomic function, controlling glands and smooth muscle

Nerve fibers under the skin include those that react to temperature, touch, pressure, and pain. The number of nerve fibers varies in different areas of the body. Some areas of the skin are highly sensitive; other areas are only mildly sensitive. The insertion of a needle in one area may cause a great deal of pain, yet another area may be virtually insensitive to pain. The inner aspect of the wrist is a highly sensitive area. Venipunctures are performed here only when other veins have been exhausted.

The anatomic divisions of the nervous system are the CNS (the brain and spinal cord) and PNS (12 cranial and 31 spinal nerves). The vagus nerve, which innervates the heart, is of prime importance. Stimulation of the vagus nerve produces a depressant effect on cardiac muscle, resulting in clinical signs such as bradycardia and hypotension. This condition is known as a **vasovagal reaction** or vasovagal syncope.

Cardiovascular System

The blood volume and distribution, for which the circulatory system is responsible, result from complex interactions among cardiac output, excretion of fluids and electrolytes by the kidneys, and hormonal and nervous system factors. Total blood volume may be enhanced by pregnancy, large varicose veins, polycythemia, and inability of the heart to pump enough blood to perfuse the kidneys.

The circulatory system is divided into two main systems, the pulmonary and the systemic, each with its own set of vessels. The pulmonary system directs the blood flow from the right ventricle of the heart to the lungs, where it is oxygenated and returned to the left atrium.

The systemic circulatory system, the larger of the two, is the one that concerns the IV nurse. It consists of the aorta, arteries, arterioles, capillaries, venules, and veins through which the blood must flow.

The blood leaves the left ventricle, flows to all parts of the body, and returns to the right atrium of the heart through the vena cava. Systemic veins are categorized as superficial and deep.

The heart is encased in the pericardium, which has two layers. The outer, fibrous layer is composed of strong collagen fibers and covers the aorta, superior vena cava, right and left pulmonary arteries, and the four pulmonary veins. The inner, serous layer is further divided into the parietal and visceral layers. A thin film of fluid between these two layers enables the heart to move.

HEART WALL

The wall of the heart consists of three layers:

- The *epicardium* is the visceral layer of the serous pericardium.
- The *myocardium* is the muscular part of the heart that consists of contracting cardiac muscle and noncontracting Purkinje fibers that conduct nerve impulses. Cardiac cells (cardiomyocytes) are in this layer.
- The *endocardium* is the thin, smooth, endothelial, inner lining of the heart, which is continuous with the inner lining of the blood vessels.

As blood travels through the heart, it enters a total of four chambers and passes through four valves. The two upper chambers, the right and left atria, are separated longitudinally by the interatrial septum. The two lower chambers, the right and left ventricles, are the pumping machines of the heart and are separated longitudinally by the interventricular septum. A valve follows each chamber and prevents the blood from flowing backward into the chamber from which the blood originated.

RIGHT SIDE OF THE HEART

The function of the right side of the heart is to collect deoxygenated blood, in the right atrium, from the body (via superior and inferior vena cavae) and pump it, via the right ventricle, into the lungs so that carbon dioxide can be dropped off and oxygen picked up (CliffsNotes, 2013).

An air embolism can develop when the right side of the heart is open to outside air through a disconnected catheter and a negative intrathoracic pressure is present, such as during inspiration. The right side of the heart is open to outside air when the catheter is first inserted and during catheter changes. The path to outside air can also be opened accidentally in three ways: if the Luer taper fitting disconnects and becomes tangled in the tubing when the patient gets out of bed or rolls over; if the stopcock is placed in the wrong position;

or if there is a crack in the hub of the catheter. When the path to the outside is open, the negative intrathoracic pressure generated by respiration can draw air into the right side of the heart through the catheter. The air passes through the pulmonary artery and, if the bubble is large enough, may cause a pulmonary infarction.

CARDIAC CONDUCTION

Unlike skeletal muscle fibers (cells), which are independent of one another, cardiac muscle fibers (contractile muscle fibers) are linked by intercalated discs, areas where the plasma membranes intermesh. Within the intercalated discs, the adjacent cells are structurally connected by tight seals that weld the plasma membranes together and electrically connected by gap junctions, ionic channels that allow the transmission of a depolarization event. As a result, the entire myocardium functions as a single unit with a single contraction of the atria followed by a single contraction of the ventricles (Noble, Johnson, Thomas, & Bass, 2010).

THE GREAT VESSELS

The pathway of blood through the chambers and valves of the heart is described as follows (see Figures 6-2 and 6-3):

- The right atrium, located in the upper right side of the heart, and a small appendage, the right auricle, act as a temporary storage chamber so that blood will be readily available for the right ventricle.

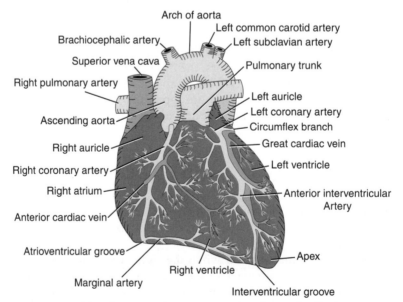

FIGURE 6-2 The heart and great vessels. (From Snell, R. (2003). *Clinical anatomy* (7th ed.). Philadelphia, PA: Lippincott Williams & Wilkins.)

Anterior view

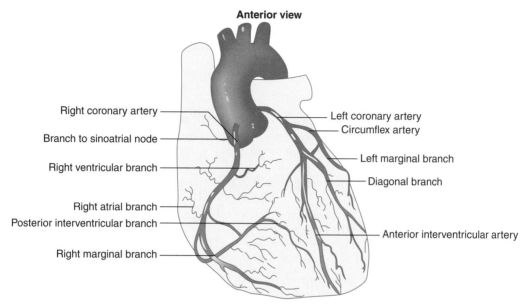

Right coronary artery

Branch to sinoatrial node

Right ventricular branch

Right atrial branch

Posterior interventricular branch

Right marginal branch

Left coronary artery

Circumflex artery

Left marginal branch

Diagonal branch

Anterior interventricular artery

FIGURE 6-3 Coronary arteries that supply the heart, or myocardium. (From Anatomical Chart Co. (2001). *Atlas of human anatomy.*)

Deoxygenated blood from the systemic circulation enters the right atrium through three veins: the superior vena cava, the inferior vena cava, and the coronary sinus. During the interval when the ventricles are not contracting, blood passes down through the right atrioventricular (AV) valve into the next chamber, the right ventricle. The AV valve is also called the tricuspid valve because it consists of three flexible cusps (flaps).

• The right ventricle is the pumping chamber for the pulmonary circulation. The ventricle, with walls thicker and more muscular than those of the atrium, contracts and pumps deoxygenated blood through the three-cusped pulmonary semilunar valve and into a large artery, the pulmonary trunk. The pulmonary trunk immediately divides into two pulmonary arteries, which lead to the left and right lungs, respectively. The following events occur in the right ventricle:

When the right ventricle contracts, the right AV valve closes and prevents blood from moving back into the right atrium. When the right ventricle relaxes, there is less pressure in the right ventricle and more pressure in the pulmonary trunk. This high pressure in the pulmonary trunk causes the valve to close, thereby preventing the backflow of blood and the return of blood to the right ventricle.

The left atrium and its auricle receive oxygenated blood from the lungs through four pulmonary veins. The left atrium, like its counterpart, is a holding chamber for blood in readiness for its flow into the left ventricle. When the ventricles relax, blood leaves the left atrium and passes through the left AV valve into the left ventricle.

Cardiac output is regulated by changes in the volume of blood flowing into the heart and control of the heart by the ANS (Noble et al., 2010).

Respiratory Anatomy

FUNCTION

The function of the respiratory system is to deliver air to the lungs. Oxygen in the air diffuses out of the lungs and into the blood, while carbon dioxide diffuses in the opposite direction, out of the blood and into the lungs.

- External respiration involves gas exchange between the atmosphere and the body tissues.
- Internal respiration is the process of gas exchange between the blood, the interstitial fluids, and the cells.

GAS EXCHANGE

Gas exchange occurs in the lungs between alveoli and blood plasma and throughout the body between plasma and interstitial fluids.

Parenteral fluid administration affects the trachea, bronchi, and lungs. Blood flows into the lungs from the pulmonary arteries, which carry deoxygenated blood. These arteries follow the path of the bronchi. Undissolved particles in infusates may enter the microcirculation of the lungs, which may lead to emboli.

Locating Important Arteries

Arteries require more protection than veins and are placed where injury is less likely to occur. Whereas veins are superficially located, most arteries lie deep in the tissues and are protected by muscle. Occasionally an artery is located superficially in an unusual place; this artery is then called an **aberrant artery**. An aberrant artery must not be mistaken for a vein. If a chemical that causes spasm is introduced into an aberrant artery, permanent damage may result.

The axillary artery extends from the first rib to the lateral edge of the chest in the axilla. The sheath is a neurovascular bundle containing the axillary artery, vein, and parts of the brachial nerve plexus controlling the arm. The continuation of the axillary artery is the brachial artery, which moves down the arm to immediately below the elbow, where it divides into the ulnar artery (medial side) and the radial artery (lateral side).

The radial artery is preferred for arterial puncture for blood withdrawal and catheter insertion because it is more superficial and is more readily stabilized. The Allen test must be performed to assess the collateral circulation. This is done by locating and compressing both arteries and noting the blanching that occurs. When only the ulnar artery is released, blood flow should return to the remainder of the hand.

Inadvertent arterial puncture can result in both acute and chronic problems; first complaints occur within seconds and range from mild irritation to intense pain distal to the injection site. Signs of vascular compromise may appear within 7 to 10 days and include pain, absence of peripheral pulses, cyanosis, and the beginning of compartment syndrome.

Tissue necrosis, complex regional pain syndrome, and sometimes amputation may result (Hadaway, 2010).

Locating Important Veins

SUPERFICIAL VEINS

The superficial or cutaneous veins are used in venipuncture. Located just beneath the skin in the superficial fascia, these veins and the deep veins sometimes unite, especially in the lower extremities. For example, the small saphenous vein, a superficial vein, drains the dorsum of the foot and the posterior section of the leg; it ascends the back of the leg and empties directly into the deep popliteal vein.

SUPERFICIAL VEINS OF THE LOWER EXTREMITIES

Before the small saphenous vein terminates in the deep popliteal, it sends out a branch that, after joining the great saphenous vein, also terminates in a deep vein, the femoral vein. Because of these deep connections, great concern arises when it becomes necessary to use the veins in the lower extremities. Thrombosis may occur, which could easily extend to the deep veins and cause pulmonary embolism. Understanding this, the nurse should refrain from using these veins.

Varicosities in the lower extremities, although readily available to venipuncture, are not a satisfactory route for parenteral administration. The relatively stagnant blood in such veins is likely to clot, resulting in a superficial phlebitis. Medication injected below a varicosity may result in another potential danger: a collection of the infused drug as a result of stagnated blood flow. This pocket of infused medication may delay the effect of the drug when immediate action is desired. Another concern is the danger of untoward reactions to the drug, which may occur when this accumulation finally reaches the general circulation.

SUPERFICIAL VEINS OF THE UPPER EXTREMITIES

The superficial veins of the upper extremities are shown in Figures 6-4 and 6-5. They consist of the digital, metacarpal, cephalic, basilic, and median veins (Table 6-3).

DEEP VEINS

Deep veins are usually enclosed in the same sheath with the arteries. Occasionally an arteriovenous anastomosis may occur congenitally or as the result of past penetrating injury of the vein and adjacent artery. When such trauma occurs, the blood flows directly from the artery into the vein. As a result, the veins draining an arteriovenous fistula are overburdened with high-pressure arterial blood. These veins appear large and tortuous. In these unusual circumstances, the nurse's quick recognition of an arteriovenous fistula may prevent pain, complications, and loss of time resulting from repeated unsuccessful attempts to start the infusion.

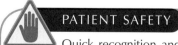

PATIENT SAFETY

Quick recognition and awareness of an arteriovenous fistula may prevent pain and complications.

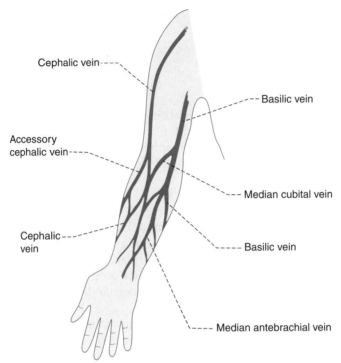

FIGURE 6-4 Superficial veins of the forearm.

STRUCTURAL DIFFERENCES BETWEEN ARTERIES AND VEINS

Possibly, the most dramatic difference between arteries and veins is that arteries pulsate and veins do not. Less apparent differences involve location and structure. Although arteries and veins are similar in structure—both comprise three layers of tissue—a close examination of these layers reveals their differentiating characteristics.

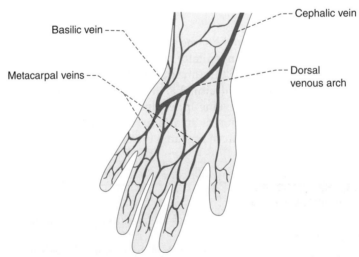

FIGURE 6-5 Superficial veins of the dorsal aspect of the hand.

TABLE 6-3	DETERMINING THE APPROPRIATE PERIPHERAL VENIPUNCTURE SITE		
Vein	Location	Advantages	Disadvantages
Digital	Along lateral–distal portion of the fingers	Ideal for short-term use	Fingers may require splinting and immobilization. Catheterization may create patient discomfort.
Metacarpal	On dorsum of the hand; formed by the union of digital veins between the knuckles	Easily accessible; lies flat on the back of the hand	Wrist movement is decreased unless a short catheter is used. Insertion is painful because of increased nerve endings. Site may become phlebitic.
Accessory cephalic	Along radial bone	Large vein ideal for venipuncture; readily accepts large-bore needle; easily stabilized	May be difficult to align catheter hub flush with the patient's skin. Catheter may impair patient mobility if placed over a point of flexion.
Cephalic	Along radial side of the forearm–upper arm	Excellent large vein; readily accessible; does not impair mobility	Proximity to elbow may compromise joint movement; site must be stabilized properly before venipuncture.
Medial antebrachial	Arises from palm and runs along ulnar side of the forearm	Easily accommodates winged infusion needle access	Proximity to nerve endings; inherent danger of infiltration
Basilic	Along ulnar side of the forearm–upper arm	Accommodates large-gauge needle; appropriate for large-gauge devices	May be difficult to position patient comfortably during insertion; penetration of dermal layer of the skin and proximity of site to nerve endings may cause pain
Antecubital	In the antecubital fossa: median cephalic (radial side); median basilic (ulnar side); median cubital (in front of elbow joint)	Large veins facilitate blood sampling; good for emergency use	Median cephalic crosses in front of brachial artery; scarred vessels owing to frequent blood draws; difficult to stabilize properly

TUNICA INTIMA: THE INNER LAYER

The first vascular layer is known as the tunica intima. It consists of an inner elastic endothelial lining, which also forms the valves in veins. Although these valves are absent in arteries, the endothelial lining is identical in the arteries and the veins, consisting of a smooth layer of flat cells.

This smooth surface allows the cells and platelets to flow through the blood vessels without interruption under normal conditions. Care must be taken to avoid roughening this surface when performing a venipuncture or removing a needle from a vein. Any trauma that roughens the endothelial lining encourages thrombin formation, a result of cells and platelets adhering or aggregating to the vessel wall.

Many veins contain valves, which are semilunar folds of the endothelium. Found in the larger veins of the extremities, these valves function to keep the blood flowing toward the heart. Where muscular pressure would cause a backup of the blood supply, these valves play an important role. They are located at points of branching and often cause a noticeable bulge in the veins. Applying a tourniquet to the extremity impedes the venous flow. When suction is applied, as occurs in the process of drawing blood, the valves compress and close the lumen of the vein, preventing the backward flow of blood. Thus, these valves interfere with the process of withdrawing blood. Recognizing the presence of a valve, the nurse may resolve the difficulty by slightly readjusting the needle.

These valves are absent in many of the small veins. However, if a thrombus obstructs an ascending vein, a small vein may be used instead. The catheter may be inserted below the thrombosis, directed toward the distal end of the extremity; this results in a rerouting of the fluid and avoidance of the thrombosed portion.

TUNICA MEDIA: THE MIDDLE LAYER

The second layer consists of muscular and elastic tissue. The nerve fibers, both vasoconstrictors and vasodilators, are located in this middle layer. These fibers, which constantly receive impulses from the vasoconstrictor center in the medulla, keep the vessels in a state of tonus. They also stimulate both arteries and veins to contract or relax.

The middle layer is not as strong and stiff in the veins as it is in the arteries. Therefore, the veins tend to collapse or distend as the pressure within falls or rises. Arteries do not collapse.

Stimulation by a change in temperature or by mechanical or chemical irritation may produce spasms in the vein or artery. For example, interrupting a continuous infusion to administer a pint of cold blood may produce vasoconstriction; this results in spasm, impedes the flow of blood, and causes pain. Application of heat to the vein promotes vasodilation, which relieves the spasm, improves the flow of blood, and relieves the pain. The same results are obtained by heat when an irritating drug has caused vasoconstriction. In this situation, heat relieves the spasm, increases the blood flow, and protects the vessel wall from inflammation caused by the medication. With heat dilating the vein and increasing the flow of blood, the drug becomes more diluted and less irritating. The use of heat to achieve vasodilation is also helpful when the nurse must use a small or poorly filled vein.

Spasms produced by a chemical irritation in an artery may have dire consequences. A single artery supplies circulation to a particular area. If this artery is damaged, the related area experiences impaired circulation, with the possible development of necrosis and gangrene. If a chemical agent is introduced into the artery, the result may be a spasm—a contraction that could shut off the blood supply completely. This problem is not as serious when veins are used because many veins supply a particular area; if one is injured, others maintain the circulation.

TUNICA ADVENTITIA: THE OUTER LAYER

The third layer, which consists of areolar connective tissue, surrounds and supports the vessel. In arteries, this layer is thicker than in veins because it is subjected to greater pressure from the force of blood.

Velocity

Velocity refers to the distance blood flows in a specific period. Under normal circumstances, blood moves through the aorta at a rate of 33 cm/second, but in capillaries, the velocity drops to 0.3 mm/second (Guyton & Hall, 2006).

The Clotting Cascade

Man's circulatory system is dependent for survival on the capacity of the circulating blood that is shed from injured vessels to clot. An understanding of the clotting cascade is imperative in dealing with the patient receiving infusion therapy.

The coagulation cascade of secondary hemostasis has two pathways leading to fibrin formation. These are the *contact activation pathway* (also known as the intrinsic pathway) and

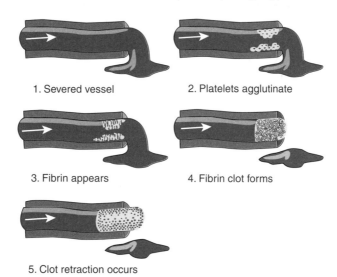

1. Severed vessel

2. Platelets agglutinate

3. Fibrin appears

4. Fibrin clot forms

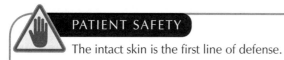

5. Clot retraction occurs

FIGURE 6-6 Clotting process in a traumatized vessel.

the *tissue factor pathway* (also known as the extrinsic pathway). The primary pathway for the initiation of blood coagulation is the *tissue factor pathway*.

The contact activation (intrinsic) pathway is initiated by activation of the "contact factors" of plasma and can be measured by the activated partial thromboplastin time test.

The tissue factor (extrinsic) pathway is initiated by release of tissue factor and can be measured by the prothrombin time (PT) test. PT results are often reported as ratio (INR values) to monitor dosing of anticoagulants (Weinstein, 1981; Hughes-Jones, Wickramasinghe, & Hatton, 2008) (Figure 6-6).

Defense Mechanisms

The body has innate defense mechanisms to control and to cope with the constant attack of microorganisms. These include the skin and respiratory tract, white blood cells, the immune system, the alimentary canal, and the mucous membranes of the eye. During the delivery of infusion therapy, skin is the first barrier to be breached. Inflammation is the body's response to injury from microorganisms, trauma, harmful chemicals, and temperature extremes.

The process of venipuncture breaks the skin, subcutaneous tissue, and the vessel wall. The degree of cellular injury is dependent on the skill used to enter the vein and advance the catheter within the vessel wall. Using peripheral veins to insert midline and peripherally inserted central catheters increases the potential for inflammation because longer vein section may be injured (Hadaway, 2010).

> **PATIENT SAFETY**
>
> The intact skin is the first line of defense.

Injury to the skin may occur from repeated application and removal of dressings and tape, securing tubing to the skin, catheter migration into or out of the insertion site, and the use of antiseptic agents. The infusion nurse should remain aware of the vulnerability of the human body and the skin's surface when selecting and accessing a site for venipuncture.

Review Questions   *Note: Questions below may have more than one right answer.*

1. Blood volume and distribution result from which of the following interactions?
   A. Interaction between cardiac output and excretion of excessive amounts of fluids and electrolytes
   B. Excretion of excess fluids and electrolytes by the kidneys, and hormonal and nervous system
   C. Neither of the above
   D. A and B

2. Total fluid volume may be enhanced by
   A. Pregnancy
   B. Large varicose veins
   C. Polycythemia
   D. Inability of the heart to pump enough blood to perfuse the kidneys

3. Which of the following statements about valves is *false*?
   A. They may be found in many veins.
   B. They are semilunar folds of the endothelium.
   C. They are found in smaller veins of the extremities.
   D. They keep the blood flowing toward the heart.

4. Stimulation of which nerve produces a depressant effect on cardiac muscle?
   A. Vagus
   B. Brachial
   C. Ulnar
   D. Radial

5. All of the following statements about the epidermis are true *except*
   A. It is the uppermost layer.
   B. It forms a protective covering.
   C. Its thickness varies.
   D. It is thinnest on the palms of the hands.

6. Which of the following veins is appropriate for peripheral access (short-term)?
   A. Digital
   B. Brachial
   C. Ulnar
   D. Femoral

7. Which vein is located on the surface of the hand?
   A. Ulnar
   B. Radial
   C. Metacarpal
   D. Brachial

8. Which of the following statements is true of an aberrant artery?
   A. It requires more protection than a vein.
   B. It lies deep in tissue.
   C. It is protected by muscle.
   D. It is located superficially in an unusual place.

9. A working knowledge of the anatomy and physiology of which systems enables the IV clinician to practice?
   A. Peripheral vasculature
   B. Neurologic and cardiopulmonary systems
   C. Neither of the above
   D. A and B

10. Which of the following contributes to arterial spasm?
    A. Chemical irritation
    B. Impaired circulation
    C. Intra-arterial injection
    D. Necrosis

References and Selected Readings *Asterisks indicate references cited in text.*

Aaronson, P.I., & Ward, J.P.T. (2007). *The cardiovascular system at a glance* (3rd ed.), Blackwell Publishing.

Pennsylvania Patient Safety Advisory. (2012). Produced by ECRI Institute and ISMP under contract to the Pennsylvania. *Patient Safety Advisory, 9*(2) 58–64.

Bullock-Corkhill, M. (2010). Central venous access devices: Access and insertion. In M. Alexander, A. Corrigan, L. Gorski, J. Hankins, & R. Perucca, eds. *Infusion nursing: An evidence-based approach* (3rd ed.). St. Louis, MO: Saunders/Elsevier, 480–494.

*CliffsNotes. (2013). *Cranial nerves.* http://www.cliffsnotes.com/study_guide/Cranial-Nerves.topicArticleId-277792,articleId-277635.html

*ECRI Institute. (1985). Air embolism through central venous catheters. *Hazard [Health Devices], 14*(14), 436–437.

*Guyton, A., & Hall, J. (2006). *Textbook of medical physiology* (11th ed.). Philadelphia, PA: Saunders.

*Hadaway, L. (2010). Anatomy and physiology related to infusion therapy. In M. Alexander, A. Corrigan, L. Gorski, J. Hankins, & R. Perucca, eds. *Infusion therapy: An evidence-based approach* (3rd ed.), St. Louis, MO: Saunders/Elsevier, 139–177.

Hall, J.E. (2011). *Guyton and Hall's textbook of medical physiology* (12th ed.). Philadelphia, PA: Saunders/Elsevier, 159–186.

*Hughes-Jones, N.C., Wickramasinghe, S.N., & Hatton, C. (2008). *Lecture notes haematology.* Cambridge, MA: Wiley-Blackwell, 145–148.

Infusion Nurses Society [position paper]. (2008). The role of the registered nurse in the insertion of external jugular peripherally inserted central catheters (EJ PICC) and external jugular peripheral intravenous catheters (EJ PIV). *Journal of Infusion Nursing, 31*(4), 226–227.

Jardin, F., & Vieillard-Baron, A. (2005). Monitoring of right-sided heart function. *Current Opinions in Critical Care, 11*(3), 271–279.

Marieb, E.N., & Hoehn, K. (2010). Human anatomy and physiology, *Cardiovascular system* (8th ed.). Benjamin Cummings.

Mirski, M.A., Lele, A.V., Fitzsimmons L., & Toung, T.J.K. (2007). Diagnosis and treatment of vascular air embolism. *Anesthesiology,* 106, 164–177.

*Noble, A., Johnson, R., Thomas, A., & Bass, P. (2010). *The cardiovascular system: Systems of body series* (2nd ed.). Churchill Livingstone.

*Standring, S. (2008). *Anatomy: The anatomical basis of clinical practice* (40th ed.). London, UK: Churchill Livingston Elsevier.

*Weinstein, S.M. (1981). Clotting cascade. *Journal of Infusion Nursing (NITA), 4*(4), 290–294.

*Williams, P.L., Warwick, R., Dyson, M., & Bannister, L.H. (1995). *Gray's anatomy* (39th ed.). London, UK: Churchill Livingstone.

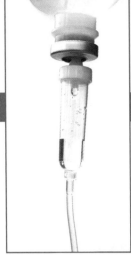

CHAPTER 7

Diagnostic Testing and Values

Abigail Ranum
Mary E. Hagle

KEY TERMS		
	Agglutination	Hemolysis
	Agglutinin	International
	Agglutinogen	Normalized Ratio
	Antibody	(INR)
	Antigen	Natural products
	Blood typing	Peak Level
	Factor V Leiden	Point-of-care testing
	Glycolysis	Postprandial
	Hematoma	Reference Range
	Hemoconcentration	Trough Level

CLINICAL SIGNIFICANCE OF BLOOD COLLECTION FOR TESTING

An important aspect of nursing care is the collection of blood samples for laboratory testing. This chapter details the most commonly performed laboratory tests—their purpose and normal values—and the collection and proper handling of blood samples. An overview of point-of-care testing as well as laboratory and nursing roles is included. Laboratory procedures are not a focus and thus are not explained.

Role of the Infusion Nurse

An IV department with responsibility for venous sampling is in a unique position to ensure adequate venous access and quality outcomes. First, the nurse, understanding the importance of preserving veins for infusion therapy, is cautious when choosing veins and in applying blood-drawing techniques. Second, the infusion nurse is skilled at using a single venipuncture to permit both the withdrawal of blood and the initiation of an infusion, thereby preserving veins, reducing discomfort, and avoiding undue patient distress. Third, patient–blood identification is of paramount importance in preventing the error of infusing incompatible blood. Because the IV department assumes responsibility for patient–blood identification before transfusion and is aware of existing hazards, its personnel are well qualified and educated in the collection of samples for typing and crossmatching. Another advantage of having infusion nurses collect blood samples is advocacy for patients to reduce blood loss due to phlebotomy: reduce unwarranted repeat testing and consolidate blood sampling.

The infusion nurse in laboratory testing adheres to the Infusion Nursing Standards of Practice for blood sampling (Infusion Nurses Society, 2011). The phlebotomy standard outlines evidence-based practices to promote patient safety, prevent infection, and reduce blood loss. All nurses should be knowledgeable and skillful in blood sampling. For example, withdrawing blood for specimen collection and safely maintaining central venous catheter patency should be a demonstrated competency outlined in institutional policy and procedure.

Laboratory Language

Clinical laboratories may be a separate business entity within a medical center or a private business contracting with an infusion center to provide services. They balance their own budget, maintain a professional environment, and aim for high customer satisfaction. In the case of the laboratory, both patients and ordering professionals are the consumers. Laboratories often operate on the premise that in order to provide a quality "product" (results), it is critical that an accurate sample is received. This begins with the correct selection and ordering of tests, proper identification of the patient, and superior sample collection. These steps enable the laboratory to provide reliable results to its customers. Understanding this information promotes a beneficial working relationship among all departments and the sharing of vital information.

PRACTICE STANDARDS IN TESTING

The nurse is responsible for maintaining the practice standard in diagnostic testing (Table 7-1). The collection of blood samples for certain tests must meet special requirements. Some tests call for whole blood, whereas others require components such as plasma, serum, or cells. The requirements must be met correctly to prevent erroneous or misleading laboratory analysis. Practice standards cover a wide range of test procedures, techniques, and circumstances.

Safety

Safety is the first priority in obtaining, handling, and processing blood samples. In the past, infusion departmental responsibilities included the collection of venous blood samples. Although collection of venous blood is usually delegated now to a team of laboratory phlebotomists or technologists, in many instances, the IV nurse will be involved in the following situations:

- When veins have become exhausted;
- When the patient is to receive an IV infusion;

TABLE 7-1	STANDARDS FOR DIAGNOSTIC TESTING[a]
Source and Standard	**Applications to Testing**
American Nurses Association Council on Cultural Diversity and Nursing Practice prescribes culturally competent care.	The nurse serves as an advocate for the patient and communicates and collaborates with health care team from a cultural perspective. The nurse tailors instructions and care to patient's cultural needs.
Individual agency has a policy statement for specimen collection and procedure statement for monitoring patient after an invasive diagnostic procedure; policy for unusual witnessed consent situations.	The nurse observes universal precautions when handling any body fluid specimens. Labeled biohazard bags are used for transport of specimens. The nurse monitors and records vital signs for specific times before, during, and after completion of certain procedures. The nurse documents any deviations from basic consent policies and employs measures to obtain appropriate consents for the procedure.
U.S. Department of Transportation requires alcohol testing in emergency rooms in special situations.	The properly trained emergency room nurse performs blood and breath alcohol testing in unresponsive people and accident victims.
OSHA standards apply to preventing transmission of hepatitis B and C and human immunodeficiency virus, safe work practices, vaccinations, and minimizing exposure to hazardous and toxic materials.	Nurses are exposed to blood-borne pathogens in the course of their work and are trained to observe universal precautions. Tasks and procedures in which occupational exposure may occur include the following: phlebotomy, injections, immunizations; handling contaminated materials, wastes, body fluids, and sharps; performing laboratory tests on body fluids; invasive procedures; vaginal exams and procedures; starting IVs; spinal taps; wound care; surgical procedures; cleaning.

[a]Nurses are accountable for safeguarding their patients within reasonable and prudent professional limits of practice.
Adapted from Dunning, M. B., & Fischbach, F. (2011). *Nurse's quick reference to common laboratory and diagnostic tests* (5th ed.). Philadelphia, PA: Wolters Kluwer/Lippincott Williams & Wilkins.

- When the specimen is to be obtained from a central venous catheter that is to be removed, from a multilumen central venous catheter, or from an implanted vascular access device.

A critical practice in blood sampling is specimen labeling. Errors can occur along the continuum from patient identification to results reporting. Use two patient identifiers when meeting the patient to collect the sample. Verify the accuracy of the labels and ensure that they are fully completed, easily read, and applied before leaving the patient and that they reflect the correct patient information.

Point-of-Care Testing

Point-of-care testing is synonymous with bedside testing or ancillary testing and is defined as medical testing at or near the site of patient care (Kost, 2002). The function of this testing is to provide rapid turnaround of test results that may directly affect patient care. Compact and mobile instruments or testing kits are employed. It is generally under the direction of the central laboratory and must adhere to the same expectations of quality involving the total testing process, covering the pre-, intra-, and postanalytic phases of testing (College of American Pathologists—Point of Care Testing Committee, 2009). Tests that may fall under this category include blood glucose, pregnancy dipstick, and fecal occult blood.

NURSING ROLE

The complexity of these tests generally falls under the *waived testing* category dictated by the Clinical Laboratory Improvement Amendments of 1988 (CLIA) law (U.S. Food and Drug Administration, 2009). Testing personnel must meet facility-defined minimum requirements and have documented training of each testing methodology. A small sample (whole blood, urine, stool, etc.) is collected and tested immediately, according to a specific procedure. In some cases, software interface may allow for integration directly into the patient's electronic medical record.

BENEFITS

Point-of-care testing can allow for swift, on-the-spot decisions and may facilitate goal-directed therapy. It generally requires a small volume sample, which is desirable for patients by reducing blood loss. This testing can increase efficiency for nurses by providing immediate information rather than waiting for clinical laboratory results. With proper monitoring and training, point-of-care testing can be a valuable nursing tool.

COLLECTING BLOOD AND BLOOD COMPONENTS

Serum consists of plasma minus fibrinogen and is obtained by drawing blood in a dry tube and allowing the blood to coagulate. Serum is required for most of the laboratory tests in common use.

Plasma consists of the stable components of blood minus the cells and is obtained by using an anticoagulant to prevent the blood from clotting. Several anticoagulants are available in color-coded tubes. Choice of the anticoagulant depends on the test to be performed. Most of the anticoagulants, including sodium or potassium oxalate, citrate, and ethylenediaminetetraacetic acid (EDTA), prevent coagulation by binding the serum calcium. Other anticoagulants, such as heparin, are valuable in specific tests but are not commonly used. Heparin prevents coagulation for only limited periods.

Whole blood is required for many tests, including blood counts and bleeding time. Potassium oxalate is commonly used to preserve whole blood.

> **PATIENT SAFETY**
>
> **Hemoconcentration** through venous stasis should be avoided to avoid inaccurate results in some tests. Hemoconcentration, which occurs when a tourniquet is applied, increases proportionally with the length of time the tourniquet is in use. Once the venipuncture has been made, the tourniquet should be removed. This is a simple but important precaution.

Carbon dioxide and pH are examples of tests in which results are affected by hemoconcentration. If the tourniquet is required to withdraw the blood, it should be noted on the requisition that the blood was drawn with stasis.

Hemolysis causes serious errors in many tests in which lysis of the red blood cells (RBCs) permits the substance being measured to escape into the serum. When erythrocytes, which are rich in potassium, rupture, the serum potassium level rises, giving a false measurement. See Box 7-1 for a summary of special precautions for avoiding hemolysis.

BOX 7-1   AVOIDING HEMOLYSIS WHEN DRAWING A BLOOD SAMPLE

1. Use dry syringes and dry tubes.
2. Avoid excess pressure on the plunger of the syringe. Such pressure collapses the vein and may cause air bubbles to be sucked from around the hub of the needle into the blood.
3. Do not shake clotted blood specimens unnecessarily.
4. Avoid using force when transferring blood to a container or tube. Force of the blood against the tube results in rupture of the cells. In transferring blood to a vacuum tube, use no needle larger than 20 gauge.

EFFECT OF INFUSION FLUIDS ON BLOOD SAMPLE

Infusion fluids may contribute to misleading laboratory interpretations. Blood samples should never be drawn proximal to an infusion but preferably from the contralateral extremity. If the fluid contains a substance that may affect the analysis, an indication of its presence should be made on the requisition—for example, "potassium determination during infusion of electrolyte solution."

SPECIAL HANDLING

Some samples require special handling when a delay is unavoidable. Some determinations, such as the pH, must be done within 10 minutes after the blood is drawn. When a delay is inevitable, the sample is placed in ice, which partially inhibits glycolysis—the production of lactic acid by the glycolytic enzymes of the blood cells—resulting in a rapid lowering of pH on standing.

   Samples for blood gas analyses also require special handling and must be analyzed as soon as blood is collected. When the carbon dioxide content of serum is to be determined, the blood must completely fill the tube or carbon dioxide will escape. Several procedures are currently in use; in each, the escape of carbon dioxide must be prevented.

FASTING

Because absorption of food may alter blood composition, test results often depend on the patient fasting. Blood glucose and serum lipid levels are increased by ingestion of food. Serum inorganic phosphorus values are depressed after meals.

TIMELY EXAMINATION

Immediate dispatch of blood samples to the laboratory is vital to accuracy of findings in some blood tests. Promptness in examining blood samples is necessary in the analysis of labile constituents of blood. In certain tests (e.g., those involving potassium), the substance being measured diffuses out of the cells into the serum being examined. The result is a false measurement. To prevent this rise in serum concentration, the cells must be separated from the serum promptly.

INFECTED SAMPLES

Special caution must be observed in the care of all blood samples because blood from all patients is considered infective. Blood samples should not be allowed to spill on the outside of the containers. Contaminated material should be placed in bags and treated according to institutional policies for disposal of infectious material. Catheters should not be recapped or broken but disposed of intact in catheter-proof containers. All personnel handling blood should wear gloves.

EMERGENCY TESTS

Blood for tests ordered on an emergency basis must be sent directly to the laboratory. Special markings or labels, according to the facility's procedures, may be used to indicate results are needed as soon as possible, or STAT, due to an emergency or crisis situation. Tests most likely to be designated as emergency tests include amylase, blood urea nitrogen (BUN), carbon dioxide, potassium, prothrombin, sodium, glucose, and blood typing.

Effective Equipment: Vacuum System

Infusion nurses are often involved in venous sampling from peripheral or long-term vascular access devices. The vacuum system, which has increased the efficiency of the blood sampling process, consists of a plastic holder into which screws a sterile, disposable, double-ended needle. A rubber-stoppered vacuum tube slips into the barrel. The barrel has a measured line denoting the distance the tube is inserted into the barrel; at this point, the needle becomes embedded in the stopper. The stopper is not punctured until the needle has been introduced into the vein. Advancing technology has made this process relatively bloodless and consistent with Occupational Safety and Health Administration (OSHA) and Centers for Disease Control and Prevention (CDC) safety standards.

After entry into the vein, the rubber-stoppered tube is pushed the remaining distance into the barrel. As the needle is pushed into the vacuum tube, a rubber sheath covering the shaft is forced back, allowing the blood to flow. The tourniquet is released, and several blood specimens may be obtained by simply removing the tube containing the sample and replacing it with another tube. As the tube is removed, the rubber sheath slips back over the needle, preventing blood from dripping into the holder (Figure 7-1).

If the vein is not located, removing the tube before the needle is withdrawn preserves the vacuum in the tube.

It sometimes is necessary to draw blood from small veins. If suction from the vacuum tube collapses the vein, drawing the blood becomes difficult. By pressing a finger against the vein beyond the point of the needle or by placing the bevel of the needle lightly against the wall of the vein, suction is reduced and the vein is allowed to fill. In the latter process, the nurse should exercise particular caution to prevent injury to the endothelial lining of the vein. The pressure is intermittently applied and released, filling and emptying the vein. A small-gauge winged infusion needle with vacuum adapter may also be used; the smaller needle reduces the amount of suction and may prevent collapse of the vein. A syringe is often used to draw blood from small veins because the amount of suction can be more easily controlled.

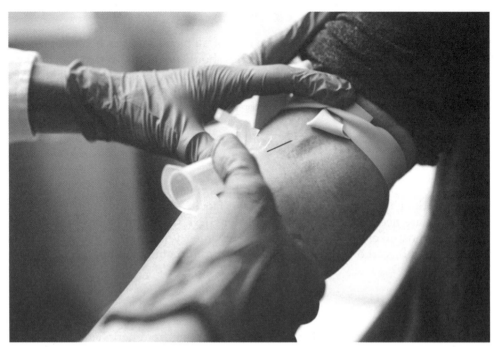

FIGURE 7-1 Nurse drawing venous sample using a vacuum system.

Skillful Technique

PERIPHERAL VENIPUNCTURES

When skillfully executed, a venipuncture causes the patient little discomfort. The numerous blood determinations necessary for diagnosis and treatment make good technique imperative. The one-step entry technique should be avoided because too often it results in through-and-through punctures, contributing to hematoma formation. The needle should be inserted under the skin and then, after relocation of the vein, into the vessel.

The veins most commonly used are those in the antecubital fossa. The median antecubital vein, although not always visible, is usually large and palpable. Because it is well supported by subcutaneous tissue and least likely to roll, it is often the best choice for venipuncture. Second choice is the cephalic vein. The basilic vein, although often the most prominent, is likely to be the least desirable. This vein rolls easily, making the venipuncture difficult, and a hematoma may readily occur if the patient is allowed to flex the arm, which squeezes the blood from the engorged vein into the tissues.

Sufficient time should be spent in locating the vein before attempting venipuncture. Whenever the veins are difficult to see or palpate, the patient should lie down. If the patient is seated, the arm should be well supported on a pillow.

CENTRAL ACCESS CATHETER BLOOD WITHDRAWAL

Venous samples are often drawn from a central line, especially because these catheters are commonly placed in patients with limited venous access. A dual-lumen catheter may facilitate this process. When multiple-lumen catheters are used for central venous blood sampling, the proximal lumen is the preferred site from which to draw the specimen. Aseptic technique is vital in preventing the introduction of bacteria into the catheter. A sterile IV catheter cap (Luer locking) reduces the risk of bacterial invasion. A recommended method is highlighted in Box 7-2. Manufacturers have kept pace with our demands for technologically advanced products that enhance the sampling process, maintain the integrity of the sample, and ensure safety for both patient and caregiver.

> ### PATIENT SAFETY
>
> Do not reinfuse the blood aspirate withdrawn prior to specimen collection ("discard specimen"). Reinfusion carries the risk of contamination and thrombotic complications (Infusion Nurses Society, 2011, pp. S77–S80).

Complications Resulting From Venipuncture and Blood Sampling

Complications related to venipuncture include hematomas, clotting, blood-borne diseases, syncope, and other problems.

HEMATOMAS

Hematomas are the most common complication of routine venipuncture for withdrawing blood, and they contribute more to the limitation of available veins than any other complication. They may result from through-and-through puncture to the vein or from incomplete insertion of the needle into the lumen of the vein, which allows the blood to leak into the tissues through the bevel of the needle. In the latter case, advancing the needle into the vein corrects the situation. At the first sign of uncontrolled bleeding, the tourniquet should be released and the needle withdrawn.

Hematomas also result from the application of the tourniquet after an unsuccessful attempt to draw blood. The tourniquet should never be applied to the extremity immediately after a venipuncture.

Hematomas most frequently result from insufficient time spent in applying pressure and from the bad habit of flexing the arm to stop the bleeding. Once the venipuncture is completed, the patient should be instructed to elevate the arm; elevation causes a negative pressure in the vein, collapsing it and facilitating clotting. With patients who have cardiac disease, elevation of the arm should be avoided. Constant pressure is maintained until the bleeding stops. The pressure is applied with a dry, sterile sponge because a wet sponge encourages bleeding. Adhesive strips do not take the place of pressure and, if ordered, are not applied until bleeding stops. Ecchymoses on the arm indicate poor or haphazard technique.

BLOOD-BORNE DISEASE

Special caution must be exercised to prevent blood-borne exposure from needle puncture or blood splash. Contaminated needles should be placed immediately in a separate container for disposal, and standard precautions should be followed. A vacuum tube with stopper provides adequate protection against accidental puncture from the contaminated needle until proper disposal can be made. Any needle puncture should be reported at once.

BOX 7-2 STEPS FOR OBTAINING BLOOD SAMPLES FROM A LOCKED (CAPPED) CENTRAL VENOUS CATHETER

Equipment

To collect a blood sample from a central venous catheter when the patient is not receiving medications, obtain the following:

Gloves

Alcohol wipes or other appropriate cleansing agent

Sterile 2" × 2" gauze sponge

Needleless injection cap, may be needed

Collection tubes

Vacutainer equipment or syringes as needed

Labels

Action	**Rationale**
Wash hands, put on gloves, and clamp the central venous catheter.	Ensures closed system. Groshong catheters do not need to be clamped.
Aseptically cleanse infusion port or injection cap: "Scrub the hub." Scrub catheter hub with alcohol wipe for 15 s before access (Gorski et al., 2010, p. 503)	Ensures aseptic technique
Access infusion port with 10 mL syringe filled with 3 mL of 0.9% normal saline. Open clamp. Flush catheter, then aspirate 4–5 mL blood. Clamp catheter. Remove syringe and discard.	To clear infusate. First sample contains flush solution, which may alter test results. Do not reinfuse blood (Infusion Nurses Society, 2011, S79).
Attach vacuum system for blood sampling with appropriate tubes. Open clamp. Obtain required quantity of blood. Clamp. Remove vacuum system. Attach syringe filled with 10–20 mL 0.9% normal saline (per agency procedure) (ONS, 2011). Unclamp. Flush catheter. Clamp.	Maintains patency and locks catheter.
Wash hands and properly dispose of all sharps and any contaminated equipment.	Promotes safety and infection control

NOTES:

- Only nurses or specified staff with delineated competencies should draw blood from central venous catheters.
- If blood withdrawal is difficult, the injection cap may need to be removed and the syringe/vacuum system attached directly to the catheter port.
- Coagulation testing through heparinized catheter or catheter used for parenteral nutrition is not recommended.

OTHER COMPLICATIONS

Other complications of venipuncture include syncope, continued bleeding, and thrombosis of the vein. Syncope is rarely encountered when the clinician is confident and skillful and when patient teaching has preceded the venipuncture process. Continued bleeding is a complication that may affect the patient receiving anticoagulants, the patient with a blood dyscrasia, or the oncology patient undergoing chemotherapy. To prevent bleeding and to preserve the vein, pressure to the site may be required for an extended period. The nurse should remain with the patient until the bleeding stops.

Thrombosis in routine venipuncture occurs from injury to the endothelial lining of the vein during the venipuncture. Antecubital veins may be used indefinitely if the clinician uses good technique.

COMMON LABORATORY TESTS

Laboratory tests are performed for several reasons:

- To indicate relatively common disorders
- To make a diagnosis
- To follow the course of a disease
- To regulate therapy

Standard laboratory values are listed in Table 7-2; examples of conversions of those values to Système International (SI) units are given in Table 7-3.

Reference Range

Although some laboratory tests offer a simple yes or no answer, for example, whether the culture was positive or negative, other results depend on their context. Results are reported in ranges, and those ranges are established by testing a large number of healthy people and observing what appears to be normal for them. The term **reference range** is preferred over *normal range* because the reference population can be clearly defined. What is normal for one group may not appear normal for another, that is, the changes that occur during pregnancy alter the body's chemistry and thus test results.

Blood Cultures

Blood cultures are performed to identify the causative microorganism when a bacteremia is suspected. Isolation of the organism facilitates appropriate treatment. Blood cultures are performed during febrile illnesses or when the patient is having chills with spiking fever. Intermittent bacteremia accompanies such infections as pyelonephritis, brucellosis, cholangitis, osteomyelitis, and others. In such cases, repeated blood cultures are usually ordered when the fever spikes.

In other infections, such as subacute bacterial endocarditis, the bacteremia is more constant during the 4 to 5 febrile days. Usually four or five cultures are obtained over a span of 1 to 2 days, and antimicrobial therapy is initiated once it is established that most cultures harbor the offending microorganism. If antimicrobial therapy is administered before the blood culture or before the patient's admittance to the hospital, the bacteremia may be suppressed, rendering isolation difficult.

TABLE 7-2 SELECTED LABORATORY VALUES

Parameter		Parameter	
Blood Chemistry/ Electrolytes	**Normal Values**	**Blood Chemistry/ Electrolytes**	**Normal Values**
BUN	10–20 mg/dL	Magnesium	1.3–2.1 mEq/L or 1.8–3.0 mg/dL
Serum creatinine	0.7–1.5 mg/dL	Chloride	97–110 mEq/L
Creatinine clearance	Male: 110–150 mL/min	Carbon dioxide	24–30 mmol/L
	Female: 105–132 mL/min	Phosphate	Adults: 2.5–4.5 mg/dL (1.8–2.6 mEq/L)
BUN: creatinine ratio	10:1		Children: 4.0–7.0 mg/dL (2.3–4.1 mEq/L)
Hematocrit	Male: 44%–52%	Zinc	77–137 µg/dL (by atomic absorption)
	Female: 39%–47%	Lithium	0.8 mEq/L (therapeutic level 8–12 h after administration)
Hemoglobin	Male: 13.5–18.0 g/dL Female: 12.0–16.0 g/dL	Serum proteins	
RBCs	Male: 4,600–6,000/mm³ Female: 4,200–5,400/mm³	Total	6.0–8.00 g/dL
Mean corpuscular volume (MCV)	80–95 mm³	Albumin	3.5–5.5 g/dL
Mean corpuscular hemoglobin	26–34 pg	Globulin	1.5–3.0 g/dL
Mean corpuscular hemoglobin concentration	32%–36%	Lactate (arterial blood)	4.5–14.4 mg/dL
		Serum ketones	Often >50 mg/dL in diabetic ketoacidosis. Usually <20 mg/dL in salicylate intoxication
Complete blood count		Serum salicylates	Therapeutic range: 20–25 mg/dL
Total leukocytes	4,500–11,000/mm³		Toxic range: >30 mg/dL
Myelocytes	0	Anion gap	12–15 mEq/L
Band neutrophils	150–400/mm³ (3%–5%)	AST	5–40 U/L
Segmented neutrophils	3,000–5,800/mm³ (54%–62%)	ALT	10–60 U/L
Lymphocytes	1,500–3,000/mm³ (25%–33%)	ALP	Varies with testing method
Monocytes	300–500/mm³ (3%–7%)	Serum bilirubin	
Eosinophils	50–250/mm³ (1%–3%)	Total	0.3–1.1 mg/dL
Basophils	15–50/mm³ (0%–0.75%)	Direct	0.1–0.4 mg/dL
Platelets	150,000–300,000/mm³	Indirect	0.2–0.7 mg/dL (total minus direct)
Reticulocytes	0.5%–1.5%	Lactate dehydrogenase (LDH)	100–190 mµ/mL

TABLE 7-2   SELECTED LABORATORY VALUES   *(Continued)*

Parameter		Parameter	
Blood Chemistry/ Electrolytes	**Normal Values**	**Blood Chemistry/ Electrolytes**	**Normal Values**
Red cell volume	Male: 20–36 mL/kg	Urine chemistry/ electrolytes[a]	
	Female: 19–31 mL/kg	Sodium	80–180 mEq/24 h (varies with Na^+ intake)
Plasma volume	Male: 25–43 mL/kg	Potassium	40–80 mEq/24 h (varies with dietary intake)
	Female: 28–45 mL/kg	Chloride	100–250 mEq/24 h
Clotting time	8–18 min	Calcium	100–150 mg/24 h (if on average diet; varies with dietary intake)
PT	11–15 s		
Iron	60–90 µg/dL	Osmolality	Typical urine is 500–800 mOsm/L (extreme range is 50–1,400 mOsm/L); usually about 1½–3 times greater than serum osmolality
Total iron-binding capacity	250–420 µg/dL	Specific gravity (SG)	1.002–1.030 (most random samples have an SG of 1.012–1.025)
		pH	4.5–8.0
Serum transferrin	>200 mg/dL (measured directly)	Arterial blood gases	
Partial thromboplastin time	Standard: 68–82 s Activated: 32–46 s	pH	7.35–7.45
Fibrinogen	160–415 mg/dL	PaO_2	80–100 mm Hg
Serum osmolality	280–295 mOsm/kg		
Serum amylase	25–125 U/L		
Serum glucose	70–110 mg/dL	$PaCO_2$	38–42 mm Hg
Serum electrolytes		Bicarbonate	22–26 mEq/L
Sodium	135–145 mEq/L		
Potassium	3.5–5.0 mEq/L	Base excess	− 2 to + 2
Calcium	Total: 8.9–10.3 mg/dL or 4.6–5.1 mEq/L Ionized: 4.6–5.1 mg/dL		

[a]Measurement of electrolytes may be of limited value because of recent administration of diuretics or lack of knowledge of dietary intake.

Penicillinase may be ordered to be added to the blood culture medium to neutralize the existing penicillinemia and recover the organism. Antimicrobial therapy usually must be withheld to await report of culture to make a precise diagnosis. The penicillinase is added to the culture medium before or immediately after the blood sample is drawn.

TABLE 7-3   **EXAMPLES OF CONVERSIONS TO SYSTÈME INTERNATIONAL (SI) UNITS**

Component	System	Present Reference Intervals	Present Unit	Conversion Factor	SI Reference Intervals	SI Unit
ALT	Serum	5–40	U/L	1.0	5–40	U/L
Albumin	Serum	3.9–5.0	mg/dL	10	39–50	g/L
ALP	Serum	35–110	U/L	1.00	35–110	U/L
AST	Serum	5–40	U/L	1.00	5–40	U/L
Bilirubin	Serum					
Direct		0–0.2	mg/dL	17.10	0–4	μmol/L
Total		0.1–1.2	mg/dL	17.10	2–20	μmol/L
Calcium	Serum	8.6–10.3	mg/dL	0.2495	2.15–2.57	mmol/L
Carbon dioxide, total	Serum	22–30	mEq/L	1.00	22–30	mmol/L
Chloride	Serum	98–108	mEq/L	1.00	98–108	mmol/L
Cholesterol	Serum					
Age < 29 y		<200	mg/dL	0.02586	<5.15	mmol/L
30–39 y		<225	mg/dL	0.02586	<5.80	mmol/L
40–49 y		<245	mg/dL	0.02586	<6.35	mmol/L
>50 y		<265	mg/dL	0.02586	<6.85	mmol/L
Complete blood count	Blood					
Hematocrit						
Men		42–52	%	0.01	0.42–0.52	1
Women		37–47	%	0.01	0.37–0.47	1
Hemoglobin						
Men		14.0–18.0	g/dL	10.0	140–180	g/L
Women		12–16	g/dL	10.0	120–160	g/L
Red cell count						
Men		$4.6–6.2 \times 10^8$	/mm^3	10^6	$4.6–6.2 \times 10^{12}$/L	
Women		$4.2–5.4 \times 10^8$	/mm^3	10^6	$4.2–5.4 \times 10^{12}$/L	
White cell count		$4.5–11.0 \times 10^3$	/mm^3	10^6	$4.5–11.0 \times 10^9$/L	
Platelet count		$150–300 \times 10^3$	/mm^3	10^6	$150–300 \times 10^9$/L	
Cortisol	Serum					
8 AM		5–25	μg/dL	27.59	140–690	nmol/L
8 PM		3–13	μg/dL	27.59	80–360	nmol/L
Cortisol	Urine	20–90	μg/24 h	2.759	55–250	nmol/24 h
Creatine kinase (CK)	Serum					
High CK group (black men)		50–520	U/L	1.00	50–520	U/L

TABLE 7-3	EXAMPLES OF CONVERSIONS TO SYSTÈME INTERNATIONAL (SI) UNITS *(Continued)*					
Component	System	Present Reference Intervals	Present Unit	Conversion Factor	SI Reference Intervals	SI Unit
Intermediate CK group (nonblack men, black women)		35–345	U/L	1.00	35–345	U/L
Low CK group (nonblack women)		25–145	U/L	1.00	25–145	U/L
Creatinine kinase isoenzyme, MB fraction	Serum	>5	%	0.01	>0.05	1
Creatinine	Serum	0.4–1.3	mg/dL	88.40	35–115	μmol/L
Men		0.7–1.3	mg/dL	88.40	60–115	μmol/L
Women		0.4–1.1	mg/dL	88.40	35–100	μmol/L
Digoxin, therapeutic	Serum	0.5–2.0	ng/mL	1.281	0.6–2.6	nmol/L
Erythrocyte indices	Blood					
MCV		80–100	μm^3	1.00	80–100	fL
Mean corpuscular hemoglobin concentration (MCHC)		27–31	pg	1.00	27–31	pg
MCHC		32–36	%	0.01	0.32–0.36	1
Ferritin	Serum					
Men		12–300	ng/mL	1.00	29–438	μg/L
Women		12–150	ng/mL	1.00	9–219	μg/L
Folate	Serum	2.5–20.0	ng/mL	2.266	6–46	nmol/L
Follicle-stimulating hormone	Serum					
Children		≤12	mIU/mL	1.00	≤12	IU/L
Men		2.0–10.0	mIU/mL	1.00	2.0–10.0	IU/L
Women, follicular		3.2–9.0	mIU/mL	1.00	3.2–9.0	IU/L
Women, midcycle		3.2–9.0	mIU/mL	1.00	3.2–9.0	IU/L
Women, luteal		2.0–6.2	mIU/mL	1.00	2.0–6.2	IU/L
Gases, arterial	Blood					
Po_2		80–95	mm Hg	0.1333	10.7–12.7	kPa
Pco_2		37–43	mm Hg	0.1333	4.9–5.7	kPa
Glucose	Serum	62–110	mg/dL	0.05551	3.4–6.1	mmol/L
Iron	Serum	50–160	μg/dL	0.1791	9–29	μmol/L
Iron-binding capacity (IBC)	Serum					
Total IBC		230–410	μg/dL	0.1791	41–73	μmol/L
Saturation		15–55	%	0.01	0.15–0.55	1

(Continued)

TABLE 7-8	EXAMPLES OF CONVERSIONS TO SYSTÈME INTERNATIONAL (SI) UNITS (Continued)					
Component	**System**	**Present Reference Intervals**	**Present Unit**	**Conversion Factor**	**SI Reference Intervals**	**SI Unit**
Lactic dehydrogenase	Serum	120–300	U/L	1.00	120–300	U/L
Luteinizing hormone	Serum					
Men		4.9–15.0	mIU/mL	1.00	4.9–15.0	IU/L
Women, follicular		5.0–25	mIU/mL	1.00	5.0–25	IU/L
Women, midcycle		43–145	mIU/mL	1.00	43–145	IU/L
Women, luteal		3.1–31	mIU/mL	1.00	3.1–31	IU/L
Magnesium	Serum	1.2–1.9	mEq/L	0.4114	0.50–0.78	mmol/L
Osmolality	Serum	278–300	mOsm/kg	1.00	278–300	mmol/kg
Osmolality	Urine	None defined	mOsm/kg	1.00	None defined	mmol/kg
Phenobarbital, therapeutic	Serum	15–40	µg/mL	4.306	65–175	µmol/L
Phenytoin, therapeutic	Serum	10–20	µg/mL	3.964	40–80	µmol/L
Phosphate (phosphorus, inorganic)	Serum	2.3–4.1	mg/dL	0.3229	0.75–1.35	mmol/L
Potassium	Serum	3.7–5.1	mEq/L g/mL	1.00	3.7–5.1	mmol/L
Protein, total	Serum	6.5–8.3	g/dL	10.0	65–83	g/L
Sodium	Serum	134–142	mEq/L	1.00	134–142	mmol/L
Theophylline, therapeutic	Serum	5–20	µg/mL	5.550	28–110	µmol/L
Thyroid-stimulating hormone	Serum	0–5	µIU/mL	1.00	0–5	mIU/L
Thyroxine	Serum	4.5–13.2	µg/dL	12.87	58–170	nmol/L
T_3 uptake ratio	Serum	0.88–1.19	—	1.00	0.88–1.19	—
Tri-iodothyronine (T_3)	Serum	70–235	ng/mL	0.01536	1.1–3.6	nmol/L
Triglycerides	Serum	50–200	mg/dL	0.01129	0.55–2.25	mmol/L
Urate (uric acid)	Serum					
Men		2.9–8.5	mg/dL	59.48	170–510	µmol/L
Women		2.2–6.5	mg/dL	59.48	130–390	µmol/L
Urea nitrogen	Serum	6–25	mg/dL	0.3570	2.1–8.9	mmol/L
Vitamin B_{12}	Serum	250–1,000	pg/mL	0.7378	180–740	pmol/L

Adapted from Fischbach, F. T., & Dunning, M. B. (2009). *A manual of laboratory and diagnostic tests* (8th ed.). Philadelphia, PA: Wolters Kluwer/Lippincott Williams & Wilkins.

Some bacteriology laboratories routinely culture blood under both aerobic and anaerobic conditions. If this is not done routinely and the clinician suspects bacteremia with strict anaerobes, the laboratory should be notified because a special culture broth is necessary.

Extreme care should be taken in ensuring a sterile field for venipuncture; the skin is a fertile field for bacterial growth. Colonization of organisms at the insertion site is associated with a high incidence of catheter-related infections. *Staphylococcus epidermidis*, diphtheroids, and yeast (common skin or environment contaminants) usually indicate contamination, whereas *Staphylococcus aureus* presents a greater problem, indicating either a contaminant or another serious pathogen.

Electrolyte Measurements

Electrolyte imbalances are serious complications in the critically ill patient and must be recognized and corrected at once. Electrolyte determinations frequently are ordered on an emergency basis. Accurate measurement is essential and to a large degree depends on the proper collection and handling of blood specimens.

POTASSIUM LEVEL

Potassium is an electrolyte essential to body function. Approximately 98% of all body potassium is found in the cells; only small amounts are contained in the serum.

The kidneys normally do not conserve potassium. When large quantities of body fluid are lost without potassium replacement, a severe deficiency occurs. Chronic kidney disease and the use of diuretics may cause a potassium deficit. Adrenal steroids play a major role in controlling the concentration of potassium: hyperadrenalism causes increased potassium loss, with deficiency resulting; steroid therapy promotes potassium excretion.

An elevated potassium level results from potassium retention in renal failure or adrenal cortical deficiency. Hypoventilation and cellular damage also result in an elevated potassium level.

Because intracellular ions are not accessible for measurement, determination must be made on the serum. Because the concentration of potassium in the cells is roughly 15 times greater than that in the serum, the blood for potassium determination must be carefully drawn to prevent hemolysis.

BLOOD COLLECTION

Blood (2 mL) is drawn in a dry tube and allowed to clot or, preferably, placed under oil, which minimizes friction and hemolysis of the RBCs. The blood should be sent to the laboratory immediately because potassium diffuses out of the cells and gives a falsely high reading.

TEST RESULT

Normal serum range is 3.5 to 5.0 mEq/L.

SODIUM LEVEL

The main role of sodium is the control of the distribution of water throughout the body and the maintenance of a normal fluid balance.

The excretion of sodium is regulated mainly by the adrenocortical hormone aldosterone. Water excretion is regulated by antidiuretic hormone, and as long as these two systems are in harmony, the sodium and water remain in isosmotic proportion. Any change in the normal sodium concentration indicates that the loss or gain of water and sodium is in other than isosmotic proportion. Increased sodium levels may be caused by excessive infusions of sodium, insufficient water intake, or excess loss of fluid without a sodium loss, as in tracheobronchitis. Decreased sodium levels may be caused by excessive sweating accompanied by intake of large amounts of water by mouth, adrenal insufficiency, excessive infusions of nonelectrolyte fluids, or gastrointestinal suction accompanied with water by mouth.

BLOOD COLLECTION

Blood (3 mL) is drawn carefully to prevent hemolysis and placed in a dry tube or a tube with oil.

TEST RESULT

Normal serum range is 135 to 145 mEq/L.

CHLORIDE LEVEL

Chlorides are usually measured along with other blood electrolytes. The measurement of chlorides is helpful in diagnosing disorders of acid–base balance and water balance of the body. Chloride reciprocally increases or decreases in concentration whenever changes in concentration of other anions occur. In metabolic acidosis, a reciprocal rise in chloride concentration occurs when the bicarbonate concentration drops.

Elevation in the blood chloride level occurs in such conditions as Cushing syndrome, hyperventilation, and some kidney disorders. A decrease in blood chloride levels may occur in diabetic acidosis and heat exhaustion and after vomiting and diarrhea.

BLOOD COLLECTION

Venous blood (5 mL) is withdrawn and placed in a dry tube to clot.

TEST RESULT

Normal serum range is 97 to 110 mEq/L.

CALCIUM LEVEL

Calcium, an essential electrolyte of the body, is required for blood clotting, muscular contraction, and nerve transmission. Only ionized calcium is useful, but because it cannot be satisfactorily measured, the total amount of body calcium is determined; 50% of the total is believed to be ionized. In acidosis, there is a higher level of ionized calcium; in alkalosis, a lower level.

Hypocalcemia (decrease in blood calcium) occurs whenever impairment of the gastrointestinal tract, such as with sprue or celiac disease, prevents absorption. Deficiency, which also occurs in hypoparathyroidism and in some kidney diseases, is characterized by muscular twitching and tetanic convulsions.

Hypercalcemia (excess of calcium in the blood) occurs in hyperparathyroidism and in respiratory disturbances in which the carbon dioxide blood content is increased, such as in respiratory acidosis.

BLOOD COLLECTION

Venous blood (5 mL) is placed in a dry tube and allowed to clot. Analysis is performed on the serum.

TEST RESULT

Normal serum range in adults is 8.9 to 10.3 mg/100 mL. The range is slightly higher in children.

PHOSPHORUS LEVEL

Phosphorus metabolism is related to calcium metabolism, and the serum level varies inversely with calcium.

Phosphorus concentrations may be increased in conditions such as hypoparathyroidism, kidney disease, or excessive intake of vitamin D. Decreased concentrations may occur in hyperparathyroidism, rickets, and some kidney diseases.

BLOOD COLLECTION

Because RBCs are rich in phosphorus, hemolysis must be avoided. Analysis is performed on the serum; 4 mL blood is placed in a dry tube to clot.

TEST RESULT

Normal serum range is 2.5 to 4.5 mg/100 mL. In infants in the 1st year, the upper limit of the range rises to 6.0 mg/100 mL.

Venous Blood Measurements of Acid–Base Balance

The body's major buffer system is the bicarbonate (HCO_3)–carbonic acid (H_2CO_3) buffer system. Normally, there are 20 parts of bicarbonate to 1 part of carbonic acid. When deviations occur in the normal ratio, the pH changes. The change is accompanied by a change in bicarbonate concentration.

CARBON DIOXIDE CONTENT

Carbon dioxide content is the measurement of the free carbon dioxide and bicarbonate content of the serum, which provides a general measure of acidity or alkalinity. An increase in carbon dioxide content usually indicates alkalosis; a decrease indicates acidosis. This test, along with clinical findings, is helpful in determining the severity and nature of the disorder. Measurement of pH is necessary for accuracy—a change in carbon dioxide does not always signify a change in pH because pH depends on the buffer ratio and not the carbon dioxide content. When the carbon dioxide and pH are known, the buffer ratio can be determined.

An elevated carbon dioxide content is present in metabolic alkalosis, hypoventilation, loss of acid secretions (such as occurs in persistent vomiting or drainage of the stomach), and excessive administration of corticotropin or cortisone. A low carbon dioxide content usually occurs in loss of alkaline secretions such as in severe diarrhea, certain kidney diseases, diabetic acidosis, and hyperventilation.

BLOOD COLLECTION

Several procedures are now used to collect blood: collection in a heparinized syringe with immediate placement on ice, collection in a heparinized vacuum tube, or collection in a dry tube without an anticoagulant. The procedure used depends on the laboratory. The containers must always be filled with blood to prevent carbon dioxide from escaping.

> **PATIENT SAFETY**
>
> In all methods, it is important that the patient avoid clenching his or her fist; excess muscular activity of the arm can increase the carbon dioxide level in the blood.

TEST RESULT

Normal serum range is 22 to 31 mEq/L.

BLOOD pH

The pH, a measure of acidity, indicates the serum concentration of hydrogen ions. The pH becomes lower in acid conditions, such as hypoventilation, diarrhea, and diabetic acidosis. The pH rises in alkaline conditions, such as hyperventilation and excessive vomiting.

BLOOD COLLECTION

The blood is collected without stasis in a heparinized 2-mL syringe; the syringe is then capped. The blood may be drawn with a small-vein needle, the needle discarded, and the tubing tied off. The specimen is left in the syringe and packed in ice. Loss of carbon dioxide from contact with the air is thus avoided, and excess production of lactic acid by enzymic reaction reduced. Blood (5 mL) may also be collected in a green-stoppered vacuum tube containing heparin.

TEST RESULT

Normal blood pH ranges between 7.35 and 7.45.

Enzyme Analyses

AMYLASE

Amylase determination is helpful in the diagnosis of acute pancreatitis or the acute recurrence of chronic pancreatitis. Amylase is secreted by the pancreas; a rise in the serum level occurs when outflow of pancreatic juice is restricted. This test is usually performed on patients with acute abdominal pain or on surgical patients in whom injury may have occurred to the pancreas. Amylase levels usually remain elevated for only a short time (3 to 6 days).

BLOOD COLLECTION

Venous blood (6 mL) is allowed to clot in a dry tube.

TEST RESULT

Normal serum range is 4 to 25 U/mL. The range may depend on the normal values established by clinical laboratories because the method may be modified.

LIPASE

Lipase determination is used for detecting damage to the pancreas and is valuable when too much time has elapsed for the amylase level to remain elevated. When secretions of the pancreas are blocked, the serum lipase level rises.

BLOOD COLLECTION

The test is performed on serum from 6 mL of clotted blood.

TEST RESULT

Normal serum level is 2 U/mL or less.

ACID PHOSPHATASE

Acid phosphatase levels are useful in determining metastasizing tumors of the prostate. The prostate gland and prostatic carcinoma are rich in phosphatase but do not normally release the enzyme into the serum. Once the carcinoma has spread, it starts to release acid phosphatase, increasing the serum concentration. In addition to carcinoma of the prostate, other conditions that produce increased serum acid phosphatase levels are Paget disease, hyperparathyroidism, metastatic mammary carcinoma, renal insufficiency, multiple myeloma, some liver disease, arterial embolism, myocardial infarction, and sickle cell crisis.

BLOOD COLLECTION

Blood (5 mL) is allowed to clot in a dry tube. Hemolysis should be avoided. Analysis should be immediate, or the serum should be frozen.

TEST RESULT

Normal serum range is 0 to 3, 1 ng/mL

ALKALINE PHOSPHATASE

Alkaline phosphatase (ALP) is a useful test in diagnosing bone diseases and obstructive jaundice. In bone diseases, the small amount of ALP usually present in the serum rises in proportion to the number of new bone cells. When excretion of ALP is impaired, as in some disorders of the liver and biliary tract, the serum level rises and may give some evidence of the degree of blockage in the biliary tract.

BLOOD COLLECTION

Blood (5 mL) is drawn, and the test is performed on the serum. Sodium sulfobromophthalein dye should be avoided.

TEST RESULT

Normal serum range is 13 to 39 U/mL.

ASPARTATE AMINOTRANSFERASE

The transaminases are enzymes found in large quantities in the heart, liver, muscle, kidney, and pancreas cells. Any disease that damages these cells results in an elevated serum transaminase level. Clinical signs and other tests are used in diagnosis.

The aspartate aminotransferase (AST; formerly known as serum glutamic–oxaloacetic transaminase) level is used to distinguish between myocardial infarction and acute coronary insufficiency without infarction. It is also useful as a liver function test to follow the progression of liver damage or ascertain when the liver has recovered.

BLOOD COLLECTION

The test is performed on serum from 5 mL clotted blood.

TEST RESULT

Normal serum range is 10 to 40 U/mL. In myocardial infarction, the level is increased 4 to 10 times, whereas in liver involvement, a high of 10 to 100 times normal may occur. The serum level remains elevated for approximately 5 days.

ALANINE AMINOTRANSFERASE

The alanine aminotransferase (ALT) (formerly known as serum glutamic–pyruvic transaminase) level is more specific for hepatic malfunction than is the AST value.

BLOOD COLLECTION

The test is performed on 5 mL of serum.

TEST RESULT

Normal serum range is 10 to 60 U/L.

SERUM LACTATE DEHYDROGENASE

The transaminase lactate dehydrogenase is present in all tissues and in large quantities in the kidney, heart, and skeletal muscles. Elevated serum levels usually parallel AST levels. Elevation occurs in myocardial infarction and may continue through the 6th day. Elevations have been found in lymphoma, disseminated carcinoma, and some cases of leukemia.

BLOOD COLLECTION

Blood (3 mL) is collected and allowed to coagulate. Care must be taken to avoid hemolysis because only a slight degree may give an incorrect reading.

TEST RESULT

Normal serum range is 60 to 120 U/mL.

Liver Function Tests

Liver function tests measure albumin, globulin, total protein levels, and the albumin/globulin ratio. These tests may be useful in diagnosing kidney and liver disease or in judging the effectiveness of treatment. The chief role of serum albumin is to maintain osmotic pressure of the blood; globulin assists. The globulin molecule, because it is larger than the albumin, is less efficient in maintaining osmotic pressure and does not leak out of the blood. With the loss of albumin through the capillary wall, the body compensates by producing more globulin. The osmotic pressure is reduced, which may result in edema. Certain conditions, such as chronic nephritis, lipoid nephrosis, liver disease, and malnutrition, result in a lowered albumin concentration.

BLOOD COLLECTION

The test is performed on serum from 6 mL of clotted blood.

TEST RESULT

Normal serum ranges:

- Total protein: 6.0 to 8.0 g/100 mL
- Albumin: 3.2 to 5.6 g/100 mL
- Globulin: 1.3 to 3.5 g/100 mL

BILIRUBIN (DIRECT AND INDIRECT)

The bilirubin test, which is becoming less common, differentiates between impairment of the liver by obstruction and hemolysis. Bilirubin arises from the hemoglobin liberated from broken-down RBCs. It is the chief pigment of the bile, excreted by the liver. Impairment by obstruction of the excretory function of the liver leads to an excess of free (non–protein-bound) circulatory bilirubin. Measurement of free bilirubin (direct) usually indicates obstruction.

When increased RBC destruction (hemolysis) occurs, the increased bilirubin is believed to be bound to protein (indirect).

A total bilirubin determination detects increased concentration of bilirubin before jaundice appears.

BLOOD COLLECTION

The test is performed on serum from 5 mL of clotted blood.

TEST RESULT

Normal serum range is 0.1 to 1.0 mg/100 mL.

CHOLESTEROL

Cholesterol, a normal constituent of the blood, is present in all body cells. In various disease states, the cholesterol concentration in the serum may rise or fall. Cholesterol is transported in the blood by the low-density lipoproteins (LDLs; 60% to 75%) and high-density lipoproteins (HDLs; 15% to 35%). A high level of HDL indicates a healthy metabolic system in a patient free of liver disease. Very–low-density lipoproteins (VLDLs) are major carriers of triglyceride. Degradation of VLDL is a major source of LDLs.

Cholesterol measurements may be part of a total lipid profile or an absolute test value. A lipid profile includes total cholesterol count.

BLOOD COLLECTION

The test is performed on serum from 5 mL of clotted blood.

TEST RESULT

Normal serum range is 120 to 260 mg/100 mL.

Peak and Trough Testing

The value of drug level testing is enhanced when those levels are obtained at the most appropriate times. The actual time the specimen was obtained must be known to interpret the level, whether the specimen was drawn at the optimal sampling time or not. The actual time of draw should be entered on the requisition by the person obtaining the specimen. This will ensure that the draw time is entered into the patient's clinical record along with the serum concentration. The lab request should also indicate whether the draw is a peak or trough. For greatest utility, the best time to draw a **trough level** is just before the next dose. For convenience, trough levels may be obtained from 0 to 30 minutes before the dose, provided the actual time of draw is indicated on the requisition. Except where otherwise indicated, **peak levels** should be drawn 30 minutes after an IV dose and 1 to 2 hours after an oral dose.

Coagulation Tests

PROTHROMBIN TIME AND INTERNATIONAL NORMALIZED RATIO

The prothrombin time (PT) is a screening test used to assess the activity of factors in the extrinsic pathway of the coagulation system and to monitor oral anticoagulant therapy. The extrinsic pathway includes factors VII, X, V, II (prothrombin), and I (fibrinogen). Long considered one of the most important screening tests in coagulation studies, PT indirectly measures the ability of the blood to clot. During the clotting process, prothrombin is converted to thrombin. It is thought that when the prothrombin level falls below normal, the tendency for the blood to clot in the blood vessel decreases. The PT is an important guide to drug therapy and is commonly used when anticoagulants are prescribed. The prothrombin content is reduced in liver diseases.

The lack of uniformity for the reporting of PT results along with variations in thromboplastin (PT reagent) sensitivities, instrumentation, and methodologies have led to interlaboratory variations in patient's PT results.

The World Health Organization (WHO) developed a protocol to standardize PT results internationally. All PT reagents and methodologies are compared with the WHO reference thromboplastin and laboratory method. The International Sensitivity Index (ISI) is a number derived from the comparison of the PT reagent with the WHO reference PT reagent. The ISI is used by the laboratory to calculate the **international normalized ratio (INR)**. The INR is the PT ratio that would have been obtained using the WHO reference PT reagent. As a result, a patient on oral anticoagulant therapy could be accurately monitored anywhere in the world providing the INR is calculated and reported (see Box 7-3.)

Currently, the Activated Partial Thromboplastin Time (aPTT) is the laboratory test most commonly used to monitor unfractionated heparin therapy. The aPTT is a measure of the integrity of the intrinsic and common pathways of the coagulation cascade. The value represents the time, in seconds, for a patient's plasma to clot after the addition of an intrinsic pathway activator, phospholipid and calcium. The APTT reagent is called a partial thromboplastin because tissue factor is not included with the phospholipid as it is with the protime (PT) reagent. The activator initiates the contact system. Then, the remaining steps of the intrinsic pathway occur in the presence of phospholipid. Reference ranges vary from one laboratory to another, but the usual range is 22 to 34 seconds.

BOX 7-3   USE OF THE COAGUCHEK PLUS SYSTEM TO ASSESS INR

The CoaguChek Plus System is a photometric system for measuring PTs on whole blood. The system is activated by inserting a reagent cartridge, encoded for calibration and test identity. The reagent cartridge contains a sample application area, a reaction chamber containing the PT reagent, and a molded capillary pathway. After applying whole blood to the sample site, capillary action draws the sample through the cartridge. A coherent laser light is focused through the reaction chamber so that the blood flowing through the cartridge causes an interference pattern. The interference pattern is measured by a photo detector and converted to an electrical signal. The instrument measures the optical patterns from the time of application of blood to the cessation of flow. The biochemical reactions of the assay create an alteration in the optical interference pattern detected, resulting in a change in the photo detector's electronic signal. This change in electronic signal is converted to a quantitative result shown on the liquid crystal display.

Specimen Requirements
1. Whole blood collected using the finger stick method or whole blood collected in a syringe
2. Test sample immediately after collection.

Interferences
1. Do not test anticoagulated samples or serum.
2. Do not test clotted samples. If the sample clots before testing, collect another sample.

Linearity
1. If the PT result is <8 seconds or >0.32 seconds, collect a citrate tube and send to the Core Laboratory for testing.

Reference Range
INR = 0.98–1.08 INR range for normal patient

INR = 2.00–3.00 INR range for anticoagulant therapy

INR = 2.50–3.50 INR range for high-intensity anticoagulant therapy for patients with mechanical valves

Adapted from http://www.coaguchek.com/com/?target=/en/professionals/products/coaguchek_xs_plus_system

Sometimes, further studies are needed, in which case the Anti-Xa test can quantitatively determine the plasma level of unfractionated heparin as well as low molecular weight heparin (LMWH). For example, the aPTT cannot monitor therapy with newer "low molecular weight heparin." LMWH effect is usually predictable from the dose and only occasionally needs to be measured, using an anti-Xa test.

aPTT THERAPEUTIC RANGE

Historically, an aPTT prolongation of 1.5 to 2.5 times the mean normal reference is desired. Recently, another method of determining the heparin therapeutic range was developed utilizing a procedure derived from Brill-Edwards et al., in which aPTT values and heparin levels are obtained from patients actually receiving heparin. Using linear regression, a graph is prepared that correlates the aPTT in seconds to the heparin anti-Xa units. The ranges established are the time in seconds equivalent to 0.1 to 0.3 and 0.3 to 0.7 anti-Xa units of heparin. See Table 7-4 for a discussion of the advantages and disadvantages of aPTT and anti-Xa monitoring.

BLOOD COLLECTION

Venous blood (4 mL) is collected, added to the coagulant, and quickly mixed. It is important to avoid clot formation and hemolysis. The blood should be examined as soon as possible.

TEST RESULT

The normal value is between 11 and 18 seconds, depending on the type of thromboplastin used.

FACTOR V LEIDEN DEFICIENCY

Hypercoagulable states can be inherited, acquired, or both. **Factor V Leiden** is the most common hereditary blood coagulation disorder in the United States (US). It is present in 5% of the White population and 1.2% of the Black population. Factor V Leiden increases the risk of venous thrombosis 3- to 8-fold for heterozygous (one bad gene inherited) and substantially more, 30- to 140-fold, for homozygous (two bad genes inherited) individuals (Weinstein, 2009).

The prothrombin 20210 mutation is the second most common inherited clotting abnormality. It is more common than protein S and C deficiency and antithrombin deficiency combined; 2% of the general population is heterozygous. It is only a mild risk factor for

TABLE 7-4 ADVANTAGES AND DISADVANTAGES OF aPTT AND ANTI-Xa MONITORING

aPTT Monitoring	Anti-Xa
Advantages	**Advantages**
– Inexpensive	– Measures actual enzyme activity
– Widely used	– Target is better defined
– Comfort zone	– Fewer errors in analysis
– 24/7 in all labs	
Disadvantages	**Disadvantages**
– Relationship of heparin dose and heparin level is not predicted reliably	– More expensive
– aPTT does not correlate to heparin blood concentration	– Not always available 24/7
– Variables	– Limited evidence based
– aPTT reagents vary in responsiveness to heparin	– Requires processing within 1 h to avoid heparin neutralization from platelet factor

Adapted from Lehman, C.M., & Frank, E.L. (2009). Laboratory monitoring of heparin therapy: Partial thromboplastic time or Anti-Xa assay? *LabMedicine*, *40*(1), 47–51.

clots, but together with other risk factors (such as oral contraceptives, surgery, trauma, high blood pressure, obesity, smoking, etc.) or combined with other clotting disorders (like Factor V Leiden), the risk of clotting increases dramatically (National Institutes of Health, 2011).

Factor V Leiden can be associated with the following complications:

- Venous thrombosis in veins, such as:
  - Deep vein thrombosis, veins in arms and legs
  - Superficial thrombophlebitis
  - Sinus vein thrombosis, veins around the brain
  - Mesenteric vein thrombosis, intestinal veins
  - Budd-Chiari syndrome, liver veins
- Pulmonary embolism, blood clots in the lungs
- Arterial clots (stroke, heart attack) in selected patients (some smokers)
- Possibly with stillbirth or recurrent unexplained miscarriage
- Preeclampsia and/or eclampsia (toxemia while pregnant)
  - Recommended laboratory evaluation for those suspected of having an underlying hypercoagulable state may be seen in Table 7-5.

Kidney Function Tests

CREATININE

The creatinine test measures kidney function. Creatinine, the result of the breakdown of muscle creatinine phosphate, is produced daily in a constant amount in each person. A disorder of kidney function prevents excretion, and an elevated creatinine value gives a reliable indication of impaired kidney function. A normal serum creatinine value does not indicate unimpaired renal function, however. Baseline creatinine should be determined.

 TABLE 7-5   **RECOMMENDED LABORATORY EVALUATION FOR SUSPECTED UNDERLYING HYPERCOAGULABLE STATE**

Screening Tests	Confirmatory Tests
• Activated protein C resistance • Prothrombin G20210A mutation testing by PCR • Antithrombin, protein C, and protein S activity (functional) levels • Factor VIII activity level • Screening tests for lupus anticoagulants (sensitive aPTT, aPTT mixing studies, dilute Russell viper venom time) • Anticardiolipin antibody testing by ELISA • Fasting total plasma homocysteine level	• Factor V Leiden PCR • Antigenic assays for antithrombin, protein C, and/or protein S • Confirmatory tests for lupus anticoagulants[a]

[a]Include at least one of the following: platelet neutralization procedure, hexagonal phase phospholipids, Textarin/Ecarin test, platelet vesicles, DVV confirm.
PCR, polymerase chain reaction; aPTT, activated partial thromboplastin time; ELISA, enzyme-linked immunosorbent assay. (From The Cleveland Clinic Foundation, 2010.)

BLOOD COLLECTION

The test is performed on serum from 6 mL of clotted blood.

TEST RESULT

Normal serum range is 0.6 to 1.3 mg/100 mL.

BLOOD UREA NITROGEN

The BUN is a measure of kidney function. Urea, the end product of protein metabolism, is excreted by the kidneys. Impairment in kidney function results in an elevated concentration of urea nitrogen in the blood. Rapid protein metabolism may also increase the BUN above normal limits. The nonprotein nitrogen is a similar test for measuring kidney function.

BLOOD COLLECTION

The test is performed on blood or serum. Blood (5 mL) is added to an oxalate tube and shaken, or placed in a dry tube to clot.

TEST RESULT

Normal range is 10 to 20 mg/100 mL.

BLOOD GLUCOSE TESTS

The tests for blood glucose detect a disorder of glucose metabolism, which may result from any one of several factors, including inability of pancreatic islet cells to produce insulin, inability of the intestines to absorb glucose, and inability of the liver to accumulate and break down glycogen.

An elevated blood glucose level may indicate diabetes, chronic liver disease, or overactivity of the endocrine glands. A decrease in blood glucose concentration may result from an overdose of insulin, tumors of the pancreas, or insufficiency of various endocrine glands.

A fasting blood glucose test requires that the patient fast for 8 hours.

BLOOD COLLECTION

Venous blood (3 to 5 mL) is collected in an oxalate tube and shaken to prevent microscopic clots.

TEST RESULT

Normal serum range is 70 to 100 mg/100 mL (true blood glucose method). The normal value depends on the method of determination. Values >120 mg/100 mL on several occasions may indicate diabetes mellitus.

POSTPRANDIAL BLOOD GLUCOSE DETERMINATIONS

The postprandial blood glucose test, which is performed approximately 2 hours after the patient has eaten, is helpful in diagnosing diabetes mellitus. If the blood glucose value is above the upper limits of normal for fasting, a glucose tolerance test is performed.

The glucose tolerance test is indicated for the following conditions:

- When the patient has glycosuria
- When the fasting or 2-hour blood glucose concentration is only slightly elevated
- When Cushing syndrome or acromegaly is a suspected diagnosis
- When the cause of hypoglycemia needs to be determined

Blood Collection

First, a sample of blood is drawn from the fasting patient. The patient then drinks 100 g of glucose in lemon-flavored water (some laboratories use 1.75 g glucose/kg of ideal body weight). Blood and urine samples are then collected at 30, 60, 90, 120, and 180 minutes after ingestion of glucose.

Test Result

Normal (true blood glucose) values are:

- Fasting blood glucose <100 mg/100 mL
- Peak <160 mg/100 mL in 30 or 60 minutes

The values depend on the standards used.

Transfusion Medicine Testing

Blood typing, which is one of the most common tests performed on blood, is required for all donors and for all patients who may need blood. The ABO system denotes four main blood groups: O, A, B, and AB. The designations refer to the particular antigen present on the RBCs: group A contains RBCs with the A antigen, B with B antigen, AB with A and B antigens, and group O erythrocytes contain neither A nor B antigens.

When erythrocytes containing antigens are placed with serum containing corresponding antibodies under favorable conditions, **agglutination** (clumping) occurs. Therefore, an **antigen** is known as an **agglutinogen** and an **antibody** as an **agglutinin**.

A person's serum contains antibodies that react with corresponding antigens not usually found on the person's own cells. For instance, serum of group O contains antibodies A and B, which react with the corresponding antigens A and B found on the RBCs of group AB.

Although agglutination occurs in antigen–antibody reactions in the laboratory, hemolysis occurs in vivo; antibody attacks RBCs, causing rupture with liberation of hemoglobin. Hemolysis results from infusion of incompatible blood and may lead to fatal consequences.

Blood Typing

Various methods are used in typing blood, but all involve the same general principle. The patient's cells are mixed in standard saline serum samples of anti-A and of anti-B. The type of serum, A or B that agglutinates the patient's cells, indicates the blood group. As a double check, the patient's serum is mixed with saline suspensions of A and of B erythrocytes. The ABO group is determined on the basis of agglutination or absence of agglutination of A and of B cells.

Rh Factor and Blood Collection

The antigens belonging to the Rh system are D, C, E, c, and e. They are found in conjunction with the ABO group. The strongest of these factors is the Rho(D) factor, found in approximately 85% of the White population. Therefore, the Rho(D) factor is often the only factor identified in Rh typing. When the Rho(D) factor is not present, further typing may be done to identify the less common Rh factors.

Venous blood is collected and allowed to clot. Usually one tube (10 mL) sets up 4 to 5 units of blood. Positive patient identification must be made before the blood is drawn; the name and number on the identification bracelet must correspond with that on the requisition and label. The label is placed on the blood tube at the patient's bedside.

Coombs Test

Not all antibodies cause agglutination in saline; some merely coat the RBCs by combining with the antigen, which is not a visible reaction. Coombs test is performed to detect antibodies that cannot cause agglutination in saline; these are known as incomplete antibodies. Anti–human globulin serum is used. This serum is obtained by the immunization of various animals, usually rabbits, against human gamma globulin by the injection of human serum, plasma, or isolated globulin. This antiserum, when added to sensitized RBCs (erythrocytes coated with incomplete antibody), causes visible agglutination.

Direct Method

Coombs test is performed in two ways. The direct Coombs test is performed when the patient's RBCs have become coated in vivo. This test is a valuable procedure in diagnosing the following:

- Erythroblastosis fetalis. The erythrocytes of the infant are tested for sensitization.
- Acquired hemolytic anemia. The patient may have produced an antibody that coats his or her own cells.
- Investigating reactions. The patient may have received incompatible blood that sensitizes the RBCs.

Indirect Method

The indirect Coombs test detects incomplete antibodies in the serum of patients sensitized to blood antigens. It tests the patient's serum, in contrast to the patient's RBCs in the direct Coombs test. When pooled, normal erythrocytes containing the most important antigens are exposed in a test tube to the patient's serum and to Coombs serum; the RBCs agglutinate, indicating the presence of incomplete antibody. This test is valuable in the following:

- Detecting incompatibilities not found by other methods
- Detecting weak or variant antigens
- Typing with certain antiserums, such as anti-Duffy or anti-Kidd, which requires Coombs serum to produce agglutination
- Detecting antiagglutinins produced by exposure during pregnancy

COMPLEMENTARY AND ALTERNATIVE MEDICINE

Complementary and alternative medicine (CAM) is a "group of diverse medical and health care systems, practices, and products that are not generally considered part of conventional medicine. Conventional medicine, also called Western or allopathic medicine, is medicine practiced by a medical doctor (M.D.) and doctor of osteopathic medicine (D.O.) and by allied health professionals, such as physical therapists, psychologists, and registered nurses" (National Center for Complementary and Alternative Medicine, 2012).

When conventional medicine is used along with some or all of the CAM practices and products not part of conventional medicine, it is referred to as integrated medicine. Alternative medicine indicates that conventional medicine is not being utilized. Natural products are part of CAM. These products include a "variety of herbal medicines (also known as botanicals), vitamins, and minerals. Many are sold over the counter as dietary supplements." Others are sold as whole food nutrition and include over 700 medicinal mushroom products. There are very high-quality dietary whole food products on the market that normalize or support the body's immune system and promote well-being. Other natural products include "live microorganisms (usually bacteria) that are similar to microorganisms normally found in the human digestive tract and that may have beneficial effects. Probiotics are available in foods (e.g., yogurts) or as dietary supplements. They are not the same thing as prebiotics—nondigestible food ingredients that selectively stimulate the growth and/or activity of microorganisms already present in the body" (National Center for Complementary and Alternative Medicine, 2012).

Whole medical systems are built upon complete systems of theory and practice. Often, these systems have evolved apart from, and are earlier than, the conventional medical approach used in the US. Examples of whole medical systems that have developed in Western cultures include homeopathic medicine and naturopathic medicine. Examples of systems that have developed in non-Western cultures include Traditional Chinese Medicine (TCM) and Ayurveda, a whole medical system that originated in India.

There is increasing use of natural products. The National Health Interview Survey (NHIS), conducted on a regular basis by the CDC, found that in 2007 almost 18% of American adults, or 42 million, used a natural product (nonvitamin/nonmineral) (NCCAM, 2012). The National Center for Complementary and Alternative Medicine (NCCAM) is now a significant part of the National Institute of Health (NIH). With more than 750 herbs on the market, Americans spend over $18 billion a year on herbal remedies and dietary supplements (Fontaine, 2011). Herbal remedies have reached their highest usage since the Food and Drug Administration's (FDA's) decision to categorize them as food supplements in 1990.

The infusion nurse needs to know if natural products are being used because of the possibility of drug interaction, enhancement, and product contamination (NCCAM, 2013), thus influencing laboratory testing , the timing of laboratory testing, and interfering with laboratory results. With increasing usage, it is imperative that nurses ask patients if they are taking any other supplements or products not prescribed by their physician/LIP. Estimates suggest that 47% to 72% of patients fail to report herbal medicine use to health care professionals. Patients may be reluctant to disclose their consumption of these products for fear of disapproval; thus a nonjudgmental attitude is important.

Health care professionals are challenged to stay current with the variety of natural and herbal products, their effects, and potential interactions. Health care professionals must

PATIENT SAFETY

Herbal medicines may affect clinical laboratory testing. Abnormal laboratory results owing to the use of herbal medicine may be classified into three categories:
1. Abnormal test results owing to direct interference of a component of the herbal medicine with the assay
2. Unexpected concentration of a therapeutic drug owing to drug–herb interactions
3. Abnormal test results owing to toxic effects of the herbal product.

continue to educate themselves and patients about herb–drug interactions and the need to make educated decisions concerning quality, safety, and efficacy.

Herbal medicines can alter test results by direct interference with certain immunoassays. Drug–herb interactions can result in unexpected concentrations of therapeutic drugs. For example, low concentrations of several drugs (e.g., cyclosporine, theophylline, and digoxin) can be observed in patients who initiated self-medication with St John's wort.

TABLE 7-6   **CLINICALLY IMPORTANT INTERACTIONS OF ST. JOHN'S WORT (SJW)**

Drug	Effect of Interaction on Drug	Suggested Management of Patients Already Taking SJW Preparations
HIV protease inhibitors (indinavir, nelfinavir, ritonavir, saquinavir)	Reduced blood levels with possible loss of HIV suppression	Measure HIV RNA viral load and stop SJW.
HIV nonnucleoside reverse transcriptase inhibitors (efavirenz, nevirapine, delavirdine)	Reduced blood levels with possible loss of HIV suppression	Measure HIV RNA viral load and stop SJW.
Cyclosporin, tacrolimus	Reduced blood levels with risk of transplant rejection	Check cyclosporin or tacrolimus blood levels and stop SJW. Levels may increase on stopping SJW. The dose may need adjusting.
Warfarin	Reduced anticoagulant effect and need for increased warfarin dose	Check INR and stop SJW. Monitor INR closely as this may rise on stopping SJW. The dose of warfarin may need adjusting.
Digoxin	Reduced blood levels and loss of control of heart rhythm or heart failure	Check digoxin levels and stop SJW. Digoxin levels may increase on stopping SJW. The dose of digoxin may need adjusting.
Theophylline	Reduced blood levels and loss of bronchodilator effect	Check theophylline levels and stop SJW. Theophylline levels may increase on stopping SJW. The dose of theophylline may need adjusting.
Anticonvulsants (carbamazepine, phenobarbitone, phenytoin)	Reduced blood levels with risk of seizures	Check anticonvulsant levels and stop SJW. Anticonvulsant levels may increase on stopping SJW. The dose of anticonvulsant may need adjusting.

Patients taking drugs listed in the table should not start taking SJW preparations.
Note: The action of many other drugs depends on their rate of metabolism, and thus, other drugs may also interact with St. John's wort preparations.

TABLE 7-7	HERB OR SUPPLEMENT AND DRUG-TYPE INTERACTIONS WITH POSSIBLE EFFECTS	
Herb/Supplement	Drug or Drug-Type	Possible Interaction Effect
Capsicum Feverfew Garlic Ginger Ginkgo biloba Goldenseal Ma huang	Anticoagulants, aspirin	Prolonged bleeding time
Garlic Ma huang	Hypoglycemics	Hypoglycemia
Licorice	Bumetanide, chlorthalidone, digoxin, furosemide, indapamide	Depletes potassium, possibly leading to hypokalemia

Adapted from Fontaine, K.L. (2011). Herbs and nutritional supplements. In *Complementary and alternative therapies for nursing practice* (3rd ed., pp. 123–144). New York: Pearson.

Herbal medicines can alter physiology, and these changes can be reflected in abnormal test results. For example, kava-kava can cause drug-induced hepatitis, leading to unexpectedly high concentrations of liver enzymes. Use of toxic herbal products such as ma huang (an ephedra-containing herbal product), Chan Su, and comfrey may cause death. Other effects of herbal medicines include cardiovascular toxic effects, hematologic toxic effects, neurotoxic effects, nephrotoxic effects, carcinogenic effects, and allergic reactions. In Table 7-6, drug interactions with St. John's wort are highlighted, along with possible management actions. Other herbs and supplements have possible interactions with drug types that then may affect laboratory results (Table 7-7).

CAM practices can be safe and provide comfort. Health care clinicians need to disclose the benefits, risks, and alternatives for any treatment, and patients, especially, need to disclose their use of natural products of all kinds. With a patient–clinician team, laboratory testing can be effective and accurate.

The goal of the infusion nurse is to be familiar with laboratory testing and the implications for practice, ensuring quality and safety for the patient.

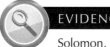

EVIDENCE FOR PRACTICE

Solomon, P.R., Adams, F., Silver, A., Zimmer, J., DeVeaux, R. Ginkgo for memory enhancement: A randomized controlled trial. *JAMA, 288*(7), 835–840.

Ginkgo leaf is often used by the older adult patient for memory disorders, Alzheimer's, migraines-headaches, dizziness, tinnitus, vertigo, glaucoma, retinopathy and macular degeneration. Over 400 clinical trials have been performed looking at a variety of medicinal properties and clinical uses. How do terpene lactones and ginkgo flavone glycosides impact the health of the older adult?

Review Questions   *Note: Questions below may have more than one right answer.*

1. A glucose tolerance test is indicated in which of the following clinical situations?
   A. When the patient shows glycosuria
   B. When fasting or 2-hour blood glucose concentration is only slightly elevated
   C. When Cushing syndrome or acromegaly is a suspected diagnosis
   D. To establish the cause of hypoglycemia

2. Blood sampling through the central venous catheter may be required in which of the following situations?
   A. When it is difficult to obtain an adequate vein
   B. When frequent sampling is required
   C. A only
   D. A and B

3. Which of the following statements is true of creatinine?
   A. Elevated creatinine level is a reliable indication of impaired kidney function.
   B. Normal serum creatinine level does not indicate normal renal function.
   C. B only
   D. A and B

4. Measurement of chlorides is effective in diagnosing which of the following types of disorders?
   A. Acid–base balance
   B. Water balance
   C. Anion concentration
   D. Hypoventilation

5. Which of the following is true of blood glucose and serum lipid levels?
   A. They are increased by ingestion of food.
   B. They are depressed after meals.
   C. They are not affected by food.
   D. None of the above

6. To prevent an elevated serum potassium concentration, which of the following is true?
   A. Avoid vigorous shaking of the specimen.
   B. Avoid forceful transfer of blood into the tube.
   C. Avoid hemolysis.
   D. All of the above

7. Complications of venipuncture (for venous sampling) include which of the following?
   A. Syncope
   B. Continued bleeding
   C. Thrombosis
   D. All of the above

8. Coombs test is valuable in which of the following clinical situations?
   A. Detecting incompatibilities not found by other methods
   B. Detecting weak or variant antigens
   C. Detecting antiagglutinins produced by exposure during pregnancy
   D. All of the above

9. All of the following statements about prothrombin are true *except*
   A. Prothrombin indirectly measures the ability of the blood to clot.
   B. Prothrombin is converted to thrombin during the coagulation cascade.
   C. A low level of prothrombin increases the blood's tendency to clot.
   D. Prothrombin is reduced in liver disease.

10. Urea is an end product of which metabolism?
    A. Carbohydrate
    B. Fat
    C. Protein
    D. Mineral

References and Selected Readings   *Asterisks indicate references cited in text.*

*Cleveland Clinic Foundation. (2010). http://www.clevelandclinicmeded.com/medicalpubs/ diseasemanagement/hematology-oncology/hypercoagulable-states/#s0035

*College of American Pathologists—Point of Care Testing Committee. (2009). *Point-of-Care Testing Toolkit.* http://www.cap.org/apps/cap.portal?_nfpb=true&cntvwrPtlt_actionOverride=/portlets/content Viewer/show&_windowLabel=cntvwrPtlt&cntvwrPtlt%7BactionForm.contentReference%7D=committees/ pointofcare/poct_toolkit.html

Commission on Laboratory accreditation. (2009). Laboratory Accreditation Program. Point-of-Care Testing Checklist. College of American Pathologists.

*Dunning, M.B., & Fischbach, F. (2011). *Nurse's quick reference to common laboratory and diagnostic tests.* (5th ed.). Philadelphia, PA: Wolters Kluwer/Lippincott Williams & Wilkins.

*Fischbach, F.T., & Dunning, M.B. (2009). *A manual of laboratory and diagnostic tests* (8th ed.). Philadelphia, PA: Wolters Kluwer/Lippincott Williams & Wilkins.

*Fontaine, K.L. (2011). Herbs and nutritional supplements. In K.L. Fontaine (Ed.). *Complementary and alternative therapies for nursing practice* (3rd ed., pp. 123–144). New York: Pearson.

Ginsberg H.N., & Fisher E.A. (2009). The ever-expanding role of degradation in the regulation of apolipoprotein B metabolism. *Journal of Lipid Research, 50,* S162–S166.

Gordan, J.D., Chay, W.Y., Kelley, R.K., Ko, A.H., Choo, S.P., & Venook, A.P. (2011). And what other medications are you taking? *Journal of Clinical Oncology 29*(11), e289-e291.

*Gorski, L., Perucca, R., & Hunter, M.R. (2010). Central venous access devices: Care, maintenance, and potential complications. In M. Alexander, A. Corrigan, L. Gorski, J. Hankins, & R. Perucca (Eds.), *Infusion nursing: An evidence-based approach* (3rd ed., pp. 495–515). St. Louis, MO: Saunders Elsevier.

Guervil, D.J., Rosenberg, A.F., Winterstein, A.G., Harris N.S., Johns, T.E., & Zumberg, M.S. (2011). Activated partial thromboplastin time versus antifactor Xa heparin assay in monitoring unfractionated heparin by continuous intravenous infusion. *The Annals of Pharmacotherapy, 45*(8), 861–868.

Kennedy, D.A., & Seely, D. (2010). Clinically based evidence of drug-herb interactions: a systematic review. *Expert Opinion on Drug Safety, 9*(1), 79–124.

Hur, M., Kim H., Park C.M., et al. (2013). Comparison of International Normalized Ratio Measurement between CoaguChek XS Plus and STA-R Coagulation Analyzers, *BioMed Research International*, vol. 2013, Article ID 213109, 6 p.

Integrative Health Forum (www.ihfglobal.com)

*Infusion Nurses Society. (2011). Infusion nursing standards of practice. *Journal of Infusion Nursing, 34,* S77–S80.

Izzo, A.A., & Ernst, E. (2009). Interactions between herbal medicines and prescribed drugs: An updated systematic review. *Drugs, 69,* 1777–1798.

*Kost, G.J. (2002). *Principles and practice of point of care testing.* Philadelphia, PA: Lippincott Williams & Wilkins.

*National Center for Complementary and Alternative Medicine. (2012). *What is complementary and alternative medicine*? http://nccam.nih.gov/health/whatiscam

*National Center for Complementary and Alternative Medicine. (2013). *Safe use of complementary health products and practices.* http://nccam.nih.gov/health/safety

*National Institutes of Health. (2011). *Factor V Leiden thrombophilia.* http://ghr.nlm.nih.gov/condition/ factor-v-leiden-thrombophilia

National Institute for Occupational Safety and Health. (1997). *NIOSH alert: Preventing allergic reactions to natural rubber latex in the workplace* (NIOSH Publication 97–135). Washington, DC: Author.

*Oncology Nursing Society (ONS)/Camp-Sorrell, D. (Ed.). (2011). *Access device guidelines: Recommendations for nursing practice and education* (3rd ed.). Pittsburgh, PA: ONS.

*U.S. Food and Drug Administration. (2009). *Medical Devices - CLIA Waivers.* http://www.fda.gov/ MedicalDevices/DeviceRegulationandGuidance/IVDRegulatoryAssistance/ucm124202.htm?utm_ campaign=Google2&utm_source=fdaSearch&utm_medium=website&utm_term=waived%20tests%20 under%20clia&utm_content=8

*Weinstein, S.M. (2009). Factor V Leiden: Impact on infusion nursing practice. *Journal of Infusion Nursing 32*(4), 219–223.

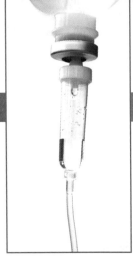

CHAPTER 8

Fluid and Electrolyte Balance

Sharon M. Weinstein

KEY TERMS		
	Active Transport	Hypokalemia
	Dehydration	Hyponatremia
	Diffusion	Metabolic Acidosis
	Filtration	Metabolic Alkalosis
	Glycosuria	Osmosis
	Homeostatic	Respiratory Acidosis
	Mechanisms	Respiratory Alkalosis
	Hyperkalemia	Stress Response
	Hypernatremia	

OVERVIEW OF PHYSIOLOGY

An imbalance of fluid or electrolyte levels is recognized as a threat to life. Never before has the nurse's responsibility for fluid and electrolyte administration and monitoring been more intense, and this applies to all clinical settings in which care is delivered. Patient outcomes depend in large part on specialty practice skills, which are based on a sound knowledge of physiology, in particular of fluid and electrolyte interplay.

Understanding fluid and electrolyte balance begins with understanding the intake, output, and utilization of water and electrolytes. Regulating mechanisms include osmosis, diffusion, filtration, and active transport, all of which affect the movement of water and electrolytes within the body.

Regulating Mechanisms

OSMOSIS

Osmosis is a passive transport mechanism that allows the movement of water freely through the semipermeable membrane. During this process, fluid moves in relation to the concentration of the solutes, taking it from an area of low solute concentration and continuing until both sides of the membrane are of equal concentration.

DIFFUSION

Diffusion is also a passive transport mechanism and represents the random movement of molecules and ions from an area of higher concentration to an area of lower concentration in a solution. An example is the exchange of oxygen and carbon dioxide between the alveoli and capillaries in the lungs (Chernecky, Macklin, & Murphy-Ende, 2002).

FILTRATION

Filtration refers to the movement of solutes and water through selectively permeable membranes, always moving from an area of higher pressure to an area of lower pressure. Filtration involves the movement of solutes and water in relation to hydrostatic pressure. While osmosis and diffusion are a response to concentrations, filtration is a response to pressure (Alexander, Corrigan, Gorski, Hankins, & Perucca, 2010).

ACTIVE TRANSPORT

Fluids passively move from higher concentrations/pressures to lower concentrations/pressure to equalize the concentrations on either side of a semipermeable membrane with osmosis, diffusion, and filtration.

At times, a higher concentration is required on one side of the membrane than on the other. Active transport is a mechanism that utilizes energy to achieve equilibrium. Particles are actually pushed out of the cells through a membrane while other particles are drawn in (Elkin, Perry, & Potter, 2007). Two types of active transport are known: primary and secondary. Adenosine triphosphate is the energy source for primary active transport, an example of which is the sodium–potassium pump. When there is an increase of sodium concentration within the cell, this usually activates the "pump" and a sodium/potassium ion exchange begins.

There are two forms of secondary active transport including cotransport and countertransport. With cotransport, the molecule or ion with a higher concentration outside the cell creates a storehouse of energy that will be used for its transport into the cell (Guyton & Hall, 2006).

Dehydration

Dehydration lowers the blood volume, decreasing renal blood flow, and the kidneys produce less of the ammonia needed to maintain acid–base balance. Severe dehydration may lower the blood volume enough to cause circulatory shock and oliguria (Collins & Claros, 2011).

Water is one of the most important nutrients for maintaining life and ensuing healthy aging. Body fluids move nutrients, gases, and wastes throughout the body; are essential in metabolizing food into energy; and assist in the body's overall functions. The body loses water from the lungs, skin, gastrointestinal tract, and kidneys on a regular basis. There is a small, but significant, amount of water lost in the stool in normal conditions. The renal and stool loss of water is known traditionally as *sensible water loss*. Although the kidney can minimize the loss of fluid, it can never totally conserve water (Klotz, 1998).

The evaporative water loss that occurs through the lungs and skin is known as *insensible water loss*. Insensible water loss is independent of the body water and solute (electrolytes) and content. It does, however, depend on the patient's body surface area and environmental temperature (Adelman & Solhung, 1996).

At least 80% of all fluids administered today contain some electrolytes. Because electrolyte therapy is often a lifesaving procedure, its safe and successful administration is essential. Knowledge of the fundamentals of fluid and electrolyte metabolism contributes to safe electrolyte therapy.

Abnormalities of body fluid and electrolyte metabolism present therapeutic problems. Treatment is complex when the mechanisms that normally regulate fluid volume, electrolyte composition, and osmolality are impaired. An understanding of these metabolic abnormalities enables the nurse to recognize the problems involved. Such clinical challenges arise in patients with renal insufficiency, adrenal insufficiency, adrenal hyperactivity, and other kinds of impaired organ function.

The two following examples illustrate how knowledge of fluid and electrolyte metabolism contributes to safe, successful therapy in the critically ill patient. Correction of a severe potassium deficit resulting from vomiting and diarrhea presents a problem in the dehydrated patient. Potassium replacement is imperative. However, potassium administered to patients with renal insufficiency results in potassium toxicity because the kidneys are unable to excrete electrolytes. The adverse effects of excess potassium on the heart muscle are arrhythmia and heart block. The nurse must recognize the importance of both hydrating the patient before potassium can be administered safely and watching for diminished diuresis that could necessitate a change in therapy. Once antidiuresis occurs, the potassium infusion must be interrupted and the physician/licensed independent practitioner (LIP) notified. Potassium is the chief cation of body cells (160 mEq/L of intracellular water) and is concerned with the maintenance of body fluid composition and electrolyte balance. Potassium participates in carbohydrate utilization and protein synthesis and is critical in the regulation of nerve conduction and muscle contraction, particularly in the heart. Chloride, the major extracellular anion, closely follows the metabolism of sodium, and changes in the acid–base of the body are reflected by changes in the chloride concentration.

Normally about 80% to 90% of the potassium intake is excreted in the urine and the remainder in the stools and, to a small extent, in the perspiration. The kidney does not conserve potassium well so that during fasting, or in patients on a potassium-free diet, potassium loss from the body continues resulting in potassium depletion. A deficiency of either potassium or chloride will lead to a deficit of the other.

Another example relates to therapeutic problems in patients with impaired liver function. When excessive loss of gastric fluid occurs, replacement fluid is necessary. Most deficits caused by gastric suction, unless severe, are treated with 0.9% sodium chloride in 5% dextrose in water or 0.33% sodium chloride in 5% dextrose in water. However, severe loss may call for gastric replacement fluids containing ammonium chloride, which can be potentially dangerous when administered to patients with impaired liver function. Ammonium chloride administered to a patient with severe liver damage may result in ammonia intoxication because of the liver's inability to convert ammonia to hydrogen ions and urea.

Fluid Content of the Body

The total body water content of a person varies with age, weight, and sex. The amount of water depends on the amount of body fat. Body fat is essentially water free; the greater the fat content, the lower the water content.

   In contrast to infants, who have a high body fluid content (approximately 70% to 80% of the body weight), approximately 60% of a typical adult's weight consists of fluid (water and electrolytes; Figure 8-1). After 40 years of age, mean values for total body fluid in percentage of body weight decrease for both men and women; a sex differentiation, however, remains. After 60 years of age, the percentage may decrease to 52% in men and 46% in women. With aging, lean body mass decreases in favor of fat (Metheny, 2012).

Fluid Compartments

The total body fluid is functionally allocated into two main compartments: the intracellular and the extracellular compartments (Figure 8-2). The intracellular compartment consists of the fluid inside the cells and comprises approximately two thirds of the body fluid, or 40% of the body weight. The extracellular compartment consists of the fluid outside the body cells—the plasma, representing 5% of the body weight, and the interstitial fluid (fluid in tissues), representing 15% of the body weight (Metheny, 2012).

   In newborn infants, the proportion is approximately three-fifths intracellular and two-fifths extracellular. This ratio changes and reaches the adult level by the time the infant is approximately 30 months of age.

   There is one additional compartment, the transcellular compartment. The transcellular fluid is the product of cellular metabolism and consists of secretions such as gastrointestinal secretions and urine. An analysis of the secretions may assist the practitioner in tracing lost electrolytes and prescribing proper fluid and electrolyte replacement. Excessive fluid and electrolyte loss must be replaced to maintain fluid and electrolyte balance in the two main

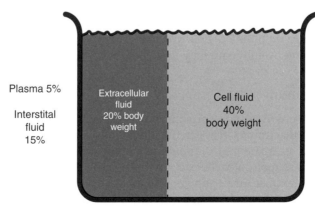

FIGURE 8-1   Total body fluid is 60% of body weight.

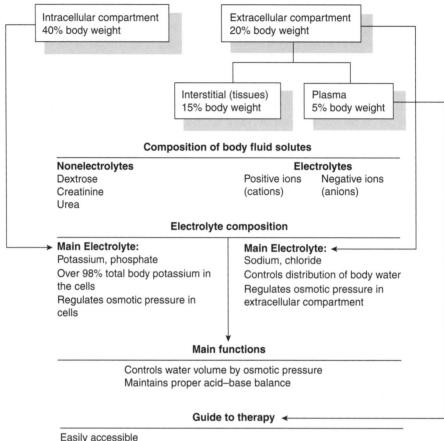

FIGURE 8-2 Total body water composition.

compartments. The amount of body water loss is easily computed by weighing the patient and noting loss of weight: 1 L body water is equivalent to 1 kg, or 2.2 lb, of body weight. Up to 5% weight loss in a child or adult may signify moderate fluid volume deficit— > 5% may indicate severe fluid volume deficit. Weight changes are also valuable as indicators of body water gains—acute weight gain may indicate water excess.

Body Fluid Composition

Body fluid contains two types of solutes (dissolved substances): the electrolytes and the nonelectrolytes. Electrolytes serve two main purposes: to act in controlling body water volume by osmotic pressure and to maintain the proper acid–base balance of the body. The nonelectrolytes are molecules that do not break into particles in solution but remain intact. They consist of dextrose, urea, and creatinine.

Electrolytes are molecules that break into electrically charged particles called *ions*. The ion carrying a positive charge is called a *cation*, and the ion with a negative charge is called an *anion*. Potassium chloride is an electrolyte that, dissolved in water, yields potassium cations and chloride anions. Chemical balance is always maintained; the total number of positive charges equals the total number of negative charges. The quantity of charges and their concentration are expressed as milliequivalents (mEq) per liter of fluid. Because the number of negative charges must equal the number of positive charges for chemical balance, the milliequivalents of cations must equal the milliequivalents of anions.

Electrolyte Composition

Each fluid compartment has its own electrolyte composition. The extracellular compartment (plasma and interstitial fluid) contains a high concentration of sodium, chloride, and bicarbonate and a low concentration of potassium. The composition of the intracellular fluid is quite different; the concentrations of potassium, magnesium, and phosphate are high, whereas the sodium and chloride concentrations are relatively low.

Electrolyte composition of the intracellular fluid is in part related to electrolyte composition of the plasma and interstitial fluids. Disturbances in the extracellular fluid (ECF) are reflected in the patient's symptoms; this information, combined with an analysis of plasma, is thus a valuable guide to therapy.

Occasionally, however, the electrolyte determination of plasma may be misleading. For example, the concentration of potassium in plasma may be high while there is a body deficit. This surplus is due to the shift of potassium from intracellular to ECF in the process of large potassium losses through the kidneys. Determination of plasma sodium may also present a false picture. In the case of an edematous cardiac patient, the plasma concentration may be low despite excess body sodium because total body sodium is equal to the sum of the products of volume times concentration in the various compartments.

Characteristics of Fluids

Fluids are described in various ways. Significant characteristics of fluids include their concentration, or osmolality, as well as their acidity or alkalinity (pH).

Osmolality

Osmolality is the total solute concentration and reflects the relative water and total solute concentration; it is expressed per liter of serum. Osmotic pressure is determined by the amount of solutes in solution. If the ECF contains a relatively large number of dissolved particles and the intracellular fluid contains a small amount of dissolved particles, the osmotic pressure causes water to pass from the less concentrated fluid to the more concentrated. Therefore, fluid from the intracellular compartment passes into the extracellular compartment until the concentration becomes equal.

The unit of osmotic pressure is the osmole, and values are expressed in milliosmoles (mOsm). Normal blood plasma has an osmolality of approximately 290 mOsm/kg water. The determination of serum osmolality is sometimes used to detect dehydration or overhydration. Measurement of sodium concentration also indicates the water needs of the body. At times, the osmolality reading may falsely indicate dehydration. Because the osmolality is the total solute concentration, nonelectrolytes are included in the reading. An elevated blood urea level can therefore increase the osmolality without exerting osmotic pressure.

A determination of blood urea nitrogen (BUN) may supply a correction to the osmolality reading in cases of increased serum urea.

CONCENTRATION AS A METRIC VALUE

Concentrations of solutes may be expressed in several ways in addition to milliequivalents per liter, such as milligrams per deciliter (mg/dL) or millimoles per liter (mmol/L). Each of these units of measure may be used in a clinical setting. A milliequivalent of an ion is its atomic weight expressed in milligrams divided by the valence. This is the measure most often used for expressing small concentrations of electrolytes in body fluids because it emphasizes the principles that ions combine milliequivalent for milliequivalent.

CONCENTRATION AS AN SI VALUE

Milligrams per 100 mL (deciliter) express the weight of the solute per unit volume. In the International System of Units (Système Internationale, SI), electrolyte content in body fluids is expressed in millimoles. For practical purposes, 1 mole (mol) of a substance has a mass equal to its atomic weight, expressed in grams. For example, a mole of sodium has a mass of 23 g (the atomic weight of sodium is 23). A millimole is one thousandth of a mole or the molecular or atomic weight expressed in milligrams. Therefore, a millimole of sodium equals 23 mg. Sometimes, it is necessary to convert from millimoles per liter to milliequivalents per liter (Figure 8-3). The following formula applies:

$$mEq / L = mmol / L \times valence$$

ACID–BASE BALANCE

The acidity or alkalinity of a solution depends on the degree of hydrogen ion concentration. An increase in the hydrogen ions results in a more acid solution; a decrease results in a more alkaline solution. Acidity is expressed by the term *pH*, which refers to the amount of hydrogen ion concentration. A solution having a pH of 7 is regarded as neutral.

The ECF has a pH ranging from 7.35 to 7.45 and is slightly alkaline. When the pH of the blood is > 7.45, an alkaline condition exists; when < 7.35, an acid condition exists.

The biologic fluids, both extracellular and intracellular, contain a buffer system that maintains the proper acid–base balance. This buffer system consists of fluid with salts of a weak acid or weak base. A base or hydroxide neutralizes the effect of an acid. These weak acids and bases maintain pH values by soaking up surplus ions or releasing them; acids yield hydrogen ions; bases accept hydrogen ions.

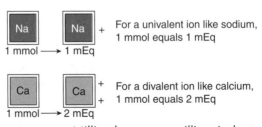

FIGURE 8-3 Millimoles versus milliequivalents for univalent and divalent ions.

The carbonic acid–sodium bicarbonate system is the most important buffer system in the extracellular compartment. The normal ratio is 1 part of carbonic acid to 20 parts of base bicarbonate, which represents 1.2 mEq carbonic acid to 24 mEq base bicarbonate.

Acid–Base Imbalance

Acid–base imbalances are normally the result of an excess or a deficit in either base bicarbonate or carbonic acid. Deviations of pH from 7.35 to 7.45 are combated by the buffer system and by the respiratory and renal regulatory mechanisms. Two types of disturbance can affect the acid–base balance: respiratory and metabolic. A diagrammatic presentation of these disturbances is presented in Figure 8-4.

PATIENT SAFETY

The patient with electrolyte imbalance may have a disturbance of sensorium, putting him or her at risk for falls. All precautions should be taken to protect the patient.

Respiratory Disturbances

Respiratory disturbances affect the carbonic side of the balance by increasing or decreasing carbonic acid; when carbon dioxide unites with ECF, carbonic acid is produced.

Respiratory alkalosis results when excess carbon dioxide is exhaled during rapid or deep breathing. Carbonic acid is depleted because of the carbon dioxide loss. Respiratory alkalosis may occur as the result of emotional disturbances, such as anxiety and hysteria, and also from lack of oxygen or from fever (Metheny, 2012).

Symptoms are convulsions, tetany, and unconsciousness. Laboratory determination is a urinary pH > 7 and a plasma bicarbonate concentration < 24 mEq/L. The body attempts to restore the ratio to normal by depressing the bicarbonate to compensate for the deficit in the carbonic acid.

Respiratory acidosis occurs when exhalation of carbon dioxide is depressed and the excess retention of carbon dioxide increases the carbonic acid. It may occur in conditions that interfere with normal breathing, such as emphysema, asthma, and pneumonia. Symptoms are weakness, disorientation, depressed breathing, and coma. Urinary pH is below 6, and plasma bicarbonate concentration is above 24 mEq/L. The bicarbonate increase is due to the body's attempt to restore the carbonic acid–bicarbonate ratio.

Metabolic Disturbances

Metabolic disturbances affect the bicarbonate side of the balance. Kidney function controls the bicarbonate concentration by regulating the amount of cations (hydrogen, ammonium, and potassium) in exchange for sodium ions to combine with the reabsorbed bicarbonate in the distal tubular lumen. As hydrogen ions are excreted, bicarbonate is generated, maintaining the proper acid–base balance of the blood. Ammonia excretion is increased in response to a high acidity; bicarbonate replaces the ammonia.

Metabolic alkalosis is a condition associated with excess bicarbonate; it occurs when chloride is lost. Chloride and bicarbonate are both anions, and the total number of anions must equal the total number of cations. When chloride anions are lost, the deficit must be

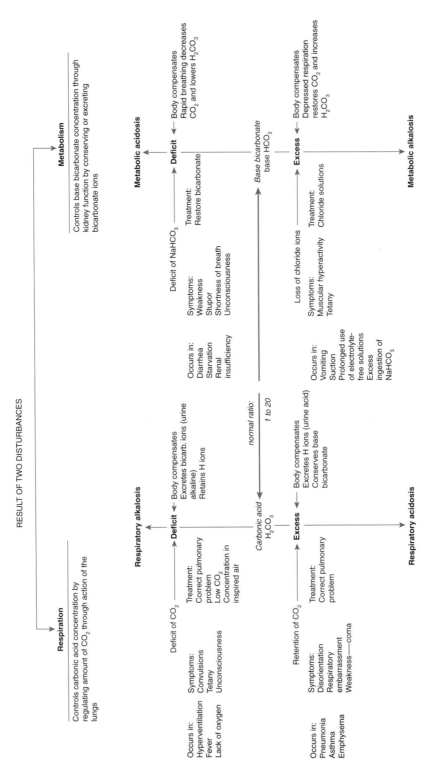

FIGURE 8-4 Acid–base imbalances resulting from respiratory or metabolic disturbances.

made up by an equal number of anions to maintain electrolyte equilibrium; bicarbonate increases in compensation and alkalosis occurs.

Metabolic alkalosis is also associated with decreased levels of intracellular potassium. Potassium escapes from the cell into the ECF and is lost through the transcellular fluid. When body potassium is lost, the shift of sodium and hydrogen ions from the ECF causes alkalosis, whereas the increase of hydrogen ions in the intracellular fluid causes cellular acidosis.

Muscular hyperactivity, tetany, and depressed respiration are symptoms of metabolic alkalosis. Muscular hyperactivity and tetany are symptoms of the deficit in ionized calcium that exists in alkalosis. Laboratory determinations are urinary pH > 7, plasma pH > 7.45, and bicarbonate level > 24 mEq/L.

Treatment consists of the administration of fluids containing chloride to replace bicarbonate ions. An excess of bicarbonate ions is accompanied by potassium deficiency, so potassium must also be replaced.

Metabolic acidosis is a condition associated with a deficit in the bicarbonate concentration. This occurs when

- Excessive amounts of ketone acids accumulate, as in uncontrolled diabetes or starvation.
- Inorganic acids, such as phosphate and sulfate, accumulate, as in renal disease.
- Excessive losses of bicarbonate occur from gastrointestinal drainage or diarrhea.

Acidosis may occur also from intravenous (IV) administration of excessive amounts of sodium chloride or ammonium chloride, causing chloride ions to flood the ECF.

Stupor, shortness of breath, weakness, and unconsciousness are the symptoms of metabolic acidosis, and laboratory determinations of metabolic acidosis are a urinary pH < 6, plasma pH < 7.35, and plasma bicarbonate concentration < 24 mEq/L.

Treatment and clinical management consist of increasing the bicarbonate level. Solutions of sodium lactate are often used, but because lactate ion must be oxidized to carbon dioxide before it can affect the acid–base balance, it is advisable to use sodium bicarbonate solutions, which are effective even when the patient is suffering from oxygen lack.

Homeostatic Mechanisms

The body uses regulating mechanisms called homeostatic mechanisms to maintain the constancy of body fluid volume, electrolyte composition, and osmolality. These mechanisms function through the renocardiovascular, endocrine (adrenal, pituitary, and parathyroid), and respiratory systems. The kidneys, skin, and lungs are the main regulating agents (Metheny, 2012).

KIDNEY FUNCTION

The kidney plays a major role in fluid and electrolyte balance. To function adequately, the kidney depends on its own soundness as well as on the coordination of all the regulating organs. The distal renal tubules in the kidney are important in regulating body fluid. They selectively retain or reject electrolytes and other substances to maintain normal osmolality and blood volume. Sodium is retained, and potassium is excreted.

The kidneys also play an important part in acid–base regulation. The distal tubule has the ability to form ammonia and exchange hydrogen ions (in the form of ammonia) for bicarbonate to maintain the carbonic acid–bicarbonate ratio.

SKIN AND LUNG FUNCTION

The skin and lungs play an important role in fluid balance—the skin in loss of fluid through insensible perspiration and the lungs in loss of fluid by expiration. Normal intake of 2,500 mL from all sources delivers a loss of approximately 1,000 mL in breath and perspiration, 1,400 mL in urine, and 100 mL in feces.

FUNCTIONS OF OTHER SYSTEMS AND ORGANS

The renocardiovascular system maintains fluid balance by regulating the amount and composition of urine. Plasma must reach the kidneys in sufficient volume to permit regulation of water and electrolyte balance. Renal disease, cardiac failure, shock, postoperative stress, and alarm impair this regulating mechanism.

The adrenal glands influence the retention or excretion of sodium, potassium, and water. These glands secrete aldosterone, a hormone that increases the reabsorption of sodium from the renal tubules in exchange for potassium, thus maintaining normal sodium concentration. Any stress, such as surgery, increases the secretion of aldosterone, thus increasing the reabsorption of sodium bicarbonate. Adrenal hyperactivity also increases the secretion of aldosterone and causes excess sodium retention. Excess loss of sodium occurs with adrenal insufficiency.

The pituitary gland is another important organ in the control of fluid and electrolyte balance. The posterior lobe of the pituitary releases antidiuretic hormone (ADH), which inhibits diuresis by increasing water reabsorption in the distal tubule. Increased concentration of sodium in the ECF stimulates the pituitary to release ADH. This hormone increases the reabsorption of water to dilute the sodium to the normal level of concentration. Increased body fluid osmolality, decreased body fluid volume, stress, and shock are conditions that increase ADH secretion. Increased body fluid volume, decreased osmolality, and alcohol inhibit ADH secretion.

The parathyroid glands, pea-sized glands embedded in the corners of the thyroid gland, regulate calcium and phosphate balance by means of parathyroid hormone (PTH). When the calcium level is low, PTH secretion is stimulated. This acts on bone to increase reabsorption of bone salts, releasing large amounts of sodium into the ECF. When the extracellular calcium concentration is too high, PTH secretion is depressed so that almost no bone reabsorption occurs (Metheny, 2012).

The pulmonary system regulates acid–base balance by controlling the concentration of carbonic acid through exhalation or retention of carbon dioxide.

Electrolytes of Biologic Fluids

Electrolyte content of the intracellular fluid differs from that of the ECF. Because specialized techniques are required to measure electrolyte concentration in the intracellular fluid, it is customary to measure the electrolytes in the ECF, chiefly plasma. Plasma electrolyte concentrations may be used to assess and manage patients with a diversity of electrolyte imbalances. Although some tests are performed on serum, the terms *serum electrolytes* and

TABLE 8-1	INTRACELLULAR AND EXTRACELLULAR CONCENTRATIONS AND RELATED SERUM VALUES		
	Normal Concentrations and Values		
	Intracellular	**Extracellular**	**Serum Laboratory Value**
Elements:			
Na^+	10 mEq/L	142 mEq/L	135–145 mEq/L
K^+	140 mEq/L	4 mEq/L	3.5–5.2 mEq/L
Ca^{2+}	> 1 mEq/L	5 mEq/L	8.5–10.5 mg/dL
Mg^{2+}	58 mEq/L	3 mEq/L	1.5–3.5 mEq/L
Cl^-	4 mEq/L	103 mEq/L	100–106 mEq/L
(HCO_3^-)	10 mEq/L	28 mEq/L	24–31 mEq/L
pH	7.0	7.4	7.35–7.45
Osmolality			280–294 mOsm/kg

plasma electrolytes are used interchangeably. Table 8-1 identifies intracellular and extracellular concentrations and serum values. Table 8-2 lists plasma electrolyte values.

POTASSIUM

Potassium is one of the most important electrolytes in the body. An excess or deficiency of potassium can cause serious impairment of body function and even result in death. Potassium is the main electrolyte in the intracellular compartment, which houses more than

TABLE 8-2	PLASMA ELECTROLYTES	
Electrolytes		**mEq/L**
Cations		
Sodium (Na^+)		142
Potassium (K^+)		5
Calcium (Ca^{2+})		5
Magnesium (Mg^{2+})		2
Total cations		154
Anions		
Chloride (Cl^-)		103
Bicarbonate (HCO_3^-)		26
Phosphate (HPO_4^{2-})		2
Sulfate (SO_4^{2-})		1
Organic acids		5
Proteinate		17
Total anions		154

From Metheny, N. M. (2012). *Fluid and electrolyte balance: Nursing considerations* (5th ed.). Sudbury, MA: Jones & Bartlett Learning.

98% of the body's total potassium. The healthy cell requires a high potassium concentration for cellular activity. When the cell dies, there is an exchange of potassium into the ECF with a transfer of sodium into the cell. This process also occurs to some degree when cellular metabolism is impaired, as in catabolism (breaking down) of cells from a crushing injury.

Serum concentration of potassium is 3.5 to 5.0 mEq/L. In the cell, the normal concentration is 115 to 150 mEq/L fluid. Variations from either of these levels can produce critical effects. When the potassium level is repeatedly > 5 to 6 mEq/L, a potassium excess is indicated; renal impairment usually is shown by renal function studies.

High serum concentrations have an adverse effect on the heart muscle and may cause cardiac arrhythmias. Serum potassium levels that are elevated two to three times normal may result in cardiac arrest. The electrocardiogram (ECG) may detect signs of potassium excess with peaked and elevated T waves, later disappearance of P waves, and finally, decomposition and prolongation of the QRS complex (Metheny, 2012).

HYPOKALEMIA

Hypokalemia refers to a serum potassium level below normal, whereas hyperkalemia denotes a serum potassium level above normal. Hypokalemia, or a serum potassium level < 4 mEq/L, may result when either of the following conditions occurs:

- Total body potassium is below normal.
- Concentration of potassium in cells is below normal.

Hypokalemia and hyperkalemia are often caused by variations in the intake or output of potassium. A decreased intake of potassium from prolonged fluid therapy (lacking potassium replacement) may result in hypokalemia. Hypokalemia also may occur during a "starvation diet" because the kidneys do not normally conserve potassium. An increased loss of potassium usually results from polyuria, vomiting, gastric suction (prolonged), diarrhea, and steroid therapy.

Potassium deficiency may be unrelated to intake and output. It can be caused by a sudden shift of potassium from the extracellular to intracellular fluid, such as that occurring from anabolism (building up of cells), healing processes, or the use of insulin and glucose in the treatment of diabetic acidosis. The shifts resulting from anabolism and healing processes are not usually of severe consequence unless accompanied by intervening factors. During treatment of diabetic acidosis, for example, the potassium shift may occur suddenly with grave consequences. When cells are anabolized, potassium shifts into the cells. When glucose is used in the treatment of diabetic acidosis, the glucose in the cells is quickly metabolized into glycogen for storage, causing a sudden shift of potassium from the extracellular to the intracellular fluid. This process results in hypokalemia.

The signs and symptoms of hypokalemia are malaise, skeletal and smooth muscle atony, apathy, muscular cramps, and postural hypotension. Treatment consists of administration of potassium orally or parenterally.

HYPERKALEMIA

Hyperkalemia may result from renal failure with potassium retention or from excessive or rapid administration of potassium in fluid therapy. It may also occur in conditions unrelated to retention or excessive intake. A sudden shift of potassium from the intracellular fluid to the ECF results when catabolism of cells occurs, as in a crushing injury; potassium shifts from cells to plasma.

The signs and symptoms of hyperkalemia are similar to those of hypokalemia. In addition to the signs already listed, the patient may experience tingling or numbness in the extremities, and the heart rate may be slow. A serum potassium level > 5.5 mEq/L confirms the diagnosis.

Treatment consists of stopping the potassium intake. Dialysis may be necessary for a long-term renal problem. If the cause is a shift of potassium from cells to plasma, glucose and insulin therapy may be used.

Sodium

Sodium is the main electrolyte in the ECF; its normal concentration is 135 to 145 mEq/L plasma. The main role of sodium is to control the distribution of water throughout the body and maintain a normal fluid balance. Alterations in sodium concentration markedly influence the fluid volume: the loss of sodium is accompanied by water loss and dehydration; the gain of sodium, by fluid retention.

The body, by regulating urine output, normally maintains a constant fluid volume and isotonicity of the plasma. Urine output is controlled by ADH, secreted by the pituitary gland. If a hypotonic concentration results from a low sodium concentration, the fluid is drawn from plasma into the cells. The body attempts to correct this process; the pituitary inhibits ADH and diuresis results, with a loss of ECF. This loss of fluid increases sodium concentration to a normal level.

If a hypertonic concentration results from increased concentration of extracellular sodium, fluid is drawn from the cells. Again the body reacts, and the pituitary is stimulated to secrete ADH. This causes a retention of fluid that dilutes sodium to normal concentrations.

Therefore, increased sodium concentration stimulates the production of ADH, with retention of water, thus diluting sodium to the normal level; a decrease in sodium concentration inhibits the production of ADH, resulting in a loss of water, which raises the concentration of sodium to the normal level.

In the kidneys, sodium is reabsorbed in exchange for potassium. Therefore, with an increase in sodium, there is loss of potassium; with a loss of sodium, there is an increase in potassium.

Hyponatremia

A sodium deficit (**hyponatremia**) may be present when the plasma sodium concentration falls below 135 mEq/L. It is caused by excessive sweating combined with a large intake of water by mouth (salt is lost and fluid increased, thus reducing the sodium concentration), excessive infusion of nonelectrolyte fluids, gastrointestinal suction plus water by mouth, and adrenal insufficiency, which causes a large loss of electrolytes.

The symptoms of a sodium deficit are apprehension, abdominal cramps, diarrhea, and convulsions. Dehydration results from loss of sodium and leads to peripheral circulatory failure. When sodium and water are lost from the plasma, the body attempts to replace them by a transfer of sodium and water from the interstitial fluid. Eventually, water is drawn from the cells and circulation fails; plasma volume cannot be sustained.

HYPERNATREMIA

Sodium excess (**hypernatremia**) may be present when the plasma sodium rises >145 mEq/L. Its causes are excessive infusions of saline, diarrhea, insufficient water intake, diabetes mellitus, and tracheobronchitis (excess loss of water from the lungs because of rapid breathing). The symptoms of sodium excess are dry, sticky mucous membranes, oliguria, excitement, and convulsions.

CALCIUM

Calcium is an electrolyte constituent of the plasma present in a concentration of approximately 4.6 to 5.1 mg/dL ionized calcium. The total calcium range is 8.5 to 10.5 mg/dL. Calcium serves several purposes. It plays an important role in formation and function of bones and teeth. As ionized calcium, it is involved in normal clotting of the blood and regulation of neuromuscular irritability.

The parathyroid glands control calcium metabolism. By acting on the kidneys and bones, PTH regulates the concentration of ionized calcium in the ECF. Impairment of this regulatory mechanism alters the calcium concentration. Hyperparathyroidism typically elevates the serum calcium level and decreases the serum phosphate level.

HYPOCALCEMIA

Calcium deficit may occur in patients who have diarrhea or problems in gastrointestinal absorption, extensive infections of the subcutaneous tissue, or burns. This deficiency can result in muscle tremors and cramps, excessive irritability, and even convulsions.

Calcium ionization is influenced by pH; it is decreased in alkalosis and increased in acidosis. With no loss of calcium, a patient in alkalosis may have symptoms of calcium deficit (e.g., muscle cramps, tetany, and convulsions). This is due to the decreased ionization of calcium caused by the elevated pH.

A patient in acidosis may have a calcium deficit with no symptoms because the acid pH has caused an increased ionization of available calcium. Symptoms of calcium deficit may appear if acidosis is converted to alkalosis.

HYPERCALCEMIA

It is estimated that 98% of patients with hypercalcemia, or calcium excess, have cancer or hyperparathyroidism or they use thiazide diuretics. Characteristics of hypercalcemia include muscular weakness, tiredness, lethargy, constipation, anorexia, polyuria, polydipsia, shortened QT interval on the ECG, and a serum calcium concentration >10.5 mg/dL.

OTHER ELECTROLYTES

The primary role of magnesium is in enzyme activity, where it contributes to the metabolism of both carbohydrates and proteins. Its serum concentration is 1.3 to 2.1 mEq/L. A magnesium deficit is a common imbalance in critically ill patients. Deficits may also occur in less acutely ill patients, such as those experiencing withdrawal from alcohol and those receiving parenteral or enteral nutrition after a period of starvation. Neuromuscular irritability, disorientation, and mood changes are indicative of hypomagnesemia. Hypermagnesemia is uncommon, but it may be seen in patients with advanced renal failure. Magnesium is excreted by the kidneys; therefore, diminished renal function results in abnormal renal magnesium retention.

Chloride, the chief anion of the ECF, has a plasma concentration of 97 to 110 mEq/L. A deficiency of chloride leads to a deficiency of potassium and vice versa. There is also a loss of chloride with a loss of sodium, but because this loss can be compensated for by an increase in bicarbonate, the proportion differs.

Phosphate is the chief anion of the intracellular fluid. Its normal level in plasma is 1.7 to 2.3 mEq/L.

OBJECTIVES OF FLUID AND ELECTROLYTE THERAPY

Parenteral therapy has three main objectives: to maintain daily body fluid requirements, to restore previous body fluid losses, and to replace present body fluid losses.

Maintenance

Maintenance therapy is aimed at providing all the nutrient needs of the patient: water, electrolytes, dextrose, vitamins, and protein. Of these needs, water is the most important. The body may survive for a prolonged period without vitamins, dextrose, and protein, but without water, dehydration and death occur.

WATER

The body needs water to replace the insensible loss that occurs with evaporation from the skin and from expired air. An average adult loses from 500 to 1,000 mL water per 24 hours through insensible loss. The skin loss varies with the temperature and humidity. Water balance is closely correlated to energy expenditure (Klotz, 1998).

Water is essential for kidney function. The amount needed depends on the amount of waste products to be excreted as well as the concentrating ability of the kidneys. Protein and salt increase the need for water.

A person's fluid requirements are based on age, height, weight, and amount of body fat. Because fat is water free, a large amount of body fat contains a relatively low amount of water; as body fat increases, water decreases in inverse proportion to body weight. The normal fluid and electrolyte requirements based on body surface area are more constant than when expressed in terms of body weight. Many of the essential physiologic processes such as heat loss, blood volume, organ size, and respiration have a direct relationship to the body surface area.

Fluid and electrolyte requirements are also proportionate to surface area, regardless of the patient's age. These requirements are based on square meters of body surface area and are calculated for a 24-hour period. Nomograms are available for determining surface area (see Chapter 12). Table 8-3 highlights maintenance requirements based on body weight (assuming that renal function, gastrointestinal status, and temperature are normal).

Balanced electrolyte fluids are available for maintenance. The average requirements of fluid and electrolytes are estimated for a healthy person and applied to a patient. The balanced fluids contain electrolytes in proportion to the daily needs of the patient, but not in excess of the body's tolerance, as long as adequate kidney function exists. When a patient's water needs are provided by these maintenance fluids, the daily needs of sodium and

TABLE 8-3 FLUID AND ELECTROLYTE MAINTENANCE REQUIREMENTS[a]	
Weight Range	**Required Volume**
Premature infant (<3 kg)	60 mL/kg
Younger patient	
0–10 kg	100 mL/kg/d
10–20 kg	1,000 mL + 50 mL/kg/d
21 kg to average adult weight	1,500 mL + 20 mL/kg/d
Adult (nonpregnant)	30–35 mL/kg/d

[a]Based on body weight.

potassium are also met. For maintenance, 1,500 mL/m² body surface area is administered over a 24-hour period.

GLUCOSE

Because it is converted into glycogen by the liver, thereby improving hepatic function, glucose has an important role in maintenance. By supplying necessary calories for energy, it spares body protein and minimizes the development of ketosis caused by the oxidation of fat stores for essential energy in the absence of added glucose.

The basic daily caloric requirement of a 70-kg adult at rest is approximately 1,600 calories. However, the administration of 100 g glucose a day is helpful in minimizing the ketosis of starvation; 100 g is contained in 2 L of 5% dextrose in water or 1 L 10% dextrose in water.

PROTEIN

Protein is another nutrient important to maintenance therapy. Although a patient may be adequately maintained on glucose, water, vitamins, and electrolytes for a limited time, protein may be required to replace normal protein losses over an extended period. Protein is necessary for cellular repair, wound healing, and synthesis of vitamins and some enzymes. The usual daily protein requirement for a healthy adult is 1 g/kg body weight. Protein is available as amino acid. Taken orally, protein is broken down into amino acids before being absorbed into the blood.

VITAMINS

Vitamins, although not nutrients in the true sense of the word, are necessary for the utilization of other nutrients. Vitamin C and the various B complex vitamins are the most frequently used in parenteral therapy. Because these vitamins are water soluble, they are not retained by the body but lost through urinary excretion. Because of this loss, larger amounts are required parenterally to ensure adequate maintenance than may be required when administered orally. The B complex vitamins play an important role in the metabolism of carbohydrates and in maintaining gastrointestinal function. Vitamin C promotes wound healing and is frequently used for surgical patients. Vitamins A and D are fat-soluble vitamins, better retained by the body and not usually required by the patient on maintenance therapy.

Restoration of Previous Losses

Restoration of previous losses is essential when past maintenance has not been met—that is, when output exceeds intake. Severe dehydration may occur from failure to replace these losses. Therapy consists of replacing losses from previous deficits in addition to providing fluid and electrolytes for daily maintenance. Kidney status must be considered before electrolyte replacement and maintenance can be initiated; urinary suppression may result from decreased fluid volume or renal impairment. A hydrating fluid such as 5% dextrose in 0.2% (34.2 mEq) sodium chloride solution is administered. Urinary flow is restored if the retention is functional. The patient must be rehydrated rapidly to establish adequate urine output. Only after kidney function proves adequate can large electrolyte losses be replaced.

Replacement of Present Losses

Replacement of present losses of fluid and electrolytes is also an objective of therapy. Accurate measurement of all intake and output is a significant means of calculating fluid loss. Fluid loss may be estimated by determining loss of body weight; 1 L body water equals 1 kg, or 2.2 lb, body weight. An osmolality determination may indicate the water needs of the body. If necessary, a corrective BUN determination may be performed with the osmolality evaluation.

The type of replacement depends on the type of fluid being lost. A choice of appropriate replacement fluids is available. For example, excessive loss of gastric fluid may be replaced by fluids resembling the fluid lost, such as gastric replacement fluids. Excessive loss of intestinal fluid must be replaced by an intestinal replacement fluid. Examples of conditions that may result from current losses are alkalosis and acidosis (Table 8-4).

FLUID AND ELECTROLYTE DISTURBANCES IN SPECIFIC PATIENTS

Understanding how the endocrine system responds to stress helps the nurse better understand the imbalances and problems associated with stress. It also contributes to safe and successful parenteral therapy. The nurse anticipates what to expect, knows the possible dangers of imbalances, and recognizes early symptoms.

TABLE 8-4	DIFFERENTIATING ACIDOSIS FROM ALKALOSIS		
Cause	Physiology	Symptoms	Intervention
Alkalosis			
Loss of NaCl/ KCl gastric fluid	Concentration of bicarbonate gastric ions; anions must equal cations.	Slow shallow respiration, pallor	Administer appropriate replacement fluids.
	Ammonia is converted into urea and hydrogen ion. If the liver fails to convert ammonia to urea, ammonia retention and toxicity result.	Sweating, tetany, coma	
Acidosis			
Excess fluid is alkaline	Intestinal secretions contain excessive bicarbonate ions; with loss, chloride ion	Shortness of breath; rapid breathing	Administer base salts; that is, sodium lactate or sodium.

The Surgical Patient

The neuroendocrine response stimulated by many anesthetic agents is further heightened by surgical stress. Apprehension, pain, and duration and severity of trauma give rise to surgical stress and contribute to an increased endocrine response during the first 2 to 5 days after surgery.

The **stress response** is normal and is nature's way of protecting the body from hypotension resulting from trauma and shock. Correction is often unnecessary and may, in fact, be harmful.

The two major endocrine homeostatic controls affected by stress are pituitary gland and adrenal gland function (Figure 8-5). The posterior pituitary controls quantitative secretions of ADH. The anterior pituitary controls secretions of corticotropin, which stimulates

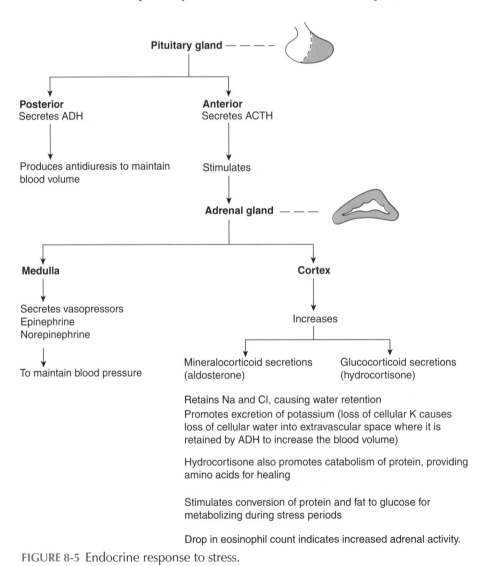

FIGURE 8-5 Endocrine response to stress.

the adrenal gland to increase mineralocorticoid secretions (aldosterone) and glucocorticoid secretions (hydrocortisone). The adrenal medulla secretes vasopressors (epinephrine and norepinephrine) to help maintain the blood pressure.

A direct physiologic effect occurs when stress increases the secretions of these various hormones. When the posterior pituitary increases ADH secretions, antidiuresis is affected, thus helping maintain blood volume. When the anterior pituitary increases corticotropin secretions, the adrenal gland is stimulated to increase aldosterone.

FLUID REPLACEMENT MECHANISMS

Adrenal hormones help maintain blood volume by causing the retention of sodium ions and chloride anions, thereby causing water retention and promoting the excretion of potassium (loss of cellular potassium ions causes loss of cellular water into extracellular space, where it is retained by ADH to maintain blood volume).

Hydrocortisone also promotes the catabolism of protein to provide necessary amino acids for healing and stimulates the conversion of protein and fat to glucose for metabolism during the stress period. This metabolic activity may elevate the blood glucose level, a finding that may mistakenly suggest diabetes mellitus. A drop in the eosinophil count and an elevated level of serum 17-hydroxycorticosteroid hormones indicate increased adrenal activity.

FLUID NEEDS

Accurate records of intake and output are important for assessing fluid requirements and preventing serious fluid imbalances during the early postoperative period. The daily requirement of 1,500 to 2,000 mL varies with the patient's needs. Caution must be taken not to overhydrate the patient—the intake should be adequate but should not exceed the fluid losses.

The adrenocortical secretions, increased by trauma and stress of surgery, cause some water and sodium retention. This retention may be severe enough to present a false picture of oliguria. Excessive quantities of nonelectrolyte fluids (such as 5% dextrose in water) administered at a time when antidiuresis is occurring may cause hyponatremia, a serious electrolyte imbalance.

In hyponatremia, the serum sodium concentration is lower than normal. Water-yielding fluids, infused in excess of the body's tolerance, expand the extracellular compartment, lowering the electrolyte concentration. By osmosis, water invades the cells, with a resulting excess accumulation of intracellular fluid. Usually, there is no edema because edema is the result of an excess accumulation of fluid in the extracellular compartment.

Symptoms of water excess include confusion, hallucinations, delirium, weight gain, hyperventilation, muscular weakness, twitching, and convulsions. If these occur during the early postoperative stages, the nurse should suspect water excess. This is of particular concern in young and elderly patients. Serious consequences, even death, can result.

Restricting the fluid intake may correct mild water excess, but for more severe cases, the administration of high concentrations of sodium chloride may be indicated. The electrolyte concentration of the plasma, increased by the concentrated saline, causes an increase in the osmotic pressure, drawing fluid from the cells for excretion by the kidneys.

Parenteral therapy during the stress period often consists of administering conservative amounts of 5% dextrose in water. Because some sodium retention results from the endocrine response to stress, care must be taken to avoid administering excessive quantities of saline at a time when there is an interference in the elimination of salt. During this early period, the physician/LIP frequently gives 5% dextrose in quarter- or half-strength saline to avoid sodium excess.

In hypernatremia, the serum sodium concentration is higher than normal. This excess may expand ECF volume or cause edema and possible disruption of cellular function (in potassium-depleted patients, the sodium may replace the intracellular potassium).

Symptoms of sodium excess include flushed skin, elevated temperature, dry and sticky mucous membranes, thirst, and a decreased or absent urine output. Treatment consists of reducing the salt and water intake and promoting diuresis to eliminate the excess salt and water from the plasma.

NUTRIENT NEEDS

Among the various nutrients needed by postsurgical patients are carbohydrates, proteins, fats, potassium, and vitamins.

CARBOHYDRATES

Carbohydrates provide an indispensable source of calories for the postoperative patient unable to receive food orally. When carbohydrate supplies are inadequate, the body uses its own fat to supply calories; the by-products are ketone bodies. These acid bodies neutralize bicarbonate and produce metabolic acidosis. The only by-products excreted in the metabolism of carbohydrates are water and carbon dioxide.

By providing calories for essential energy, carbohydrates also reduce catabolism of protein. During the stress response, the renal excretion of nitrogen (from the catabolism of protein) exceeds the intake. By reducing the protein breakdown, glucose helps prevent a negative nitrogen balance.

Carbohydrates do not provide adequate calories for the patient receiving prolonged therapy. Approximately 1 L of 5% dextrose in water provides 170 calories. Many liters, a volume too great for most patients to tolerate, would be required to provide a patient with 1,600 calories. Greater concentrations of glucose, 20% and 50%, may be administered to provide calories for patients unable to tolerate large volumes of fluid (e.g., patients with renal insufficiency). The concentrated fluids must be administered slowly for glucose utilization to occur. Rapid administration results in diuresis; the concentrated glucose acts as a diuretic, drawing interstitial fluid into the plasma for excretion by the kidneys.

ALCOHOL

Alcohol fluids may be administered to the postoperative patient for nutritional and physiologic benefits. Nutritionally, the alcohol supplements calories provided by the glucose, with 1 g ethyl alcohol yielding 6 to 8 calories. Because alcohol is quickly and completely metabolized, it provides calories for essential energy, sparing fat and protein. Metabolized in preference to glucose, alcohol allows the infused glucose to be stored as glycogen.

Physiologically, alcohol produces a sedative effect, reducing pain; 200 to 300 mL of a 5% solution per hour produces sedation without intoxication in the average adult. Alcohol also inhibits the secretion of ADH, promoting water excretion.

Fluids containing alcohol, particularly hypertonic fluids, can cause phlebitis. These fluids, if allowed to infiltrate, may cause tissue necrosis. The IV catheter should be carefully inserted within the lumen of the vessel and inspected frequently to detect any infiltration.

PROTEIN

Patients who receive parenteral fluid therapy for a prolonged time require protein for cellular repair, wound healing, and growth. Stress states accompanying surgical procedures and trauma frequently result in protein deficiency.

During the stress period, increased secretions of glucocorticoids from the adrenal cortex cause protein breakdown and the conversion of protein and fat to glucose for energy. More urinary nitrogen is lost than normal. When nitrogen loss exceeds intake, the patient is said to be in a negative balance. This response to stress is normal. However, protein losses must be counteracted; preservation of body cell mass is essential. A depleted body cell mass can be restored only by parenteral nutrition. Approximately 1 g/kg body weight is required by a healthy adult to replace normal protein loss.

Because of their high ammonia level, extreme caution is required if proteins are administered to patients with hepatic insufficiency or emaciation. Organ-specific formulas have been developed for the patient with renal or hepatic disease.

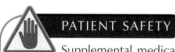

PATIENT SAFETY

Supplemental medications added to the fluid may result in incompatibilities. Always check with the pharmacist before adding any medication to fluids.

Fluids, once opened, must be used immediately. Storing a partially used container of fluid in the refrigerator for future use provides a culture medium for the growth of bacteria. No fluids that are cloudy or contain precipitate should be used.

LIPID EMULSIONS

Lipid emulsions offer calories and essential fatty acids for metabolic processes. They are rich in calories, yielding 9 kcal/g, compared with 4 kcal/g from carbohydrates.

POTASSIUM

Once the stress period passes, adrenal activity decreases and diuresis begins. At this time, usually after the 2nd to the 5th postoperative day, potassium is given daily to prevent a deficit. Potassium is not conserved by the body but is lost in the urine. Electrolyte maintenance fluids may be used or potassium may be added to parenteral fluids. When potassium is added to parenteral fluids, the container, bag, or bottle should be thoroughly shaken to mix and dilute the potassium. Potassium should never be added to a hanging container while the infusion is running. Such an action could result in a bolus injection of the drug. Rapid injection, which increases the drug concentration in the plasma, can result in trauma to the vessel wall and even in cardiac arrest. Potassium should never be given by IV push or bolus administration.

The status of the kidneys must be considered. If kidney function is inadequate, the patient must be rehydrated. During this infusion, the nurse must watch for diminished diuresis and notify the physician/LIP if antidiuresis occurs.

PATIENT SAFETY

Potassium chloride must be used with caution and is considered potentially dangerous if administered when renal function is impaired. A buildup of potassium, caused by the kidney's inability to excrete salts, can prove hazardous; arrhythmia and heart block can result from the effect of excess potassium on the heart muscle.

An amount of 40 mEq/L usually is sufficient to replace normal potassium loss. It is usually infused over an 8-hour period. Premixed potassium replacement fluids are available in a variety of strengths.

In extreme cases of hypokalemia, when the serum potassium concentration is <2.0 mEq/L, the nurse may need to infuse potassium at a much faster rate—but not faster than 40 mEq/hour. When the serum potassium concentration reaches 2.5 mEq/L and ECG manifestations of hypokalemia diminish, the rate should be decreased to no more than 10 mEq/hour, using a fluid that contains no more than 30 mEq/L.

Continuous ECG monitoring is required when high doses of potassium are infused. The fluid containing potassium should be conspicuously labeled and must never be used when positive pressure is indicated—rapid infusion may result in cardiac arrest.

Potassium is irritating to the vein and may cause a great deal of discomfort, especially if infused into a vein where a previous venipuncture has been performed. Slowing the rate may decrease the pain.

VITAMINS

The B complex vitamins and vitamin C are usually added to parenteral fluids if, after 2 or 3 days, the patient cannot take fluids orally. Vitamin C is important in promoting healing in the surgical patient, and B complex vitamins aid carbohydrate metabolism.

NURSING DIAGNOSES

Nursing diagnoses for the postsurgical patient should address relevant fluid and electrolyte disturbances. Table 8-5 lists selected nursing diagnoses.

The Burn Patient

The patient with burns presents special clinical challenges (Table 8-6). The rule of nines (Table 8-7) is commonly used to estimate burned area. The body's surface area is divided into sections equal to 9% or multiples of 9% of total body area. The portion of the areas sustaining second- or third-degree burns is identified, and the percentages are totaled to represent the full percentage of body surface area burned. This method may be inaccurate in children, and other charts are available for accurately determining percentage of body surface area burned.

TABLE 8-5	SELECTED NURSING DIAGNOSES FOR POSTOPERATIVE PATIENT AFTER ABDOMINAL SURGERY	
Nursing Diagnosis	**Etiologic Factors**	**Defining Characteristics**
Fluid volume deficit related to actual fluid loss and third-space fluid shift during surgical procedure	Vomiting after reaction to anesthesia GI suction. Third-space fluid shift at surgical site	Postural tachycardia; postural hypotension initially; later, low blood pressure in all positions; decreased skin turgor; decreased capillary refill time; oliguria (<30 mL/h in adult); weight change depends on cause (decreased if actual fluid loss, as in GI suction; usually increased if fluid loss is due to third-space shift, provided parenteral fluids are given in an attempt to correct hypovolemia)
Altered tissue perfusion (renal) related to hypotension during surgical procedure	Hypotensive effects of anesthesia. Hypovolemia due to direct or indirect loss of fluid. Hypovolemia due to inadequate parenteral fluid replacement	Oliguria or polyuria in the presence of elevated serum creatinine
Alteration in sodium balance (hyponatremia) related to excessive ADH activity	Major surgery with its premedication, anesthesia, decreased blood volume, and postoperative pain results in increased ADH release (causing water retention with sodium dilution)	Serum sodium <135 mEq/L; may be asymptomatic if Na > 120 mEq/L; lethargy, confusion, nausea, vomiting, anorexia, abdominal cramps, muscular twitching
Alteration in acid–base balance (metabolic alkalosis) related to vomiting or gastric suction	Vomiting after reaction to anesthesia. Gastric suction, particularly if patient is allowed to ingest ice chips freely	Tingling of fingers, toes, and circumoral region, due to decreased calcium ionization pH > 7.45, bicarbonate above normal, chloride below normal
Altered nutrition (less than body requirements) related to negative nitrogen balance after surgical stress, and inadequate caloric intake	Catabolic response to stress of surgery. Inability to tolerate oral feedings during first few postoperative days due to decreased GI motility, anorexia, nausea, and general discomfort. Failure of health care providers to administer sufficient calories via the parenteral route	Weight loss of approximately ¼ to ½ lb/d in adult (provided fluids are not abnormally retained). Perhaps a decrease in serum albumin, transferrin, and retinol-binding protein levels (although delivery of a large volume of blood products or the long half-life of certain secretory proteins can interfere with correct interpretation)

ADH, antidiuretic hormone; GI, gastrointestinal.
From Metheny, N.M. (2012). *Fluid and electrolyte balance: Nursing considerations* (5th ed.). Sudbury, MA: Jones & Bartlett Learning.

FORMULAS FOR FLUID REPLACEMENT

Fluid requirements for the first 24 hours after burn injury range from 2 to 4 mL/kg body weight depending on percentage of body surface area burned. Several factors must be considered, including age of the patient, size and depth of the burn, type of fluid, and complication factors such as inhalation injury, electrical burns, or multiple trauma. Numerous formulas

TABLE 8-6	THE BURN PATIENT RECEIVING PARENTERAL FLUID THERAPY	
	Objectives/Mechanisms	Intervention
First 48 h	Maintain fluid volume relative to loss and third spacing	Ensure venous access; administer fluids consistent with clinical condition and physician/LIP's orders
Intravascular to interstitial shift	Treat volume depletion	Administer albumin as ordered to correct third-space shifts; maintain fluid status and IV access
Shock perfusion	Re-establish adequate tissue protein (from skin). Deliver oxygen to metabolically active cells	Replace fluid and electrolytes
Dehydration	Water and electrolyte loss are less than protein loss. Osmotic pressure draws fluid from undamaged tissues	Determine replacement needs and administer fluids adequate to restore perfusion. Administer colloids to draw fluid in from other compartments, thus increasing vascular volume
Hypovolemia	Exudate from burned area, water (as vapor), and blood loss occur	Ensure adequate venous access to provide fluid volume
Decreased urine output	Ensure that the kidneys are working before administration of potassium replacement. ADH exceeds water reabsorption by the kidneys	Replace blood volume and maintain kidney output. Monitor intake and output to ensure elimination of wastes
Potassium excess	Hyperkalemia; cells release potassium, and decreased renal flow obstructs normal excretion of potassium	Initiate fluid replacement with albumin, dextran, hetastarch
Sodium deficit	Due to edema and loss of exudate	Administer nonelectrolyte solution to replace insensible losses
Metabolic acidosis	Due to accumulation of fixed acids released from tissue	Administer only enough fluid to maintain blood volume/urine output
2nd to 3rd day	Shift from interstitial fluid to plasma	Reduce parenteral fluids accordingly; excess urinary output is evidence of need to decrease fluid therapy
	Avoid circulatory overload	Maintain fluid volume and monitor patient for hypophosphatemia

have been developed for this purpose, but an ideal rate of infusion is one that maintains perfusion, as reflected by a urinary output of 0.5 mL/kg body weight per hour in the adult patient.

ASSESSMENT

Ongoing assessment of the patient is needed to tailor fluid replacement to individual patient needs. Monitoring parameters include urine volume, sensorium, vital signs, and central venous pressure.

Urine output is the best indicator of adequate fluid resuscitation. Adult output should be 30 to 50 mL/hour. Lack of urine output or a substantial decrease in volume may be attributed to inadequate fluid replacement, gastric dilation, or renal failure. Daily weights are a

TABLE 8-7	RULE OF NINES FOR ESTIMATING BURNED BODY AREA IN ADULTS
Body Parts	**Percentage of Body**
Head and neck	9
Anterior trunk	18
Each arm	9
Posterior trunk	18
Genitalia	1
Each leg	18

helpful tool for monitoring the burned patient. A weight gain of 15% to 20% may indicate fluid retention. Adequacy of tissue perfusion is measured by assessing the patient's sensorium. Sensorium should remain normal with appropriate fluid replacement unless other factors, such as head injury, are present.

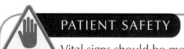

PATIENT SAFETY

Vital signs should be monitored hourly in the burn patient.

Blood pressure should remain at near normal values with consideration given to the patient's baseline pressure. Temperature may be elevated and tachycardia may be present. Rate and character of respirations should be evaluated. Peripheral pulses and capillary refill times should be monitored. Vasoconstriction of unburned skin is a compensatory response to help preserve normal blood flow in the hours immediately after a severe burn. Hence, unburned skin may be cool to the touch and appear pale at first.

Central venous and arterial pressure monitoring may be used to evaluate the effects of fluid replacement. Signs of inadequate fluid replacement are decreased urine output, thirst, restlessness and disorientation, hypotension, and increased pulse rate. Circulatory overload may be suspected with an elevated central venous pressure reading (15 to 20 cm H_2O), shortness of breath, and moist crackles when auscultating the lungs.

The Diabetic Patient

Diabetic acidosis is an endocrine disorder causing complex fluid and electrolyte disturbances. It occurs when a lack of insulin prevents the metabolism of glucose, and essential calories are provided instead by the catabolism of the patient's own fat and protein. Acidosis results from the accumulation of acid by-products. Understanding the physiologic changes in diabetic acidosis aids the nurse in detecting early imbalances and the subsequent treatment.

PHYSIOLOGIC CHANGES IN DIABETIC ACIDOSIS

Lack of insulin prevents cellular metabolism of glucose and its conversion into glycogen. Glucose accumulates in the bloodstream (hyperglycemia). When the blood glucose level rises >180 mg/100 mL, glucose spills over into the urine (**glycosuria**). The kidneys require 10 to 20 mL water to excrete 1 g glucose; water excretion increases (polyuria).

The body's fat and protein are used to provide necessary calories for energy. Ketone bodies, metabolic by-products, reduce plasma bicarbonate, and acidosis occurs.

FLUID AND ELECTROLYTE DISTURBANCES

Dehydration results from excessive fluid and electrolyte losses. Cellular fluid deficit occurs when water is drawn from the cells by the hyperosmolality of the blood. ECF deficit occurs when

- Glycosuria increases the urinary output.
- Ketone bodies raise the load on the kidneys and increase the water to excrete them.
- Vomiting causes loss of fluid and electrolytes.
- Oral intake falls because of the patient's condition.
- Hyperventilation is induced by the acidotic state.

KETOSIS

Ketosis is the excessive production of ketone bodies in the bloodstream. Ketone bodies are the end products of oxidation of fatty acids. Ketosis occurs when a lack of insulin results in excessive fatty acids being converted by the liver to ketones and the decreased utilization of ketones by the peripheral tissues. Electrolytes and ketone bodies, retained in high serum concentration, increase the acidosis; the increase in the number of hydrogen ions, from the retention of ketone bodies, may drop the blood pH to 7.25 and lower. The bicarbonate anions decrease to compensate for the increase in ketone anions and may drop the bicarbonate level to 12 mEq/L or less.

HYPERGLYCEMIC HYPEROSMOLAR NONKETOTIC COMA

Hyperglycemic hyperosmolar nonketotic coma (HHNC) is a syndrome that may develop in the middle-aged or elderly type 2 diabetic patient. The condition is often associated with the stress of cardiovascular disease, infection, or pharmacologic treatment with steroids or diuretics. It is also precipitated by too-rapid infusion of parenteral nutrition fluid. Blood glucose levels may reach 4,000 mg/dL but without the ketosis of diabetic ketoacidosis. Fluid volume deficit is profound and may lead to death. Underlying factors contributing to development of diabetic ketoacidosis or HHNC are found in Table 8-8. Signs and symptoms of diabetic acidosis are summarized in Box 8-1.

PARENTERAL THERAPY

Insulin is given to metabolize the excess glucose and combat diabetic acidosis. Because absorption is quickest by the bloodstream, insulin is administered IV. When given subcutaneously or intramuscularly, the slower rate of absorption of insulin may be further decreased by peripheral vascular collapse in the presence of shock. The dose of insulin, when administered by continuous infusion, is usually 4 to 8 U/hour. Many types of infusion pumps are available to ensure accurate and continuous administration of medications.

TABLE 8-8 FACTORS CONTRIBUTING TO DEVELOPMENT OF DKA OR HHNC IN SUSCEPTIBLE PERSONS

DKA	HHNC
Infections, illness	Chronic renal disease
Physiologic stresses (e.g., trauma, surgery, myocardial infarction, dehydration, pregnancy)	Chronic cardiovascular disease Acute illness, infection Surgery burns, trauma
Psychologic/emotional stress	Parenteral nutrition, tube feedings
Omission/reduction of insulin	Peritoneal dialysis
Failure of insulin delivery system (pump)	Mannitol[a] therapy
Excess alcohol intake	Pharmacologic agents
	Chlorpromazine
	Cimetidine
	Diazoxide
	Diuretics (thiazide, thiazide-related, and loop diuretics)
	Glucocorticoids and immunosuppressive agents
	L-Asparaginase
	Phenytoin
	Propranolol

[a]Mannitol does not cross the blood–brain barrier, so an elevated plasma osmolality due to an infusion of hypertonic mannitol is effective in removing fluid from the brain and is known as "mannitol osmotherapy."
DKA, diabetic ketoacidosis; HHNC, hyperglycemic hyperosmolar nonketotic coma.
From Metheny, N.M. (2012). *Fluid and electrolyte balance: Nursing considerations* (5th ed.). Sudbury, MA: Jones & Bartlett Learning.

Parenteral fluids are administered to increase the blood volume and restore kidney function. Early treatment of the hypotonic patient usually consists of the administration of 0.9% sodium chloride solution to replace sodium and chloride losses and to expand the blood volume. Later, hypotonic fluids with sodium chloride may be used. Bicarbonate replacement may be necessary in severe acidosis.

Potassium administration is contraindicated in the early treatment of diabetic acidosis. During the later stages (10 to 24 hours after treatment), the plasma potassium level falls; improved renal function increases potassium excretion, and, in anabolic states, as the glucose is converted into glycogen, a sudden shift of potassium from ECF to intracellular fluid further lowers the plasma potassium level. If the patient is hydrated, potassium should be administered when the plasma potassium concentration falls.

A severe potassium deficit may occur if symptoms are not recognized and early treatment begun. Symptoms include weak grip, irregular pulse, weak picking at the bedclothes, shallow respiration, and abdominal distention.

SUMMARY

Under normal circumstances, the body is able to maintain a state of equilibrium or homeostasis. Various checks and balances contribute to the process. It is essential that the nurse responsible for infusion therapy have a solid understanding of fluid and electrolyte levels

---

BOX 8-1 SIGNS AND SYMPTOMS OF DIABETIC KETOACIDOSIS

Infusion nurses need to become familiar with the signs and symptoms that characterize diabetic acidosis. By recognizing impending diabetic acidosis, early treatment may be initiated and complications prevented.

Hyperglycemia—When a lack of insulin prevents glucose metabolism, glucose accumulates in the bloodstream.

Glycosuria—When the accumulation of glucose exceeds the renal tolerance, glucose spills over into the urine.

Polyuria—Osmotic diuresis occurs when the heavy load of nonmetabolized glucose and the metabolic end products increase the osmolality of the blood. In turn, the increased renal solute load requires more fluid for excretion.

Thirst—Cellular dehydration, arising from the osmotic effect produced by hyperglycemia, prompts thirst.

Weakness and fatigue—The body's inability to use glucose and a potassium deficit lead to weakness and fatigue.

Flushed face—Flushing results from the acid condition.

Rapid, deep breathing—The body's defense against acidosis, expiration of large amounts of carbon dioxide reduces carbonic acid and increases the pH of the blood.

Acetone breath—Increased accumulation of acetone bodies results in acetone-scented breath.

Nausea and vomiting—Distention resulting from atony of gastric muscles causes nausea and vomiting.

Weight loss—An excess loss of fluid (1 L body water equals 2.2 lb, or 1 kg, body weight) and a lack of glucose metabolism contribute to weight loss.

Low blood pressure—Severe fluid deficit leads to low blood pressure.

Oliguria—Decreased renal blood flow that results from a severe deficit in fluid volume produces oliguria.

---

and their importance to the outcome of care. When recognized and treated promptly, most imbalances may be resolved and the body returns to homeostasis.

Review Questions   *Note: Questions below may have more than one right answer.*

1. Which of the following contributes to respiratory alkalosis?

   A. Inhalation of excess carbon dioxide

   B. Shallow breathing

   C. Depletion of carbon monoxide

   D. Increased oxygenation

2. Symptoms associated with respiratory alkalosis include all of the following *except*

   A. Tetany

   B. Unconsciousness

   C. Convulsions

   D. Lethargy

3. Respiratory acidosis is associated with all of the following *except*
   A. Diabetes
   B. Emphysema
   C. Asthma
   D. Pneumonia

4. Kidney function controls which of the following?
   A. Bicarbonate concentration
   B. Sodium exchange
   C. Intracellular potassium
   D. Acidity

5. Symptoms associated with metabolic alkalosis include
   A. Muscular hyperactivity
   B. Tetany
   C. Depressed respirations
   D. Increased respirations

6. Metabolic acidosis is associated with a deficit of
   A. Bicarbonate ion
   B. Carbon dioxide
   C. Sodium
   D. Chloride

7. Symptoms of metabolic acidosis include which of the following?
   A. Stupor and shortness of breath
   B. Weakness and unconsciousness
   C. A plasma pH below 7.35
   D. Plasma bicarbonate concentration below 24 mEq/L

8. Regulating mechanisms that maintain the constancy of body fluid volume, electrolyte composition, and osmolality are functions of which of the following?
   A. Renocardiovascular system
   B. Endocrine system
   C. Respiratory system
   D. Kidneys

9. Normal intake of 2,500 mL from all sources is estimated to deliver a loss of approximately how many milliliters in breath and perspiration?
   A. 1,000 mL
   B. 1,400 mL
   C. 1,500 mL
   D. 1,800 mL

10. Which of the following is the major electrolyte of the intracellular compartment?
    A. Calcium
    B. Potassium
    C. Sodium
    D. Bicarbonate

References and Selected Readings   *Asterisks indicate references cited in text.*

*Adelman, R.D., & Solhung, M.J. (1996). Pathophysiology of body fluids and fluid therapy. In R.E. Behrman, R.M. Kliegman, & A.M. Arvin (Eds.), *Nelson textbook of pediatrics* (15th ed., pp. 185–222). Philadelphia, PA: W.B. Saunders.

*Alexander, M., Corrigan, A., Gorski, L., Hankins, J., & Perucca, R. (2010). *Infusion nursing: An evidence-based approach* (3rd ed., pp. 178–203). St. Louis, MO: Saunders.

*Chernecky, C., Macklin, D., & Murphy-Ende, K. (2002). *Real world nursing survival guide: Fluids & electrolytes*. Philadelphia, PA: Saunders.

*Collins, M., & Claros, E. (2011). Recognizing the face of dehydration. *Nursing* , 41(8), 26–31.

*Elkin, M.K., Perry, A.G., & Potter, P.A. (2007). *Nursing interventions and clinical skills* (4th ed.). St. Louis, MO: Mosby.

Foley, M. (1998). *Lippincott's need-to-know nursing reference facts* (pp. 107–148). Philadelphia, PA: Lippincott-Raven.

*Guyton, A.C., & Hall, J.E. (2006). *Textbook of medical physiology* (11th ed.). Philadelphia, PA: Saunders.

Kee, J., Paulanka, B., & Purnell, L. (2004). *Fluids and electrolytes with clinical applications: A programmed approach* (7th ed.). Clifton Park, NY: Delmar Learning.

*Klotz, R. (1998). The effects of infusion solutions on fluid and electrolyte balance. *Journal of Infusion Nursing, 21*, 20–24.

*Metheny, N.M. (2012). *Fluid and electrolyte balance: Nursing considerations* (5th ed.). Sudbury, MA: Jones & Bartlett Learning.

Porth, C.M. (2011). *Essentials of pathophysiology* (3rd ed.). Philadelphia, PA: Wolters Kluwer.

*Smeltzer, S.C., Bare, B.G., Hinkle, J.L., et al. (2008). *Brunner and Suddarth's textbook of medical-surgical nursing* (11th ed.). New York: Lippincott Williams & Wilkins.

Taylor, C., Lillis, C., & LeMone, P. (2007). *Fundamentals of nursing* (7th ed.). Philadelphia, PA: Lippincott Williams & Wilkins, Chapters 12 and 40.

CHAPTER 9

Principles of Parenteral Administration

Sharon M. Weinstein

PARENTERAL FLUIDS

To help enhance patient outcomes, knowledge of parenteral fluids is essential when delivering infusion therapy. This is particularly important because rapid and critical changes in fluid and electrolyte balance may be caused by infusates.

Until the 1930s, intravenous (IV) fluids consisted of dextrose and saline solutions. Little was known about electrolyte therapy. Today, however, more than 200 types of commercially prepared fluids are available. The great increase in their use leads to a more common occurrence of fluid and electrolyte disturbances. Moreover, with the increased administration of fluids in alternative care settings, nurses must know the chemical composition and the physical effects of the infusions they administer.

> ### PATIENT SAFETY
>
> Nurses have a legal and professional responsibility to know the
> - Normal amount of any IV infusion they administer
> - Desired and untoward effects of any IV infusion
> - Type of fluid, the amount, and the rate of flow, determined only after the physician/ licensed independent practitioner (LIP) has carefully assessed the patient's clinical condition

Intravenous Infusion

Today, methods of infusion have changed dramatically, and small-volume parenteral *fluids* may be administered as a secondary infusate or in a volume-controlled reservoir for electronic drug delivery.

An infusion is usually regarded as an amount of fluid > 100 mL designated to be infused parenterally because the volume must be administered over a long period. However, when medications are administered as a *piggyback* (secondary to and delivered with the initial infusion) small-volume (50 to 100 mL) parenteral infusion, a shorter period (usually 30 to 60 minutes) may be required, whereas volumes of 150 to 200 mL may require > 1 hour. Today, methodologies have changed to be consistent with the clinical needs of patients, and alternate delivery systems are readily available.

IV fluids are mistakenly referred to as *IV solutions*. The term *solution* is defined in the *United States Pharmacopeia* (USP) as a liquid preparation that contains one or more soluble chemical substances usually dissolved in water. Solutions are distinguished from injections, for example, because they are not intended for administration by infusion or injection. Moreover, methods of preparation may vary widely. The USP refers to parenteral fluids as injections, and methods of preparation must follow standards for injection. IV injections must meet the tests, standards, and all specifications of the USP applicable to injections. This includes quantitative and qualitative assays of infusions, including tests for pyrogens and sterility (McEvoy, 2007).

Particulate Matter

Each fluid container must be carefully examined to detect cracks. The fluid must be examined for cloudiness or particles. The final responsibility falls on the pharmacist and the nurse who administers the fluid. Tests to detect particulate matter, and standards for an acceptable limit of particles, have been established by the USP. A large-volume injection for single-dose infusion meets the requirements of the test if it contains not more than 50 particles per milliliter that are ≥ 10.0 μm and not more than 5 particles per milliliter that are ≥ 25.0 m in effective linear dimension.

pH Value

The pH indicates hydrogen ion concentration or free acid activity in solution. All IV fluids must meet the pH requirements set forth by the USP. Most of these requirements call for a fluid that is slightly acid, usually ranging in pH from 3.5 to 6.2. Dextrose requires a slightly acid pH to yield a stable fluid. Heat sterilization, used for all commercial fluids, contributes to the acidity. It is important to know the pH of the commonly used IV fluids because it may affect the stability of an added drug and cause the drug to deteriorate. The acidity of dextrose fluids has been criticized for its corrosive effect on veins.

Water

The cell wall separates the intracellular compartment from the extracellular compartment. The capillary endothelium and the arterial and venous walls divide the extracellular compartment into the intravascular and interstitial compartments. Water flows freely through cell and vessel calls and is distributed throughout these compartments. (Grocott, Mythen, & Gan, 2005).

Osmosis

Osmosis is the process by which a solvent, usually water, moves through a semipermeable membrane from a solution of lower concentration to a solution of higher concentration. The osmotic pressure exerted by particles in solution is determined by the number of particles per volume of fluid versus the mass or size of the particles (Phillips, 2005).

Capillary pressure has a tendency to force fluid and dissolved substances through the capillary pore into the interstitial spaces.

Tonicity

A change in water content causes cells to swell or shrink. Tonicity refers to the tension or effect that the osmotic pressure of a solution, with impermeable solutes, exerts on cell size due to water movement across the cell membrane.

Solutions are classified according to the tonicity of the fluid in relation to normal blood plasma. The osmolality of blood plasma is 290 mOsm/L. Fluid that approximates 290 mOsm/L is considered isotonic. IV fluids with an osmolality significantly > 290 mOsm (+50 mOsm) are considered hypertonic, whereas those with an osmolality significantly < 290 mOsm (–50 mOsm) are hypotonic.

Parenteral fluids usually range from approximately one-half isotonic (0.45% sodium chloride) to 5 to 10 times isotonic (25% to 50% dextrose). The tonicity of the fluid infused into the circulation affects fluid and electrolyte metabolism and may result in disastrous clinical disturbances (see Table 9-1 for more information on the effects of isotonic, hypertonic, and hypotonic fluids).

Knowing the osmolality of the infusion and the physical effect it produces alerts the nurse to potential fluid and electrolyte imbalances. The choice of veins used for an infusion is affected by the tonicity of the fluid; hyperosmolar fluids, for example, must be infused

TABLE 9-1   RESULTS OF INFUSION OF FLUIDS WITH DIFFERENT TONICITIES

Tonicity	Effect
Hypertonic fluid	Increases osmotic pressure of plasma Draws fluid from the cells
Hypotonic fluid	Lowers the osmotic pressure of plasma Causes fluid to invade the cell
Isotonic fluid	Increases extracellular volume

through veins that carry a large blood volume to dilute the fluid and prevent trauma to the vessel.

The tonicity of the fluid also affects the rate at which it can be infused. Hypertonic dextrose infused rapidly may result in diuresis and dehydration.

Because of the direct and effective role osmolality plays in IV therapy, the nurse involved in administering IV fluids needs to be familiar with various terms and calculations. For instance, the *osmotic pressure* is proportional to the total number of particles in the fluid. The *milliosmole* (mOsm) is the unit that measures the particles or the osmotic pressure. By converting milliequivalents to milliosmoles, an approximate osmolality may be determined.

FLUIDS CONTAINING UNIVALENT ELECTROLYTES

Each milliequivalent is approximately equal to a milliosmole because univalent electrolytes, when ionized, carry one charge per particle. An injection of normal saline (0.9% sodium chloride) contains 154 mEq sodium and 154 mEq chloride per liter of fluid, making a total of 308 mEq/L, or approximately 308 mOsm/L.

FLUIDS CONTAINING DIVALENT ELECTROLYTES

Because each particle carries two charges when ionized, the milliequivalents per liter of fluid or the number of electrical charges per liter when divided by the charge per ion (2) gives the approximate number of particles or milliosmoles per liter. As an example, when 20 mEq magnesium sulfate is introduced into a liter of fluid, each ionized particle carries two charges. By dividing 20 mEq or 20 charges by 2, an approximate 10 particles or 10 mOsm/L is reached for each component, or 20 mOsm/L total.

The osmolality of electrolytes in solution may be accurately computed but involves using the atomic weight and the concentration of the given electrolytes in milligrams per liter. The methods for accurately computing the osmolality of an electrolyte, such as potassium (K), in solution follow:

$$\frac{\text{milligrams of electrolyte / L}}{(\text{Atomic weight})(\text{valance})} = \text{milliosmoles / L}$$

$$\text{Example} : 35 \,\text{mg K / L}$$

$$\frac{35}{35 \times 1} = 0.5 \,\text{mOsm / L}$$

$$\text{Example} : 40 \,\text{mg K / L}$$

$$\frac{40}{40 \times 2} = 1 \,\text{mOsm / L}$$

KINDS AND COMPOSITION OF FLUIDS

Various kinds of fluids are used for parenteral injections. These fluids are composed of dextrose in water, sodium chloride in water, sodium bicarbonate, ammonium chloride, and other substances.

Premixed Solutions

A significant number of solutions are available premixed. Premixed solutions have been sterilized following the admixture process, ensuring longer shelf life. The pH has already been adjusted to enhance stability, and the correct amount of medication has been added to the proper volume and type of solution.

Care should be taken in selecting premixed solutions when multiple types are available. For example, premixed solutions with potassium chloride are available in several concentrations. Other premixed solutions include heparin sodium, theophylline, lidocaine hydrochloride, and dopamine hydrochloride. Antibiotics are often premixed in small-volume parenterals. In addition to premixed solutions, some products allow the medication container to be connected to the IV solution. In general, premixed solutions tend to increase cost.

Dextrose in Water

When glucose is part of parenteral injections, it is usually referred to as *dextrose*, a designation by the USP for glucose of requisite purity. Dextrose is available in concentrations of 2.5%, 5%, 10%, 20%, and 50% in water. To determine the osmolality or the caloric value of a dextrose fluid, the nurse needs to know the total number of grams or milligrams per liter. Because 1 mL water weighs 1 g, and 1 mL is 1% of 100 mL, milliliters, grams, and percentages can be used interchangeably when calculating solution strength. Thus, dextrose 5% in water equals 5 g dextrose in 100 mL, or 50 g dextrose in 1 L. The metabolic effects of dextrose are listed in Box 9-1.

CALORIES

Hexoses (glucose or dextrose and fructose) do not yield 4 calories per gram, as do dietary carbohydrates (e.g., starches). Each gram of hydrous or anhydrous dextrose provides approximately 3.4 or 3.85 calories, respectively. One liter of 5% glucose infusion yields 170 calories; 1 L of 10% glucose infusion yields 340 calories (USP, 2012).

TONICITY OF DEXTROSE 5% IN WATER

Dextrose 5% in water is considered an isotonic fluid because its tonicity approximates that of normal blood plasma, or 290 mOsm/L. Because dextrose is a nonelectrolyte and the total number of particles in solution does not depend on ionization, the osmolality of dextrose

---

BOX 9-1   METABOLIC EFFECTS OF DEXTROSE

- Provides calories for essential energy
- Improves hepatic function because glucose is converted into glycogen by the liver
- Spares body protein (prevents unnecessary breakdown of protein tissue)
- Prevents ketosis or excretion of organic acid (which may occur when fat is burned by the body without an adequate supply of glucose)
- Stored intracellularly in the liver as glycogen, causes the shift of potassium from the extracellular to the intracellular fluid compartment (*Note: This effect is desired as treatment for hyperkalemia. It is achieved by infusing dextrose and insulin.*)

fluids is determined differently from that of electrolyte fluids. One millimole (one formula weight in milligrams) of dextrose represents 1 mOsm (unit of osmotic pressure). One millimole of monohydrated glucose is 198 mg, and 1 liter of dextrose 5% in water contains 50,000 mg. Thus:

$$\frac{50,000 \text{ mg}}{198} = 252 \text{ mOsm / L}$$

pH VALUE

The USP requirement for the pH of dextrose fluids is 3.5 to 6.5. This broad range may at times contribute to an incompatibility in one bottle of dextrose and not in another when an additive is involved.

INDICATIONS FOR USE

Dextrose fluids are used for patients with dehydration, hyponatremia, and hyperkalemia. They are also vehicles for drug delivery and nutrition.

DEHYDRATION

In cases of dehydration, dextrose 2.5% in water and dextrose 5% in water provide immediate hydration for medical as well as surgical patients. Dextrose 5% in water is considered isotonic only in the bottle. Once infused into the vascular system, the dextrose is rapidly metabolized, leaving water. The water decreases the osmotic pressure of the blood plasma and invades the cells, providing immediately available water to dehydrated tissues.

HYPERNATREMIA

If the patient is not in circulatory difficulty with extracellular expansion, dextrose 5% in water may be administered to decrease the concentration of sodium.

MEDICATION ADMINISTRATION

Many of the drugs for IV therapy are added to infusions of dextrose 5% in water.

NUTRITION

Concentrations of dextrose 20% and 50% in conjunction with electrolytes provide long-term nutrition. Insulin is frequently added to prevent overtaxing the islet tissue of the pancreas.

PATIENT SAFETY

Because the kidneys do not store potassium, prolonged fluid therapy with electrolyte-free fluids may result in hypokalemia. This happens when cells are anabolized by the metabolism of glucose and potassium shifts from the extracellular to the intracellular fluid. Conversely, when renal function is impaired, IV potassium should be used cautiously. Remain alert for signs of hyperkalemia. If such signs develop, notify the physician/LIP and be prepared to replace fluid components with more appropriate electrolytes.

HYPERKALEMIA

Infusions of dextrose in high concentration with insulin cause anabolism (buildup of body cells), which results in a shift of potassium from the extracellular to the intracellular compartment, thereby lowering the serum potassium concentration.

DANGERS OF USE

Among abnormalities resulting from infusion of dextrose are dehydration, hypokalemia, hyperinsulinism, and water intoxication.

DEHYDRATION

Osmotic diuresis occurs when dextrose is infused at a rate faster than the patient's ability to metabolize it. A heavy load of nonmetabolized glucose increases the osmolality of the blood and acts as a diuretic; the increased solute load requires more fluid for excretion. A normal, healthy person with a urine specific gravity of 1.029 to 1.032 requires 15 mL water to excrete 1 g solute, whereas people with poor kidney function or low concentrating ability of the kidneys require much more water to excrete the same amount of solute (Metheny, 2012).

HYPERINSULINISM

A rapid infusion of hypertonic carbohydrate solutes may result in hyperinsulinism. In response to a rise in blood glucose level, extra insulin pours from the beta cells of the pancreatic islets in an attempt to metabolize the infused carbohydrate. Terminating the infusion may leave excess insulin in the body, resulting in symptoms such as nervousness, sweating, and weakness caused by the severe hypoglycemia that may be induced. Typically, after infusion of hypertonic dextrose, a small amount of isotonic dextrose is administered to cover the excess insulin (Metheny, 2012).

WATER INTOXICATION

An imbalance resulting from an increase in the volume of the extracellular fluid from water alone is known as water intoxication. Prolonged infusions of isotonic or hypotonic dextrose in water may cause this condition, which is compounded by stress and leads to inappropriate release of antidiuretic hormone (ADH) and fluid retention. The average adult can metabolize water at a rate of approximately 35 to 40 mL/kg/day, and the kidney can safely metabolize only approximately 2,500 to 3,000 mL/day in an average patient receiving IV therapy (Metheny, 2012). Under stress, the patient's ability to metabolize water decreases (Box 9-2).

BOX 9-2   POTENTIAL CONSEQUENCES OF INFUSING SPECIFIC FLUIDS

- *Cellular dehydration* may result from excessive infusions of hypertonic fluids.
- *Water intoxication* results when hypotonic fluid is infused beyond the patient's tolerance for water.
- *Circulatory overload* can result from isotonic fluid administration.

Isotonic dextrose may be administered through a peripheral vein. Hyperosmolar fluids, such as dextrose 50% in water, should be infused into the superior vena cava through central venous access. Hypertonic dextrose administered through a peripheral vein with small blood volume may traumatize the vein and cause thrombophlebitis. Infiltration can result in tissue necrosis.

Sodium-free dextrose injections should not be administered by **hypodermoclysis** (direct administration into subcutaneous tissue to enhance hydration). Dextrose fluids, by attracting body electrolytes in the pooled area of infusions, may cause peripheral circulatory collapse and anuria in sodium-depleted patients.

Electrolyte-free dextrose injections should not be used in conjunction with blood infusions. Dextrose mixed with blood causes **hemolysis** of the red blood cells.

The amount of water required for hydration depends on the clinical condition and the needs of the patient. The average adult patient requires 1,500 to 2,500 mL water each day. In patients with prolonged fever, however, the water requirement depends on the degree of temperature elevation. For example, the 24-hour fluid requirement for a patient with a body temperature between 101°F and 103°F increases by at least 500 mL; the fluid requirement for a prolonged temperature above 103°F increases by at least 1,000 mL.

The rate of administration depends on the patient's condition and the purpose of therapy. When the infusion is used to supply calories, the rate must be slow enough to allow complete metabolism of the glucose (0.5 g/kg/hour in normal adults). The maximum rate usually should not exceed 0.8 g/kg/hour. When the infusion is used to produce diuresis, the rate must be fast enough to prevent complete metabolism of the dextrose, thereby increasing the osmolality of the extracellular fluid.

Isotonic Sodium Chloride Infusions

Sodium chloride injection (0.9%), USP (normal saline), contains 308 mOsm/L (sodium, 154 mEq/L; chloride, 154 mEq/L). It has a pH between 4.5 and 7.0 and is usually supplied in volumes of 1,000, 500, 250, and 100 mL. The term *normal* (or *physiologic*) is misleading because the chloride in normal saline is 154 mEq/L, compared with the normal plasma chloride value of 103 mEq/L, whereas the sodium is 154 mEq/L, or approximately 9% higher than the normal plasma value of 140 mEq/L. Because normal saline lacks the other electrolytes present in plasma, the isotonicity of the fluid depends on the sodium and chloride ions, resulting in a higher concentration of these ions (USP, 2012).

INDICATIONS FOR USE

Normal sodium chloride injection is indicated for the following:

- Extracellular fluid replacement when chloride loss is relatively greater than or equal to sodium loss.
- Treatment of metabolic alkalosis in the presence of fluid loss; the increase in chloride ions provided by the infusion causes a compensatory decrease in the number of bicarbonate ions.

- Sodium depletion. When there is an extracellular fluid volume deficit accompanying the sodium deficit, an isotonic solution of sodium chloride is used to correct the deficit (Metheny, 2012).
- Initiation and termination of blood transfusions. When 0.9% sodium chloride is used to precede a blood transfusion, the hemolysis of red blood cells, which occurs with dextrose in water, is avoided.

PATIENT SAFETY

Sodium chloride 0.9% solution (normal saline) provides more sodium and chloride than the patient needs. Marked electrolyte imbalances have resulted from the almost exclusive use of normal saline. Hypernatremia, acidosis, and circulatory overload may result when normal saline is administered in excess of the patient's tolerance.

Dangers of Use

An adult's dietary requirement for sodium is approximately 90 to 250 mEq/day, with a minimum requirement of 15 mEq and a maximum tolerance of 400 mEq (United States Pharmacopeia [USP], 2012). When 3 L of 0.9% sodium chloride or dextrose 5% in 0.9% sodium chloride is administered, the patient receives 462 mEq sodium (154 mEq/L), a level that exceeds normal tolerance.

Hypernatremia

Infusion of saline during a period of sodium retention—for example, during stress—can result in hypernatremia. The danger of hypernatremia increases in the elderly, in patients with severe dehydration, and in patients with chronic glomerulonephritis; these patients require more water to excrete the salt than do patients with normal renal function. Isotonic saline does not provide water but requires most of its volume for the excretion of salt.

Acidosis

One liter of 0.9% sodium chloride solution contains one third more chloride than is present in the extracellular fluid. When infused in large quantities, the excess chloride ions cause a loss of bicarbonate ions and result in acidosis.

Hypokalemia

Infusion of saline increases potassium excretion and at the same time expands the volume of extracellular fluid, further decreasing the concentration of the extracellular potassium ion.

Circulatory Overload

Continuous infusions of isotonic fluids expand the extracellular compartment and lead to circulatory overload.

Requirements

In an average adult, the daily requirements of sodium chloride are met by infusing 1 L of 0.9% sodium chloride or 1 to 2 L of 4.5% sodium chloride, but the dosage depends on the patient's age, weight, clinical condition, and fluid, electrolyte, and acid–base status.

Dextrose 5% in 0.9% Sodium Chloride

Dextrose 5% in 0.9% sodium chloride (normal or isotonic saline solution), which contains 252 mOsm dextrose (chloride, 154 mEq/L; sodium, 154 mEq/L), has a pH of 3.5 to 6.0 and is available in volumes of 1,000, 500, 250, and 150 mL. When normal saline is infused, the addition of 100 g dextrose prevents both the formation of ketone bodies and the increased demand for water the ketone bodies impose for renal excretion. The dextrose prevents catabolism and, consequently, loss of potassium and intracellular water.

INDICATIONS FOR USE

Isotonic saline with dextrose injection is indicated for the following:

- Temporary treatment of circulatory insufficiency and shock caused by hypovolemia in the immediate absence of a plasma expander
- Early treatment along with plasma or albumin for replacement of loss caused by burns
- Early treatment of acute adrenocortical insufficiency

DANGERS OF USE

The hazards are the same as those for normal saline injection (see preceding section).

Dextrose 10% in 0.9% Sodium Chloride

Dextrose 10% in 0.9% sodium chloride contains 504 mOsm/L dextrose (sodium, 154 mEq/L; chloride, 154 mEq/L), has a pH of 3.5 to 6.0, and is usually supplied in volumes of 1,000 and 500 mL.

INDICATIONS FOR USE

This fluid is used as a nutrient and an electrolyte (sodium and chloride) replenisher.

ADMINISTRATION

Dextrose 10% in 0.9% sodium chloride, because of its hypertonicity, must be administered IV, preferably through a wide vein to dilute the fluid and reduce the risk of trauma to the vessel. Close observation and precautions are necessary to prevent infiltration and damage to the tissues.

Hypertonic Sodium Chloride Infusions

These infusions include 3% sodium chloride (sodium, 513 mEq/L; chloride, 513 mEq/L) and 5% sodium chloride (sodium, 850 mEq/L; chloride, 850 mEq/L).

INDICATIONS FOR USE

Infusion of hypertonic sodium is indicated for

- Severe dilutional hyponatremia (water intoxication). Hypertonic sodium chloride, on infusion, increases the osmotic pressure of the extracellular fluid, drawing water from the cells for excretion by the kidneys.
- Severe sodium depletion. Infusions of hypertonic saline replenish sodium stores. An estimate of the sodium deficit can be made by taking the difference between the normal sodium concentration and the patient's current sodium concentration and multiplying the difference by 60% of the body weight in kilograms; sodium depletion is based on total body water and not on extracellular fluid.

ADMINISTRATION

Hypertonic sodium chloride injection must be administered with great caution to prevent pulmonary edema. Cautions include frequent reevaluation of the patient's clinical and electrolyte status during administration. A 3% or 5% solution of sodium chloride is used to correct the deficit, providing the fluid volume is normal or excessive; the amount of sodium administered depends on the sodium deficit in the plasma (Metheny, 2012).

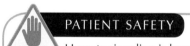

PATIENT SAFETY

Hypertonic saline is harmful to local tissues and could contribute to necrosis.

Hypertonic saline solutions should be infused slowly (e.g., 200 mL over a minimum of 4 hours), and the patient should be observed constantly. The fluid must be infused with great care taken to prevent infiltration and trauma to the tissues. Box 9-3 summarizes the important nursing considerations in the administration of hypertonic saline infusion.

Hypotonic Sodium Chloride in Water

One-half hypotonic saline (0.45% saline containing sodium, 77 mEq/L, and chloride, 77 mEq/L) is used as an electrolyte replenisher. When there is a question regarding the amount of saline fluid required, hypotonic saline is preferred over isotonic saline. In general, 0.45% sodium chloride is preferable to 0.9% sodium chloride.

Hydrating Fluids

Because fluids consisting of dextrose with hypotonic saline provide more water than is required for excretion of salt, they are useful as hydrating fluids. These fluids include dextrose 2.5% in 0.45% saline (dextrose, 126 mOsm/L, with sodium, 77 mEq/L, and chloride, 77 mEq/L), dextrose 5% in 0.45% saline (dextrose, 252 mOsm/L, with sodium, 77 mEq/L,

---

BOX 9-3   NURSING CONSIDERATIONS FOR ADMINISTERING HYPERTONIC (3% AND 5%) SALINE SOLUTION

- Check the serum sodium level before administering the solution and frequently thereafter.
- These solutions are dangerous and should be used only in critical situations in which the serum sodium level is very low (i.e., <110 mEq/L) and the patient exhibits neurologic signs.
- Administer the solution only in intensive care settings where the patient can be closely monitored. Watch for signs of pulmonary edema and worsening of neurologic signs. Use with great caution in patients with congestive heart failure or renal failure.
- Only small volumes are needed (e.g., 5 or 6 mL/kg body weight of 5% sodium chloride) to elevate the serum sodium level by 10 mEq/L. For example, elevating the serum sodium level of a 70-kg patient from 110 to 120 mEq/L requires approximately 350 to 420 mL.
- The serum sodium should not rise more rapidly than 2 mEq/L/hour unless the clinical state of the patient indicates the need for more rapid treatment.
- The fluid can be administered with an electronic infusion device. The device should be monitored closely because no instrument is foolproof.
- Therapy aims to elevate the serum sodium level enough to alleviate neurologic signs—not to raise the serum sodium level to normal quickly. Recommendations include raising the serum concentration no higher than 125 mEq/L with hypertonic saline. The health care provider may prescribe furosemide to promote water loss and prevent pulmonary edema. Urine should be saved because renal sodium and potassium losses may need to be measured to allow for replacement.

---

and chloride, 77 mEq/L), and dextrose 5% in 0.2% saline (dextrose, 252 mOsm/L, with sodium, 34.2 mEq/L, and chloride, 34.2 mEq/L).

INDICATIONS FOR USE

Commonly called *initial hydrating fluids*, hypotonic saline dextrose infusions are indicated as follows:

- To assess the status of the kidneys before electrolyte replacement and maintenance is initiated
- To provide hydration for medical and surgical patients
- To promote diuresis in dehydrated patients

ADMINISTRATION

To assess the status of the kidneys, the fluid is administered at the rate of 8 mL/m² body surface area (BSA) per minute for 45 minutes. The restoration of urine flow shows that the kidneys have begun to function. The hydrating fluid then may be replaced by more specifically needed electrolytes. If after 45 minutes the urine flow is not restored, the rate of infusion is reduced to 2 mL/m² BSA per minute for another hour. If this does not produce diuresis, renal impairment is assumed (Metheny, 2012).

Initial hydrating fluids must be used cautiously in edematous patients with cardiac, renal, or hepatic disease. Once good renal function is obtained, appropriate electrolytes should be administered to prevent hypokalemia.

Hypotonic Multiple-Electrolyte Fluids

Hypotonic multiple-electrolyte fluids are patterned after the type devised by Butler and colleagues at Massachusetts General Hospital, who were the first to emphasize that basic water and electrolyte requirements are proportionate to the BSA. Butler-type fluids are one third to one half as concentrated as plasma. They provide fluid to meet the patient's fluid volume requirement. In so doing, they provide cellular and extracellular electrolytes in quantities balanced between the minimal needs and the maximal tolerance of the patient. These fluids, because of their hypotonicity, provide water for urinary elimination and metabolic needs and take advantage of the body's homeostatic mechanisms to retain the electrolytes and reject those not needed, thereby maintaining water and electrolyte balance.

Hypotonic fluids should contain 5% dextrose for its protein-sparing and antiketogenic effect. The dextrose increases the tonicity of the fluid in the container, but once infused, the dextrose is metabolized, leaving the water and salt. Whether the patient has received too much or too little water depends on the tonicity of the electrolyte and not the osmotic effect of dextrose.

A balanced solution of hypotonic electrolytes is ideal for routine maintenance. Of the various modifications of the Butler-type fluids, those containing 75 mEq total cations per liter are used for older infants, children, and adults.

ADMINISTRATION

A useful formula for maintenance water requirements, based on studies by Crawford, Butler, and Talbot, is the following: maintenance water equals 1,600 mL/m² BSA per day. For obese or edematous patients, this should be calculated on ideal weight rather than actual weight. The water requirement must be patterned after the condition of the patient.

When infection, trauma involving the brain, or stress lead to inappropriate release of ADH, maintenance requirements are less. Excessive fluid losses through urine, stool, expired air, and so forth require increased water. The rate of infusion is usually 3 mL/m² BSA per minute.

DANGERS OF USE: WATER INTOXICATION

The patient's tolerance limits for water can be exceeded. Care should be exercised in maintaining the prescribed flow rate and in ensuring that the patient receives the prescribed volume of fluid. Water intoxication is more likely to occur when inappropriate release of ADH, in response to stress, causes water retention. These patients should be carefully watched to detect any early signs of an imbalance so that a change in therapy can be initiated before the condition becomes precarious. Weighing the patient is the best way to monitor the status of water balance. Daily weights are extremely important in following the state of hydration in extremely ill patients.

Isotonic Multiple-Electrolyte Fluids

Many types of commercial replacement fluids are available. When severe vomiting, diarrhea, or diuresis result in a heavy loss of water and electrolytes, replacement therapy is necessary. Balanced fluids of isotonic electrolytes with an ionic composition similar to plasma are used.

Rapid initial replacement is seldom necessary. However, if a severely dehydrated patient shows signs of impaired circulation and renal function and it is necessary to restore the patient's blood pressure quickly, 30 mL/kg of an isotonic fluid may be provided in the first 1 or 2 hours.

Fluid overload must be prevented. Central venous pressure monitoring is especially helpful in elderly patients and in those with renal or cardiovascular disorders.

Extracellular replacement can usually be assumed to be complete after 48 hours of replacement therapy unless proved otherwise by clinical or laboratory evidence. To continue replacement fluids after deficits have been corrected may result in sodium excess, leading to pulmonary edema or heart failure. Patients receiving replacement therapy should be observed closely to detect any signs of circulatory overload.

Gastric replacement fluids provide the usual electrolytes lost by vomiting or gastric suction. They contain ammonium ions, which are metabolized in the liver to hydrogen ions and urea, replacing the hydrogen ions lost in gastric juices. They are useful in metabolic alkalosis caused by excessive ingestion of sodium bicarbonate. The usual adult dose is 500 to 2,000 mL, and the rate should be consistent with the patient's clinical condition but not >500 mL/hour.

Gastric replacement fluids are contraindicated in patients with hepatic insufficiency or renal failure. They require the same precautions as any fluid containing potassium and should be avoided in patients with renal damage or Addison disease. Also, the low pH causes incompatibilities with many additives.

Lactated Ringer injection is considered safe in certain conditions. Because the electrolyte concentration closely resembles that of the extracellular fluid, it may be used to replace fluid loss from burns and fluid lost as bile and diarrhea. Lactated Ringer injection has been useful in mild acidosis, the lactate ion being metabolized in the liver to bicarbonate.

PATIENT SAFETY

Three liters of lactated Ringer injection contain approximately 390 mEq sodium, which can quickly elevate the sodium level in a patient who is not sodium deficient. Lactated Ringer injection is contraindicated in severe metabolic acidosis or alkalosis and in liver disease or anoxic states that influence lactate metabolism.

Alkalizing Fluids

When anesthesia or disorders, such as dehydration, shock, liver disease, starvation, and diabetes, cause a patient to retain chlorides, ketone bodies, or organic salts, or when a patient loses excessive bicarbonate, metabolic acidosis occurs. Treatment consists of infusing an appropriate alkalizing fluid. These fluids include one-sixth molar isotonic sodium lactate (1.9%, with sodium, 167 mEq/L, and lactate ions, 167 mEq/L, and a pH of 6.0 to 7.3), one-sixth molar sodium bicarbonate injection, USP (1.5%, with sodium, 178 mEq/L, and bicarbonate, 178 mEq/L, and a pH of 7.0 to 8.0), and hypertonic sodium bicarbonate injection (7.5% or 5%).

One-Sixth Molar Sodium Lactate

The lactate ion must be oxidized in the body to carbon dioxide before it can affect acid–base balance; the complete conversion of sodium lactate to bicarbonate requires approximately 1 to 2 hours.

INDICATIONS FOR USE

One-sixth molar sodium lactate is used when acidosis results from a sodium deficiency in such disorders as vomiting, starvation, uncontrolled diabetes mellitus, acute infection, and renal failure.

DANGERS OF USE

Because oxidation is necessary to increase the bicarbonate concentration, sodium lactate is not used for patients experiencing oxygen lack, as in shock or congenital heart disease with persistent cyanosis. It is also contraindicated in liver disease because the lactate ions are improperly metabolized.

ADMINISTRATION

The usual dose is 1 L of a one-sixth molar solution, but the dosage depends on the patient's condition and the serum sodium level. One-sixth molar infusion may be administered by venoclysis or hypodermoclysis and usually at a rate not greater than 300 mL/hour. The patient should be observed closely for any evidence of alkalosis.

Sodium Bicarbonate Injection

Sodium bicarbonate injection, USP (1.5%, with sodium, 178 mEq/L, and bicarbonate, 178 mEq/L), is an isotonic fluid that provides bicarbonate ions for conditions of excess depletion.

IV sodium bicarbonate therapy increases plasma bicarbonate, buffers excess hydrogen ion concentration, raises blood pH, and reverses the clinical manifestations of acidosis.

Sodium bicarbonate in water dissociates to provide sodium (Na^+) and bicarbonate (HCO_3^-) ions. Sodium (Na^+) is the principal cation of the extracellular fluid and plays a large part in the therapy of fluid and electrolyte disturbances. Bicarbonate (HCO_3^-) is a normal constituent of body fluids, and the normal plasma level ranges from 24 to 31 mEq/L. Plasma concentration is regulated by the kidney through acidification of the urine when there is a deficit or by alkalinization of the urine when there is an excess. Bicarbonate anion is considered "labile" since at a proper concentration of hydrogen ion (H^+), it may be converted to carbonic acid (H_2CO_3) and thence to its volatile form, carbon dioxide (CO_2) excreted by the lung. Normally, a ratio of 1:20 (carbonic acid; bicarbonate) is present in the extracellular fluid. In a healthy adult with normal kidney function, practically all the glomerular filtered bicarbonate ion is reabsorbed; < 1% is excreted in the urine.

INDICATIONS FOR USE

Sodium bicarbonate injection, USP, is indicated in the treatment of metabolic acidosis that may occur in severe renal disease, uncontrolled diabetes, circulatory insufficiency due to shock or severe dehydration, extracorporeal circulation of blood, cardiac arrest, and severe primary lactic acidosis. Sodium bicarbonate is further indicated in the treatment of certain drug intoxications, including barbiturates (where dissociation of the barbiturate–protein complex is desired), in poisoning by salicylates or methyl alcohol, and in hemolytic reactions requiring alkalinization of the urine to diminish nephrotoxicity of hemoglobin and its breakdown products. Sodium bicarbonate also is indicated in severe diarrhea, which is often accompanied by a significant loss of bicarbonate.

Treatment of metabolic acidosis should, if possible, be superimposed on measures designed to control the basic cause of the acidosis—for example, insulin in uncomplicated diabetes, blood volume restoration in shock. But since an appreciable time interval may elapse before all of the ancillary effects are brought about, bicarbonate therapy is indicated to minimize risks inherent to the acidosis itself.

Vigorous bicarbonate therapy is required in any form of metabolic acidosis where a rapid increase in plasma total CO_2 content is crucial—for example, cardiac arrest, circulatory insufficiency due to shock or severe dehydration—and in severe primary lactic acidosis or severe diabetic acidosis. Sodium bicarbonate injection is used for severe hyperpnea early in the treatment of severe acidosis until the signs of dyspnea and hyperpnea subside. The bicarbonate ion is released in the form of carbon dioxide through the lungs, leaving an excess of sodium cation behind to exert its electrolyte effect (Phillips, 2010).

Recommendations and practice related to pharmacologic management of cardiopulmonary resuscitation suggest a cautious use of sodium bicarbonate to manage acidosis (Metheny, 2012).

ADMINISTRATION

The usual dose is 500 mL in a 1.5% solution. The dosage depends on the patient's weight, condition, and carbon dioxide content. If the isotonic infusion is not available, it may be made by adding two 50-mL ampules containing 3.75 g each of sodium bicarbonate to 400 mL hypotonic saline.

The fluid should be infused slowly IV. Rapid injection may induce cellular acidity and death.

The patient should be watched for signs of hypocalcemic tetany, and calcium supplement should be administered if required; calcium does not ionize well in an alkaline medium. Extravasation of hypertonic sodium bicarbonate injections must be avoided. Bicarbonate therapy should cease when the pH reaches 7.2.

Acidifying Infusions

Normal saline (0.9% sodium chloride injection, USP) is not usually listed among the **acidifying infusions**. However, because metabolic alkalosis is a condition associated with excess bicarbonate and loss of chloride, isotonic saline provides conservative treatment. When the chloride ions are infused, the bicarbonate decreases in compensation and the alkalosis is relieved.

Ammonium chloride, the usual acidifying agent, is available as isotonic 0.9% ammonium chloride injection (ammonium, 167 mEq/L; chloride, 167 mEq/L) and hypertonic 2.14% ammonium chloride injection (ammonium, 400 mEq/L; chloride, 400 mEq/L). The pH range is 4.0 to 6.0. Both concentrations are supplied in 1-L bottles.

INDICATIONS FOR USE

Ammonium chloride is used as an acidifying infusion in severe metabolic alkalosis caused by loss of gastric secretions, pyloric stenosis, or other causes. Ammonium ions are converted by the liver to hydrogen ions and to ammonia, which is excreted as urea.

ADMINISTRATION

The 2.14% ammonium chloride is usually used in the treatment of the adult patient; 0.9% ammonium chloride is used for children.

The dosage depends on the condition of the patient and on an accurate chemical picture, including plasma carbon dioxide–combining power. Ammonium chloride must be infused at a very slow rate to enable the liver to metabolize the ammonium ions, not to exceed 5 mL/ minute in adults. Rapid injection can result in toxic effects, causing irregular breathing, bradycardia, and twitching (USP, 2012). See Table 9-2 for more information on contents of fluids.

PATIENT SAFETY

Because its acidifying effect depends on the liver for conversion, ammonium chloride must not be administered to patients with severe hepatic disease or renal failure. It is contraindicated in any condition in which the patient has a high ammonium level.

TABLE 9-2   CONTENTS OF SELECTED WATER AND ELECTROLYTE SOLUTIONS

Solution	Cautions and Considerations
Dextrose 5% in water (D_5W): No electrolytes	Supplies approximately 170 cal/L and free water to aid in renal excretion of solutes
50 g of dextroses	Should not be used in excessive volumes in patients with increased ADH activity or to replace fluids in hypovolemic patients
0.9% NaCl (isotonic saline): Na^+ 154 mEq/L	Isotonic fluid commonly used to expand the extracellular fluid in presence of hypovolemia
Cl^- 154 mEq/L	Because of relatively high chloride content, can be used to treat mild metabolic alkalosis
0.45% NaCl (½-strength saline): Na^+ 77 mEq/L	A hypotonic solution that provides N^+, Cl^-, and free water; Na^+ and Cl^- provided in fluid allows kidneys to select and retain needed amounts
Cl^- 77 mEq/L	Free water desirable as aid to kidneys in elimination of solutes
0.33% NaCl (⅓-strength saline):	A hypotonic solution that provides Na^+, Cl^-, and free water
Na^+ 56 mEq/L Cl^- 56 mEq/L	Often used to treat hypernatremia (because this solution contains a small amount of N^+, it dilutes the plasma sodium while not allowing it to drop too rapidly)

(Continued)

TABLE 9-2	CONTENTS OF SELECTED WATER AND ELECTROLYTE SOLUTIONS *(Continued)*
Solution	**Cautions and Considerations**
3% NaCl: Na⁺ 513 mEq/L	Grossly hypertonic solutions used only to treat severe hyponatremia
Cl⁻ 513 mEq/L	See Box 9-3 summary of important nursing considerations in administration of dangerous solutions

5% NaCl:
  Na⁺ 855 mEq/L
  Cl⁻ 855 mEq/L	

Lactated Ringer solution:
  Na⁺ 130 mEq/L
  K⁺ 4 mEq/L
	A roughly isotonic solution that contains multiple electrolytes in approximately the same concentrations as found in plasma (note that this solution is lacking in Mg and PO₄)

Ca²⁺ 3 mEq/L Cl⁻ 109 mEq/L	Used in the treatment of hypovolemia, burns, and fluid lost as bile or diarrhea
Lactate (metabolized to bicarbonate) 28 mEq/L	Useful in treating mild metabolic acidosis

Sodium lactate solution, 1/6 M:
  N⁺ 167 mEq/L
  Cl⁻ 167 mEq/L
	A roughly isotonic solution used to correct severe metabolic acidosis (lactate is metabolized to bicarbonate in 1–2 h by the liver)

	Not used in patients with liver disease (lactate cannot be converted to bicarbonate in such patients); also not used in patients with oxygen lack (unable adequately to convert lactate to bicarbonate)
Sodium bicarbonate, 5%: Na⁺ 595 mEq/L	A very hypertonic solution used to correct severe metabolic acidosis
Cl⁻ 595 mEq/L	Should be cautiously administered at a slow rate, using electronic infusion device (EID)
	Should be administered only with extreme caution to salt-retaining patients (e.g., those with cardiac, renal, or liver damage)
Ammonium chloride, 2.14%:	Acidifying solution used to correct severe metabolic alkalosis
	Because of high ammonium content, must be administered cautiously in those with compromised hepatic function

Potassium chloride, 0.15%:
  K⁺ 20 mEq/L
  Cl⁻ 20 mEq/L
	Premixed potassium chloride solution

Potassium chloride, 0.30%:
  K⁺ 40 mEq/L
  Cl⁻ 40 mEq/L
	Premixed potassium chloride solution

NURSING FOCUSED ASSESSMENT

Assessment of a patient for parenteral fluid therapy includes collecting a nursing history, performing a focused physical assessment, review of pertinent laboratory tests, and evaluating intake and output. The two systems with the most direct impact on fluid balance are the renal and cardiovascular systems. Box 9-4 summarizes laboratory findings for monitoring effective parenteral fluid therapy.

BOX 9-4 LABORATORY VALUES ASSESSED DURING PARENTERAL FLUID THERAPY

Renal function and fluid volume changes
- Blood urea nitrogen to assess renal function
- Creatinine
- Specific gravity
- Urine osmolarity

Deviations from normal serum values
- Serum electrolytes

Prior to replacement of RBC, WBC, and platelets or ECF expansion
- Complete blood count

Acid–base balance assessment
- Blood gases

Evaluation prior to plasma volume expanders
- Coagulation studies

Osmotic diuresis

Serum glucose

A rational approach is necessary if the patient is to receive safe and successful IV therapy. In the past, the nurse's technical responsibility in maintaining the infusion and patent venous access were emphasized. Changes in the patient's status can occur quickly and in the absence of the physician/LIP. Today, the nurse's responsibility consists of monitoring the fluid and electrolyte status of the patient as well as the progress of the infusion. Greater emphasis must be placed on the causes and effects of fluid and electrolyte abnormalities so that these imbalances may be anticipated and recognized before they become disastrous. Further assessment includes specific monitoring parameters.

Monitoring Parameters

The nurse should be familiar with the parameters used in evaluating fluid and electrolyte imbalances and in supplying fluid and electrolyte requirements.

CENTRAL VENOUS PRESSURE

Central venous pressure monitoring provides a simple, accurate, and valuable guide in detecting changes in blood volume and assessing fluid requirements. It is particularly valuable in assessing the ability of the heart to tolerate the infusion. Many erroneous conclusions are drawn from false values recorded when the infusion line is not properly responsive to right atrial pressures.

Normal venous pressure indicates an adequate circulatory blood volume; elevated venous pressure may mean an increase in circulatory volume and right heart pressure, with the possibility of circulatory overload. It may also indicate other problems such as a pulmonary embolus, myocardial infarction, or lack of digitalis. Determination of the hematocrit value supplements clinical information.

A low venous pressure, too low to measure, indicates that the patient has probably lost fluid or blood. The nurse must not overlook the fact that fluid loss can result from drug-induced vasodilation or improper administration of IV fluids. If rapid infusion of dextrose exceeds the patient's tolerance, massive diuresis with dehydration and diminished circulatory volume may occur. The decreased venous blood return into the right atrium is reflected by a decrease in the central venous pressure.

PULSE

The pulse quality and rate provide valuable clinical information for assessing fluid and electrolyte changes in the patient. A high pulse pressure, bounding and not easily obliterated by pressure, indicates a high cardiac output caused by circulatory overload. A regular pulse, easily obliterated by pressure, indicates low cardiac output resulting from a lowered blood volume.

A bounding, easily obliterated pressure signifies a drop in blood pressure with a wide pulse pressure, indicative of impending circulatory collapse. As the patient's condition deteriorates, the pulse becomes rapid, weak, thready, and easily obliterated, signifying circulatory collapse.

HAND VEINS

Examination of the hand veins provides a means of evaluating the plasma volume. The hand veins usually empty in 3 to 5 seconds when the hand is elevated and fill in the same length of time when the hand is lowered to a dependent position. Peripheral vein filling takes longer than 3 to 5 seconds in patients with sodium depletion and extracellular dehydration.

Slow emptying of the hand veins indicates overhydration and excessive blood volume; slow filling indicates a low blood volume and often precedes hypotension. Hand veins that become engorged and clearly visible indicate an increase in plasma volume secondary to an interstitial-to-vascular fluid shift or an increase in extracellular fluid volume (Metheny, 2012). A rapid guide for fluid assessment is found in Table 9-3.

NECK VEINS

Changes in fluid volume are reflected by changes in neck vein filling, provided the patient is not in heart failure. In the supine position, the patient's external jugular veins fill to the anterior border of the sternocleidomastoid muscle. Flat neck veins in the supine position indicate a decreased plasma volume.

WEIGHT

A sudden gain or loss in weight is a significant sign of a change in the fluid volume. A change in the volume of body fluid can be computed by weighing the patient daily at the same time of day, on the same scales, with the same amount of clothing. A loss or gain of 1 kg body weight reflects a loss or gain of 1 L body fluid. A rapid 2% loss of total body weight indicates mild fluid volume deficit, and a rapid loss of 8% or more represents severe fluid volume deficit. Conversely, weight gain occurs when total fluid intake exceeds total

TABLE 9-3	RAPID FLUID IMBALANCE ASSESSMENT GUIDE	
Assessment Focus	Fluid Volume Excess (Hypervolemia)	Fluid Volume Deficit (Hypovolemia)
Cardiovascular system	Bounding pulse	Decreased blood pressure
	Elevated pulse rate	Decreased pulse rate
	Jugular distention	Flat neck veins
	Overdistended hand veins	Narrow pulse pressure
		Slow hand vein filling
Integumentary system	Warm, moist skin	Decreased turgor over sternum/forehead
	Sternal fingerprinting	
		Lowered skin temperature
Neurologic system	—	Altered orientation: confusion
Respiratory system	Moist crackles	Clear lungs
	Respiratory rate >20/min	
	Dyspnea	
	Pulmonary edema	
Eyes	Periorbital edema	Dry conjunctiva
		Sunken eyes
		Decreased tearing
Lips	—	Dry and cracked
Mouth	—	Dry mucous membranes
Tongue	—	Dry, leathery texture
		Longitudinal furrows
Weight	Mild: 2% above normal	Mild: <2% below normal
	Moderate: 5% above normal	Moderate: 5% below normal
	Severe: >8% above normal	Severe: >8% below normal

fluid output. A rapid 2% gain of total body weight indicates mild fluid volume excess; a 5% gain represents a moderate fluid volume excess; and 8% or greater indicates a severe fluid volume excess.

THIRST

Thirst is an important symptom denoting a deficit in body fluid or, more specifically, cellular dehydration. This type of dehydration occurs when the extracellular fluid becomes hypertonic, either as a result of water deprivation or the infusion of hypertonic saline. The increase in osmotic pressure causes fluid to be drawn from the cells, resulting in cellular dehydration, the stimulus to thirst. Normally, thirst governs the need for water, but, in certain conditions, the lack of thirst may accompany dehydration. This is especially true in the aged, in whom thirst is not urgent. These patients may lose their thirst and as a result become severely dehydrated before the condition is recognized. In the severely burned patient, the great thirst experienced may lead to ingestion of excess water and to a serious sodium deficit.

INTAKE AND OUTPUT

Water intake and output should be carefully measured and recorded. Hourly urine output measurements may be particularly important. A urine output of 200 mL/hour indicates that too much water is being infused too rapidly. By regulating the urine output between 30 and 50 mL/hour, the patient receives at least enough fluid for the kidneys to work efficiently.

A decreased urinary output accompanies a decreased blood volume; changes in the arterial pressure and pressure in the glomeruli result in the oliguria or anuria of profound shock. The increase in urinary output accompanying an increase in blood volume is primarily caused by changes in arterial pressure and pressure in the glomeruli. Output should include urine, vomitus, diarrhea, drainage from fistulas, and drainage from suction apparatus.

SKIN TURGOR

Observing changes in skin turgor (elasticity) and texture is helpful in assessing the state of water balance. To test skin turgor, the skin is pinched over the sternum, inner aspect of the thigh, or forehead in the adult or the medial aspects of the thigh or abdomen in the child and then released; in the normal person, the pinched skin returns to its original position. Skin that remains in a raised position for several seconds indicates a deficit in fluid volume. Decreased skin turgor is a late sign in dehydration. It occurs with moderate-to-severe dehydration. Fluid loss of 5% of the body weight is considered mild dehydration, 10% is moderate, and 15% or more is severe dehydration.

TONGUE TURGOR

A dry, leathery tongue may indicate a fluid volume deficit or mouth breathing. To differentiate between the two, the mucous membrane may be checked for moisture by running the finger between the gums and the cheek; dryness indicates a fluid volume deficit.

Normally, the tongue has one longitudinal furrow. In the patient with fluid volume deficit, additional longitudinal furrows are present, and the tongue is smaller because of the fluid loss. Not significantly affected by age, the tongue is a good parameter to measure in all age groups.

EDEMA

Edema reflects an increase in the extracellular fluid volume outside the circulating intravascular compartment. It depends on an imbalance or a disturbance in the exchange of water and electrolytes between the patient and the environment or the exchange of water and electrolytes between the compartments of the body. The fluid and electrolyte exchange between the body compartments may be affected by an alteration in the circulatory system, the lymphatic system, or the concentration of albumin in the serum; water and electrolytes escape from the circulation faster than they enter, and edema ensues.

Edema may be generalized, as in congestive failure; localized, as with ascites; or peripheral. By detecting edema early, a clinical imbalance may be corrected before the patient's condition deteriorates. Early peripheral edema may be detected by fingerprinting, a procedure

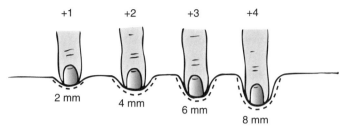

FIGURE 9-1 Edema scale. Severity of edema is ranked on a scale of +1 to +4, with +1 being barely perceptible and +4 being visible and remarkable.

in which the finger is rolled over the bony prominence of the sternum or tibia. As edema increases, pitting edema occurs and may be detected by pressure of the fingers on the subcutaneous tissue. Figure 9-1 shows the degrees of edema.

In generalized edema, such as that seen in cardiac failure, total extracellular water volume as well as interstitial edema increase. Symptoms such as venous engorgement, restlessness, dyspnea, cyanosis, and pulmonary rales indicate generalized edema.

Laboratory Values

Laboratory values, when used to supplement clinical observations, aid in forming diagnostic and therapeutic guidelines. Electrolyte studies (serum sodium, potassium, chloride, bicarbonate, and pH) performed daily are important in assessing the fluid and electrolyte status of the patient receiving IV fluids. In patients with massive electrolyte losses, such studies may be required two or three times a day. Blood cell count and hematocrit determinations are helpful in detecting hemoconcentration or hemodilution; *hemoconcentration* reflects a diminished plasma volume caused by dehydration, and *hemodilution*, an increased volume from overtreatment with water.

Measurement of serum protein with the albumin/globulin ratio helps in detecting a change in fluid volume; large quantities of rapidly administered parenteral fluid dilute and decrease the serum protein concentration. This determination is helpful when used to supplement clinical observation—otherwise; it may be misleading and interpreted as showing actual depletion. A decrease in serum protein reduces the osmotic pressure of the extracellular compartment, causing some edema and loss of plasma volume. Blood urea nitrogen should be measured frequently to evaluate kidney function, an important parameter in treating fluid and electrolyte imbalances.

CLINICAL DISTURBANCES OF WATER AND ELECTROLYTE METABOLISM

Most of the common clinical disturbances in water and electrolyte balance result from changes in the volume of total body water or in one or more of the fluid compartments of the body. Clinical disturbances in water and electrolyte metabolism have been classified into six types: isotonic, hypertonic, and hypotonic expansion and isotonic, hypertonic, and hypotonic contraction. These are discussed in the following sections.

Isotonic Expansion

Isotonic expansion (circulatory overload) occurs when fluids of the same tonicity as plasma are infused into the vascular circulation. Because fluids isotonic to plasma do not affect the osmolality, water does not flow from the extracellular to the intracellular compartment. The extracellular compartment expands in proportion to the fluid infused and is the only compartment affected. The increase in the volume of fluid dilutes the concentration of hemoglobin and lowers the hematocrit and total protein levels, but the serum sodium level remains the same.

Isotonic expansion is a critical complication of IV therapy. Patients who receive isotonic fluids around the clock are at particular risk and should be observed closely for early signs of circulatory overload. Sodium chloride (0.9%) or fluids containing balanced isotonic multiple electrolytes are used for preexisting or continuing fluid and electrolyte losses and are not the ideal fluids for maintenance therapy. The electrolyte isotonicity of these fluids causes expansion of the extracellular compartment and does not provide the extra water that balanced hypotonic fluids provide for the kidney to retain or secrete as needed. The early postoperative or posttrauma patient is susceptible to this critical complication. The increased endocrine response to stress during the first 2 to 5 days after surgery results in retention of sodium chloride and water. When a patient under stress is receiving isotonic infusions, the nurse must anticipate and watch for signs of circulatory overload.

Elderly patients receiving isotonic fluids must be carefully monitored because they have a lower tolerance for fluids and electrolytes. Because they are also likely to have some degree of cardiac and renal impairment, the ability of the kidneys to eliminate fluid is likely to be diminished. The status of these patients can change quickly. In the patient who has had a craniotomy, large-volume isotonic infusions can increase the intracranial pressure and prove detrimental.

Patients who are potential candidates for isotonic expansion must be watched carefully and turned frequently to prevent fluid from settling in the lungs. Pulmonary edema can result from the cardiac and pulmonary side effects of IV therapy. The apices of the lungs, which are high, tend to be fairly dry, but the bases of the lungs, posteriorly and inferiorly, can be fairly wet (Metheny, 2012). As a result, hypostatic pneumonia secondary to gravity may develop.

MANIFESTATIONS

The nurse who monitors IV infusions must be familiar with the early clinical manifestations that accompany isotonic expansion to recognize and prevent its development; mild pulmonary edema progressing to severe pulmonary edema is a late stage that must be prevented. Early clinical manifestations include (a) weight gain; (b) increased fluid intake over output; (c) high pulse pressure; (d) increase in central venous pressure; (e) peripheral hand vein emptying time; (f) peripheral edema; and (g) hoarseness. If IV therapy is allowed to continue, isotonic expansion becomes more apparent and dangerous, with easily recognized signs: cyanosis, dyspnea, coughing, and neck vein engorgement. Laboratory characteristics include a drop in the hematocrit value and reduced concentrations of hemoglobin and total protein.

TREATMENT

Treatment for circulatory overload when detected early is relatively simple and consists of withholding all fluids until excess water, and electrolytes have been eliminated by the body. After the condition is rectified, hypotonic maintenance fluids provide the patient with fluid and a minimum daily requirement of electrolytes. The hypotonicity of the fluid allows the kidneys to maintain the needed amount and selectively retain or excrete the excess.

Isotonic Contraction

Isotonic contraction occurs when there is loss of fluid and electrolytes isotonic to the extracellular fluid, such as whole blood or large volumes of fluid from diarrhea or vomiting. The extracellular compartment contracts. Because the fluid lost is isotonic, the osmolality of the extracellular compartment remains unchanged and no movement of water occurs between the compartments; only the extracellular volume is affected.

MANIFESTATIONS

Because of the loss of fluid, the hematocrit level and the concentrations of hemoglobin and total protein are increased. The serum sodium concentration does not change. Clinical manifestations include

- Weight loss
- Negative fluid balance (a decrease in urinary output but a greater output than total fluid intake)
- Regular pulse rate, easily obliterated by pressure, and, as the patient's condition deteriorates, becoming weak and thready
- Possible increase in peripheral hand vein filling time above the normal 3 to 5 seconds when the hand is moved from an elevated to a dependent position

TREATMENT

Treatment consists of replacing the fluid loss with isotonic fluids containing balanced electrolytes.

Hypertonic Expansion

Hypertonic expansion occurs when the volume of body water is increased by the IV infusion of hypertonic saline. Sodium chloride 3% or 5% is used to replace a massive sodium loss or remove excess accumulation of body fluids, but, if the infusion is administered rapidly, hypertonic expansion can result. The saline increases the osmotic pressure of the extracellular compartment, causing water to be drawn from the intracellular compartment until both compartments are isosmotic. The volume of the extracellular compartment increases and that of the intracellular compartment decreases. The osmolality of the extracellular fluid is higher than before the infusion but lower than the high level after the infusion because of the increased extracellular fluid volume.

Caution must be used in the IV administration of hypertonic saline fluid. Circulatory overload with hypernatremia can occur. An understanding of the reason for the infusion, the condition of the patient, the proper rate of administration, and the signs and symptoms of hypertonic expansion provides a basis for sound IV practice.

MANIFESTATIONS

Clinical manifestations include a gain in body weight dependent on the volume infused. A small volume (500 mL) does not contribute to a significant weight gain (Metheny, 2012).

An increased sodium load results in a decreased rate of water excretion; however, the abrupt increase in plasma volume may cause an increase in the rate of water excretion as the body attempts to excrete the excess salt and water. The degree of thirst depends on the hypertonicity of the plasma and consequently the amount of cellular dehydration.

Peripheral hand vein emptying time may be increased beyond the normal 5 seconds when the hand is elevated but depends on the degree of expansion of the extracellular compartment. A bounding pulse is significant in detecting hypertonic expansion. The serum sodium concentration is increased. The hematocrit level and the concentrations of hemoglobin and total serum protein are decreased as a result of the expanded fluid volume in the extracellular compartment.

TREATMENT

Treatment consists of stopping the infusion to allow the kidneys to eliminate the overload of salt and water. If no cardiovascular side effects are noted, dextrose 5% in water may be infused slowly to reduce the tonicity of the extracellular fluid and replace body water.

Hypertonic Contraction

Hypertonic contraction (hypertonic dehydration) occurs when water is lost without a corresponding loss of salt. This condition occurs in patients who are unable to take sufficient fluid for a prolonged period or in patients with excess insensible water loss through the lungs and skin.

In elderly patients, hypertonic dehydration is a common clinical disturbance; they frequently experience a decrease in the thirst stimuli in response to hypertonicity of body fluids, and adequate intake of fluid is not met. In the unconscious or incontinent patient, frequency and excess urination may go undetected or may be interpreted as a sign of good renal function. A loss of tubular ability to concentrate urine in the aged results in a large urinary volume when an increased solute load is presented to the patient (Metheny, 2012).

Elderly patients also have a diminished response to ADH. Large amounts of dilute urine may be lost, resulting in hypertonic dehydration. To prevent fluid imbalance, the nurse must recognize that individuals differ widely in the water they require; patients whose kidneys do not concentrate urine well require more water than those whose kidneys do concentrate urine well.

The daily fluid requirement must be met. In hypertonic contraction, the loss of water from the extracellular compartment results in an increase in the osmolality, causing water to flow from the cells to the extracellular compartment. Dehydration occurs as water leaves the cellular compartment to replace the plasma volume.

Both the intracellular and the extracellular compartments are affected by the water loss; there is a decrease in volume and an increase in osmolality in both compartments. In contrast, in isotonic contraction, only the extracellular compartment is affected, and the contraction is more serious. Because signs of hypertonic contraction are not obvious in the early stages, the nurse must anticipate such an imbalance and be alert to any changes.

MANIFESTATIONS

Clinically, thirst is an early and reliable sign of hypertonic contraction, but it may be absent in the elderly, complicating early recognition of this imbalance. Weight loss occurs. Negative fluid balance (output greater than intake) is present. Hourly output measurements show a decrease in the rate of excretion of water.

The pulse has a normal quality and is regular in the early stages of hypertonic contraction. The hand vein filling time may be within the normal limits; cellular fluid has partly replenished the plasma.

Irritability, restlessness, and possibly confusion may be present. Skin turgor diminishes and is a sign of dehydration in the later stages. A dry mouth with a furrowed tongue indicates dehydration. Laboratory studies show an increase in serum sodium concentration, hematocrit level, hemoglobin concentration, and total serum protein concentration.

TREATMENT

Treatment consists of hydrating the patient by administering a balanced hypotonic fluid such as the Butler-type fluids: 2,400 mL/m² BSA per day for moderate preexisting deficit and 3,000 mL/m² BSA per day for severe preexisting deficit. The usual rate for IV administration is 3 mL/m² BSA. A therapeutic test for functional renal depression may be necessary before infusing water and electrolytes for maintenance.

Hypotonic Expansion

Hypotonic expansion (water intoxication, dilutional hyponatremia) occurs when the increase in the volume of body fluids is caused by water alone. Water expands the extracellular compartment, causing a decrease in the concentration. Water then diffuses into the cells until both compartments are isosmotic. Both the extracellular and the intracellular compartments are affected; the volume is increased, and the concentration is decreased.

The serum sodium concentration and the hematocrit, hemoglobin, and total serum protein levels are reduced. Hypotonic expansion occurs in patients who are receiving large quantities of electrolyte-free water to replace excessive fluid and electrolytes lost from gastric suction, vomiting, diarrhea or diuresis, or insensibly through the skin.

Patients receiving continuous infusion of dextrose 5% in water are particularly susceptible to water intoxication. This fluid contains 252 mOsm dextrose per liter, making it an isotonic fluid in the container. Once introduced into the circulation, the dextrose is quickly metabolized, leaving the water free to dilute and expand the extracellular compartment. With the decreased osmolality of the extracellular fluid, water diffuses into the cells and hypotonic expansion occurs. The patient's tolerance to water can be exceeded by infusion of excess amounts of hypotonic fluids. The kidneys of the normal adult can metabolize water in amounts of 35 to 45 mL/kg/day, but the kidneys of the average patient can metabolize only 2,500 to 3,000 mL/day; above these volumes, abnormal accumulation of water occurs (Metheny, 2012).

Hypotonic expansion is more likely to occur during the early postoperative period, when retention of water is affected by the response to stress, particularly in the elderly patient, in whom the response to stress is compounded by impairment in renal function.

Small amounts of adjusted hypotonic saline (sodium, 90 mEq/L; chloride, 60 mEq/L; and lactate, 30 mEq/L) may be used in the early postoperative management of the aged.

MANIFESTATIONS

When acute onset of behavioral changes, such as confusion, apathy, and disorientation, occurs in the elderly postoperative patient, overhydration should be suspected.

Central nervous system disturbances such as weakness, muscle twitching, and convulsions are seen, as are headaches, nausea, and vomiting. Fluid intake is increased over fluid output. Weight gain is always present.

Blood pressure usually is normal but may be elevated. Peripheral hand veins are usually full, and hand emptying time is increased beyond the normal 5 seconds when the hand is elevated from a dependent position. The pulse may be regular and not easily obliterated when pressure is applied.

TREATMENT

Treatment consists of withholding all fluids until the excess water is excreted. In severe hyponatremia, it may be necessary to administer small quantities of hypertonic saline to increase the osmotic pressure and the flow of water from the cells to the extracellular compartment for excretion by the kidneys. Hypertonic saline must be used cautiously and must not be administered to patients with congestive heart failure.

Hypotonic Contraction

Hypotonic contraction (hypotonic dehydration) occurs when fluids containing relatively more salt than water are lost from the body. This loss results in a decrease in the effective osmolality of the extracellular compartment. Water is drawn into the cells until osmotic equilibrium is established. Because of the invasion of water, the intracellular compartment is expanded and the extracellular compartment is contracted. This imbalance may result from the loss of salt from any one of several sources: urine of patients receiving diuretics, fistula drainage, severe burns, vomitus, and sweat. The elderly are affected by the loss of small quantities of sodium.

MANIFESTATIONS

Clinical manifestations include weight loss; negative fluid balance; pulse rate that is increased, weak or thready, and easily obliterated; increased hand filling time; and decreased skin turgor. Laboratory studies show a decrease in serum sodium concentration and an increase in hematocrit, hemoglobin, and total serum protein levels.

TREATMENT

Treatment of hypotonic contraction consists of replacing the fluids and electrolytes that have been lost. Because other electrolytes are usually lost along with the sodium loss, a balanced electrolyte fluid may be administered.

Parenteral fluid therapy is a complex treatment modality and an important responsibility of the nurse caring for a patient with potential fluid imbalances.

Review Questions   *Note: Questions below may have more than one right answer.*

1. Which of the following IV dextrose fluids is considered isotonic?
   A. 2.5%
   B. 5%
   C. 0%
   D. 20%

2. A teaching plan for a patient diagnosed with hypermagnesemia should include
   A. Preventing injury due to hypotension or weakness
   B. Availability of an antacid to prevent gastric acidity or reflux
   C. Preventing constipation by routine laxative administration
   D. Restricting fluid intake

3. Edema is the result of excess fluid in which of the following areas?
   A. Interstitial space
   B. Intracellular space
   C. Intrathecal space
   D. Intravascular space

4. One-sixth molar sodium lactate may be infused by which of the following methods?
   A. IV push
   B. Hypodermoclysis
   C. Venoclysis
   D. Syringe pump

5. The electrolyte concentration of Lactated Ringer injection closely resembles that of
   A. Extracellular fluid
   B. Intracellular fluid
   C. Pericardium
   D. Intravascular compartment

6. Which of the following is true of high pulse pressure?
   A. Indicates high cardiac output
   B. Indicates reduced cardiac output
   C. Indicates impending circulatory collapse
   D. Indicates low cardiac output

7. Hypotonic expansion may also be known as which of the following?
   A. Dilutional hyponatremia
   B. Water intoxication
   C. A only
   D. A and B

8. Slow filling of the hand veins indicates which of the following?
   A. Excessive blood volume
   B. Low blood volume
   C. Increased plasma volume
   D. Increased extracellular fluid volume

9. Gastric replacement fluids are contraindicated in patients with
   A. Renal failure
   B. Hepatic insufficiency
   C. Increased pulse pressure
   D. Isotonic expansion

10. Which of the following is not true of hypertonic fluid?
    A. Lowers osmotic pressure of plasma
    B. Causes fluid to invade the cell
    C. Increases extracellular volume
    D. Draws fluid from the cells

References and Selected Readings   *Asterisks indicate references cited in text.*

American Society of Health-System Pharmacists [AHFS DI]. (2013). Bethesda, MD: American Hospital Formulary Service Drug Information.

McIntyre, L. (2012). Developing a bundle to improve fluid management. *Nurs Times*, Nursingtimes.net. http://www.nursingtimes.net/nursing-practice/clinical-zones/management/developing-a-bundle-to-improve-fluid-management/5046817.article

Farrell, D.J., & Bower, L. (2003). Fatal water intoxication. *Journal of Clinical Pathology, 56*(10), 803–804.

Gahart, L., & Nazareno, A.R. (2008). *Intravenous medications* (24th ed.). St. Louis, MO: Mosby.

*Grocott, M., Mythen, M.G., & Gan, T.J. (2005). Perioperative fluid management and clinical outcomes in adults. *International Anesthesia Research Society, 100*, 1093–1106.

Haut, E.R., Kalish, B.T., Cotton, B.A., Efron, D.T., Haider, A.H., Stevens, K.A., & Chang, D.C. (2011). Prehospital intravenous fluid administration is associated with higher mortality in trauma patients: a National Trauma Data Bank analysis. *Annals of Surgery, 253*(2), 371.

*McEvoy, G.K. (2007). *AHFS drug information*, Bethesda, MD: American Society of Health System Pharmacists.

*Metheny, N.M. (2012). *Fluid and electrolyte balance: nursing considerations* (5th ed.). Sudbury, MA: Jones & Bartlett Learning.

Phillips, L.D. (2005). *Manual of IV therapeutics* (4th ed.). Philadelphia, PA: FA Davis.

Shamsuddin, A.F., & Shafie, S.D. (2012). Knowledge of nurses in the preparation and administration of intravenous medications. *Procedia-Social and Behavioral Sciences, 60*, 602–609.

Stopyra, A., Jalynski, M., Sobiech, P., Chyczewski, M., Holak, P., & Lew, M. (2010). The effect of isotonic multiple electrolyte infusions during anesthesia on blood gas values. *Polish Journal of Veterinary Science, 13*(2), 287–292.

*Phillips, L. (2010). Parenteral fluids. In M. Alexander, A. Corrigan, L. Gorski, J. Hankins, & R. Perucca. (Eds.), *Infusion Nursing: an evidence-based approach*. Philadelphia, PA: W.B. Saunders.

United States Pharmacopeia [USP]. (2012). *NF 31* (36th ed.). Easton, PA: Mack Publishing.

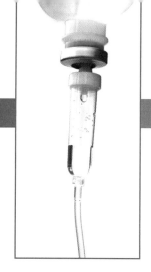

CHAPTER 10

Complications and Nursing Interventions

Sharon M. Weinstein
Mary E. Hagle

KEY TERMS

Air Embolism
Catheter Embolism
Cellular Toxicity
Debridement
Ecchymosis
Extravasation
Hematoma
Infiltration

Ischemia
Necrosis
Phlebothrombosis
Reflex Sympathetic
   Dystrophy (RSD)
Thrombogenicity
Thrombophlebitis
Thrombosis

UNDERSTANDING COMPLICATIONS

As many as 90% of all hospitalized patients in the United States receive some form of infusion therapy, and the number of patients in non–acute care settings continues to proliferate. Although most infusion therapy is administered without problems, some complications, ranging from minor to more serious, do occur. Such complications increase hospital length of stay, length of therapy, and may put the patient at risk for additional problems. Fortunately, most of these complications are preventable. A comprehensive knowledge of the inherent risks and measures to prevent their occurrence may eliminate many of the hazards associated with infusion therapy. The infusion nurse needs to recognize complications and respond with appropriate nursing interventions to ensure quality of care. Complications are varied and may be local or systemic. Local complications occur frequently but are rarely serious. Systemic complications, although more rare, are serious and frequently life threatening. They require immediate recognition and medical attention. Sentinel events, as defined by

The Joint Commission (TJC), are unexpected occurrences involving death or serious physical or psychological injury, or the risk thereof. Tracking, reporting, and analyzing complications are critical to prevention.

LOCAL COMPLICATIONS

Local complications are those seen at or near the catheter insertion or exit site as a result of trauma to the vessel wall or as a result of mechanical failure. In general, they are easily corrected and are associated with no serious problems when appropriate interventions are initiated. Occasionally, local complications are not recognized until considerable damage occurs, making early recognition of complications a key factor in infusion therapy. Early recognition may prevent the following:

- Extensive edema that deprives the patient of urgently needed fluid and medications
- Necrosis (localized death of tissue)
- Thrombophlebitis with the subsequent danger of embolism

Local complications that are mechanical in nature are generally resolved by correction of the mechanical failure, such as adjusting a tourniquet, insertion site, cannula, container, tubing, or patient position. Local complications may also occur as the result of trauma to the wall of the vein. Among the common local complications are ecchymosis or hematoma, infiltration, extravasation, phlebitis, postinfusion phlebitis, thrombosis, thrombophlebitis, and phlebothrombosis.

Ecchymosis/Hematoma

Ecchymosis denotes the infiltration of blood into the tissues; hematoma usually refers to uncontrolled bleeding at a venipuncture site, generally creating a hard, painful lump. Both are commonly associated with venipunctures that are performed by unskilled professionals or on elderly patients who have a tendency to bruise easily. Ecchymosis and hematomas often occur when multiple entries are made into a vein or when attempts are made into veins that are not easily palpated. These injuries may limit veins for future use.

PATIENT SAFETY

If ecchymosis occurs during venipuncture, the cannula should be removed and light pressure should be applied. If hematoma occurs during a venipuncture attempt, the cannula is immediately removed, direct pressure is applied to the area, catheter integrity is assessed, and the extremity is elevated until bleeding has stopped. A dry, sterile dressing is applied to the site, and the area is monitored for signs of breakthrough bleeding. Ice may be applied, and the area is observed for circulatory, neurologic, and motor function (INS, 2011).

Infiltration

Dislodgment of the catheter with consequent infiltration of fluid is common and frequently is considered of minor significance. In 1998, the Infusion Nurses Society (INS) published an infiltration scale as a part of the Revised Intravenous Nursing Standards of

Practice. The scale was revised in 2010 to include psychometric properties. The tool was edited for pediatric use by researchers from Children's Medical Center of Dallas; Box 10-1. The infiltration scale was removed from the Standards of Practice, and a recommended scale is now available in INS' Policies and Procedures for Infusion Nursing. (www.ins1.org/onlinestore)

With the increasing numbers of irritating solutions and the frequency with which potent drugs are infused in intravenous (IV) solutions, serious problems may occur when the fluid invades the surrounding tissues. Hypertonic, acid, and alkaline fluids are contraindicated for hypodermoclysis and are not intended for other than venous infusions. If they are allowed to infiltrate, necrosis may occur.

If necrosis is avoided, edema may nevertheless

- Deprive the patient of fluid and drug absorption at the rate essential for successful therapy
- Limit veins available for venipuncture, complicating therapy
- Predispose the patient to infection

BOX 10-1   PEDIATRIC PERIPHERALLY INSERTED IV (PIV) INFILTRATION SCALE

Grade	Appearance
0	Asymptomatic Flushes easily
1	Localized swelling Flushes with difficulty Discomfort at site
2	Evidence of slight swelling at site or below site Redness Discomfort at site
3	Moderate swelling Pain at site Skin cool to touch Blanching present Diminished pulse below the site
4	Severe swelling Infiltration Skin cool to touch Blanching Necrosis Blistering Diminished or absent pulses Pain at site Capillary refill > 4 seconds

Adapted from Pop, R. (2012). A pediatric peripheral intravenous infiltration assessment tool. *Journal of Infusion Nursing, 35*(4), 243–248.

> ### ✋ PATIENT SAFETY
>
> To confirm an infiltration, apply a tourniquet proximal to the injection site tightly enough to restrict the venous flow. If the infusion continues regardless of this venous obstruction, infiltration is evident.

Extravasation

Extravasation is the infiltration of a medication that causes tissue necrosis or damage. Edema may be present, due to infiltration or tissue damage. Comparing the infusion area with the identical area in the opposite extremity can help the nurse identify swelling.

In many cases, the edema is allowed to increase to great proportions because of the misconception that backflow of blood into the adapter is significant proof that the infusion is entering the vein. This is not a reliable method for detecting possible infiltration because the point of the IV catheter may puncture the posterior wall of the vein, leaving the greater portion of the bevel in the lumen of the vein. Blood return is obtained on negative pressure, but if the infusion is allowed to continue, fluid seeps into the tissues at the point of the catheter, thereby increasing the edema.

Occasionally, a blood return is not obtained on negative pressure. This may occur when the needle occludes the lumen of a small vein, obstructing the flow of blood. Evidence of backflow should not be the sole criterion for confirming extravasation.

Drugs that contribute to necrosis as a result of extravasation are most often osmotically active or ischemia-inducing or they cause direct cellular toxicity. Mechanical compression in the infiltrated tissue can increase the extent of damage, as can infection of the resulting wound. If only superficial tissue loss occurs and the area remains free of infection, debridement yields a clean bed capable of granulation. If deep structures are involved, however, spontaneous wound healing may be averted, resulting in the need for wide excision, debridement, and grafting or amputation to restore tissue integrity.

Phlebitis

Phlebitis, or inflammation of the intima of the vein, is a commonly reported complication of infusion therapy. The inflammatory process occurs as a result of irritation to the endothelial cells of the vein intima, creating a rough cell wall where platelets readily adhere. Phlebitis is characterized by pain and tenderness along the course of the vein, erythema, and inflammatory swelling with a feeling of warmth at the site.

An intact skin surface is the first line of defense, and when it has been violated, patients are at risk for bacterial infection. Hand hygiene is the most important preventive activity, followed by thorough cleaning of the site prior to cannulation and applying a sterile dressing after insertion. Maintenance of the site and the peripheral IV (PIV) catheter also involves good handwashing prior to dressing or tubing changes. Manipulation of the PIV catheter during patient movement or dressing/tubing changes can be a key factor in the development of phlebitis (Washington & Barrett, 2012). Phlebitis may be mechanical, chemical, or bacterial. See Box 10-2, Factors Contributing to Venous Inflammation; Box 10-3, Phlebitis Rating Scale; and Figure 10-1, Visual Infusion Phlebitis (VIP) score.

Mechanical phlebitis is associated with cannula placement; cannulas placed in areas of flexion may result in mechanical phlebitis. As the extremity is mobilized, the cannula may

---

BOX 10-2 FACTORS CONTRIBUTING TO VENOUS INFLAMMATION

Inflammation of the vein can occur from any foreign body and is mediated by the following:

- Duration of the infusion
- Composition of the solution
- Site of the infusion
- Venipuncture technique
- Method used for cleansing the skin

---

irritate the vein intima, causing injury and resultant phlebitis. The cannula should closely approximate the lumen of the vessel to avoid mechanical phlebitis. Proper taping and securement are essential.

PATIENT SAFETY

To evaluate a mechanical phlebitis, check the dressing securement device, site, cannula, tubing, and involved extremity.

Bacterial phlebitis is an inflammation of the vein intima associated with a bacterial infection. The condition may be serious and predispose the patient to systemic complications addressed later in this chapter. Handwashing is the single most important procedure for preventing nosocomial infections, and aseptic technique is essential in the preparation and care of venipuncture sites (APIC, 2011).

Chemical phlebitis is associated with a response of the vein intima to chemicals producing inflammation. The inflammatory response is created by the administration of solutions or medications or as a result of certain cannula materials. We know that the normal blood pH is 7.35 to 7.45 and is slightly alkaline. The normal pH for solutions is 7.0, which is neutral. The pH of dextrose solutions ranges from 3.5 to 6.5. Acidity is needed to prevent caramelization of the dextrose

---

BOX 10-3 PHLEBITIS RATING SCALE

Grade 0 No symptoms

Grade 1 Erythema at access site with or without pain

Grade 2 Pain at access site with erythema and/or edema

Grade 3 Pain at access site with erythema and/or edema, streak formation, palpable venous cord

Grade 4 Pain at access site with erythema and/or edema, streak formation, palpable venous cord > 1 inch in length; purulent drainage

From Infusion Nurses Society. (2011). Infusion nursing standards of practice. *Journal of Infusion Nursing, 34*(1 Suppl), S47.

Visual Infusion Phlebitis Score

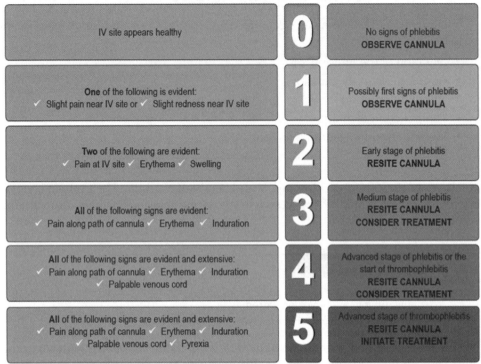

Adapted with permission from Andrew Jackson IV Nurse Consultant, The Rotherham NHS Foundation Trust, UK © Andrew Jackson 1997.

FIGURE 10-1 Visual Infusion Phlebitis scale. (From Gallant, P., & Schultz, A.A. (2006). Evaluation of a visual infusion phlebitis scale for determining appropriate discontinuation of peripheral intravenous catheters. *Journal of Infusion Nursing, 29*(6), 338–345.)

during sterilization and to maintain the stability of the solution during storage. Solutions and medications with a high pH or osmolality predispose the vein intima to irritation. The more acidic an IV admixture, the greater the risk. In addition, additives such as potassium chloride, vancomycin hydrochloride, and many antineoplastic agents can contribute to chemical phlebitis.

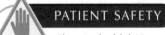

PATIENT SAFETY

Chemical phlebitis may be caused by irritating medications or solutions, medications improperly diluted or administered too rapidly, particulate matter, cannula material, or extended dwell time.

Postinfusion Phlebitis

Postinfusion phlebitis refers to inflammation of the vein that usually presents within 48 to 96 hours of cannula removal or after administration of a specific drug. Factors contributing to the development of postinfusion phlebitis include the following: poor cannula insertion technique, a debilitated patient, poor vein condition, hypertonic or acidic solutions,

BOX 10-4   MEASURES FOR PREVENTING POSTINFUSION PHLEBITIS

- Ensure that a skilled clinician is performing venipuncture.
- Apply antiseptic technique.
- Check compatibility of solutions and medications prior to mixing/administering.
- Use filters to prepare medications and solutions.
- Use final filtration, as recommended, for administering medications and solutions.
- Add a buffer agent to known irritants.
- Rotate peripheral infusion sites.
- Change the solution container per INS recommendations.
- Change accessories, including caps and needleless devices, at the time of peripheral catheter change and as needed.

ineffective filtration, placement of a large-gauge cannula in a small vessel, and failure to change tubings, dressing, injection site caps, and cannulas consistent with the INS Standards of Practice. Measures for preventing postinfusion phlebitis are provided in Box 10-4.

Thrombosis

Any injury that roughens the endothelial cells of the venous wall allows platelets to adhere and a thrombus to form (Figure 10-2). Because the point of the IV catheter traumatizes the wall of the vein where it touches, a thrombus or thrombi form on the vein and at the tip of the catheter. The result of local thrombi obstructing the circulation of blood is thrombosis. Thrombi not only

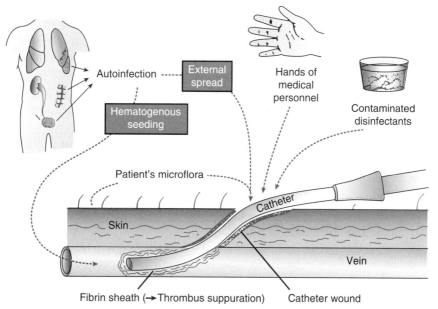

FIGURE 10-2 Sources of vascular catheter–related infection.

obstruct circulation but also form an excellent trap for bacteria, whether the bacteria are carried by the bloodstream from an infection in a remote part of the body or enter the body through a subcutaneous orifice. Khalidi, Kovacevich, Papke-O'Donnell, and Btaiche (2009) found that *"The use of needleless positive pressure connector valves (PPVs) on venous access devices (VADs) has helped to decrease VAD occlusion rates, but catheter-related bloodstream infections (CRBSI) rates vary."*

Occlusion remains a concern for short- and long-term catheters, including peripherally inserted central catheters (PICCs). Occluded catheters place the patient at risk for mechanical complications, including pneumothorax and hematoma as well as delays in treatment.

Thrombosis of the deep veins (axillary, subclavian, innominate, internal jugular, and superior vena cava) and subsequent risk of infection occur when catheters are placed in the venous system. The device that poses the greatest risk of iatrogenic bloodstream infection is the central venous catheter (CVC) in its numerous forms (Centers for Disease Control and Prevention [CDC], 2011). Bennett and Brachman's classic studies addressed patients with PICCs, implanted venous access ports, and CVCs (Jarvis, 2013).

Bloodstream infection remains the most common life-threatening complication associated with central venous access (Sadfar, Jacobs, & Gaines, 2012). Central line bundles are groupings of best practices that individually improve care but when applied together result in substantially greater improvement. According to the Institute for Healthcare Improvement (2013), the science supporting the bundle components is sufficiently established to be considered standard of care.

Risk of bloodstream infection associated with various devices may be found in Table 10-1. See Chapter 14 for detailed information regarding central venous access.

Thrombophlebitis

Thrombophlebitis denotes a twofold injury—thrombosis plus inflammation. The development of thrombophlebitis is easily recognized. Classic symptoms of tenderness, erythema, and swelling are seen the longer a catheter remains in place. A painful inflammation develops along the length of the vein. If the infusion is allowed to continue, the thrombosis progressively obstructs the circulation and the vein becomes hard, tortuous, tender, and painful. Early detection may prevent an obstructive thrombophlebitis that can slow and eventually stop the infusion. This condition, which is painful, may persist indefinitely, incapacitating the patient and limiting available veins for future therapy.

CONTRIBUTING FACTORS

Any irritation involving the wall of the vein predisposes the patient to thrombophlebitis. *Duration of the infusion* is a significant factor in the development of thrombophlebitis. As the duration increases, so do the incidence and degree of inflammation.

EVIDENCE FOR PRACTICE

Bartock, L. (2010). *An Evidence-Based Systematic Review of Literature for the Reduction of PICC Line Occlusions.* Additional research is needed concerning the impact of standardized tools to predict PICC occlusions or protocols recommended to prevent occlusions.
Journal of the Association of Vascular Access Nurses, 15(2), 58–63.

TABLE 10-1	APPROXIMATE RISKS OF BLOODSTREAM INFECTION ASSOCIATED WITH VARIOUS TYPES OF ACCESS DEVICES		
Type of Device		Representative Rate	Representative Range
Short-term temporary access[a]			
Peripheral IV cannulas			
Winged steel needles		<0.2	0–1
Peripheral IV catheters			
Percutaneously inserted		0.2	0–1
Cutdown		6	0–1
Midline catheters		0.7	0.7–0.8
Arterial catheters		1	—
Central venous catheters			
All-purpose, multilumen		3	1–7
Pulmonary artery		1	0–5
Hemodialysis		10	3–18
Long-term indefinite access[b]			
Peripherally inserted, CVCs		0.20	—
Cuffed central catheters		0.20	0.10–0.53
Subcutaneous central venous ports		0.04	0.00–0.10

Based on data from recently published, prospective studies.
[a]Number of bloodstream infections per 100 devices.
[b]Number of bloodstream infections per 100 device–days.
IV, intravenous.
From Bennett, J.V., & Brachman, P.S. (2007). *Hospital infections* (5th ed.). Philadelphia, PA: Lippincott Williams & Wilkins.

The *composition of the solution* may play a role. Venous irritation and inflammation may result from the infusion of hypertonic glucose solutions, certain drug additives, or solutions with a pH significantly different from that of the plasma. Dextrose solutions are irritating to the vein. The *United States Pharmacopeia* (USP) specifications for pH of dextrose solutions range from 3.5 to 6.5; acidity is necessary to prevent caramelization of the dextrose during autoclaving and to preserve the stability of the solution during storage. Studies show a significant reduction in thrombophlebitis when buffered glucose solution has been infused. Neut, a sodium bicarbonate 1% solution, may be added to increase the pH of acid IV solutions. This additive, however, poses a problem of incompatibility when added to solutions containing drugs. The greatest number of incompatibilities may be produced by changes in pH (Bennett & Brachman, 2007). As an example, tetracycline hydrochloride, with a pH of 2.5 to 3.0, is unstable in an alkaline environment.

The *infusion site* can be a factor contributing to thrombophlebitis. The veins in areas over joint flexion undergo injury when motion of the catheter irritates the venous wall. The veins in the lower extremities are especially susceptible to trauma, which may be enhanced by stagnant blood in varicosities and stasis in peripheral venous circulation.

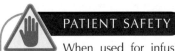

PATIENT SAFETY

When used for infusing an irritating solution, small veins are more susceptible to inflammation.

The *infusion catheter* may occlude the entire lumen of the vein, obstructing the flow of circulating blood; the solution then flows undiluted, irritating the wall of the vein.

Venipuncture technique can mean the difference between a successful infusion and the complication of thrombophlebitis. Only minimal trauma results from a skillfully executed venipuncture, whereas a carelessly performed venipuncture may seriously traumatize the venous wall. Phlebitis associated with sepsis may be related to the technique of the clinician. Infection is always a risk if sterile technique is not zealously observed. Thorough cleansing of the skin is important in preventing infections. Maintenance of asepsis is essential during long-term therapy, particularly in the use of the through-the-needle catheter.

Infusion methods for parenteral solutions may foster septic thrombophlebitis. This complication is most often associated with the through-the-needle catheter. Infrequently used, the catheter threaded through the needle remains sterile and does not come in contact with the skin but provides a large subcutaneous orifice facilitating entry of bacteria around the catheter and seepage of fluid.

The over-the-needle catheter is not without fault because it comes in direct contact with the skin before being introduced into the vein. However, the tight fit through the skin may bar further bacterial entry.

TREATMENT

Most cases of superficial thrombophlebitis respond to prompt removal of the IV catheter and local application of heat, although the affected vein may remain firm for several months.

A sterile inflammation usually develops from a chemical or mechanical irritation. When the inflammation is the result of sepsis, however, the condition is much more serious and carries with it the potential danger of septicemia and acute bacterial endocarditis. Additional treatment measures are required, possibly including excision of the infected vein. The wound is then left to heal secondarily. Antibiotic therapy then begins and continues for 7 to 10 days.

An additional complication is embolism when thrombosis occurs. The more pronounced the inflammation and the more intense the pain, the more organized the thrombus is likely to become. Embolism is less likely to occur from the well-attached clot of thrombophlebitis than from phlebothrombosis.

PREVENTIVE MEASURES

In performing venipunctures, the nurse exercises every caution to avoid injuring the wall of the vein needlessly. Multiple punctures, through-and-through punctures, and damage to the posterior wall of the vein with the point of the catheter can lead to thrombosis. The nurse can minimize the risk of phlebitis by implementing these measures:

- Refrain from using veins in the lower extremities.
- Select veins with ample blood volume when infusing irritating substances.
- Avoid veins in areas over joint flexion and use an arm board if the vein must be located in an area of flexion.

• Anchor the catheter securely with a stabilization device to prevent motion, which may loosen the catheter.

To prevent septic phlebitis, thorough preparation of the skin, together with aseptic technique and maintenance of asepsis during infusion, is imperative. Periodic inspection of the injection site will detect developing complications before serious damage occurs.

Complaints of a painful infusion make it necessary to differentiate between early phlebitis and venospasm from an irritating solution. In the case of venospasm, slowing the infusion and applying heat to the vein dilates the vessel and increases the blood flow, thereby diluting the solution and relieving the pain. After a hypertonic solution infusion, infusion with an isotonic fluid flushes the vein of irritating substances.

If inflammation accompanies the pain, a change in the injection site should be considered. Continuing the infusion leads to progressive trauma and limits available veins. Adherence to routine replacement time limits for removal of the catheter reduces the incidence of phlebitis (INS, 2011). During removal of the infusion catheter, care must be taken to prevent injury to the wall of the vein; the catheter should be removed at an angle nearly flush with the skin. Pressure should be applied for a reasonable length of time to prevent extravasation of blood.

Phlebothrombosis

Phlebothrombosis denotes thrombosis and usually indicates that the inflammation is relatively inconspicuous. It is thought to give rise to embolism because the thrombus is poorly attached to the wall of the vein. Both thrombophlebitis and phlebothrombosis have a degree of inflammation and are associated with potential embolism. Factors that promote thrombosis are summarized in Table 10-2.

SYSTEMIC COMPLICATIONS

Serious, even life-threatening systemic complications range from septicemia to embolism to shock and infection. These complications need to be prevented or identified as soon as possible and treatment interventions begun.

Septicemia

Septicemia is caused by invasion of the bloodstream by microorganisms or their by-products, including bacteria, fungi, mycobacteria, and, rarely, viruses. Clinical manifestations of septicemia include chills, fever, general malaise, and headache (see Chapter 14).

TABLE 10-2	GENESIS OF THROMBOSIS	
Type	**Clinical Manifestation**	**Contributing Factors**
Fibrin sheath thrombosis	Inability to aspirate blood; catheter occlusion	Thrombogenic catheter material
Vascular mural thrombosis	Vein obstruction; classic symptoms of thrombosis	Difficult insertions; multiple attempts at venipuncture; sustained contact of the catheter with the venous wall

CONTRIBUTING FACTORS

Certain predisposing factors put the infusion therapy patient at risk:

- Age younger than 1 year or older than 60 years
- Granulocytopenia
- Immunocompromised state
- Loss of skin integrity
- Distant infection that might contribute to hematogenous seeding.

Also contributing to the development of septicemia are catheter-related factors, such as the size of the catheter, number of lumens, function and use of the catheter, catheter material, bacterial adherence, and **thrombogenicity**.

TREATMENT

Supportive therapy for the patient with septicemia includes fluid replacement, blood pressure maintenance, oxygenation, cardiac output maintenance, nutritional support, and preservation of acid–base balance. Ancillary treatments involve administration of steroids, antibiotics, and endotoxin vaccination.

PREVENTIVE MEASURES

Because intravascular systems should be considered potential portals for infection, prevention programs support the use of 0.2-μm air-eliminating, bacterial-retentive filters. In addition, good handwashing techniques, line care protocols, and adherence to the INS Standards of Practice for monitoring, maintenance of infusion, tubing changes, and catheter care all contribute to an environment that does not readily support development of septicemia in patients receiving infusion therapies.

Pulmonary Embolism

Pulmonary embolism occurs when a substance, usually a blood clot, dislodges and floats freely, propelled by the venous circulation to the right side of the heart and into the pulmonary artery (Metheny, 2012). Emboli may obstruct the main pulmonary artery or the arteries to the lobes, occluding arterial apertures at major bifurcations. Obstruction of the main artery then results in circulatory and cardiac disturbances. Recurrent small emboli may eventually result in pulmonary hypertension and right heart failure (Metheny, 2012). See Chapter 14.

Precautions for preventing this serious complication include the following:

- Filter infusions of blood or plasma through an adequate filter to remove any particulates that could promote small emboli formation.
- Do not perform venipuncture in the veins of the lower extremities. These veins are particularly susceptible to trauma that predisposes the patient to thrombophlebitis. Although superficial veins rarely seem to

be the source of emboli (INS, 2011), a thrombus may extend into the deep veins, resulting in a potentially viable clot; superficial and deep veins unite freely in the lower extremities.

• Avoid applying positive pressure to relieve clot formation.

PATIENT SAFETY

Avoid irrigating a plugged catheter. Doing so may embolize small catheter thrombi, some of which are infected.

• Check for patency of the lumen of the catheter by kinking the infusion tubing approximately 8 inches from the catheter. Then, kink and release the tubing between the catheter and the pinched tubing. If the tubing becomes hard and meets with resistance, obstruction is evident. The catheter should be removed and the infusion reinstated.
• Take special precautions with drug additives. Reconstituted drugs must be completely dissolved before being added to parenteral solutions because it is the inherent nature of red blood cells to adhere to particles, adding to the danger of clot formation.
• Examine fluids to detect particulate matter.

Air Embolism

Although **air embolism** is a significant possible complication with air-dependent containers, it is more frequently associated with central venous lines. There is a potential risk for air embolism to result from the insertion of a CVC, inadequate sealing of the tract before disconnecting a CVC, disconnection of central lines, and bypassing the pump housing of an electronic volumetric pump with an IV piggyback connection. Smart pump technology has eliminated some of the potential for error.

PATIENT SAFETY

A fatal embolism may occur when small bubbles accumulate dangerously and form tenacious bubbles that block the pulmonary capillaries. Recognition of the circumstances that contribute to this hazard and measures taken to prevent its occurrence are imperative for safe fluid therapy.

Symptoms associated with air embolism arising from sudden vascular collapse include cyanosis, drop in blood pressure, weak, rapid pulse, rise in venous pressure, and loss of consciousness.

PATIENT SAFETY

If air embolism occurs, the source of air entry must be immediately rectified. The patient should be turned on the left side with his or her head down. This causes the air to rise in the right atrium, preventing it from entering the pulmonary artery. Oxygen is then administered and the physician/licensed independent practitioner (LIP) notified.

CONTRIBUTING FACTORS: GRAVITY INFUSIONS

If a vented container is allowed to run dry, air enters the tubing, and the fluid level drops to the proximity of the patient's chest. The pressure exerted by the blood on the walls of the veins controls the level to which the air drops in the tubing. A negative pressure in the vein may allow air to enter the bloodstream. Negative pressure occurs when the extremity receiving the infusion is elevated above the heart (Metheny, 2012).

Infusions flowing through a CVC carry an even greater risk of air embolism as the container empties than when infusions flow through a peripheral vein. Because the central venous pressure is lower than the peripheral venous pressure, a negative pressure that could suck air into the circulation is more likely. The nurse needs to take precautions while changing the administration set of a central venous infusion.

Running solutions simultaneously is a key factor. One empty vented container becomes the source of air for the flowing solution. This happens because the atmospheric pressure is greater in the open tubing to the empty container than below the partially restricted clamp on the infusion side. Recurrent small air bubbles are constantly aspirated into the flowing solution and on into the venous system. The introduction of air may be prevented by running one solution at a time. Vigilance is imperative if vented solutions are prescribed to run simultaneously. The tubing must be clamped off completely before the solution container is allowed to empty.

This principle is also involved in the piggyback setup for secondary infusions. The potential danger of air embolism exists whenever solutions from two vented sets run simultaneously through a common catheter. Again, advanced technologies have minimized the use of piggyback setups.

All connections of an infusion set must be tight. Any faulty opening or defective hole in the set allows air to be emitted into the flowing solution. If a stopcock is used, the outlets not in use must be completely shut off.

The regulating clamp on the infusion set should be located no higher than the patient's chest. Because the pressure exerted by the blood on the venous wall normally raises a column of water from 4 to 11 cm above the heart, a restricting clamp placed above this point results in a negative pressure in the tubing. If great enough, the pressure can suck air into the flowing solution should a loose connection or a faulty opening exist between the clamp and the catheter. The lower the clamp, the greater the chance of defects occurring above the clamp, where positive pressure can force the solution to leak out.

If the fluid container on a continuous infusion should empty, fresh fluid will force trapped air into the circulation and air embolus may result. Table 10-3 addresses the method to help ensure that air does not enter the patient's system during administration.

An infusion set long enough to drop below the extremity gives added protection against air being drawn into the vein should the infusion bottle empty. In-line pressure chambers on administration sets should be kept filled at all times. Manual compression of an empty chamber forces air into the bloodstream.

CONTRIBUTING FACTORS—CATHETER REMOVAL

Venous air embolism (VAE) is a complication that occurs when atmospheric gas is introduced into the systemic venous system. Previously associated with neurosurgical procedures conducted in the sitting position, it is now recognized as a complication of

TABLE 10-3   **REMOVING AIR FROM THE INFUSION SET**

1. Immediately before and during the time that the catheter will be open to the air, assist the patient to lie flat and supine in bed and perform the Valsalva maneuver (forced expiration with the mouth closed).
2. To remove the air from the administration set, first place a hemostat (clamp) close to the infusion catheter and hang the fresh solution container.
3. With an antiseptic agent, clean the section of the tubing proximal to the hemostat and below the air level in the tubing.
4. Insert a sterile needle to allow the air to escape.
5. Unclamp the hemostat and readjust flow.
6. A. When the infusate container runs dry during simultaneous infusion of fluids through a Y-type administration set; pressure below the partially constricted clamp is lower than the atmospheric pressure, allowing air from the empty container (atmospheric) to enter the infusion.
   B. Without an automatic shutoff valve on a secondary infusion piggybacked through the injection site of a primary IV set, air from the empty infusate container will enter the patient's circulation.

The Y-type infusion set used with vented containers is a less obvious source of air embolism but one by which unknown quantities of air can be drawn into the bloodstream.

central venous catheterization. Catheter-associated VAE mortality rates have reached 30%. Symptoms include

- Acute dyspnea
- Continuous cough
- "Gasp" reflex (a classic gasp at times reported when a bolus of air enters the pulmonary circulation and causes acute hypoxemia)
- Dizziness/light-headedness/vertigo
- Nausea
- Substernal chest pain
- Agitation/disorientation/sense of "impending doom"

VAE is a potentially life-threatening and underrecognized complication of central venous catheterization (CVC), including central lines, pulmonary catheters, hemodialysis catheters, and Hickman (long-term) catheters.

The frequency of VAE associated with CVC use ranges from 1 in 47 to 1 in 3,000. The emboli may occur at any point during line insertion, maintenance, and/or removal. Failure to occlude the needle hub and/or catheter during insertion or removal is a contributing factor. Other factors are upright positioning of the patient, which reduces central venous pressure, deep inspiration during insertion or removal (which increases the degree of negative pressure), and fracture or detachment of catheter connections. Catheter removal should be performed with the patient supine or in a Trendelenburg position while holding his/her breath at the end of inspiration or during a Valsalva maneuver (Natal & Brown, 2012). In a classic citation, Boer and Hene (1999) state, *During the procedure, the patients are placed in the head-down position, making sure that the exit site is well below the right atrium. They are specifically instructed to inhale and hold their breath for a few seconds until the catheter has been removed and are warned not to cough, talk or make a deep inspiration during the actual catheter removal. The gauze used to occlude the exit site while the catheter is being pulled out is covered with a generous amount of an inert ointment to provide an instantaneous air seal. After application of local pressure for 10 minutes, the absence of bleeding is checked and an air-occlusive dressing is rapidly applied with the patient still in the head-down position.*

There is a plethora of literature describing best practice, complications, and treatment of VAE associated with central line catheter use. The infusion nurse has the responsibility to ensure that practice guidelines and protocols are met consistently.

Catheter Embolism

Catheter embolism may occur during the insertion of a through-the-needle catheter if part of the catheter breaks off, which may happen if the proper procedure is not strictly followed. The catheter should never be pulled back through the needle. If it becomes necessary to remove the catheter, the entire unit should be removed and a new catheter inserted. Catheter embolism may also occur during the insertion of an over-the-needle catheter if the needle is either partially or totally withdrawn or then reinserted. If the catheter shears off into circulation, fluoroscopic cardiac catheterization may be necessary to visualize and remove the embolus. See Chapter 14.

Pulmonary Edema

Overloading the circulation is hazardous to any patient but especially to elderly patients and to patients with impaired renal and cardiac function. Infusing fluids too rapidly increases the venous pressure, with the possibility of consequences such as cardiac dilation and pulmonary edema.

Signs and symptoms such as venous dilation with engorged neck veins, increased blood pressure, and a rise in venous pressure should alert the nurse to the danger of pulmonary edema. Rapid respiration and shortness of breath may occur.

TREATMENT

With signs of circulatory overload, the infusion should be slowed to a minimal rate and the physician/LIP notified. Raising the patient to a sitting position may facilitate breathing.

PREVENTIVE MEASURES

Several preventative measures may reduce the likelihood of pulmonary edema:

- Maintain infusions at the prescribed flow rate.
- Avoid applying positive pressure using the pressure–chamber administration sets to infuse solutions. If the patient requires fluids so rapidly that positive pressure is required, infusion then becomes the physician/LIP's responsibility.
- Use of a controlled-volume infusion set often provides additional protection. These sets control the volume from 10 to 150 mL and prevent large quantities of fluid from being accidentally infused.
- Discard solutions not infused within the 24-hour period prescribed. Do not infuse them with the following day's fluids. Fluids administered in excess of the quantity ordered can overtax the homeostatic controls, thereby increasing the danger of pulmonary edema.

Allergic Reactions

An allergic reaction is a response to the medication or infusate to which the patient is sensitive. Such reactions may occur from the passive transfer of sensitivity to the patient from a blood donor or sensitivities to substances normally present in the blood, as seen in transfusion reactions.

PATIENT SAFETY

If an allergic reaction is suspected, the infusion should be stopped immediately, the tubing and solution container changed, and the vein kept open to permit treatment of possible anaphylactic shock. Notify the physician/LIP and initiate appropriate interventions as ordered.

Catheter-Associated Infection

Intravascular infection is related to many factors, such as the intravascular device (catheter/cannula), contaminated solution or other substances, and blood-borne pathogens, among others.

Intravascular device–related bloodstream infections are perhaps the least frequently recognized nosocomial infection. Catheter-related infections are those that originate from the catheter material itself or from migration of organisms through the open skin along the catheter. Solution-related infections are those that result from contamination of IV solutions, either in the manufacturing process or in use.

SOURCES OF INFECTION

Bacteria responsible for IV-associated infection come from three main sources: air, skin, and blood. Microorganisms (flora and fauna) characteristic of a given location are referred to accordingly, hence the terms *skin flora*, *intestinal flora*, and so on. Table 10-4 identifies microbial pathogens associated with infusion-related septicemia.

AIR

The number of microbes per cubic foot of air varies depending on the particular area involved. Where infection is present, bacteria escape in bodily discharges, contaminating clothing, bedding, and dressings. Activity, such as making a bed, sends bacteria flying into the air on particles of lint, pus, and dried epithelium (Bennett & Brachman, 2007). Increased activity raises the number of airborne particles and provides an environment that interferes with aseptic technique and potentially contributes to contamination. Airborne microorganisms may be plentiful in patient areas and utility rooms. These contaminants find easy access to unprotected IV fluids.

SKIN

The skin is the source of bacteria mainly responsible for IV-associated infection. The bacteria found on the skin are referred to as resident or transient. Resident bacteria are those normally present, and they are relatively constant in a given individual. They adhere tightly to

TABLE 10-4	MICROORGANISMS MOST FREQUENTLY ENCOUNTERED IN VARIOUS FORMS OF INTRAVASCULAR LINE–RELATED INFECTION
Source	**Pathogens**
Catheter-related	
Peripheral IV catheter	Coagulase-negative staphylococci[a]
	Staphylococcus aureus
	Candida spp.[a]
Central venous catheters	Coagulase-negative staphylococci
	Staphylococcus aureus
	Candida spp.
	Corynebacterium spp. (especially JK-1)
	Klebsiella and *Enterobacter* spp.
	Mycobacterium spp.
	Trichophyton beigelii
	Fusarium spp.
	Malassezia furfur[a]
Contaminated IV infusate	Tribe *Klebsiella*
	Enterobacter cloacae
	Enterobacter agglomerans
	Serratia marcescens
	Klebsiella spp.
	Burkholderia cepacia
	Burkholderia acidovorans, Burkholderia pickettii
	Stenotrophomonas maltophilia
	Citrobacter freundii
	Flavobacterium spp.
	Candida tropicalis
Contaminated blood products	*Enterobacter cloacae*
	Serratia marcescens
	Ochrobactrum anthropi
	Flavobacterium spp.
	Burkholderia spp.
	Yersinia spp.
	Salmonella spp.

[a]Also seen with peripheral IV catheters in association with the administration of lipid emulsion for parenteral nutritional support.
IV, intravenous.
From Bennett, J.V., & Brachman, P.S. (2007). *Hospital infections* (5th ed.). Philadelphia, PA: Lippincott Williams & Wilkins.

the skin and usually include *Staphylococcus albus* as well as diphtheroids and *Bacillus* species (Bennett & Brachman, 2007). Because not all bacteria are removed by scrubbing, meticulous care must be observed to avoid touching sterile equipment.

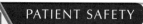

PATIENT SAFETY

Quaternary ammonium compounds such as aqueous benzalkonium chloride are inactivated by organic debris. Therefore, they are ineffective against gram-negative organisms and should not be used for skin disinfection.

The transient bacteria are responsible for infection carried from one person to another. Touch contamination is a potential hazard of infection because hospital personnel move about frequently, touching patients and objects. Frequent hand hygiene is imperative.

The patient's skin is fertile soil for bacterial growth. Organisms such as gram-positive *Staphylococcus epidermidis*, *Staphylococcus aureus*, gram-negative bacilli (especially *Klebsiella*, *Enterobacter*, and *Serratia*), and enterococci are ubiquitous on the skin of hospitalized patients (Bennett & Brachman, 2007).

Blood

Like the skin, the blood may harbor potentially dangerous microorganisms. Therefore, care must be taken to prevent bacterial or other contamination from blood spills when drawing blood samples and performing venipunctures. Refer to Chapter 17 for a discussion of blood-borne pathogens.

Survivability of Bacteria and Other Contaminants

Infection depends on the ability of bacteria to survive and proliferate. The factors that influence their survival are the specific organisms present, the number of such organisms, the resistance of the host, and the environmental conditions (CDC, 2011).

Specific Organisms

Bacteria are referred to as pathogenic or nonpathogenic. Pathogenic bacteria are capable of producing disease. All bacteria should be considered pathogenic because current data show that bacteria previously considered nonpathogenic may produce infection. In one study, *Serratia* species were implicated in 35% of cases of gram-negative septicemia resulting from IV therapy (Bennett & Brachman, 2007).

Bacteria are classified as gram positive and gram negative. In recent years, gram-negative bacteria have replaced gram-positive bacteria as the leading cause of death from septicemia (CDC, 2011; INS, 2011). The single most important reason for the intensity of the problem is probably the increased use of antibiotics that are highly effective against gram-positive organisms but only selectively effective against gram-negative organisms. With the competitive inhibition of gram-positive bacteria eliminated, the more resistant gram-negative organisms have proliferated in the hospital environment (Metheny, 2012).

Number of Organisms

The number of contaminants present influences the probability of an infection arising. The power of bacteria to proliferate must not be underestimated. It is simply not true that small amounts of bacteria from touch contamination are harmless. Contamination of IV fluids and bottles with even a few organisms is extremely dangerous because some fungi and many bacteria can proliferate at room temperature in a variety of IV solutions to more than 105 organisms per mL within 24 hours (Bennett & Brachman, 2007).

HOST RESISTANCE

The resistance of the host influences the development and course of infection, particularly septicemia. Underlying conditions such as diabetes mellitus, chronic uremia, HIV, cirrhosis, cancer, and leukemia may adversely affect the patient's capacity to resist infection. Treatment with immunosuppressive drugs, corticosteroids, anticancer agents, and extensive radiation therapy may depress immunologic response and permit the invasion of infection. Therapy may mask infection so that serious infection remains unrecognized until autopsy.

ENVIRONMENTAL CONDITIONS

Environmental conditions that affect the survival and propagation of bacteria in IV fluids are the pH, temperature, and the presence of essential nutrients in the infusion.

Some organisms grow rapidly in a neutral solution and are less likely to grow in an acid medium. Buffering of acidic dextrose solutions has been recommended for preventing phlebitis, although the neutral environment provided by the buffer may enhance the survival and proliferation of bacteria.

The temperature of the fluid may affect the ability of bacteria to multiply. At room temperature, strains of *Enterobacter cloacae*, *Enterobacter agglomerans*, and other members of the tribe *Klebsiella* proliferate rapidly in commercial solutions of 5% dextrose in water.

Total parenteral nutrition fluids should be used as soon as possible after preparation. When they must be stored temporarily, they should be refrigerated at 4°C. At this temperature, growth of *Candida albicans* is suppressed (Bennett & Brachman, 2007).

Certain nutrients must be present to support bacterial growth. Blood and crystalloid solutions provide nutrients that broaden the spectrum of pathogens capable of proliferation. Maki and associates stated that the administration of blood or reflux of blood into the infusion system may provide sufficient nutrients to broaden this spectrum. Accordingly, the American Association of Blood Banks requires blood to be stored at a constant controlled refrigeration of 1°C to 6°C.

Saline fluids are likely to contain enough biologically available carbon, nitrogen, sulfur, phosphate, and traces of other material to support, under favorable conditions, the survival and multiplication of any gram-negative bacillus introduced to as many as 1 million organisms per milliliter.

CONTRIBUTORS TO CONTAMINATION AND INFECTION

Extrinsic contamination and other factors that contribute to infection range from faulty handling of fluids to faulty devices and techniques.

FAULTY HANDLING AND FLAWED PROCEDURES

Containers of parenteral fluid are accepted as being sterile and nonpyrogenic on arrival from the manufacturer. The potential risk of contamination occurring in transit or in use is frequently overlooked by hospital personnel. However, through faulty handling or carelessness, glass containers may become cracked or damaged and plastic bags punctured. Bacteria and fungi may penetrate a hairline crack in an IV container, even though the crack is so fine that fluid does not leak from the container.

Besides providing carbon and energy, IV solutions of dextrose include the extra nutrients needed to support the growth of 10 million organisms per milliliter of fluid. If the fluid is not examined closely, its opalescence may be overlooked, and subsequent infusion of a few hundred milliliters of such contaminated fluid results in deep shock or possibly death.

The nurse is responsible for examining containers of fluid before their use. They should be inspected against a light and dark background for cracks, defects, turbidity, and particulates. Plastic containers should be squeezed to detect any puncture hole. Accidental puncture may occur without being evident and provide a port for entry for microorganisms (Bennett & Brachman, 2007). Any container with a crack or defect must be regarded as potentially contaminated and unusable. Similarly, any glass container lacking a vacuum when opened should not be used.

UNSTERILE CONDITIONS

When a 1-L glass container is opened, approximately 100 mL of air rushes in to fill the vacuum. In areas with a high concentration of airborne particles, contamination of unprotected fluids is a potential risk. The sterile environment of a laminar flow hood prevents this problem.

OUTDATED SOLUTIONS

The longer the container is in use, the greater the proliferation of bacteria and the greater the risk of infection should contamination inadvertently occur. The risk of infusing outdated fluids can be avoided by adhering to special limits, supported by a strong monitoring policy. Every container should be labeled with the time it is opened. The guidelines of the CDC and INS Standards of Practice should be followed, in addition to institutional or organizational policy.

IMPROPERLY PREPARED ADMIXTURES

Allowing untrained hospital personnel to add drugs to IV containers contributes to the potential for contamination. This risk is reduced when admixtures are prepared under laminar flow hoods by skilled personnel adhering to strict aseptic technique in accord with a pharmacy additive program.

Nurses and physicians/LIPs who have to prepare admixtures in an emergency, and other personnel involved in the preparation and administration of IV drugs, should receive special training in the preparation of admixtures and the handling of IV fluids and equipment. Adherence to strict aseptic methods is vital. It must be emphasized that touch contamination is the primary source of infection. Although laminar flow hoods prevent airborne contamination, they do not ensure sterility when a break in aseptic technique occurs.

MANIPULATION OF EQUIPMENT

Infusion fluids can be inadvertently contaminated by faulty techniques in manipulating the equipment. In open systems, in which fluids are not protected by air filters, the simple procedure of hanging the container may be taken for granted and the risk of contamination overlooked.

When an administration set is inserted into the container and the container is inverted, the fluid tends to leak out the vent onto the unsterile surface of the container. Regurgitation of the contaminated fluid into the container occurs when the container vents. Instructions in the use of the equipment often go unread and unheeded. Squeezing the drip chamber of the administration set before inserting it into the container and releasing it when the container is inverted prevents regurgitation of fluid and minimizes the risk of contamination.

EXPOSURE OF INJECTION PORTS AND STOPCOCKS

Meticulous aseptic technique must be observed in using injection ports because they are a potential source of contamination when used to piggyback infusions. The injection port location, at the distal end of the tubing, exposes it to patient excreta and drainage, which enhance the growth of microorganisms.

The injection port must be scrubbed at least 1 minute with an accepted antiseptic, such as 70% isopropyl alcohol. Scrubbing the injection cap for 30 seconds with an antimicrobial (e.g., povidone–iodine) fluid provides good protection.

Today's use of needleless systems has minimized the risk associated with connecting a needle to an injection port. The Bloodborne Pathogens Act of the Occupational Safety and Health Administration requires health care facilities *to use needle-free systems whenever possible for the collection or withdrawal of bodily fluids after initial venous or arterial access is established, the administration of medication, or any other procedure involving the potential for occupational exposure to bloodborne pathogens due to percutaneous injuries from contaminated sharps* (Smith et al., 2012). However, when a needle must be used, it should be firmly engaged up to the hub in the injection site and securely taped to prevent any in-and-out motion of the needle from introducing bacteria into the infusion.

Similarly, three-way stopcocks are potential mechanisms of bacterial transmission because their ports, unprotected by sterile coverings, are open to moisture and other contaminants. Connected to CVCs and arterial lines, they are still used in some settings for drawing blood samples. Accordingly, aseptic practices are vital in preventing bacteria from being introduced into the IV line. Attaching a sterile catheter plug when the stopcock is added and changing the devices after each use reduce the risk of contamination. Whenever fluid leakage is discovered at injection sites, connections, or vents, the IV set should be replaced.

CATHETER INSERTION

Within 24 to 48 hours after a plastic catheter is inserted into a vessel, a loosely constructed fibrin sheath develops around the intravascular portion of the device, forming a nidus within which microorganisms can multiply. The nidus shields them to an extent from host defenses and antibiotics. The thrombus or thrombi generated by the catheter material may play a role in systemic infection.

INFECTION PREVENTION

Catheter care and antibiotic lock technique are two interventions used to prevent catheter-related infection. Additional preventive measures involve careful adherence to policies and procedures based on INS standards with respect to rotating the infusion site and limiting the time that the catheter dwells in the vessel (indwell time). This may reduce the inherent problems of catheter-associated infection, even though most device-related septicemias are actually caused by the patient's own skin flora or by microorganisms transmitted from the hands of the health care professional.

The antibiotic lock technique has been used to reduce the potential for CVC-related infection in the immunocompromised patient. Vancomycin, amphotericin B, and fluconazole have all been successfully used as flush solutions. A small amount of concentrated antibiotic or antifungal agent is instilled in the catheter, and the distal portion of the catheter is capped. Al-Hwiesh and Abdul-Rahman (2007) reported successful use of the lock technique, a therapeutic modality that permits the in situ prophylaxis against tunneled, cuffed central vein catheter infections, improves outcomes, and reduces the risk of antibiotic side effects. The technique is also known as intraluminal therapy and has wide acceptance in dialysis patients.

The CDC recommends the following: "Use prophylactic antimicrobial lock solution in patients with long-term catheters who have a history of multiple CRBSI despite optimal maximal adherence to aseptic technique."

SKIN PREPARATION

Microbes on the hands of health care personnel contribute to hospital-associated infection. Too often, breaks in sterile technique occur from failure to wash the hands before changing containers or administration sets or preparing admixtures. Besides the usual skin flora, antibiotic-resistant gram-negative organisms frequently contaminate the hands of hospital personnel.

To maintain asepsis, the CDC recommends that the hands be thoroughly washed before insertion of CVCs. Furthermore, guidelines support the use of sterile gloves:

"Prepare clean skin with an antiseptic (70% alcohol, tincture of iodine, or alcoholic chlorhexidine gluconate solution) prior to peripheral venous catheter insertion. Too frequently, alcohol use consists of a quick wipe, which fails to reduce the bacterial count significantly. Prepare clean skin with a >0.5% chlorhexidine preparation with alcohol before central venous catheter and peripheral arterial catheter insertion and during dressing changes. If there is a contraindication to chlorhexidine, tincture of iodine, an iodophor, or 70% alcohol can be used as alternatives. No comparison has been made between using chlorhexidine preparations with alcohol and povidone–iodine in alcohol to prepare clean skin. Antiseptics should be allowed to dry according to the manufacturer's recommendation prior to placing the catheter" (CDC, 2011).

Frequently, the question arises of whether to shave the insertion site. The need to remove hair is not substantiated by scientific evidence. Antiseptics used to clean the skin also clean the hair. Moreover, shaving may produce microabrasions, which can enhance the proliferation of bacteria.

EQUIPMENT PREPARATION

The tourniquet itself may be a source of cross-infection and contamination owing to its potential for reuse from patient to patient. Using an IV start kit with a disposable tourniquet minimizes the problem. However, if reusable tourniquets are consistent with clinical practice, the tourniquet should be disinfected frequently.

Once the venipuncture is completed and the catheter is in the lumen of the vein, the catheter must be securely anchored. To-and-fro motion of the catheter in the puncture wound may irritate the intima of the vein and introduce cutaneous bacteria.

Thought should be given next to the possible contamination of the securement method used to secure the catheter. Because rolls of tape last indefinitely, they may harbor contaminants; they are transported from room to room, placed on patients' beds and tables, and frequently roll to the floor. Furthermore, before venipuncture, strips of tape often are torn off the roll and placed in convenient locations on the bed, table, and uniform. These facts should be kept in mind. Adhesive tape should not be applied over the puncture wound. The puncture wound must be considered an open wound, and asepsis must be maintained.

ACCESS DEVICE AND SITE CARE

The CDC recommends using either a sterile gauze or sterile, transparent, semipermeable dressing to cover the catheter sites. Do not use topical antibiotic ointment or creams on insertion sites because of their potential to promote fungal infections and antimicrobial resistance. Frequent observations should be made for signs of malfunction of the catheter, infiltration, and phlebitis characterized by erythema, induration, or tenderness. According to CDC recommendations, monitor the site visually when changing the dressing or by palpation through an intact dressing on a regular basis, depending on the clinical condition of the patient. If there is a sign of tenderness, fever without obvious source, or other indication of a local or bloodstream infection, the dressing must be removed to permit thorough examination.

In addition to monitoring for signs of catheter malfunction, the nurse needs to monitor the condition of the catheter. Contamination may result from a break in aseptic technique, from contaminated fluid or administration set, from bacterial invasion of the puncture wound, or from clinically undetected bacteremia arising from an infection in a remote area of the body, such as a tracheostomy, the urinary tract, or a surgical wound. The clot around or in the catheter serves as an excellent trap for circulatory microorganisms and as a source of nutrients for bacterial proliferation. *Staphylococcus aureus* is the second most common cause of hospital-acquired bloodstream infection (Trinh et al., 2011), and it is the pathogen most often associated with serious and costly CRBSI. Refer to the CVC research display (Table 10-5).

CONFIRMATION OF INFECTION

Infusion-associated sepsis is not always accompanied by phlebitis. Symptoms of infection consist of chills and fever, gastric complaints, headache, hyperventilation, and shock. Should infection develop from an unknown source in a patient receiving IV therapy, the IV

EVIDENCE FOR PRACTICE

Krein, S.L., Hofer, T.P., Kowalski, C.P., et al. (2007). Use of central venous catheter-related bloodstream infection prevention practices by US hospitals. *Mayo Clinic Proceedings, 82,* 672–678.

Emphasis on the care and maintenance of catheters once they are in place should be a focus of performance improvement and quality assurance in all programs. A study to assess practice and staff knowledge of CVC postinsertion care and identify aspects of CVC care with potential for improvement revealed several areas of opportunity to improve postinsertion care. Data were recorded on 151 CVCs in 106 patients giving a total of 72. In all cases, 323 breaches in care were identified giving a failure rate of 44.8%, with significant differences between intensive care unit (ICU) and non-ICU wards. Dressings (not intact) and caps (incorrectly placed) were identified as the major lapses in CVC care with 158 and 156 breaches per 1,000 catheter days, respectively. Interventions to improve reliability of care should focus on making the implementation of best practice easier to achieve.

TABLE 10- PHLEBITIS SIGNS AND SYMPTOMS AS NOTED IN A NATIONAL GUIDELINE AND TWO SCALES

Signs/Symptoms	Signs of Phlebitis (CDC, 2011)	Phlebitis Scale (INS, 2011)	VIP Scale (Jackson, 1998)
Erythema	X	X *At access site with/without pain	X *Slight redness near IV site *Erythema
Pain	X *Tenderness	X *At access site with erythema and/or edema *At access site with erythema	X *Slight pain near IV site *Pain along path of cannula
Streak formation		X	
Palpable venous cord	X	X *More than 1 inch in length	X
Purulent drainage		X	
Induration			X
Pyrexia			X
Swelling			X
Warmth	X		

"X" indicates sign or symptom is included in the list or tool.
*Indicates clarification to sign or symptom noted.
From Jackson, A. (1998). Infection control: A battle in the vein. *Nursing Times*, 94(4), 68, 71.
Note: The Phlebitis Scale and VIP both have scoring guidelines associated with the signs and symptoms; these values are not reflected in this table.

system should be suspected and the entire system, including the catheter, removed. The catheter and the infusion fluid should then be cultured.

All containers of fluid previously administered to the patient should be suspected and, if possible, retained and cultured. All information and identification, including the lot number of the suspected fluid, should be recorded on the culture requisition and the patient's chart. The U.S. Food and Drug Administration, the CDC, and the local health authorities should be notified if contamination during manufacturing is suspected; fluids bearing implicated lot numbers should be stored for investigation.

CULTURES AND CULTURE PROFILES

Culture results identify microorganisms in suspected IV infections. Before removing a catheter for culture, the surrounding skin should be cleaned with 70% isopropyl alcohol and allowed to air dry. If purulent drainage is present, a specimen of the drainage should be obtained before the skin is cleaned.

When line sepsis is suspected, three blood culture specimens should be drawn, ideally from separate venipuncture sites. Deep candidal sepsis (systemic candidiasis) is often associated with negative culture results. It is common practice in a number of clinical settings, such as ICUs, to develop a culture profile for the patient with suspected sepsis and routinely to culture the blood of patients receiving multiple infusion therapies. Quantitative blood cultures, using pour plates, are an excellent tool for diagnosing catheter-related infection.

SEMIQUANTITATIVE TECHNIQUE FOR CULTURING CATHETERS

In the presence of purulent drainage, before removing a catheter, the nurse cleans the skin around the insertion site with an alcohol-impregnated pad to reduce contaminating skin flora and to remove any residual antibiotic ointment. After the clean area dries, the nurse withdraws the catheter, taking care to avoid contact with the surrounding skin. If pus can be expressed from the catheter wound, it is prepared for Gram staining and culture separately. For short indwelling catheters, the entire length of the catheter is cut from the skin–catheter junction (Figure 10-3) using sterile scissors. With longer catheters, a 2-inch segment that includes the tip and the intracutaneous segment is cultured. Segments are cultured as soon as possible after removal and within 2 hours. In the laboratory, the segment is rolled back and forth across the surface of a 100-mm 5% blood agar plate four times. Plates are then incubated aerobically at 37°C for at least 72 hours. This technique has outstanding sensitivity and specificity in diagnosing catheter-related infections. Box 10-5 lists criteria for defining a laboratory-confirmed bloodstream infection. Table 10-6 addresses the process for culturing the catheter or infusate.

ADDITIONAL HAZARDS: PARTICULATES

Particulate matter comprises the mobile, undissolved substances unintentionally present in parenteral fluids. Such foreign matter may consist of rubber, glass, cotton fibers, drug particles, molds, metal, or paper fibers.

The pulmonary vascular bed acts as a filter for infused particles. Particles introduced into the vein travel to the right atrium of the heart, through the tricuspid valve, and into the right ventricle. From there, they are pumped into the pulmonary artery and on through branches of arteries that decrease in size until the particles are trapped in the massive capillary bed of the lungs, where the capillaries measure 7 to 12 µm in diameter.

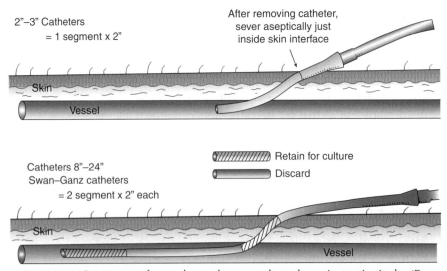

FIGURE 10-3 Segments of vascular catheters cultured semiquantitatively. (From Maki, D.G. (1986). Infection due to infusion therapy. In J.V. Bennett & P.D. Brachmann (Eds). *Hospital infections*. Boston, MA: Little, Brown.)

BOX 10-5	LABORATORY-CONFIRMED BLOODSTREAM INFECTION CRITERIA
Criterion	**Laboratory-Confirmed Bloodstream Infection (LCBI)** *Comments and reporting instructions that follow the site-specific criteria provide further explanation and are integral to the correct application of the criteria.* Must meet one of the following criteria:
LCBI 1	Patient has a recognized pathogen cultured from one or more blood cultures *and* organism cultured from blood is not related to an infection at another site.
LCBI 2	Patient has at least one of the following signs or symptoms: fever (>38°C), chills, or hypotension *and* positive laboratory results are not related to an infection at another site *and* common commensal (i.e., diphtheroids [*Corynebacterium* spp. not *C. diphtheriae*], *Bacillus* spp. [not *B. anthracis*], *Propionibacterium* spp., coagulase-negative staphylococci [including *S. epidermidis*], viridans group streptococci, *Aerococcus* spp., and *Micrococcus* spp.) is cultured from two or more blood cultures drawn on separate occasions. Criterion elements must occur within a time frame that does not exceed a gap of 1 calendar day. (See complete list of common commensals at http://www.cdc.gov/nhsn/XLS/master-organism-Com-Commensals-Lists.xls)
LCBI 3	Patient ≤1 year of age has at least one of the following signs or symptoms: fever (>38°C core), hypothermia (<36°C core), apnea, or bradycardia *and* positive laboratory results are not related to an infection at another site *and* common skin commensal (i.e., diphtheroids [*Corynebacterium* spp. not *C. diphtheriae*], *Bacillus* spp. [not *B. anthracis*], *Propionibacterium* spp., coagulase-negative staphylococci [including *S. epidermidis*], viridans group streptococci, *Aerococcus* spp., *Micrococcus* spp.) is cultured from two or more blood cultures drawn on separate occasions. Criterion elements must occur within a time frame that does not exceed a gap of 1 calendar day. (See complete list of common commensals at http://www.cdc.gov/nhsn/XLS/master-organism-Com-Commensals-Lists.xlsx))

BOX 10-5	**LABORATORY-CONFIRMED BLOODSTREAM INFECTION CRITERIA** *(Continued)*

Criterion	**Mucosal Barrier Injury Laboratory-Confirmed Bloodstream Infection (MBI-LCBI)**
	In 2013, when reporting an LCBI, it is optional to indicate which of the underlying conditions of the MBI-LCBI criterion was met, if any. However, all CLABSI, whether LCBI or MBI-LCBI, must be reported if CLABSI is part of your Monthly Reporting Plan.
	Must meet one of the following criteria:
MBI-LCBI 1	Patient of any age meets criterion 1 for LCBI with at least one blood culture growing any of the following intestinal organisms *with no other organisms isolated*: *Bacteroides* spp., *Candida* spp., *Clostridium* spp., *Enterococcus* spp., *Fusobacterium* spp., *Peptostreptococcus* spp., *Prevotella* spp., *Veillonella* spp., or Enterobacteriaceae*
	and
	patient meets at least one of the following:
	1. Is an allogeneic hematopoietic stem cell transplant recipient within the past year with one of the following documented during same hospitalization as positive blood culture:
	a. Grade III or IV gastrointestinal graft versus host disease (GI GVHD)
	b. ≥1 L diarrhea in a 24-hour period (or ≥20 mL/kg in a 24-hour period for patients <18 years of age) with onset on or within 7 calendar days before the date the positive blood culture was collected.
	2. Is neutropenic, defined as at least 2 separate days with values of absolute neutrophil count (ANC) or total white blood cell (WBC) count <500 cells/mm^3 on or within 3 calendar days before the date the positive blood culture was collected (day 1).
MBI-LCBI 2	Patient of any age meets criterion 2 for LCBI when the blood cultures are growing only viridans group streptococci *with no other organisms isolated*
	and
	patient meets at least one of the following:
	1. Is an allogeneic hematopoietic stem cell transplant recipient within the past year with one of the following documented during same hospitalization as positive blood culture:
	a. Grade III or IV GI GVHD

BOX 10-5 LABORATORY-CONFIRMED BLOODSTREAM INFECTION CRITERIA *(Continued)*

	b. ≥ 1 L diarrhea in a 24-hour period (or ≥20 mL/kg in a 24-hour period for patients <18 years of age) with onset on or within 7 calendar days before the date the first positive blood culture was collected. 2. Is neutropenic, defined as at least 2 separate days with values of ANC or total WBC count <500 cells/mm^3 on or within 3 calendar days before the date the positive blood culture was collected (day 1).

MBI-LCBI 3	Patient ≤1 year of age meets criterion 3 for LCBI when the blood cultures are growing only viridans group streptococci *with no other organisms isolated*
	and
	patient meets at least one of the following:
	
	1. Is an allogeneic hematopoietic stem cell transplant recipient within the past year with one of the following documented during same hospitalization as positive blood culture:
	  a. Grade III or IV GI GVHD
	  b. ≥20 mL/kg in a 24-hour period with onset on or within 7 calendar days before the date the first positive blood culture is collected.
	
	2. Is neutropenic, defined as at least 2 separate days with values of ANC or total WBC count <500 cells/mm^3 on or within 3 calendar days before the date the positive blood culture was collected (day 1).

Comments	1. In LCBI criterion 1, the phrase "one or more blood cultures" means that at least one bottle from a blood draw is reported by the laboratory as having grown at least one organism (i.e., is a positive blood culture). 2. In LCBI criterion 1, the term "recognized pathogen" does not include organisms considered common commensals (see criteria 2 and 3 for the list of common commensals). A few of the recognized pathogens are *S. aureus, Enterococcus* spp., *Escherichia coli, Pseudomonas* spp., *Klebsiella* spp., *Candida* spp., etc. 3. In LCBI criteria 2 and 3, the phrase "two or more blood cultures drawn on separate occasions" means (1) that blood from at least two blood draws were collected within 2 calendar days of each other (e.g., blood draws on Monday and Tuesday would be acceptable for blood cultures drawn on separate occasions, but blood draws on Monday and Wednesday would be too far apart in time to meet this criterion) and (2) that at least one bottle

---

BOX 10-5   LABORATORY-CONFIRMED BLOODSTREAM INFECTION CRITERIA   *(Continued)*

---

from each blood draw is reported by the laboratory as having grown the same common commensal (i.e., is a positive blood culture).

a. For example, an adult patient has blood drawn at 8 AM and again at 8:15 AM of the same day. Blood from each blood draw is inoculated into two bottles and incubated (four bottles total). If one bottle from each blood draw set is positive for coagulase-negative staphylococci, this part of the criterion is met.

b. For example, a neonate has blood drawn for culture on Tuesday and again on Thursday, and both grow the same common commensal. Because the time between these blood cultures exceeds the 2-day period for blood draws stipulated in LCBI and MBI-LCBI criteria 2 and 3, this part of the criterion is not met.

c. "Separate occasions" also means blood draws collected from separate sites or separate accesses of the same site, such as two draws from a single-lumen catheter or draws from separate lumens of a catheter. In the latter case, the draws may be just minutes apart (i.e., just the time it takes to disinfect and draw the specimen from each lumen). For example, a patient with a triple lumen central line has blood drawn from each lumen within 15 minutes of each other. Each of these is considered a separate blood draw.

d. A blood culture may consist of a single bottle for a pediatric blood draw due to volume constraints. Therefore, to meet this part of the criterion, each bottle from two or more draws would have to be culture positive for the same commensal.

4. If the pathogen or common commensal is identified to the species level from one blood culture, and a companion blood culture is identified with only a descriptive name (e.g., to the genus level), then it is assumed that the organisms are the same. The organism identified to the species level should be reported as the infecting organism along with its antibiogram if available.

5. Only genus and species identification should be utilized to determine the sameness of organisms (i.e., matching organisms). No additional comparative methods should be used (e.g., morphology or antibiograms) because laboratory testing capabilities and protocols may vary between facilities. This will reduce reporting variability, solely due to laboratory practice, between facilities reporting LCBIs meeting criterion 2. Report the organism

BOX 10-5   LABORATORY-CONFIRMED BLOODSTREAM INFECTION CRITERIA   *(Continued)*

to the genus/species level only once, and if antibiogram data are available, report the results from the most resistant panel.

6. LCBI criteria 1 and 2 and MCI-LCBI criteria 1 and 2 may be used for patients of any age, including these patients ≤1 year of age.

7. Specimen Collection Considerations: Ideally, blood specimens for culture should be obtained from two to four blood draws from separate venipuncture sites (e.g., right and left antecubital veins), not through a vascular catheter. These blood draws should be performed simultaneously or over a short period of time (i.e., within a few hours). If your facility does not currently obtain specimens using this technique, you must still report blood stream infections (BSIs) using the criteria and comments above, but you should work with appropriate personnel to facilitate better specimen collection practices for blood cultures.

8. "No other organisms isolated" means that there is not isolation in a blood culture of another recognized pathogen (e.g., *S. aureus*) or common commensal (e.g., coagulase-negative staphylococci) other than listed in MBI-LCBI criterion 1, 2, or 3 that would otherwise meet LCBI criteria. If this occurs, the infection should not be classified as MBI-LCBI.

9. Grade III/IV GI GVHD is defined as follows:
   - In adults: ≥1 L diarrhea/day or ileus with abdominal pain
   - In pediatric patients: ≥20 cc/kg/day of diarrhea

REPORTING INSTRUCTIONS

1. Report organisms cultured from blood as BSI–LCBI when no other site of infection is evident.

2. Catheter tip cultures are not used to determine whether a patient has a primary BSI.

3. When there is a positive blood culture and clinical signs or symptoms of localized infection at a vascular access site, but no other infection can be found, the infection is considered a primary BSI.

4. Purulent phlebitis confirmed with a positive semiquantitative culture of a catheter tip, but with either negative or no blood culture is considered a CVS-VASC, not a BSI nor an SST-SKIN or ST infection.

5. Occasionally, a patient with both peripheral and central IV lines develops a primary bloodstream infection (LCBI) that can clearly be attributed to the peripheral line (e.g., pus at the insertion site and matching pathogen from pus and blood). In this situation,

---

BOX 10-5   LABORATORY-CONFIRMED BLOODSTREAM INFECTION CRITERIA *(Continued)*

enter "Central Line = No" in the NHSN application. You should, however, include the patient's central line days in the summary denominator count.

6. If your state or facility requires that you report health care–associated BSIs that are not central line associated, enter "Central Line = No" in the NHSN application when reporting these BSIs. You should, however, include all of the patient's central line days in the summary denominator count.

Adapted from Centers for Disease Control and Prevention. (2013). April 2013 CDC/NHSN Protocol Corrections, Clarification, and Additions. http://www.cdc.gov/nhsn/pdfs/pscmanual/4psc_clabscurrent.pdf.

Five micrometers, the size of an erythrocyte suspended in fluid, has been suggested as the largest allowable size for a particle in the pulmonary capillary bed. Particles >5 μm are recognized as potentially dangerous because they are likely to become lodged. Particles as large as 300 μm can pass through an 18-gauge catheter, and much larger particles may pass through an indwelling catheter with a larger lumen. Table 10-7 lists particle size comparisons.

If the occlusion of a small arteriole inhibits oxygenation or normal metabolic activities, cellular damage or tissue death may result. Where there is ample collateral circulation, the occlusion would have no appreciable biologic effect. However, a particle that is

---

TABLE 10-6   CULTURING THE CATHETER AND INFUSATE

Catheter	*Steps* – Disinfect site with alcohol and permit to air dry – Place a sterile towel adjacent to the catheter–skin junction – Remove the catheter, avoiding contact with the surrounding skin – Uncap the culture tube – Drop the catheter into the tube. If peripheral short, cut entire length of catheter from hub using sterile scissors. For longer catheters, cut a 2-inch segment from catheter tip with sterile scissors.
Infusate	*Steps* – Disinfect the injection port of the infusion container with alcohol. – Uncap the needle with the syringe intact. – Insert needle into injection port of infusion bag. – Withdraw 5 mL of infusate into the syringe. – Remove the needle from the infusion container. – Uncap the culture tube. – Inject the contents of the syringe into the culture tube. – Recap the culture tube. – Discard the syringe in the designated waste container.

TABLE 10-? PARTICLE SIZE COMPARISONS	
Micrometers	Inches
175	0.007
150	0.006
125	0.005
100	0.004
75	0.003
50	0.002
25	0.001

not biologically inert may incite an inflammatory reaction, a neoplastic response, or an antigenic, sensitizing response.

Particles may gain access to the systemic circulation, where occlusion of a small arteriole in the brain, kidney, or eye can be serious, for the following reasons:

- The pulmonary vascular bed cannot filter out all particles. Prinzmetal and associates demonstrated that glass beads up to 390 μm may pass through the pulmonary capillary bed and reach the systemic circulation (CDC, 2011).
- Large arteriovenous shunts exist in the human lung. Particles may bypass the pulmonary capillary bed and enter the systemic circulation, where a systemic occlusion could be serious.
- Particles >5 μm may reach the systemic circulation by way of interarterial injection or infusion.

Sources of Particulates

The USP sets the acceptable limit of particles for single-dose infusion at not more than 50 particles per mL that are ≥10.0 μm and not more than 5 particles per mL that are ≥25.0 μm in effective linear dimension.

Over the years, manufacturers have made great efforts to produce high-quality products, but these efforts may be negated by manipulating the products before their infusion.

Medication Additives

Drugs constitute a major source of particulate matter. Improper technique in preparing drugs may result in the formation of insoluble particles. Use of an IV additive service precludes the need to mix drugs on the nursing unit other than in an emergency situation.

Glass Ampules

Glass ampules have been responsible for the injection of thousands of glass particles into the circulation. Turco and Davis, in a classic study prompted by the frequency of high-dose administration of furosemide, showed that a dose of 400 mg, which at that time required the breaking of 20 ampules, could add 1,085 glass particles >5 μm to the injection. A dose of 600 mg, requiring 30 ampules, could result in 2,387 particles >5 μm.

ANTIBIOTIC INJECTABLES

Particulate contamination of bulk-filled antibiotics may be 2 to 10 times greater than that of stable antibiotic solutions and lyophilized antibiotics. Filtration is impossible because packaging by the sterile bulk-fill method involves extracting and processing the antibiotic in sterile bulk powder form and then aseptically placing the bulk antibiotic into dry, presterilized vials.

In the lyophilized and the stable liquid packaging processes, the particulate matter can be terminally removed by filtration directly into presterilized vials. Most antibiotics are packed by the bulk-fill method, however.

Particulate matter in IV injections may be responsible for much of the phlebitis that so often occurs with the infusion of these drugs. Studies demonstrate that the major pathologic conditions caused by particulate matter are direct blockage of vessels, platelet agglutination leading to formation of emboli, local inflammation caused by impaction of particles, and antigenic reactions with subsequent allergic consequence.

Reducing the Particulate Level

Because particulate matter infused through IV fluids may produce pathologic changes that can have an adverse effect on critically ill patients, every effort is taken to reduce the particulate count in IV injections. In general, nurses and physicians/LIPs have been unaware of the potential dangers that exist and have unknowingly added to the contamination. To promote awareness, official agencies have developed standards for an acceptable particulate limit in IV fluids, and industry has provided the health care profession with filters to limit direct access of particulates, bacteria, fungi, and other contaminants to the bloodstream.

FILTERS

A filter aspiration needle specially designed to remove particulate matter from IV medications is available. With this device attached to a syringe, the medication is drawn from the vial or glass ampule, and the particles are filtered out. The filter needle must then be discarded to prevent the particles trapped on the filter from being injected when the medication is added to the infusate.

FINAL FILTERS

The INS policy advocates the routine use of 0.2-μm air-eliminating filters in delivering routine IV therapy because these filters remove particulates, bacteria, and air, and some remove endotoxins as well (INS, 2011).

Filters are manufactured in a variety of forms, sizes, and materials. Some block the passage of air under normal pressure when wet. Used with electronic infusion devices, they play an important role in preventing air from being pumped into the bloodstream should the fluid container empty.

Knowledge of filter characteristics, use, and proper handling is important for patient safety. Faulty handling can result in occlusion of the filter, with the patient not receiving prescribed fluids. In addition, the infusion may need to be discontinued and venipuncture repeated to insert a new line. Moreover, a ruptured filter may go undetected and introduce filter fragments, bacteria, and possibly air into the IV system.

ONGOING MONITORING AND PRECAUTIONS

The practice setting in which care is delivered has no relevance to the level of diligence needed to provide high-quality infusion therapy. This theory is based on the fact that the patient is accustomed to the flora in his or her own environment. In any clinical environment, principles of asepsis must be adhered to in an effort to minimize the risk of IV catheter–related infection and to ensure a high level of IV patient care.

Extensive guidelines for monitoring infusion therapy and preventing catheter-related infection have been published (CDC, 2011). Preventive measures described throughout this chapter should be adhered to. In addition, any device intended for vascular access must be thought of in fundamental terms as a direct conduit between the external world and the patient's bloodstream (CDC, 2011; INS, 2011).

Inappropriate catheter care and lack of monitoring and nursing interventions may contribute to catheter-related infections. The use of specialty IV teams to ensure a high level of aseptic technique during and after catheter insertion has been associated with substantially lower rates of catheter-related infection (Phillips, 2010).

Sentinel Events

We know that a sentinel event refers to an unexpected occurrence involving death or serious physical or psychological injury or the risk thereof. Serious injury specifically includes loss of limb or function. The phrase "or the risk thereof" includes any process variation for which a recurrence would carry a significant chance of a serious adverse outcome. Such events are called "sentinel" because they signal the need for immediate investigation and response (TJC, 2012; Box 10-6).

ROOT CAUSE ANALYSIS

Root cause analysis is a process for identifying the basic or causal factors that underlie variation in performance, including the occurrence or possible occurrence of a sentinel event. A root cause analysis focuses primarily on systems and processes, not individual performance. It progresses from special causes in clinical processes to common causes in organizational processes and identifies potential improvements in processes or systems that would tend to decrease the likelihood of such events in the future, or determines, after analysis that no such improvement opportunities exist (TJC, 2011).

Previously, if a surveyor identified a sentinel event in the course of conducting an on-site survey, he or she would review the root cause analysis on site, often affecting the flow and focus of the survey and introducing a potential variation in the root cause analysis review process. Currently, if during the course of a survey, a reviewer identifies a potentially reviewable sentinel event that has not previously been reported to TJC, he or she will take the following steps:

BOX 10-6   GOALS OF THE SENTINEL EVENT POLICY—HOSPITALS

Goals of the Policy

The policy has four goals:

- To have a positive impact in improving patient care, treatment, and services and preventing sentinel events
- To focus the attention of a hospital that has experienced a sentinel event on understanding the factors that contributed to the event (such as underlying causes, latent conditions and active failures in defense systems, or organizational culture) and on changing the hospital's culture, systems, and processes to reduce the probability of such an event in the future
- To increase the general knowledge about sentinel events, their contributing factors, and strategies for prevention
- To maintain the confidence of the public and accredited hospitals in the accreditation process

From Joint Commission Resources. (2012). *Sentinel events (SE)*. Oakbrook Terrace, IL: Joint Commission on Accreditation of Healthcare Organizations. Reprinted with permission.

- Inform the chief executive officer (CEO) that the event has been identified
- Inform the CEO that the event will be reported to TJC for further review and follow-up under the provisions of the Sentinel Event Policy

During the on-site survey, the surveyor(s) will assess the organization's compliance with sentinel event–related standards in the following ways:

- Review the organization's process for responding to a sentinel event
- Interview the organization's leaders and staff about their expectations and responsibilities for identifying, reporting, and responding to sentinel events
- Ask for and review an example of a root cause analysis that has been conducted in the past year to assess the adequacy of the organization's process for responding to a sentinel event. Additional examples may be reviewed if needed to more fully assess the organization's understanding of, and ability to conduct, root cause analyses. In selecting an example, the organization may choose a closed case or a "near miss" to demonstrate its process for responding to a sentinel event (TJC, 2011).

Rare Complications

Reflex Sympathetic Dystrophy

Reflex sympathetic dystrophy (RSD) is a condition of burning pain, stiffness, swelling, and discoloration of the hand (Figure 10-4). RSD includes other medical diagnoses such as causalgia, Sudeck atrophy, and shoulder–hand syndrome. RSD occurs from a disturbance in the

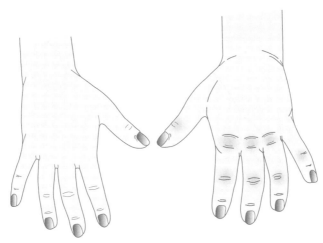

FIGURE 10-4 On the right, the swollen, painful hand of early RSD with reddened joints.

sympathetic (unconscious) nervous system that controls the blood flow and sweat glands in the hand and arm. When the nervous system becomes overactive, burning pain is felt and swelling and warmth are left in the affected arm. If untreated, RSD can cause stiffness and loss of use of the affected part of the arm.

In some cases, the cause of RSD is unknown. Often an injury can cause RSD, or the symptoms may appear after a surgery or sometimes insertion of an IV cannula (Weinstein, 2012). Other causes include pressure on a nerve, infection, cancer, neck disorders, stroke, or heart attack. These conditions can cause pain, which sets off the sympathetic reflex causing RSD symptoms. Nerve injuries may change the way the nerve impulses are sent, causing a "short circuit" (Figure 10-5).

Signs and Symptoms

The pain associated with RSD is often described as burning. Swelling can cause painful joints and stiffness. RSD has three stages:

1. Stage I (acute) may last up to 3 months. During this stage, the symptoms include pain and swelling, increased warmth in the affected part/limb, and excessive sweating. There may be faster-than-normal nail and hair growth and joint pain during movement of the affected area.
2. Stage II (dystrophic) can last 3 to 12 months. Swelling is more constant, skin wrinkles disappear, skin temperature becomes cooler, and fingernails become brittle. The pain is more widespread, stiffness increases, and the affected area becomes sensitive to touch.
3. Stage III (atrophic) occurs from 1 year on. The skin of the affected area is now pale, dry, tightly stretched, and shiny. The area is stiff, pain may decrease, and there is less hope of getting motion back.

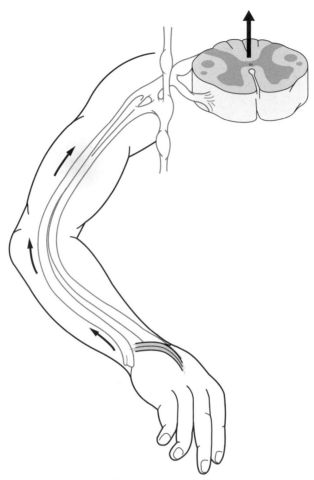

FIGURE 10-5 This illustration shows how a nerve injury may cause a "short circuit" in the nervous system, resulting in sympathetic overactivity in the hand with burning pain, swelling, and increased sweating.

DIAGNOSIS

The diagnosis usually is made when at least three of the following symptoms are present: pain and tenderness, signs of changed blood flow (either increased or decreased), swelling with joint stiffness, or skin changes.

TREATMENT

Early diagnosis and treatment are important. Three forms of treatment may be combined: medication, physical therapy, and surgery. Medication taken by mouth can help decrease the symptoms. To reduce symptoms and provide long-term relief, local anesthetics may be injected into a nerve bundle at the base of the neck (stellate ganglion block). In some cases, a tourniquet is applied to the arm, and medication can be injected into a vein along with an anesthetic. A hand surgeon may recommend therapy by a hand, occupational, or physical therapist, or by a physiatrist. Therapy is important to regain function and reduce discomfort caused by RSD. Successful treatment depends on the patient's full and active effort in therapy (AAOS, 2010).

COMPLEX REGIONAL PAIN SYNDROME

Complex regional pain syndrome (CRPS) is a chronic pain condition. The key symptom of CRPS is continuous, intense pain out of proportion to the severity of the injury, which gets worse rather than better over time. CRPS most often affects one of the arms, legs, hands, or feet. Often the pain spreads to include the entire arm or leg. Typical features include dramatic changes in the color and temperature of the skin over the affected limb or body part, accompanied by intense burning pain, skin sensitivity, sweating, and swelling. The cause of CRPS is unknown, but a proliferation of infusion-related injury cases cause one to suspect IV-related injuries (Weinstein, 2012). In some cases, the sympathetic nervous system plays an important role in sustaining the pain. Another theory is that CRPS is caused by a triggering of the immune response, which leads to the characteristic inflammatory symptoms of redness, warmth, and swelling in the affected area.

Often the pain spreads to include the entire arm or leg, even though the initiating injury might have been only to a finger or toe. Pain can sometimes even travel to the opposite extremity. It may be heightened by emotional stress.

Certification

Professional certification validates competence; it is the process through which an organization grants recognition to an individual who meets certain established criteria. A voluntary process, the gold standard for infection control is the infection preventionist who has board certification in infection control and prevention. The Certification Board of Infection Control and Epidemiology, Inc. (CBIC) is a voluntary, autonomous multidisciplinary board that provides direction for and administers the certification process for professionals in infection control and applied epidemiology (CBIC, 2013).

Competence on the part of all professionals involved in the administration of infusion therapy will ensure positive outcomes and prevent otherwise avoidable complications of this complex modality.

Review Questions   *Questions below may have more than one right answer.*

1. Gram-negative organisms include all of the following *except*
   A. *Staphylococcus aureus*
   B. *Pseudomonas aeruginosa*
   C. *Klebsiella*
   D. *Escherichia coli*

2. Which of the following microorganisms is *not* associated with IV infusate contamination?
   A. *Coccidioides immitis*
   B. *Enterobacter cloacae*
   C. *Klebsiella pneumoniae*
   D. *Serratia marcescens*

3. A diagnosis of RSD may include all of the following *except*
   A. Sudeck atrophy
   B. Causalgia
   C. Finger–hand compression
   D. Shoulder–hand syndrome

4. In the event of a suspected air embolism, the appropriate nursing intervention is to
   A. Turn patient on left side, head down
   B. Turn patient on right side, head down
   C. Turn patient on left side, head raised
   D. Turn patient on right side, head raised

5. Which of the following is *not* a sign of impending pulmonary edema?
   A. Venous dilation
   B. Increased blood pressure
   C. Engorged neck veins
   D. Slow, shallow respirations

6. Which of the following statements is true of catheter-related infection?
   A. Originates from the catheter material itself
   B. Stems from migration of organisms through the open skin along the catheter
   C. A only
   D. A and B

7. Classic symptoms of air embolism include all of the following *except*
   A. Cyanosis
   B. Dyspnea
   C. Churning over precordium
   D. Increase in pulse pressure

8. Which of the following is true concerning central line bundles?
   A. They are groupings of best practices.
   B. They individually improve care.
   C. When applied together, they result in substantially greater improvement.
   D. All of the above

9. Factors influencing the survival of bacteria include all of the following *except*
   A. Number and type of organisms present
   B. Environmental conditions
   C. Resistance of the host
   D. Use of filtration

10. Clinical manifestations of septicemia include which of the following?
    A. Chills and fever
    B. Chills and fever, headache, and general malaise
    C. General malaise only
    D. Fever and headache only

References and Selected Readings   *Asterisks indicate references cited in text.*

*Al-Hwiesh, A.K., & Abdul-Rahman, I.S. (2007). Successful prevention of tunneled, central catheter infection by antibiotic lock therapy using vancomycin and gentamycin. *Saudi Journal of Kidney Disease and Transplantation, 18*(2), 239–247.

Alexander, M., Corrigan N., Gorski, L., Hankins, J., & Perucca, R. (2010). *Infusion nursing: An evidence–based practice approach* (3rd ed.). St. Louis, MO: Saunders Elsevier.

Ajenjo, M., Morley, J.C., Russo, A. J., McMullen, K.M., Robinson, C., & Williams, R.C., et al. (2011). Peripherally inserted central venous catheter–associated bloodstream infections in hospitalized adult patients. *Infection Control and Hospital Epidemiology, 32*(2), 125–130.

Alhimyary, A., Fernandez, C., Picard, M., Tierno, K., Pignatone, N., & Chan, H.S., et al. (1996). Safety and efficacy of total parenteral nutrition delivered via a peripherally inserted central venous catheter. *Nutrition in Clinical Practice, 11*, 199–203.

*Association for Practitioners in Infection Control and Epidemiology. (2011). http://www.apic.org/Professional-Practice/Scientific-guidelines

*American Academy of Orthopaedic Surgeons. (2010). http://orthoinfo.aaos.org/topic.cfm?topic=a00021

Bennett, J.V., & Brachman, P.S. (2007). *Hospital infections* (5th ed.). Philadelphia, PA: Lippincott Williams & Wilkins.

*Boer, W.H., & Hene, R.J. (1999). Lethal air embolism following removal of a double lumen jugular vein catheter. *Nephrology Dialysis Transplantation, 14*(8), 1850–1852.

Bowers, L., Speroni, K.G., Jones, L., & Atherton, M. (2008). Comparison of occlusion rates by flushing solutions for peripherally inserted central catheters with positive pressure Luer-activated devices. *Journal of Infusion Nursing, 31,* 22–27.

Bravery, K., Dougherty, L., Gabriel, J., Kayley, J., Malster, M., & Scales, K. (2006). Audit of peripheral venous cannulae by members of an IV therapy forum. *British Journal of Nursing, 15,* 1244–1249.

Broom, J., Woods, M., Allworth, A., Mccarthy, J., Faoagali, J., & Macdonald, S., et al. (2008). Ethanol lock therapy to treat tunnelled central venous catheter-associated blood stream infections: Results from a prospective trial. *Scandinavian Journal of Infectious Diseases, 40*(5), 399–406.

*Centers for Disease Control and Prevention (CDC). (2011). Guidelines for the prevention of intravascular catheter-related infections. http://www.cdc.gov/hicpac/pdf/guidelines/bsi-guidelines-2011.pdf

*Certification Board of Infection Control and Epidemiology, Inc. (CBIC). (2013). http://www.cbic.org/about-cbic

Gallant, P., & Schultz, A. (2006). Evaluation of a visual infusion phlebitis scale for determining appropriate discontinuation of peripheral intravenous catheters. *Journal of Infusion Nursing, 29*(6), 338–345.

Groll, D., Davies, B., MacDonald, J., Nelson, S., & Virani, T. (2010). Evaluation of the psychometric properties of the phlebitis and infiltration scales for the assessment of complications of peripheral vascular access devices. *Journal of Infusion Nursing, 33*(6), 385–390.

Gura, K.M. (2004). Incidence and nature of epidemic nosocomial infections. *Journal of Infusion Nursing, 27*(3), 175–178.

Hadaway, L. (2007). Infiltration and extravasation: Preventing a complication of IV catheterization. *American Journal of Nursing, 107*(8), 64–72.

*Infusion Nurses Society. (2011). Infusion nursing standards of practice. *Journal of Infusion Nursing, 34*(1 Suppl), S1–S110.

*Institute for Healthcare Improvement (IHI). (2013). Knowledge center. http://www.ihi.org/knowledge/Pages/Changes/ImplementtheCentralLineBundle.aspx

Jarvis, W. (Ed.). (2013). *Bennett and Brachman's hospital infections* (6th ed.). Philadelphia, PA: Lippincott Williams & Wilkins.

*The Joint Commission. (2011). National patient safety goals. www.jointcommission.org/standards_information/npsgs.aspx

*The Joint Commission. (2012). Sentinel events. http://www.jointcommission.org/assets/1/6/CAMH_2012_Update2_24_SE.pdf

*Khalidi, N., Kovacevich, D., Papke-O'Donnell, L., & Btaiche, I. (2009). Impact of the positive pressure valve on vascular access device occlusions and bloodstream infections. *Journal of the Association for Vascular Access, 14*(2), 84–91.

Lee, W., Chen, H., Tsai, T., Lai, I., Chang, W., & Huang, C., et al. (2009). Risk factors for peripheral intravenous catheter infection in hospitalized patients: A prospective study of 3165 patients. *American Journal of Infection Control, 37*(8), 683–686.

Lee, J.Y., Ko, K.S., Peck, K.R., Oh, W.S., & Song, J.H. (2006). In vitro evaluation of the antibiotic lock technique (ALT) for the treatment of catheter-related infections caused by staphylococci. *Journal of Antimicrobial Chemotherapy, 57*(6), 1110–1115.

Mermel, L.A., Allon, M., Bouza, E., Craven, D.E., & Flynn, P. (2009). Clinical practice guidelines for the diagnosis and management of intravascular catheter-related infection: 2009 update by the Infectious Diseases Society of America. *Clinical Infectious Diseases, 49,* 1–45.

*Metheny, N.M. (2012). *Fluid and electrolyte balance* (5th ed.). Sudbury, MA: Jones & Bartlett Learning.

*Natal, B.L., & Brown, D.F.M. (2012). Venous air embolism treatment and management. http://emedicine.medscape.com/article/761367-treatment#a1126

Niel-Weise, B.S., Stijnen, R., Peterhans, J., & van den Broek, M. (2010). Should in-line filters be used in peripheral intravenous catheters to prevent infusion-related phlebitis? *Anesthesia Patient Safety Foundation, 110*(6), 1624–1629.

Paolucci, H., Nutter, B., & Albert, N.M. (2011). RN knowledge of vascular access devices management. *Journal of the Association for Vascular Access, 16*(4), 221–225.

*Phillips, L. (2010). State of the society. *Journal of Infusion Nursing, 33*(4), 206–208.

Pronovost, P.J., Wu, A.W., & Sexton, J.B. (2004). Acute decompensation after removing a central line: Practical approaches to increasing safety in the intensive care unit. *Annals of Internal Medicine, 140*(12), 1025–1033. [Medline].

*Sadfar, N., Jacobs, E., & Gaines, M. (2012). Patient awareness of the risks of CVS in outpatient settings: Letter to the editor. *American Journal of Infection Control, 40,* 80–89.

*Smith, J.S., Irvin, G., Viney, M., Watkins, L., Morris, S., Kirksey, K., et al. (2012). Optimal disinfection times for needleless intravenous connectors. *Journal of the Association for Vascular Access, 17*(3), 137–143.

Sviri, S., Woods, W.P., & van Heerden, P.V. (2004). Air embolism—A case series and review. *Critical Care Resuscitation, 6*(4), 271–276. [Medline].

*Trinh, R.T., Chan, P., Edwards, O., Hollenbeck, B., Huang, B., Burdick, N., et al. (2011). Peripheral venous catheter-related *Staphylococcus aureus* bacteremia. *Infection Control and Hospital Epidemiology, 32*(6), 579–583.

*Washington, G., & Barrett, R. (2012). Peripheral phlebitis: A point-prevalence study. *Journal of Infusion Nursing, 35*(4), 252–258.

*Weinstein, S.M. (2012). Reflex sympathetic dystrophy: Cause and effect of infusion-related complications. White Paper.

Weinstein, S.M. (2009). Factor V Leiden: Impact on infusion nursing practice. *Journal of Infusion Nursing, 32*(4), 219–223.

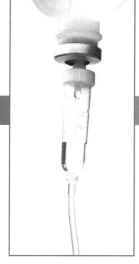

CHAPTER 11

Evidence-Based Infusion Practice

Mary E. Hagle
Beth Ann Taylor

KEY TERMS

Clinical Decision
  Making
Evidence-Based
  Practice
Outcome Indicators

Process Indicators
Professional Practice
  Model
Research
Structure Indicators

PRACTICE BASED ON EVIDENCE

Nursing practice based on best evidence is a defined, specific, and dynamic process that draws upon the latest research findings, clinical data, or, if necessary, expert opinion to drive clinical and leadership improvements in health care. Simply put, this process requires nurses to use evidence rather than tradition or personal opinion in their approach to providing care to patients. Florence Nightingale used statistics to influence changes in how British soldiers were cared for during the Crimean War (Stanley & Sherratt, 2010), and thus was born the foundation of nursing practice based on the effective use of data to ensure better health outcomes. Using evidence to inspire changes in practice is neither a new nor novel idea but rather a fundamental tenet of professional nursing.

Infusion nurses, along with other nursing specialties, share the common challenge of staying current with the rapidly growing and changing information base in their area of practice. The American Nurses Association (ANA, 2010) and Infusion Nurses Society (INS, 2011) professional standards call for infusion nurses to use research findings and to practice with the current best evidence, "The registered nurse integrates evidence and research findings into practice" (ANA, 2010, p. 51). "The nurse shall use research findings and current best evidence to expand nursing knowledge in infusion therapy, to validate and improve practice, to advance professional accountability, and to enhance evidence-based

245

decision making" (INS, 2011, p. S13). These standards are inclusive of all roles in professional nursing, and at all levels; the novice nurse understands that institutional policies and procedures are based on best evidence, while the infusion team manager plans and executes a budget for staffing based on sound administrative principles and analysis of patient needs.

For example, the Centers for Disease Control and Prevention (CDC, 2011) strongly recommended that only trained personnel with demonstrated competence manage peripheral and central venous catheters (CVCs); this was based on the evidence of 14 studies. The authors in three of the more recent studies described the initiation of infusion teams with measurable outcomes or quantified the infusion therapy procedure for average nursing times and costs (Brunelle, 2003; Hawes, 2007; Pierce & Baker, 2004), providing evidence for the manager and administrator on budgeting, staffing, and quality outcomes for patients (Box 11-1). These studies also provide evidence for any nurses, leaders, or managers who wish to compare their outcomes with another agency reporting quality practice. One more strong recommendation was to ensure that intensive care units are staffed at appropriate levels, and with nurses who regularly work for the institution, in order to prevent central line–associated blood stream infection (CLABSI) (CDC, 2011). This evidence is from two separate yet classic studies (Alonso-Echanove et al., 2003; Robert et al., 2000). Besides implementing best evidence, this is an example of the need for additional studies to provide a more robust body of evidence that drives staffing with measurable outcomes.

EVIDENCE-BASED PRACTICE

The INS Standard of Practice for Research and Evidence-based practice (EBP) states, "The nurse shall integrate evidence-based nursing knowledge with clinical expertise and the patient's preferences and values in the current context when providing infusion therapy" (INS, 2011, p. S13). The infusion nurse exemplifies this standard by basing his or her practice on the best evidence, through lifelong learning to advance one's clinical expertise, and by centering the focus of care on the patient. EBP occurs at the intersection of the three circles shown on the Venn diagram (Figure 11-1).

EBP is not simply the application of the latest research findings; it goes beyond seeking the best evidence related to a clinical or leadership question. It incorporates the best available evidence with the expertise of the nurse and the patient preferences in the context of care delivery. Therefore, the application of evidence is not done in isolation of the desires and goals of the patient, it is dependent upon the expertise of the individual nurse, and it is accomplished in the context of the care environment. For example, in home care, this context reflects the resources the nurse brings as well as what the patient has in his or her home and who can help. Additionally, context incorporates the professional practice model of the nurse and organization (Hoffart & Woods, 1996). It might be relationship-based care (Koloroutis, 2004), partnership (Jonsdottir, Litchfield, & Pharris, 2004), or caring science (Drenkard, 2008). The American Nurses Credentialing Center (ANCC) defines a professional practice model as a schematic or diagram, sometimes with descriptions, of the theory or system that "depicts how nurses practice, collaborate, communicate, and develop professionally to provide the highest quality care for those served by the organization" (ANCC, 2011). All of these components provide support for the infusion nurse making the best decision at the time.

BOX 11-1 SELECTED STUDIES CITED BY CDC (2011) AS SUPPORT FOR THE RECOMMENDATION THAT ONLY TRAINED PERSONNEL SHOULD MANAGE PERIPHERAL AND CENTRAL VENOUS CATHETERS

Source	Assessment	Intervention	Outcomes
Brunelle (2003)	• Identified problems: "(1) below-standard practice for bedside care, (2) multiple use of the same catheter, (3) staff shortage, (4) below-standard education for staff, and (5) growing number of elderly patients who are more susceptible to infection" (p. 362) • Prevalence survey to provide systematically gathered data on infection source, insertion and management practices	Develop IV team to • Educate staff • Serve as a resource Track patients with CVCs for maintenance of devices and clinical outcomes	Process outcome: • IV team does all CVC dressing changes; serves as resource to nurses Clinical outcome: • Catheter-related bloodstream infections (year/frequency): 1996/45 2001/19
Hawes (2007)	Problem identified of: • Inadequate peripheral veins for peripherally inserted central catheter (PICC) placement • Unnecessary "urgent" placement requests at end of week	Develop infusion team to: • "Increase number of PICCs placed at the bedside. • Improve patient outcomes related to infusion therapy. • Improve patient satisfaction related to infusion therapy" (p. 35)	Clinical outcomes: • Increase from 50% to over 80% PICCs placed at bedside at consistent rate • All levels of phlebitis decreased from 24% to less than 5% over 18 mo • Less than 10% PIVs infusing irritants • Increase of 7% for patient satisfaction with "Courtesy of the person that started your IV"

BOX 11-1	SELECTED STUDIES CITED BY CDC (2011) AS SUPPORT FOR THE RECOMMENDATION THAT ONLY TRAINED PERSONNEL SHOULD MANAGE PERIPHERAL AND CENTRAL VENOUS CATHETERS *(Continued)*		
Pierce and Baker (2004)	• Quantify time and effort involved in service provision for infusion therapy procedures of nonchemotherapeutic agents in outpatient infusion centers • Data collected through direct observation and staff interviews of 78 patients in 75 different offices	Not applicable	Process outcomes: • Average nursing time, average labor costs, and average time for each phase of infusion therapy were calculated and reported

EBP is the "right thing to do" for many reasons (Melnyk & Fineout-Overholt, 2011):

- It leads to best patient outcomes.
- It reduces health care costs (Hollenbeak, 2011).
- It supports clinicians feeling empowered and more satisfied in their roles.

The critical nature of nurses understanding and using evidence to drive practice is underscored by Institute of Medicine's goal proposing, "By 2020, 90% of clinical decisions will be supported by accurate, timely, and up-to-date clinical information and will reflect the best available evidence" (Institute of Medicine, 2007, p. ix). To meet this goal, EBP must be an integral part of the organization's culture. Each organization will have to evaluate their current state and identify needs of the staff. Based on a recent national survey of ANA members, work remains to be done. Less than 54% of 876 RNs strongly agreed/agreed that EBP was consistently implemented in their setting and less than 47% strongly agreed/agreed that findings from research are routinely implemented to improve patient outcomes (Melnyk, Fineout-Overholt, Gallagher-Ford, & Kaplan, 2012). In the same study, nurses' beliefs about their own practice demonstrated moderate agreement with the statement, "I consistently implement evidence-based practice with my patients"; that is, nurses rated their agreement with this

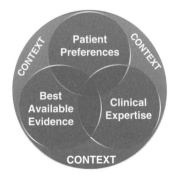

FIGURE 11-1 Components of evidence-based practice. (From Veterans Health Administration, Office of Nursing Services, Evidence-Based Practice Resource Center.)

statement an average 3.82 (standard deviation 0.883), on a scale of 1 to 5, strongly disagree to strongly agree (ibid p. 412). Interpreting this finding means there are opportunities for leaders at all levels to facilitate nurses consistently implementing EBP with their patients.

CREATING A CULTURE OF EVIDENCE-BASED PRACTICE

Effective nursing leadership is essential at all levels of the organization to create a culture that values and supports nurses in developing a spirit of inquiry, generating and answering relevant clinical questions, and making recommendations that can be operationalized (Newhouse, 2007). A robust EBP culture shortens the time between the emergence of new research findings and their implementation in clinical settings (Brady & Lewin, 2007). Adopting a model for EBP, identified and selected by all staff, may initiate a culture change. There are several models that outline steps, provide a decision tree, or give broad concepts to the process (Table 11-1). Staff nurses and organizations are varied in how they approach change, thus an open and ongoing dialogue about EBP models may be helpful.

Additionally, there are generational differences, learning differences, and attitudes that affect how a culture changes to being evidence-based. Providing options for learning about EBP will appeal to a wider variety of learners. A variety of online tutorials are available (Box 11-2), numerous texts, and summer courses across the United States, as well as those offered by the international Joanna Briggs Institute. An increasing number of journals focus solely on reports of literature synthesis and research translation projects, in addition to journals focused on infusion therapy but publishing literature syntheses, such as the *Journal of Infusion Nursing* and *Journal of the Association for Vascular Access*. Learning more about EBP was the most common response to the question, "What one thing would help to implement EBP in your daily practice?" (Melnyk et al., 2012, p. 414). Having access to information was the second request. Advocating for resources is an accountability of leaders, in partnership with staff for appropriate materials and strategies to make these accessible.

Evidence-based leadership in nursing makes each experience count. EBP gathers the wide array of skill sets that each participant brings to the health care setting and influences decisions related to patient care. Essential components for the creation of an EBP culture include institutional support, strong clinical leadership, availability of resources, and feedback on outcomes (Newell-Stokes, 2004). Enabling nurses to consistently use best evidence at the point of care with their patients means that systems need to be in place for best evidence to be easily available, or, a culture of EBP.

STEPS FOR PRACTICE BASED ON EVIDENCE

Type of Evidence

At the organizational level, there are several elements to promote EBP. Having a model is one element that may be helpful, as it guides the team along the journey of discovery. Another element is understanding what constitutes evidence. Nurses may actively seek evidence, but just as likely, they will be provided with evidence for support of some policy, procedure, or recommendation. Whether part of a team or not, each infusion nurse must be able to recognize what type of evidence is being submitted. As shown in the evidence pyramid in Figure 11-2, there are a wide variety of sources of evidence, and it is important to note that not all evidence is obtained from research. At the lowest level of evidence is nonresearch. Examples of nonresearch sources of evidence are as follows:

TABLE 11-1	MODELS OF EVIDENCE-BASED PRACTICE	
Name of Model	**Reference**	**Brief Description**
ACE Star Model of Knowledge Transformation	Stevens, K.R. (2004). *ACE Star Model of EBP: Knowledge transformation*. Academic Center for Evidence-Based Practice. The University of Texas Health Science Center at San Antonio. www.acestar.uthscsa.edu	Five stages of transforming knowledge into the clinical setting for practice use. Circular model.
Iowa Model of Evidence-Based Practice to Promote Quality Care	Titler, M.G., Kleiber, C., Steelman, V.J., Rakel, B.A., Budreau, G., Everett, L.Q., et al. (2001). The Iowa model of evidence-based practice to promote quality care. *Critical Care Nursing Clinics of North America*, 13(4), 497–509.	Decision tree starting with triggers to action. Facilitates decisions to use the evidence or to conduct research.
Johns Hopkins Evidence-Based Practice Model	Dearholt, S., & Dang, D. (2012). *Johns Hopkins nursing evidence based practice model and guidelines* (2nd ed.). Indianapolis, IN: Sigma Theta Tau.	Focuses on best available evidence; multidisciplinary approach. Provides tools for EBP use.
Model for Change to Evidence-Based Practice	Rosswurm, M.A., & Larrabee, J.H. (1999). A model for change to evidence-based practice. *Image: Journal of Nursing Scholarship, 31,* 317–322.	Linear model of six steps is explained to guide nurses through the EBP process.
PARiHS (Promoting Action on Research Implementation in Health Services)	National Collaborating Centre for Methods and Tools. (2011). *PARiHS framework for implementing research into practice*. Hamilton, ON: McMaster University. http://www.nccmt.ca/registry/view/eng/85.html. Based on: Kitson, A., Harvey, G., & McCormack, B. (1998). Enabling the implementation of evidence based practice: A conceptual framework. *Quality in Health Care, 7,* 149–158.	Provides a method to implement research into practice. Identifies three key elements for knowledge translation: Evidence (E), Context (C), and Facilitation (F). It emphasizes that successful implementation of evidence into practice is related to context or the setting where the new evidence is being introduced as the quality of the evidence.
Steps of the EBP Process Leading to High-Quality Healthcare and Best Patient Outcomes	Melnyk, B., & Fineout-Overholt, E. (2011). *Evidence-based practice in nursing & healthcare: A guide to best practice* (2nd ed.) (p. 16). New York, NY: Wolters Kluwer/Lippincott Williams & Wilkins.	Decision tree with six key steps for implementing an EBP project.
Stetler Model	Stetler, C.B. (2001). Updating the Stetler model of research utilization to facilitate evidence-based practice. *Nursing Outlook, 49,* 272–279.	Model helps to "focus on a series of judgmental activities about the appropriateness, desirability, feasibility, and manner of using research findings in an individual's or group's practice" (p. 272).

BOX 11-2   ONLINE TUTORIALS FOR EVIDENCE-BASED PRACTICE

University of Illinois at Chicago: *EBP in the Health Sciences*	http://ebp.lib.uic.edu/
University of Minnesota: *Welcome to Evidence-Based Practice: An Inter-professional Tutorial*	http://hsl.lib.umn.edu/learn/ebp/
University of North Carolina at Chapel Hill Duke University: *Introduction to Evidence-Based Practice*	http://www.hsl.unc.edu/Services/Tutorials/EBM/welcome.htm
University of Texas Health Science Center at San Antonio: *Academic Center for Evidence-Based Practice*	http://www.acestar.uthscsa.edu/

- *Expert Opinion*: An individual or professional organization that has experience and expertise in a particular area of practice. Editorials or opinion papers are examples of this type of evidence.
- *Clinical Textbooks*: Similar to expert opinion, this is a compilation of expertise regarding a topic or series of topics.
- *Quality/Performance Improvement Data*: This facility or system data may be instructive and used as process or outcome indicators of the efficacy of nursing care.

The next level of the pyramid is research. Desired sources of evidence are research reports. There are various levels of research studies such as qualitative or descriptive studies, case studies, controlled trials without randomization, with the most robust type of research being randomized controlled trials (RCTs). RCTs may not always be feasible for clinical research as they require some study subjects to receive an intervention and others not, based on random selection and therefore may not be ethical. Consider a study that would require a number of patients to receive treatment and another group that does not. If we know that the treatment is essential to thwart the advancement of disease, we are ethically obligated to provide it, and thus, many clinical studies are not well suited for RCTs.

However, RCTs are often needed, as in the case of the study by Rickard et al. (2012). This study examined the rates of phlebitis and other catheter-related outcomes when the peripheral IV catheter (PIV) was left in place until signs or symptoms of phlebitis appeared or was replaced every 3 days routinely. Patients were randomized between the two planned replacement options. Current practice is to replace PIV at a set interval in order to prevent infection. Yet, nurses can obtain orders to leave the PIV in place when there is no other access or the treatment will be ending soon. Additionally, PIVs are left in place in pediatric patients until there are signs or symptoms of phlebitis or the treatment is completed. For this practice, the best research design was an RCT, and it was done ethically, since PIVs were often left in place for many days. For the study patients' protection, a monitoring board was in place that oversaw the study, so that if the experimental intervention (leave the PIV in place until signs or symptoms of phlebitis appeared) was causing an increase in infection, the study would be stopped. Results from this study found no difference between the two

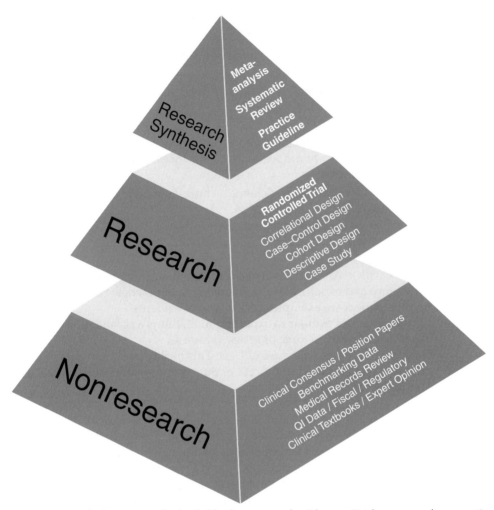

FIGURE 11-2 Rating system for individual sources of evidence. Evidence may be quantitative or qualitative. (From Veteran's Health Administration, Office of Nursing Services, Evidence-Based Practice Resource Center. Clement J. Zablocki VA Medical Center, Milwaukee, WI.)

types of replacement. Thus, the conclusion is that PIVs may be left in place until signs or symptoms of phlebitis appear.

Finally, the top of the pyramid represents research that reviews multiple studies on the same topic and determines whether the findings are similar. In essence, it is research on research. These works can be found by accessing such sites as the Cochrane Collaboration (http://www.cochrane.org/cochrane-reviews) or Joanna Briggs Institute (http://www.joannabriggs.edu.au/Home). Practice guidelines are also found at the top of the evidence pyramid, and examples can be found at such sites as the Agency for Healthcare Research and Quality (AHRQ, http://guideline.gov/) as well as published by several professional organizations, such as the INS *Standards of Practice* (2011) and the Oncology Nursing Society (ONS) *Access Device Guidelines* (Camp-Sorrell, 2011). All of these sites provide a comprehensive review of research related to specific topics and provide a summary of recommendations for practice if available.

Refine the Clinical Question or Problem

As individual clinicians, how does evidence influence and shape the interventions that we provide? This question is necessary for each of us to answer if we strive to have a practice based on evidence. As infusion nurses providing care, using a framework to structure clinical practice questions will create an approach to look for evidence that will ultimately answer the question. This is the first step in having an infusion therapy practice based on evidence. One such format is known by the acronym PICOT and is a consistent, systematic way to identify the components of a clinical issue (Stillwell, Fineout-Overholt, Melnyk, & Williamson, 2010):

- Patient/population
- Intervention
- Comparison group
- Outcome
- Time

A sample PICOT question is as follows: In adult medical/surgical acute care patients with a short-term CVC (P), does flushing with heparinized saline every day (I) versus twice a day (C) maintain the same rate of patency (O) until removed (T)? This may seem like a research question, but the intent is to look for research reports (publications) that examined this question. Structuring a clinical question using PICOT takes some practice, but once mastered, it allows the nurse to clearly communicate an inquiry to a librarian or EBP resource who may assist with an evidence (literature) search. In addition, a well-structured question will allow for a more focused review of evidence, for example, this question addresses adult medical/surgical acute care patients, not pediatric patients and not critical care patients.

Pull a Team Together

A nurse may be very interested in a clinical question, yet colleagues are wary. When a question is formulated, it may be easier to find interested partners to answer the question. It is especially important to reassure the wary bystander that such a team is not a permanent commitment. Thus, the second step is mobilizing a team. Answering the clinical question can move as fast or as slow as the clinical need or the team motivation. Minimally, the team usually consists of two to three or more clinical nurses, the librarian, and an expert in reading research. Determining a regular time to meet, with the supervisor's approval, is helpful in setting schedules. When the team is assembled, it is a good idea to revisit the clinical question or problem so that everyone understands what is being asked and that terms are clear. This keeps the project focused.

Discussion with the supervisor or manager may be helpful in determining if the clinical question is a priority for the unit or organization. For example, a question about using an essential oil to prevent the spread of methicillin-resistant *Staphylococcus aureus* may be less important than ensuring that all appropriate prevention practices are in place and the rate of contamination is low.

Search for and Assemble the Evidence

The librarian is an expert at searching for evidence, in the third step of practice based on evidence. Having the clinical question in the PICOT format ensures that the searching process is efficient and appropriate evidence is retrieved. Generally, the librarian, or the infusion nurse, would start looking for evidence at the top of the pyramid, such as a meta-analysis, systematic review, or clinical guideline. If this type of evidence is available, the next step is in order. If no guidelines were found, the search would continue for research evidence. Sources of evidence are listed in Box 11-3.

Essentially, the highest level of evidence is sought. If a good research article is found, the reference list of that article is reviewed to identify other possible sources of evidence. It is helpful to record how the literature search was done, including the dates of the search; what databases were searched, for example, the Cumulative Index to Nursing and Allied Health Literature (CINAHL) or PubMed; the key words or subject terms used; and the references that were found. This enables the nurse to repeat the search if at a later date, more information is needed. Titles and abstracts are usually reviewed first, to determine if the report meets the population of interest, and the intervention and comparison focus. When key articles are identified, these are retrieved and saved to an electronic file as well as printed as needed. When the team and librarian believe all the relevant evidence is obtained, the team examines the evidence.

Appraise the Evidence

Infusion nurses should consider the level of evidence and the quality of evidence, as well as the body of evidence obtained. Nurses are encouraged to seek the highest level of evidence first, as systematic reviews and guidelines are already critically appraised and provide a

---

BOX 11-3 SOURCES OF EVIDENCE

Collaboratives for Systematic Reviews:
- Cochrane Collaboration: http://www.cochrane.org/cochrane-reviews
- Joanna Briggs Institute: http://www.joannabriggs.edu.au/Home

Guidelines
- Agency for Healthcare Research and Quality: http://guideline.gov/
- Professional organizations, such as INS, Oncology Nursing Society, American Association of Critical-Care Nurses

Databases
- CINAHL, PubMed, MEDLINE, PsycINFO

Journals
- *Evidence-Based Nursing, Worldviews on Evidence-Based Nursing*
- *Nursing Research, Research in Nursing and Health, Western Journal of Nursing Research*
- Professional journals in topic area

great resource. Once obtained, each article, or the review or guideline, needs to be read, deemed applicable to the clinical question, and critically appraised.

Regardless of the level of evidence, the professional nurse is urged to determine whether the study and its methods are valid and reliable. Reliability refers to the degree to which a measure gives the same result two or more times under similar circumstances. Essentially, can the data be replicated by following the same approach? Validity, in simple terms, is the ability of a study to measure what it is intended to measure. The process of not only reviewing the evidence but also assessing the strength of evidence as well as the reliability and validity of the research study design is all part of finding the best available evidence.

Working with a research expert to analyze the studies is essential. There are several methods to review a study; the reader is referred to one of the many research and EBP texts listed in the reference list for critically appraising the evidence. One method answers questions about the study, while another method outlines the study on an evidence table. One or both methods may be used to understand a study. Organizing each study on an evidence table is helpful to visually gauge the body of evidence. An example of a brief evidence table was assembled based on evidence to answer the question, "What are adult patients' experiences during insertion of an implanted or tunneled vascular access device?" This table outlines the findings from two qualitative studies that involved 38 patients who reported their sensory, clinical, and psychosocial experiences during insertion or living with an implanted or tunneled vascular access device (VAD) (Table 11-2).

When the body of evidence is assembled, it is important to evaluate the strength of that evidence. This answers the question of whether there is sufficient quality and strength to make a practice change. The INS developed a rating scale to quantify the quality of the body of evidence, as illustrated in Table 11-3. This schema was used to rate each Practice Criteria in the INS *Standards of Practice* (2011). Using the evidence in Table 11-2 on patient's experiences during insertion of an implanted VAD and living with a tunneled VAD, the body of evidence could be rated level V. There often is no absolute answer; in this case, the studies include adults, but two different devices and different times of experiencing the device.

Of note, Newhouse (2007) differentiates research utilization from EBP by stating that research utilization "begins with the publication of research with a clinical application," while EBP "begins when an important clinical question emerges from practice, education, or research." Therefore, with the nurse seeking the best evidence to answer a practice question, the nurse is actively pursuing the applicable evidence and making a judgment regarding its quality and potential impact on the issue. This is different from simply applying a recommended intervention found in a research publication (research utilization).

Recommend a Change or Keep Current Practice

When all the evidence is in, and rated, the team needs to decide if there is sufficient evidence of quality to recommend a practice change. Or, is there insufficient evidence to change practice and the current practice needs to remain? Referring to Table 11-2, should a practice change be made as to what is taught to patients in preparing them for this procedure? The answer is, only change with caution in this case. The evidence did not address just the insertion procedure but also living with a tunneled device. Thus, there is only one study that addresses the question. The team could discuss further with the librarian if there was more evidence, or the decision could be made that there is insufficient evidence to recommend

TABLE 11-2	EVIDENCE TABLE OF QUALITATIVE FINDINGS FROM STUDIES OF PATIENTS' PERCEPTIONS AND EXPERIENCES WITH IMPLANTED OR TUNNELED VADs					
Citation and Country	Type of Evidence or Study Design	Research Question or Purpose	Sample and Setting	Theoretical Framework	Rigor Established	Findings
Goossens et al. (2011) Belgium	Qualitative, exploratory study using semistructured interviews; three-stage approach utilized, called sensory information grid (SIG), which used patient's five senses: hearing, sight, touch, smell, and taste	To assess the sensory perceptions of patients who had an implantable venous access device (TIVAD) placed under local anesthesia	Twenty patients, ages from 28–73 y, from a tertiary health care setting, diagnosed with oncologic or hematologic disease	Self-regulation Theory for study framework because patients have increased understanding of what to expect during procedures and positive effect on coping results	Diary used to document decision trail and reflections on collected data Peer review of interviewing technique and critical linguistic analysis performed Demographic and clinical characteristics were asked SIG questionnaire did not make a distinction between sensory perceptions and emotions No validity established with the SIG questionnaire	Most sensations dealt with touch, sight, and hearing. Most sensory perceptions occurred during the surgical prep. Both sensory and emotional experiences were described by patients
Moller and Adamsen (2010) Denmark	An exploratory, nonexperimental design using phenomenological–hermeneutic analysis; secondary study as part of another study	To explore experiences of patients who were trained and assumed self-care for their CVC compared to patients whose CVC cares remained the responsibility of health professionals	Eighteen hematologic patients; interviews ranged between 45 and 105 min in length, average was 75 min Patients were purposefully selected	Gadamer's hermeneutical framework used. Interview guide consisting of 10 themes. Banduras' Social Cognition theory used to help patients identify goals and release them from dependence on health care personnel	Educational program began 1 and 6 wk postinsertion. CNS developed step-by-step program and performed sessions, divided into four levels of patient learning (sterile technique, flushing technique) No limitations on the number of sessions available; patient assumed care when they reached the fourth level Two concepts used in analysis, "clinical management situation" and "private daily life"	No differences between groups regarding fear of catheter-related infections; differences between groups regarding CVC technique mastery Control group experienced feelings of insecurity and loss of control during conflict involving care with hospital personnel. Interviewees experienced negative self-concepts of their bodies that affected their social and sexual relationships

TABLE 11-3	STRENGTH OF THE BODY OF EVIDENCE
Strength of the Body of Evidence	Evidence Description[a]
I	Meta-analysis, systematic literature review, guideline based on RCTs, or at least three well-designed RCTs.
I A/P	Includes evidence from anatomy, physiology, and pathophysiology as understood at the time of writing.
II	Two well-designed RCTs, two or more multicenter, well-designed clinical trials without randomization, or systematic literature review of varied prospective study designs.
III	One well-designed RCT, several well-designed clinical trials without randomization, or several studies with quasi-experimental designs focused on the same question.
	Includes two or more well-designed laboratory studies.
IV	Well-designed quasi-experimental study, case–control study, cohort study, correlational study, time series study, systematic literature review of descriptive and qualitative studies, or narrative literature review, psychometric study.
	Includes one well-designed laboratory study.
V	Clinical article, clinical/professional book, consensus report, case report, guideline based on consensus, descriptive study, well-designed quality improvement project, theoretical basis, recommendations by accrediting bodies and professional organizations, or manufacturer recommendations for products or services.
	Includes standard of practice that is generally accepted but does not have a research basis (e.g., patient identification).
Regulatory	Regulations and other criteria set by agencies with the ability to impose consequences, such as the AABB, Centers for Medicare & Medicaid Services, Occupational Safety and Health Administration, and State Boards of Nursing.

[a]Sufficient sample size is needed with preference for power analysis adding to the strength of evidence.
From Infusion Nurses Society. (2011). Infusion nursing: Standards of practice—Strength of the body of evidence. *Journal of Infusion Nursing, 34*(Suppl.), S5.

a change in teaching content and practice. If that is the case, the step following insufficient evidence is to discuss a research project.

If the decision is made that there is sufficient evidence to recommend a practice change, several actions may be needed. The first may be to consult with the unit's or nursing department's shared governance practice council. When recommending a change in practice, it affects all nurses on that team, unit, or department. Shared governance promotes accountability by all nurses to have a voice in their practice. Procedures or bylaws may state that practice changes are put forth to shared governance first, before a pilot is undertaken, or a pilot may be approved.

A pilot of the proposed change is often helpful to determine how the practice will work in the nurse's setting. With varied electronic medical records, or patient teaching tools, or nurse practice acts, a pilot helps to assess the process needed to implement the change. It may identify if education is needed. In the case of changing patient teaching, there may be a committee that approves all patient education so that it meets health literacy guidelines. A pilot of the change often takes the form of a quality improvement project; the Plan-Do-Study-Act process of quality improvement provides a template to ensure that all components of a change are addressed. Confusion sometimes arises as to whether the team is conducting a quality improvement project or a research project, particularly when an individual refers to the project as a research project. Newhouse, Pettit, Poe, and Rocco (2006) address the differences between the quality improvement process and the research process:

- Quality improvement is the process "by which individuals work together to improve systems and processes with the intention to improve outcomes."
- Research is "a systematic investigation, including research development, testing and evaluation, designed to develop or contribute to generalizable knowledge" (p. 212).

If the pilot is successful and the change is approved by shared governance, the next step is to make the change part of nursing practice. Does the change need to be incorporated into a policy, procedure, or IV team/unit practice standard? Is education needed? What dissemination is needed to share the results of the team's work? This could involve the nursing newsletter or presentation to a quality improvement council, innovation council, or EBP council. Consider sharing the team's work outside the organization, such as through a professional conference or journal publication. At some point after decisions have been made, remember to celebrate the team's accomplishment. Whether the decision was made to change practice or maintain current practice, the decision was made based on evidence!

Evaluate the Practice Change

A step that is often forgotten is the quiet work after the celebration of accomplishment. This step is the evaluation of the practice change. There are possibly three parts to this evaluation, following Donabedian's quality model of structure, process, and clinical outcomes (Donabedian, 2005). Evaluation would examine if the change has occurred as planned throughout the team, unit, or organization; if the change is sustained as it was planned; if there were any unintended consequences of the change (something that may not have been anticipated); and what are the outcomes for patient care? For example, if the central line bundle for preventing CLABSI was implemented, the anticipated patient outcomes would be a decrease in the rate of CLABSI. Results of the evaluation would be reported to the shared governance council, quality improvement council, or EBP council. Regular monitoring and reporting of data promote accountability and provide evidence for sustaining the change.

Implement Practice Based on Evidence with the Patient

Reflecting on the EBP graphic (Figure 11-1), any evidence must be used with the expertise of the nurse, with patient preferences in mind, and in the context of the organization or situation presented. Effective use of evidence in answering a clinical or leadership question will assist the professional nurse in driving practice changes forward.

As mentioned, an important element of EBP is the patient's preferences. While the evidence may be unequivocal regarding a certain habit such as smoking and health outcomes, even the most expert nurse may be unsuccessful in assisting a patient with a behavior change (smoking cessation) if the patient believes this habit helps him to remain calm in psychologically stressful situations. In the same scenario, an expert nurse may be more adept at having an effective conversation with a patient about smoking cessation than a novice, even though they both have the same evidence as a foundation from which to work.

EVIDENCE-BASED PRACTICE AND OUTCOMES

The quality of information that nurses demand and how effectively they evaluate and apply it for clinical decision making influences patient outcomes and, ultimately, demonstrates the value of professional nursing in the health care delivery system. Measuring outcomes is a method of documenting the efficacy of practice and practice changes. Using evidence to influence practice is linked to reductions in patient morbidity, mortality, medical errors, and geographic variation in health care (Melnyk et al., 2012). Nurses constitute the greatest number of health care professionals in most practice settings and, collectively, have immense potential to impact the patient care provided and quality outcomes realized. The recognition of the power of applying evidence to guide clinical practice is compelling when considering the patient populations who might benefit from each practice improvement.

Nurses know that patients benefit from the care they provide, yet it is imperative to correlate patient outcomes with nursing interventions to assess the effectiveness of care. Outcomes are the consequences of a treatment or intervention. Outcome indicators, or measures, gauge how patients are affected by their nursing care. Infusion infection rates, hospital-acquired pressure ulcer rates, and falls with injury are examples of such measures. Process indicators reflect how the care was delivered or what may affect the outcomes, such as the use of central line bundles or skin cleansing solutions. For example, is the skin cleansing solution allowed to dry before venipuncture? This may affect the clinical outcome and could be assessed. Structure indicators assess the organization and the delivery of nursing care from the standpoint of staffing or policy. These measures help determine the influence of the resource infrastructure on patient care.

Quality Measurement

The Joint Commission (TJC) introduced the ORYX measures several years ago as an approach to measure patient outcomes and health care organizational performance. These measures are integrated into the accreditation process. The long-range goal of this program is to establish a data-driven continuous survey process to complement the standards-based assessment. Although accreditation is still based on standards, trends in data and in an organization's response to its data are being used as a part of TJC's overall assessment as the performance measures database expands (http://www.jointcommission.org/facts_about_oryx_for_hospitals/).

Other organizations have initiated or changed measures to reflect the care that patients receive and the outcomes from that care. Some of these organizations and descriptions are outlined in Table 11-4. By measuring patient outcomes, nurses can respond to two pivotal questions: Do our patients benefit from our care? And if so, how? A focus on outcomes may

TABLE 11-4	NATIONAL QUALITY INDICATORS	
Organization	Initiative	Description
American Nurses Association	Nursing-sensitive indicators	Provides indicators and measurement tools for evaluating quality of nursing care in acute care and other settings, for adult and pediatric populations
Centers for Medicare & Medicaid Services	OASIS (Outcome and Assessment Information Set)	Provides core comprehensive assessment questions for adult home care that form the basis for measuring patient outcomes for the purpose of outcome-based quality improvement
The Joint Commission	ORYX	Integrates use of outcomes and performance measures
National Committee for Quality Assurance	Healthcare Effectiveness Data and Information Set	Targets effectiveness of care, access and availability, patient satisfaction, and costs
National Quality Forum	Performance measures and quality standards	Provides measures for health care processes, outcomes, patient perceptions, and organizational structure and/or systems that are associated with the ability to provide quality care

help nurses survive an unstable job market, evaluate the efficacy of infusion teams, and ensure that the nursing perspective regarding outcome management is represented.

In closing, evidence-based nursing integrates the best evidence from research findings with clinical expertise, patient preferences, and existing resources to form decision-making tools about the health care of individual patients (DiCenso, Guyatt, & Ciliska, 2005). It is this process that provides nurses with the science for practice and the art for caring.

Review Questions *Note: Questions below may have more than one right answer.*

1. Outcomes can best be described as which of the following?
   A. Use of protocols to render health care
   B. Ability to provide consistent care in all regions of the country
   C. End results of treatment or intervention
   D. Use of less invasive and less costly procedures

2. One of the CDC (2011) well-supported recommendations, which included studies of IV Teams, was that only trained personnel with demonstrated competence manage peripheral and central venous catheters.
   A. True
   B. False

3. A model for evidence-based practice may initiate a
   A. Change in the organization's culture
   B. Discussion about patients' having access to their medical records
   C. New policy about infusion therapy
   D. Discussion of developing an Infusion Team

4. Which of the following is *not* an example of a useful outcome indicator to measure quality of nursing care?
   A. Functional status
   B. Patient satisfaction
   C. Patient discomfort
   D. Health insurance plan

5. Patient outcomes are influenced by which of the following?
   A. Effectiveness of care
   B. How information is used in clinical decision making
   C. A only
   D. A and B

6. Evidence-based practice supports the direct care nurse to use the best available evidence with his or her expertise in the context of care delivery, taking into account the patient's preferences and values.
   A. True
   B. False

7. One step of the process for practice based on evidence is to:
   A. Appraise the evidence critically
   B. Seek organizational approval
   C. Develop a nursing sensitive indicator
   D. Evaluate research authors

8. Reliability refers to
   A. Validity of the measurements
   B. Degree to which the same results are achieved two or more times
   C. Degree to which results are achieved under same circumstances
   D. Determining what is important to measure

9. Types of evidence include
   A. Expert opinion
   B. Research reports
   C. Staff assignments
   D. Quality data about central line infections

10. The INS Standard of Practice (2011) states, "The nurse shall use research findings and current best evidence to"
   A. Conduct research
   B. Improve practice
   C. Expand professional and ancillary knowledge
   D. Expand infusion therapy nursing knowledge

References and Selected Readings   *Asterisks indicate references cited in text.*

Alexander, M., Corrigan, A., Gorski, L., Hankins, J., & Perucca, R. (2010). *Infusion nursing: An evidence based approach* (3rd ed.). St. Louis, MO: Mosby-Elsevier.

*Alonso-Echanove, J., Edwards, J.R., Richards, M.J., Brennan, P., Venezia, R.A., Keen, J., et al. (2003). Effect of nurse staffing and antimicrobial-impregnated central venous catheters on the risk for bloodstream infections in intensive care units. *Infection Control and Hospital Epidemiology*, 24(12), 916–925.

*American Nurses Credentialing Center. (2011). *The Magnet Model components and sources of evidence: Magnet Recognition Program®*. Silver Spring, MD: Author.

*ANA (American Nurses Association). (2010). *Nursing: Scope and standards of practice* (2nd ed.). Silver Spring, MD: Author.

*Brady, N., & Lewin, L. (2007). Evidence-based practice in nursing: Bridging the gap between research and practice. *Journal of Pediatric Health Care*, 21(1):53–56.

*Brunelle, D. (2003). Impact of a dedicated infusion therapy team on the reduction of catheter-related nosocomial infections. *Journal of Infusion Nursing*, 26, 362–366.

Bucknall, T., Rycroft-Malone, J., Dobbins, M., & Titler, M. (2004). Implementation of research evidence into practice: International perspectives and initiatives. *Worldviews on Evidence-Based Nursing*, 1(4), 234–236.

*Camp-Sorrell, D. (Ed.). (2011). *Access Device Guidelines: Recommendations for nursing practice and education* (3rd ed.). Pittsburgh, PA: Oncology Nursing Society.

*Centers for Disease Control and Prevention (CDC). (2011). Guidelines for the prevention of intravascular catheter-related infections. http://www.cdc.gov/hicpac/pdf/guidelines/bsi-guidelines-2011.pdf

*DiCenso, A., Guyatt, G., & Ciliska, D. (2005). *Evidence-based nursing: A guide to clinical practice*. St. Louis, MO: Elsevier Mosby.

*Donabedian, A. (2005). Evaluating the quality of medical care. *The Milbank Quarterly, 83*(4), 691–729.

*Drenkard, K.N. (2008). Integrating human caring science into a professional nursing practice model. *Critical Care Nursing Clinics of North America, 20*, 403–414.

Goossens, E., Goossens, G.A., Stas, M., Janssens, C., Jerome, M., & Moons, P. (2011). Sensory perceptions of patients with cancer undergoing surgical insertion of a totally implantable venous access device: A qualitative, exploratory study. *Oncology Nursing Forum, 38*(1), E20–E26.

Grove, S., Burns, N., & Gray, J. (2013). *The practice of nursing research: Appraisal, synthesis, and generation of evidence* (7th ed.). St. Louis, MO: Elsevier Saunders.

*Hawes, M.L. (2007). A proactive approach to combating venous depletion in the hospital setting. *Journal of Infusion Nursing, 30*, 33–44.

*Hoffart, N., & Woods, C.Q. (1996). Elements of a nursing professional practice model. *Journal of Professional Nursing, 12*(6), 354–364.

*Hollenbeak, C.S. (2011). The cost of catheter-related bloodstream infections. *Journal of Infusion Nursing, 34*, 309–313.

*Infusion Nurses Society. (2011). Infusion nursing standards of practice. *Journal of Infusion Nursing, 34*(1 Suppl.), S1–S110.

*IOM (Institute of Medicine). (2007). *The learning healthcare system: Workshop summary*. Washington, DC: National Academies Press.

*Jonsdottir, H., Litchfield, M., & Pharris, M.D. (2004). The relational core of nursing practice as partnership. *Journal of Advanced Nursing, 47*(3), 241–250.

*Koloroutis, M. (Ed.). (2004). *Relationship-based care: A model for transforming practice*. Minneapolis, MN: Creative Health Care Management.

Leeman, J., & Sandelowski, M. (2012). Practice-based evidence and qualitative inquiry. *Journal of Nursing Scholarship, 44*(2), 171–179.

LoBiondo-Wood, G., & Haber, J. (2010). *Nursing research: Methods and critical appraisal for evidence-based practice* (7th ed.). St. Louis, MO: Mosby Elsevier.

Mateo, M., & Kirchhoff, K. (2009). *Research for advanced practice nurses: From evidence to practice*. New York, NY: Springer.

*Melnyk, B., & Fineout-Overholt, E. (2011). *Evidence-based practice in nursing & healthcare: A guide to best practice* (2nd ed.). New York, NY: Wolters Kluwer/Lippincott Williams & Wilkins.

*Melnyk, B., Fineout-Overholt, E., Gallagher-Ford, L., & Kaplan, L. (2012). The state of evidence-based practice in US nurses. *Journal of Nursing Administration, 42*, 410–417.

Melnyk, B., Fineout-Overholt, E., & Mays, M. (2008). The evidence-based practice beliefs and implementation scales: Psychometric properties of two new instruments [corrected] [published erratum: 2009, 6(1), 49]. *Worldviews on Evidence-Based Nursing, 5*(4), 208–216.

Moller, T., & Adamsen, L. (2010). Hematologic patients' clinical and psychosocial experiences with implanted long-term central venous catheter: Self-management versus professionally controlled care. *Cancer Nursing, 33*(6), 426–435.

*Newell-Stokes, G. (2004). Applying evidence-based practice: A place to start. *Journal of Infusion Nursing, 27*, 381–385.

*Newhouse, R. (2007). Creating infrastructure supportive of evidence-based nursing practice: Leadership strategies. *Worldviews on Evidence-Based Nursing, 4*(1), 21–29.

*Newhouse, R.P., Pettit, J.C., Poe, S., & Rocco, L. (2006). The slippery slope: Differentiating between quality improvement and research. *Journal of Nursing Administration, 36*(4), 211–219.

*Pierce, C.A., & Baker, J.J. (2004). A nursing process model: Quantifying infusion therapy resource consumption. *Journal of Infusion Nursing, 27*, 232–244.

Polit, D.F., & Beck, C.T. (2012). *Nursing research: Generating and assessing evidence for nursing practice* (9th ed.). New York, NY: Wolters Kluwer/Lippincott Williams & Wilkins.

Polit, D.F., & Tatano Beck, C. (2010). *Essentials of nursing research: Appraising evidence for nursing practice* (7th ed.). New York, NY: Wolters Kluwer/Lippincott Williams & Wilkins.

*Rickard, C.M., Webster, J., Wallis, M.C., Marsh, N., McGrail, M.R., French, V., et al. (2012). Routine versus clinically indicated replacement of peripheral intravenous catheters: A randomised controlled equivalence trial. *Lancet, 380*, 1066–1074.

*Robert, J., Fridkin, S.K., Blumberg, H.M., Anderson, B., White, N., Ray, S.M., et al. (2000). The influence of the composition of the nursing staff on primary bloodstream infection rates in a surgical intensive care unit. *Infection Control and Hospital Epidemiology, 21*(1), 12–17.

Sackett, D.L., Straus, S.E., Richardson, W.S., Rosenberg, W., & Hayes, R.B. (2000). *Evidence-based medicine: How to practice and teach EBM*. London, UK: Churchill Livingstone.

*Stanley, D., & Sherratt, A. (2010). Lamp light on leadership: Clinical leadership and Florence Nightingale. *Journal of Nursing Management, 18*, 115–121.

*Stillwell, S.B., Fineout-Overholt, E., Melnyk, B.M., & Williamson, K.M. (2010). Evidence-based practice, step by step: Asking the clinical question: A key step in evidence-based practice. *The American Journal of Nursing, 110*(3), 58–61.

Titler, M. (2010). Translation science and context. *Research and Theory for Nursing Practice, 24*(1), 35–55.

Williamson, K.M., Fineout-Overholt, E., Kent, B., & Hutchinson, A.M. (2011). Teaching EBP: Integrating technology into academic curricula to facilitate evidence-based decision-making. *Worldviews on Evidence-Based Nursing, 8*(4), 247–251.

Winters, C.A., & Echeverri, R. (2012). Academic Education. Teaching strategies to support evidence-based practice. *Critical Care Nurse, 32*(3), 49–54.

PART 3

CLINICAL DECISION MAKING

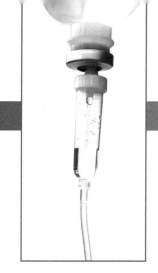

CHAPTER 12

Infusion Delivery Systems and Safety

Sharon M. Weinstein

Absorption	Hydrostatic
Adverse Drug Events (ADEs)	Hypovolemia
Alarm Fatigue	Medical Device Reporting (MDR)
Bubble point	Osmolality
Elastomeric	Pressure Pump
Good Manufacturing Process (GMP)	Psi
Gravity	Ramping
Hemorepellant	Smart Technology
Hydrophilic	Surveillance
Hydrophobic	Wetted

FROM IDEA TO INCEPTION

As technology has continued to keep pace with advances in medical science, the delivery of patient care has improved, and more sophisticated devices and innovative equipment have become available for administering infusion therapy. Many of these product concepts have evolved as a result of focus groups or nursing input; those in the field, regardless of the setting in which care is delivered, know what is needed, and nurses are willing to share those concepts. Those who design and manufacture devices do so with outcomes in mind; they are our partners and colleagues.

BOX 12-1   ROLE OF THE CENTER FOR DEVICES AND RADIOLOGIC HEALTH

- Reviews requests to research medical devices
- Collects and acts on information related to safety and possible injury
- Sets and enforces good manufacturing processes (GMP) and performance standards
- Monitors compliance and surveillance programs
- Provides technical support to small manufacturers of medical devices

Source: U.S. Food and Drug Administration, 2012.

Nurses, as gatekeepers, play an active role in making product selections that are appropriate for the patient across the continuum of infusion care. Nurses rely on best manufacturing processes, product information, the existing evidence base, and clinical research in making recommendations. As an advocate for patient safety, the nurse responsible for infusion care understands the role of safety and the need to ensure safe use of medical devices and equipment.

Equipment used to deliver infusion therapy is regulated by the Center for Devices and Radiologic Health (CDRH) at the U.S. Food and Drug Administration (FDA). The organization is a huge asset to the process of care delivery. Its roles are outlined in Box 12-1. Simply stated, a medical device is an instrument, apparatus, implement, machine, implant, or other similar article recognized in the official National Formulary of the United States Pharmacopoeia intended for use in diagnosis or treatment.

Government Regulations

Before any device may be sold in the United States, it must have FDA approval. Class I devices have nominal risk and include catheter stabilization devices, tape, pressure infusors, and IV poles. Class II devices have a moderate degree of risk and include solution containers, catheters, vessel dilators, introducers, guidewires, and stylet wires. Class III devices are more invasive and carry the greatest amount of risk. Within this category, we find cardiac pacemakers, replacement heart valves, and other surgical devices.

The classification is consistent with the level of review; for example, class I devices must demonstrate "general controls" including proper labeling, adherence to **good manufacturing processes (GMP)**, and adequate packaging/storage.

INSTITUTE OF MEDICINE AND POSTMARKET SURVEILLANCE

In the hallmark report entitled "Medical Devices and the Public's Health: The FDA 510(k) Clearance Process at 35 Years," published in July 2011, the Institute of Medicine recommended that the FDA develop and implement a comprehensive medical device postmarket **surveillance** strategy to collect, analyze, and act on medical device postmarket performance information. The FDA's postmarket surveillance system specifications are listed in Box 12-2. Once the device has been introduced and used in the clinical setting, postmarket surveillance begins. The system, known as **medical device reporting (MDR)**, involves the

> ## BOX 12-2 FDA POSTMARKET SURVEILLANCE SYSTEM SPECIFICATIONS
>
> - Establish a unique device identification system and promote its incorporation into electronic health information
> - Promote the development of national and international device registries for selected products
> - Modernize adverse event reporting and analysis
> - Develop and use new methods for evidence generation, synthesis, and appraisal

manufacturers, institutions, and professionals and is aimed at reducing possible adverse effects. Specifically, medical device postmarket surveillance should

- Provide timely, accurate, systematic, and prioritized assessments of the benefits and risks of medical devices throughout their marketed life using high-quality, standardized, structured, electronic health-related data
- Identify potential safety signals in near real time from a variety of privacy-protected data sources
- Facilitate the clearance and approval of new devices or new uses for existing devices

> ### EVIDENCE FOR PRACTICE
>
> Will quantitative decision analysis help evaluate benefits and risks of medical devices? Will this system be reliable and affect transparency to health care providers, industry, and the public?

A companion to the Institute of Medicine's 1999 Report, *To Err is Human*, is *Keeping Patients Safe: Transforming the Work Environment of Nurses* (Institute of Medicine, 2004). This report identifies solutions to problems in hospital, nursing home, and other health care organization work environments that threaten patient safety through their effect on nursing care. The report's findings and recommendations address the related issues of management practices, workforce capability, work design, and organizational safety culture. Actions needed from the federal and state governments and from coalitions of parties involved in shaping the work environments of nurses also are specified.

Medical Product Safety Network (MedSun)

The Medical Product Safety Network (MedSun) is an adverse event reporting program launched in 2002 by the CDRH. MedSun works collaboratively with the clinical community to identify, understand, and solve problems with the use of medical devices. Once a problem is identified, MedSun researchers work with each facility's representatives to clarify and understand the problem. Reports and lessons learned are shared with the clinical community and the public, without facility and patient identification, so that clinicians nationwide may take necessary preventive actions.

The Safe Medical Devices Act defines "user facilities" as hospitals, nursing homes, and outpatient treatment and diagnostic centers. They are required to report medical device problems that result in serious illness, injury, or death. By monitoring reports about problems and concerns before a more serious event occurs, the FDA, manufacturers, and clinicians work together proactively to prevent serious injuries and death (FDA, 2013).

Nongovernmental Organizations

Nongovernmental agencies play a key role in ensuring safety through oversight and creation of product standards. Appropriate use of devices is critical in ensuring patient safety; the nurse plays an important role in utilizing good technique. Professional nursing societies, such as the Infusion Nurses Society (INS), often provide feedback to manufacturers to initiate change as needed. Nongovernmental organizations (NGOs) and their contact information are listed in Box 12-3.

SAFETY PRINCIPLES AND SELECTION OF EQUIPMENT

General infusion equipment includes durable medical equipment (DME), single-use devices, and reprocessed single-use devices. A working knowledge of the selection and use of these devices is vital for the nurse who must provide infusion therapy and ensure the patient's safety and comfort. *DME* is equipment that is used for an extensive period of time; examples include IV poles, electronic infusion devices (EIDs), and ultrasound or infrared devices used to enhance vascular visualization. *Single-use devices* are discarded after initial use and include solution containers, administration sets, catheters, and dressing materials. *Reprocessed single-use devices* are those that are labeled for single use but reprocessed for use on multiple patients (e.g., angiography catheters and implantable infusion pumps). The practice is controversial but accepted within the industry (Nelson, 2006).

Although purchasing decisions continue to be made with a group purchasing contract in mind, nurses should be involved in selecting infusion equipment as members of a product evaluation committee, equipment task force, or safety committee. Product decisions

---

BOX 12-3   NONGOVERNMENTAL ORGANIZATIONS

- International Organization for Standardization (ISO)
  http://www.iso.org/iso/home.html
- Association for the Advancement of Medical Instrumentation (AAMI)
  http://www.aami.org/
- Emergency Care Research Institute (officially known as ECRI)
  https://www.ecri.org
- Advanced Medical Technology Association (AdvaMed) and formerly the Health Industry Manufacturers Association
  http://advamed.org/

may be made in an effort to solve a patient safety issue or as a cost-containment initiative. Such decisions include the following factors: cost, quality, efficacy, safety, and availability.

The concept of safety will always have a profound impact on practice. Worker safety, in particular, is a top priority for health care institutions today (Pugliese, 2013). Sharps safety is also part of a larger discussion among health care leaders and professionals about what a culture of safety means, and whether it means combining all health care safety efforts, such as employee, environmental, and patient safety. Much of the time, the efforts for improvement are similar across all categories, requiring the same culture in the same care environment. Protecting health care workers from injury is essential, especially in infusion therapy, where injuries resulting from sharp objects and devices are more prevalent than in other areas of nursing practice. Sharps injuries are related not only to needles but also to any sharp objects and devices that have the potential to cause harm by exposing the nurse or others to the blood and body fluid of patients. Box 12-4 lists examples of these objects.

Safety Devices and Programs

Many infusion nurses find that gathering information concerning the availability and use of safety devices in an institution or agency is helpful in implementing safety programs. The Centers for Disease Control and Prevention (CDC) estimates that about 385,000 sharps-related injuries occur annually among health care workers in hospitals. More recent data from the EPINet suggest that these injuries can be reduced, as sharps-related injuries in non-surgical hospital settings decreased 31.6% during 2001 to 2006 (following the Needlestick Safety and Prevention Act of 2000). It has been estimated that about half or more of sharps injuries go unreported. Most reported sharps injuries involve nursing staff, but laboratory staff, physicians/licensed independent practitioners (LIPs), housekeepers, and other health care workers are also injured (CDC, 2011).

Because of the high-risk nature of intravenous medications, the potential for harm is greatly enhanced over oral medications. A systems approach to medical safety is needed to ensure positive outcomes related to patient care.

BOX 12-4   SHARPS USED IN IV PRACTICE AND ASSOCIATED INJURY RATE

Disposable syringes (31%)
Syringe, prefilled cartridge (3%)
IV catheter (3%)
Other needles (4%)
Winged infusion needle (5%)
Other sharp items (22%)
Suture needles (24%)
Reusable scalpel (4%)
Disposable scalpel (4%)
Exposure to other sharp products includes glass infusion containers, glass vacuum blood tubes, and pipettes

Source: Exposure Prevention Information Network (EPINet) (2009).

EVIDENCE FOR PRACTICE

Whittington, J., Cohen, H. (2004). OSF Healthcare's journey in patient safety. *Quality Management in Health Care*, *13*(1), 53–59.

This article describes OSF Healthcare's recent journey in patient safety. It discusses the involvement of its six hospitals in collaboration with each other and the Institute for Healthcare Improvement. OSF focused on a strategy for decreasing **adverse drug events (ADEs)**. What has been your institution's role in ensuring patient safety, and has it been documented in the literature?

Systems Approach to Safety

The literature is replete with articles addressing patient safety related to medication administration. Common barriers to safe medication administration are divided into five categories and presented in Table 12-1 (Burke, 2005). Public awareness has pushed this effort forward, and a mandate for reform has involved clinicians, researchers, manufacturers,

TABLE 12-1	COMMON BARRIERS TO SAFE MEDICATION ADMINISTRATION

Research
Outcomes not easily adapted to practice
Lack of recognition of impact and limitations of technology
Lack of funding

Education
Knowledge deficit
Insufficient clinical practice
Lack of training on-site

Policy
Lack of nurse involvement
Lack of standardization
Practice/policy implications

Practice
Lack of best practices
Lack of standardization
Lack of focus on safety and fatigue management
Excessive nonnursing responsibilities
Inadequate/inaccurate reporting
Technology and practice failures

Administration
Lack of administrative support for safety initiatives
Integration challenges
Lack of nursing involvement at all levels
Inadequate allocation of financial resources

Adapted from Burke, K.G. (2005). The state of the science on safe medication administration symposium. *American Journal of Nursing, 105*(Suppl.), 4–9.

TABLE 12-2 STAKEHOLDERS IN INTRAVENOUS MEDICATION-RELATED EVENTS	
Internal	**External**
Patients/clients	The Joint Commission
Nurses	Boards of Pharmacy and Nursing
Pharmacists	U.S. Food and Drug Administration
Physicians/LIPs	Government: CMS, AHRQ, state regulations
Other members of multidisciplinary team	Professional advisory groups
Leadership	Patient advocacy groups
Risk management	Pharmaceutical industry
Quality	Infusion device industry
Finance	ISMP and ECRI
Board	Professional health care organizations

pharmacists, and biomedical engineers in an effort to manage the challenge and develop a system approach to safety. Stakeholders in IV medication–related events are listed in Table 12-2.

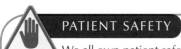

PATIENT SAFETY

We all own patient safety! We must all assume responsibility for the safe administration of infusion therapies.

The advent of **smart technology** assists in averting infusion errors at the point of care, thus creating an additional layer of safety for patients (ISMP, 2005). These technologies embed computer chips that gather information and respond within a range of preset parameters. Known as smart technology, because it performs a task we think an intelligent person can do, it includes smart IV pumps, smart beds, and smart cards. Smart beds are able to monitor patients' vital signs and mobility without using electrodes. Smart beds can interface with information systems to transfer information collected and alert health care providers when a patient is getting out of bed unattended. Smart cards collect and store information about patients that is crucial to providing safe care to that individual patient.

The role of smart technology is to recall whatever rules apply, that is, dosing limits and clinical advisories for a particular clinical area, by incorporating the rules within the software. Nurses believe it is essential to have smart, portable, point-of-care solutions for capturing and transmitting data, as well as routine communication. They want technology to reduce demand on nursing time by eliminating waste in care resulting from inefficient workflows. Reducing the opportunity for error improves patient safety. Technology driving medication administration systems, improved communications, timely acquisition of equipment and supplies, and fool-proof patient identification are just some applications that improve safety (Bolton, Gassert, & Cipriano, 2008). Smart infusion pumps provide substantial safety features during the infusion process. However, nurses need to

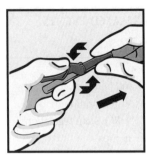

- Holding both colored shields, twist and remove white shield

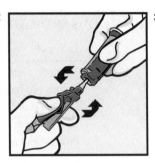

- Screw on holder (if using Pronto™, hold white tab while screwing in needle)

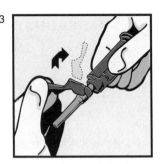

- Rotate safety shield back

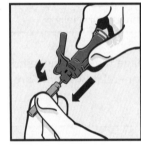

- Twist and pull needle shield straight off

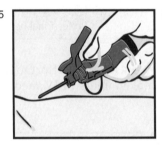

- Perform venipuncture

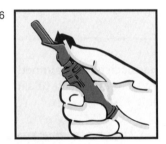

- Firmly push forward on the safety shield, lock into place and inspect

Things to Remember:
- Handle all biologic samples and blood collection sharps (lancets, needles, luer adapters and blood collection sets) according to the policies and procedures of your facility
- Obtain appropriate medical attention in the event of any exposure to biologic samples (for example, through a puncture injury) since they may transmit viral hepatitis, HIV (AIDS) or other infectious diseases
- Utilize any built-in needle protector if the blood collection device provides one
- BD does not recommend reshielding used needles, but the policies and procedures of your facility may differ and must always be followed
- Discard BD Vacutainer Brand Eclipse Blood Collection Needle in the nearest sharps collector. Follow your institution's policy for safe disposal of all medical waste

FIGURE 12-1 Vacutainer Eclipse blood collection needle, economical needle-based safety device for injection in a variety of sizes. (Adapted from BD Vacutainer Eclipse Blood Collection Needle Quick Reference Card. Courtesy of and © Becton, Dickinson and Company.)

understand the requisite education necessary to fully benefit from and improve IV smart pump use and clinical integration. Failure to use IV smart pumps places the nurse and patient at increased risk (Harding, 2013).

Infusion Safety

Manufacturers have met our demands for safer technology by providing equipment to meet complex clinical needs and to enhance patient outcomes. See Figures 12-1 to 12-3 for detailed information on how these products are used in the clinical setting. Key features of B-D's Vacutainer Push Button Collection Set are included in Box 12-5 as an example of the types of features available.

1

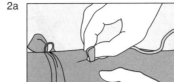

To use the BD Vacutainer® Push Button Blood Collection Set, peel off the paper backing and remove the device. Avoid contact with the activation button during the removal of the device.

2a

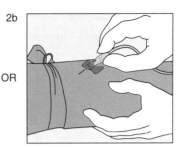

With thumb and index finger, grasp the wings together and access vein using standard needle insertion technique.

2b

OR

If preferred by your institution, the body of the device can be held, instead of the wings, during insertion.

3

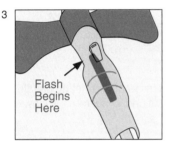

Proper access to the vein will be indicated by the presence of "flash" directly behind and below the button.

4a

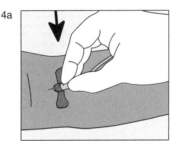

The device is designed to be activated while the needle is still in the patient's vein. Following the collection procedure, and while the needle is still in the vein, push the button to retract the needle into the body of the device.

4b

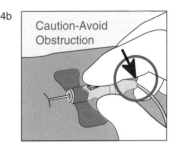

To ensure complete and immediate retraction of device, make sure to keep fingers and hands away from the end of the blood collection set during retraction. Do not impede retraction.

4c

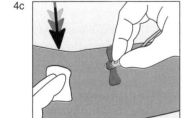

Apply pressure to the venipuncture site in accordance with your facility's protocol.

5

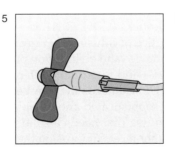

Confirm that the needle is in the shielded position prior to disposal.

6

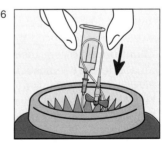

Discard the entire shielded blood collection set and holder into an approved sharps disposal container.

FIGURE 12-2 BD Vacutainer push-button blood collection/in-vein needle activation. (Adapted from BD Vacutainer Push Button Blood Collection Set InService Poster. Courtesy of and © Becton, Dickinson and Company.)

1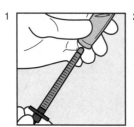

Aspiration
Draw up medication
in accordance with
established protocol.

2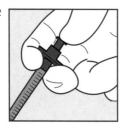

Injection
Administer medication
in accordance with
established protocols,
making sure that all
medication has been
dispensed.

3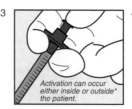

Activation can occur
either inside or outside*
the patient.

Activation
Push plunger rod to
activate the safety
mechanism. Depress until
you sense two "clicks."
If Activation is performed
before needle is withdrawn
from patient, do not
advance needle while
depressing plunger rod.

* If Activation is performed
after needle is withdrawn
from patient, minimal
splatter may occur. When
activating the device outside
of the patient, hold the
device downward at arm's
length, and activate while
pointing away from self and
others. Keep device within
sight at all times to avoid
accidental needlestick injury.

4

Retraction
The needle will disappear
into the syringe and the
plunger will be recessed
into the barrel when
activation is complete.
There is no exposure to the
used needle. Immediately
discard into an approved
sharps container.

Things to Remember:
• BD Integra Needle
  and Syringe are not a
  standard luer connection.
• After pressurizing the
  medication vial, do not
  continue to press the
  plunger rod past the
  point of resistance, as
  this may cause premature
  activation.

FIGURE 12-3 BD Integra 3-mL syringe, a low-waste space syringe with detachable retracting needle. (Adapted from BD Integra 3 mL Syringe Quick Reference Card. Courtesy of and © Becton, Dickinson and Company.)

SAFETY ASSESSMENT

Safety assessment should include the number of sharps-related injuries and the type of devices involved. The global focus on safety devices continues to proliferate. Again, smart infusion systems may avert high-risk errors and provide previously unavailable data for continuous quality improvement efforts.

NEEDLELESS SYSTEMS

In a study by the CDC, 89% of occupational exposures to HIV were caused by percutaneous injuries; most were needlesticks (CDC, 2011). In today's practice arena, the needleless system has advanced the practice of infusion therapy. In general, the product consists of a blunt-tipped plastic insertion device and an injection port that opens to reduce the incidence of accidental needlestick injuries and to promote safety in infusion practice. Again, diverse systems are available to meet clinical needs in many settings.

However, no matter how sophisticated and reliable or easy to use infusion devices and accessories are, the infusion nurse first needs a solid understanding of the physical principles that govern flow and other facets of infusion therapy.

Flow Dynamics and the Physiology of Flow

Pressure, a principle of physics underlying infusion therapy, is the force that overcomes the natural resistance to flow created by infusion equipment, such as the IV administration set, in-line filters, and narrow-gauge needles, and by venous or arterial back pressure.

BOX 12-5	B-D'S VACUTAINER PUSH BUTTON COLLECTION SET: KEY FEATURES

- Intended for blood collection and short-term infusion
- Facilitates the prevention of accidental needlestick injury
- Ease-of-use reduces training time while improving activation compliance
- Easily activated without patient discomfort
- Ideal for use in high-risk environment
- Latex-free
- Flash visualization confirms venous access prior to collection of specimen
- Blood flashback is seen clearly through the translucent body
- One-handed safety activation also allows attention to the patient and venipuncture site

Courtesy of and © Becton, Dickinson and Company.

Fortunately, the human body readily adapts to changes in pressure, which enables clinicians to deliver IV therapy safely.

PRESSURE

Pressure in the arterial system ranges from 80 mm Hg in the aorta to a low of 5 to 10 mm Hg in the venous return system. Intravenous pressure is created by the weight of a column of fluid in the catheter tubing—the weight is due to gravity—and we refer to it as **hydrostatic** pressure. Fluid always flows from an area of higher pressure to one of lower pressure. For a fluid to infuse by gravity, it is necessary to create a pressure only slightly more than normal or 40 mm Hg in a peripheral line.

A number of resistance factors may interfere with or inhibit fluid flow. These factors include the patient's vascular pressure, internal diameter of the tubing, in-line filters, viscosity of the fluid, narrow-gauge needles, and the length of the tubing. Resistance to flow is determined by the smallest component in the IV system; this is usually the catheter. An example of equipment that incorporates principles of pressure for delivery of precise amounts of drugs and fluids is the EID, which is discussed later in this chapter.

GRAVITY

Gravity is the physical force that propels the flow of the infusate, although this flow also depends on head pressure. Roller clamps and screw clamps used to adjust and maintain rates of flow on gravity infusions vary considerably in their efficiency and accuracy. Rate minders or flow-control mechanisms may also be used to regulate and adjust flow. When a rate minder is added to an infusion set, the desired flow rate may be preset. Levels of accuracy vary with the type of device used. Factors such as venous spasm, venous pressure changes, patient movement, manipulations of the clamp, and bent or kinked tubing may cause variations in the flow rate. To monitor consistency of the flow rate, preprinted or self-made time tapes may be attached to the IV container. The time tape, or pharmacy-provided monitoring strip, should be attached to the container and hourly increments marked on the tape or strip, beginning with the time the infusion began.

FLOW

To accurately determine the flow rate, the nurse must have knowledge of parenteral solutions, their effect, and the rate of administration. The nurse must also understand other factors that influence the speed of the infusion. These factors include the patient's body surface area (BSA), condition, age, and tolerance to the infusion. The composition of the fluid is also a factor in the rate of administration.

BODY SURFACE AREA

The BSA is proportionate to many essential physiologic processes (organ size, blood volume, respiration, and heat loss) and, therefore, to total metabolic activity. Knowing the BSA helps the nurse determine fluid and electrolyte amounts and compute infusion rates. The larger the person, the more fluid and nutrients are required and the faster they can be used. The usual infusion rate is 3 mL/m^2 BSA/min (see nomograms in Figure 12-4). This rate applies to maintenance and replacement fluids. However, the speed must be adjusted carefully to each individual.

PATIENT'S CLINICAL CONDITION AND AGE

Because the heart and kidneys play a vital role in using infused solutions, the cardiac and renal status of the patient affect the desired rate of administration. Blood volume may expand when rapidly infused fluids overtax an impaired heart and when renal damage causes retention of fluid. Patients with hypovolemia must receive plasma and blood rapidly, but the desired rate of the infusion should be specified by the LIP. Vital signs must be carefully observed and the speed of the infusion decreased as the blood pressure rises.

PATIENT'S TOLERANCE

Tolerance to fluids varies among individuals and influences the rate of infusion. A 5% infusion of alcohol has been administered at the rate of 200 to 300 mL/h to sedate without intoxicating an average adult. However, when such a fluid is to be administered, the rate must be titrated to the individual and prescribed by the LIP. The infusion should be checked frequently to maintain the required rate of flow. Because of certain factors, the rate is subject to change.

COMPOSITION OF SOLUTION

The composition of the fluid may affect the rate of flow. When the solution is used as a vehicle for administering drugs, the speed of the infusion depends on the drug and the desired clinical effect. Because of its deleterious effect on the heart when infused at a rapid rate, potassium should be administered with caution. Approximately 20 to 40 mEq potassium in a liter of fluid infused over an 8-hour period is an average rate for administering potassium parenterally.

Concentration of solutions must be considered because the flow rate may alter the desired effect. When dextrose is administered for caloric benefits, it is infused at a rate that ensures complete utilization. Dextrose has been administered at a maximum rate of 0.5 g/kg body weight/h without producing glycosuria in a normal person. At this rate, it

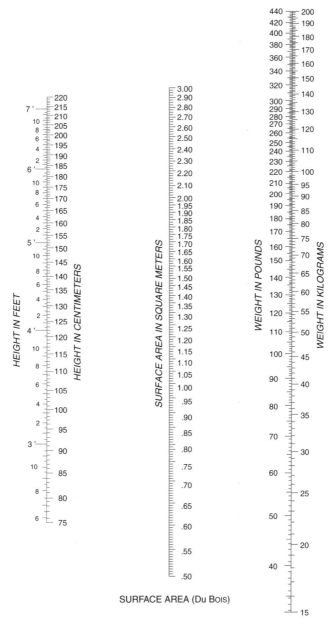

FIGURE 12-4 A nomogram.

would take approximately 1.5 hours to administer 1 L of 5% dextrose to a person weighing 70 kg or twice as long for 1 L of 10% dextrose. This maximum rate is faster than usual and is not customarily used except in an emergency.

When a diuretic effect is desired, a more rapid infusion is necessary. If the fluid is too rapidly infused for complete metabolism, the glucose accumulates in the bloodstream, increases the osmolality, and acts as a diuretic.

When oliguria or anuria occurs, the status of the kidneys must be determined before fluids containing potassium can be administered. Urinary suppression may be caused by blood volume deficit or kidney damage. An initial hydrating fluid, to test kidney function, is usually administered at a rate of 8 mL/m² BSA/min for 45 minutes. If urine does not flow, the rate is slowed to approximately 2 mL/m² BSA/min for another hour. If urine output does not occur after this period, kidney damage is likely to be present (Metheny, 2012).

HEIGHT OF THE INFUSION CONTAINER

Intravenous fluids are propelled by gravity. Any change in gravity induced by raising or lowering the infusion container, relative to the patient's position, alters the rate of flow. When patients receiving infusions are ambulatory or transported to ancillary departments, the containers should be retained at the same height or the speed of the infusion should be readjusted to maintain the prescribed rate of flow.

CLOT IN THE CATHETER

Any temporary stoppage of the infusion, such as a delay in hanging subsequent fluids, may cause a clot to form in the lumen of the catheter, partially or completely obstructing it. Clot formation may also occur when an increase in venous pressure in the extremity receiving the infusion forces blood back into the catheter. This results from restriction of the venous circulation. In arm infusion sites, this is most commonly caused by the blood pressure cuff on the infusion arm; restraints placed on or above the infusion catheter; and the patient lying on the arm receiving the infusion.

CHANGE IN CATHETER POSITION

A change in the catheter's position may push the bevel of the catheter against or away from the wall of the vein. Special precautions should be taken to prevent speed shock or vascular overload by making sure that the fluid flows freely before adjusting the rate.

OTHER CHANGES

Stimulation of vasoconstrictors from any infusion of cold blood or irritating fluid may cause venous spasm, impeding the rate of flow. A warm pack placed on the vein proximal to the infusion catheter offsets spasms. Any injury, such as phlebitis or thrombosis that reduces the lumen of the vein decreases the flow of the fluid. In addition, a clogged air vent in the administration set used with air-dependent containers causes the infusion to stop.

If the nurse has any question as to the rate of administration, the LIP should be consulted. This applies particularly to IV administration of drugs in fluid. The rates should also be established for patients receiving two or more infusions simultaneously. Any change in the rate from that normally used should be prescribed by the attending LIP.

Computation of Administration Rate

When determining drops per minute, the nurse rounds the drop rate to a whole number. The milliliters per hour also are rounded to a whole number when gravity infusion sets are being used. Flow rate calculations require the following base of information: amount of fluid to be infused, duration of the administration, and drop factor of the set to be used.

Calculating the appropriate infusion rate is easy. The nurse must first know the drop factor of the set that is being used; then, he or she can set up a fraction showing the volume of infusate over the number of minutes in which the volume should be infused. For example, if the patient is to receive 100 mL of fluid within 1 hour, the fraction would be

$$\frac{100\,\text{mL}}{60\,\text{minutes}}$$

The fraction is multiplied by the drop factor to determine the number of drops per minute to be infused, using this simple equation:

$$\text{Drops per minute} = \frac{\text{total mL}}{\text{total minutes}} \times \text{drop factor}$$

If 1,000 mL of fluid is ordered over an 8-hour period, the equation is modified as follows:

$$\text{Flow rate} = \frac{1,000\,\text{mL}}{8\,\text{hours}} = 125\,\text{mL}\,/\,\text{hour}$$

For microdrip or pediatric systems, the equation is
mL/h = drop factor
A simple, computer-generated table is presented in Figure 12-5.

Venous Access Devices (VADS)

Innovations in catheter technology have produced devices to meet the patient's every need, from routine peripheral infusion to the most sophisticated therapy. Catheters vary in gauge, length, design, and composition. Thin-walled catheters promote increased flow rates, which allow smaller catheters to be used.

Some products have wings, which confer all the advantages of a small-vein needle for insertion and taping. In these devices, the adapter of the IV set connection is located a few inches from the catheter, which provides ease and smoother technique when changing sets, thereby reducing the potential for mechanical phlebitis and contamination. Such catheters are available with injection sites as an integral part of the catheter; the mixing of drugs or blood components with primary parenteral fluid is reduced to a minimum (0.4 mL), minimizing the potential for incompatibilities.

Product Selection and Evaluation Criteria

A multidisciplinary health care team that includes front-line health care workers should be involved in selecting safety products. Other potential team members include infection control, safety, quality improvement, occupational health, materials management, medical, emergency/trauma, surgical, anesthesia, diagnostic radiology, home care, critical care, and laboratory staff. The infusion specialist must be included in the team that assesses products used in infusion therapy.

In determining the criteria for selecting IV safety devices, design and performance should be considered. The suggested FDA criteria for selecting a safety device are given in Box 12-6.

Dynamic Drip Rate Table Creation Tool

Patient: [   ] Weight: [   ] [Kg ⬍]
[If drug is not on list – Add to comments section below ⬍]

Add any comments you would like to the finished table: Maximum recommended dose, bolus dose information, usual dosing range, provider information, person who generated this table etc.
(If drug was not available in the drop down list above, add it here.)

[   ]

(1) Describe infusion solution:
Amount of drug added: [   ] [milligrams ⬍] Volume of solution: [   ] ml
(2) Select units for drug dosing: [mcg/kg/min ⬍]
(3) Select increments for table (see note) [1 ⬍] [Help?]
(4) Number of rows the completed table will contain: [10 ⬍] [Hint]
(5) Select number of decimals for program output: [0 ⬍] 🔢

[Generate Table] [Reset]

Sample of the programs output:

Table Information

Patient Name: Samuel Jackson.   **Weight (kg):** 75
Drug: Dopamine **Solution:** 400 mg/ 250 ml
Concentration of solution: 1.6 mg/ml

mcg/kg/min	ml/hr
1	3
2	6
3	8
4	11
5	14
6	17

Last updated Wed Dec 8 00:41:49 2004

FIGURE 12-5 Program for calculating flow rates. (IV drip calculator, courtesy of Globalrph, www.globalrph.com).

Consideration should be given to latex-free components of a device that may have prolonged contact with a patient, such as an IV catheter. To avoid giving a false sense of security to those who are allergic to natural rubber latex, the FDA recommends that manufacturers of FDA-regulated medical products stop using statements on labels such as "latex free" or "does not contain latex." The problem with that language is that the FDA is aware of no tests that can show a medical product is completely without the natural rubber latex proteins that can cause allergic reactions. Without a way to verify that a product is free of these proteins, claims that a product is "latex free" may be misleading. FDA wants to promote scientifically accurate labeling (FDA, 2013). The Occupational Safety and Health Administration (OSHA) and the CDC recommend the following steps to prevent allergic reactions to natural rubber latex in the workplace:

- Avoid using gloves with natural rubber latex for activities that are unlikely to involve contact with infectious materials.

BOX 12-6   FDA-SUGGESTED CRITERIA FOR SELECTING A SAFETY DEVICE

- Device provides a barrier between the hands and the needle following use.
- Device allows or requires worker's hands to remain behind the needle at all times.
- Safety constitutes an integral part of the device and is not an accessory.
- Safety features are effective before disassembly and remain in effect after disposal.
- Device should be simple and easy to use, requiring little or no training.

Adapted from U.S. Food and Drug Administration. (1995). Supplementary guidance on the content of premarket notification (510 K) submission for medical devices with sharps injury prevention features (draft). Rockville, MD: General Hospital Device Branch, Pilot Device Evaluation Division, Office of Device Evaluation.

- If you need such gloves, use powder-free gloves labeled as having reduced protein content, and when wearing them, do not use oil-based lotions. Natural rubber latex proteins can become attached to powder used to lubricate gloves; when the gloves are removed, the particles become airborne and can be inhaled, which is another form of exposure. Oil-based lotions can cause deterioration of the gloves.
- After use, wash your hands with a mild soap and dry thoroughly.
- Learn to recognize the symptoms of a natural rubber latex allergy and take any training offered by your employer.

PATIENT/STAFF SAFETY

Case Study
A 41-year-old female registered nurse suffered multiple, unidentified allergic reactions at work that continued for years. Her first severe reaction occurred after visiting a family member in the hospital. She developed breathing difficulties so intense that she was required to spend 3 days on a ventilator. At that time, it was assumed that her reaction was due to the cleaning agents used in the hospital. It was later determined that the cleaning agents had only served to make latex particles more airborne, therefore contributing to her allergic reaction. Whenever she changed jobs, she informed her supervisors of her allergy and was supplied with nonlatex gloves. Her coworkers, however, continued to use latex gloves throughout the hospital. At times, she would run out of the hypoallergenic gloves and revert to latex gloves, which always provoked an allergic reaction. Her last episode occurred after she wore latex gloves and developed anaphylaxis. She was rushed to the emergency room, where she informed medical personnel that she was latex sensitive. The staff treating her continued using the latex gloves, resulting in the death of the patient 40 minutes after first entering the emergency room. Postmortem blood tests found high levels of latex antibodies in her bloodstream.

(From Dermatology Nursing. (1997). Latex as killer: one nurse's story. *Dermatology Nursing, 9,* 348.)

INFUSION CATHETERS

Most IV catheters consist of flexible, nonthrombogenic tubing that remains within the lumen of the vessel, negating many of the formerly routine complications associated with infusion therapy. The gold standard is the over-the-needle catheter (ONC). Once the venipuncture is made, the catheter is slipped off the needle into the vein and the steel needle removed.

Most of the materials currently in use are polymers indicative of "many parts." Small molecules are chemically linked together to form a long chain or a large molecule with a thread-like appearance. Adding more molecules changes the properties of the material. Polytetrafluoroethylene (Teflon) is a carbon-based polymer. Fluorinated ethylene propylene is more flexibility as well as more compatible with tissues and drugs. These materials are generally used for short peripheral catheters (Hadaway, 2010).

Polyurethane may be formulated in various ways and is used for peripheral and central catheters. Its strength permits it to be manufactured with thin walls, allowing for great fluid flow. Some formations of polyurethane have an ultrasmooth microsurface, an exclusive lubrication process, and the ability to soften up to 70% while in the vessel. This biomaterial decreases the chance of irritation to the vessel wall, thereby reducing the potential or mechanical phlebitis. These catheter characteristics allow for ease of insertion, kink resistance, and reduced risk of phlebitis and infiltration, and also translate into optimum dwell times.

Silicone elastomer material is used for catheters due to its flexibility. Ideally, to reduce the risk of thrombus formation on the catheter, the catheter should be made of a **hemorepellant** material, such as silicone. All materials are tested for biocompatibility. Catheters should be radiopaque for detection by imaging equipment in the event the catheter is severed and lost in the circulation (INS, 2011).

Making a wise choice of a catheter for an infusion is a relatively straightforward process. Although the number and types of lines have increased dramatically, several factors remain considerations in all choices (Table 12-3). All products used should pass safety criteria.

WINGED INFUSION NEEDLES

The winged infusion device or small-vein needle is similar to the steel cannula, with the hub replaced with two flexible wings. The small-vein needle with the resealable injection site allows the intermittent administration of medications or fluids. Variations of the winged infusion needle are available for short-term infusion use. A dilute solution of heparinized saline or saline solution maintains patency of the needle when it is not in use. Winged infusion needles also enhance safety and protection (Figure 12-6).

MIDLINE CATHETERS

The introduction of the midline catheter provided an alternative to central line catheter placement for prolonged IV access. Today's midline catheter utilizes the same insertion technique as the peripherally inserted central catheter (PICC). Midline catheters are made of polyurethane or silicone and are usually 8 inch (20 cm) long. They may be single or double lumen. Advantages of using the product include reduction of peripheral IV restarts, elimination of the need for central IV lines with their associated complications, and ease of midline insertion. Professionals are encouraged to develop policies and procedures relevant to indwell time and consistent with INS standards and institutional guidelines (INS, 2011).

TABLE 12-3	PERIPHERAL VADS AND THEIR USE		
Device	Description	Advantages	Disadvantages
Short-length catheter	ONC catheter Variety of sizes and lengths Radiopaque	Easily inserted	Short-term use; site should be rotated consistent with institutional policy and Standards of Practice
Midline catheter	A midcatheter device usually placed in either the basilic or cephalic vein	ONC: Useful in acute, subacute, and home care settings. Appropriate for all intravenous fluids that would otherwise be administered through a short-length peripheral catheter; longer indwell time	Inherent risk of puncturing and shearing the catheter during insertion
Winged infusion needle	Steel needle or flexible catheter with fixed extension set	Easily inserted and secured with wings; extension set ensures access	May infiltrate easily if a rigid needle winged infusion device is used

Consistent with State Nurse Practice Act.
ONC, over-the-needle catheter.
Adapted from Prue-Owens, K.K. (2006). Use of peripheral venous access devices. *Critical Care Nurse, 28*(1), 30–38; Ludeman, K. (2008). I.V. Essentials: Which vascular access device is right for your patient? *Nursing Made Incredibly Easy, 6*(4), 7–11.

CENTRAL VENOUS AND PERIPHERALLY INSERTED CATHETERS (PICC)

Device manufacturers have designed central venous catheters with a wide variety of features and insertion methods suitable for insertion into many different anatomical sites (Hadaway, 2010). PICCs are made of polyurethane and silicone. These products, as well as nontunneled, percutaneous centrally inserted catheters, tunneled (cuffed) catheters, and ports, are addressed in the chapters on Peripheral and Central Venous Access.

FLUID CONTAINERS

Sterile glass containers first became available in 1929. Although currently used much less frequently, glass remains the container of choice for those fluids that, because of their characteristics, may not be administered in plastic containers. For example, nitroglycerin can be

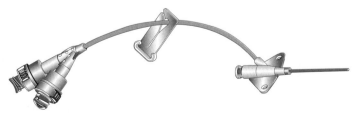

FIGURE 12-6 Winged infusion needle.

absorbed into plastic containers and tubing, and lipid emulsions can absorb certain plastics from the container into the fluid.

GLASS CONTAINERS

At manufacture, glass IV containers are sealed under vacuum and therefore must be vented when delivered to the patient. The air vent on the administration set (typically as part of the piercing pin) should have an air filter to prevent the ingress of microbes as the fluid is vented. If a nonvented administration set is used with a glass container, the fluid will not flow. Air must displace the fluid in the container for flow to occur. The venting mechanism provided by the manufacturer is intended to allow air to enter without allowing fluid to leak from the venting device.

Medications should be added to glass containers through a designated stopper with a filter needle. Glass is also an absolute barrier to gases such as carbon dioxide and oxygen.

PLASTIC CONTAINERS

Baxter Healthcare (Deerfield, IL) was the first manufacturer to develop plastic containers for parenteral fluids. Plastic containers are easily transported, minimize the risk of damage to the container, and are easily disposed of. Air venting is not required because the container collapses as the fluid is delivered. This in turn reduces the risk of air embolism and airborne contamination. Because plastic containers do not have stoppers or bushings, the risk of coring and particulate matter is eliminated. Plastic IV containers range in size from 25 to 1,000 mL for IV infusion. There have been environmental concerns with plastic IV containers containing di-2-ethylhexyl phthalate (DEHP), a plasticizer used to increase pliability.

SYRINGES AND SAFETY SYRINGES

A syringe may be a fluid container, especially when used with an infusion device that accommodates syringe delivery. Delivery of fluid or medication from a syringe is well suited to patient care areas in which small volumes of medication or fluid are required. The limiting feature of the syringe is its volume capacity. Using standard syringes, delivery times vary from 15 to 60 minutes with an accuracy rate of ± 15%.

The development of safety syringes has contributed greatly to practice. Several manufacturers provide safety syringes with needle guards to protect the health care worker and patient.

DRUG DELIVERY SYSTEMS

Drug delivery systems that enhance safety include manufacturer-prepared IV delivery systems, point-of-care–activated IV delivery systems, and pharmacy-based IV admixture programs.

MANUFACTURER-PREPARED SYSTEMS

Manufacturer-prepared fluids have revolutionized practice because increasing numbers of medications are marketed in this way. Premixed fluids are prepared under sterile conditions in the designated diluent and container with specific instructions for use. Easily transported and stable, manufacturer-prepared fluids have changed the way in which home care is delivered.

Point-of-Care System

A use-activated (point-of-care) container is compartmentalized, with premeasured drug in one compartment and the required fluid in another compartment. To activate the container for infusion, the nurse must remove or dislodge a diaphragm or seal between the compartments. This simplifies drug delivery by allowing the drug and the fluid to mix. It also eliminates the need for separate drug and diluent vials and yields an appropriate admixture for delivery.

Nurse managers are often the first to appreciate the ramifications of improved safety measures at the bedside and are the first to recommend point-of-care technology for medication administration. If nursing finds a system with a device that they find effective and easy to use while allowing for more time with patients, they will become one of the most vocal champions for implementation.

The best practices in point-of-care technology reflect significant change for hospital management. There are major implications for increased reporting capabilities and visibility into nursing metrics, such as: Are medications being given on time? What types of errors is the point-of-care system catching? What are the workload statistics by nurse? What should productivity expectations be? The technology is able to provide these metrics and usher in a new era of accountability, as well as the ability to document every step in medication administration and more generally in nurse workflow. The data available to hospital management from such a system provide useful information on the 24/7 operation of a hospital unit that has been unavailable to date without extreme monitoring and collection measures. This information on operational variability among units and various shifts can be used to determine and proliferate best practices, thus improving operations in areas beyond medication administration (Swenson, 2007).

Pharmacy-Based Infusion Admixture

Although many medications come in a prefilled container for secondary IV administration, some medications must be added to fluid before administration. Methods for adding medications to fluid containers vary with each system, and safety parameters have been added to currently available devices. The plastic bag contains a resealable medication port through which the medication is injected, although some products permit needleless access to the container.

When medications are added to the plastic containers during an infusion, care must be taken to ensure that the clamp on the administration set is closed and the flow interrupted before the medication is added. This prevents inadvertent administration of an undiluted and potentially toxic dose of medication that has not been fully diluted in the IV container. Medications and fluids should always be mixed thoroughly before administration, regardless of the system used. Most drug delivery systems use universal piercing pins. Use of such products eliminates the need to remove an existing air vent from the piercing pin.

Infusion Administration Sets

An important factor in the administration set is the rate of flow the given set is gauged to produce. Commercial sets vary, delivering anywhere from 10 to 15 drops/mL, depending on the nature of the fluid. The nurse must be aware of the drop factor to set the rate of flow correctly. Increased fluid viscosity may slow the rate of infusion but does not affect the drop factor.

Most conventional sets use the roller clamp or slide clamp for controlling the flow rate. Fluid temperature, room temperature, height of the fluid container, and the patient's catheter size all affect flow rate. The nurse should recheck the infusion rate regularly to ensure that the prescribed flow rate is maintained.

A primary set is the main administration set used for infusion therapy. Primary sets may be a gravity set, an infusion pump set, or a microbore–syringe pump set if the main infusate is being administered with a syringe pump. Ideally, the IV filter is incorporated within the set, rather than used as an add-on device.

SPECIALTY-USE SETS

Non-PVC IV administration sets are available for gravity and volumetric EIDs. Nitroglycerin and other drugs can be administered without altering the dosage of the drug through **absorption** into the walls of PVC tubing. Fat emulsion leaches plasticizers from the PVC tubing; these specialty sets may have non-PVC layers in fluid contact or use plasticizers that do not leach as easily.

In many cases, the flow must be maintained at a minimal rate. One method is to reduce the drop size by using a microdrip set. These sets deliver 60 drops/mL. At the rate of 60 drops/min, it would take 1 hour to infuse 60 mL. A variety of commercial sets are available for alternate or simultaneous infusion of two fluids. Some sets contain a filter. Positive pressure sets are designed to increase the rate of infusion and are an asset when rapid replacement of fluid becomes necessary. When used with the collapsible plastic fluid container, the danger of air embolism is minimal because as the bag collapses, the risk of air in the system is reduced. In contrast to the collapsible plastic container, glass containers must be vented to allow the fluid to flow, and air is thus present in the system. As the last portion of fluid from the glass container is delivered to the patient, the air under pressure may rapidly enter the vein before the clamp can be applied, resulting in an embolus. The nurse should never apply positive pressure to infuse fluids.

SECONDARY ADMINISTRATION SETS

Secondary sets with check valves were traditionally used to administer secondary medications as a piggyback into the injection site located below the valve. The valve automatically shut off the main-line infusion while the admixture was running and automatically allowed the main infusion to start when the medication had run in.

The connection may be made with one of several types of needleless systems. The secondary set should remain connected to the primary set, with both being changed simultaneously at the designated time. Variations of this set are available for use with electronic flow control devices (EIDs), which enable the user to back-prime the small-volume container (piggyback) with primary fluid (see Electronic Infusion Devices).

METERED VOLUME-CONTROLLED SETS

Accuracy in controlling the volume of IV fluids has always been facilitated by using a metered volume-controlled set or burette. Used less frequently today because of the plethora of EIDs available on the market and market pricing of those devices, the volume-controlled set still maintains a place in the clinical setting. Sets contain vented, calibrated burette chambers that control the volume from 100 to 150 mL. The chamber of some sets contains a rubber float that prevents air from entering the tubing once the infusion is completed; these sets are made for gravity flow and electronic infusion delivery systems (see Figure 12-7).

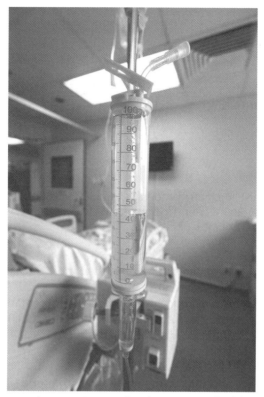

FIGURE 12-7 Metered volume-controlled set (burette).

ELECTRONIC INFUSION DEVICE–SPECIFIC SETS

Some administration sets are made specifically for use with EIDs. These sets also come in a number of configurations. Such sets and their respective electronic delivery systems ensure safe delivery of infusion therapy to patients of all ages in a variety of clinical settings. By extracting fluid from the IV container and ejecting it at predetermined intervals through the administration set, the EID delivers the appropriate preset amount of diluent.

FINAL INFUSION FILTERS

Filters prevent passage of undesirable substances into the vascular system (Figure 12-8). Particulate filters of 1 or 5 μm are recommended when IV medications are being prepared. A bacteria-retentive filter of approximately 0.2 μm is recommended for the routine delivery of IV therapies. Ideally, the filter should be an integral part of the primary administration set, rather than an add-on device to ensure sterility and avoid cross-contamination. Because all infusates cannot be filtered, administration sets without integral filters are also available.

The industry standard is a membrane filter. Membrane filters are screen-type filters with uniformly sized pores that provide an absolute rating. A 0.2-μm screen-type filter retains on the flat surface membrane all particles larger than 0.2 μm. A 0.2-μm filter is considered an

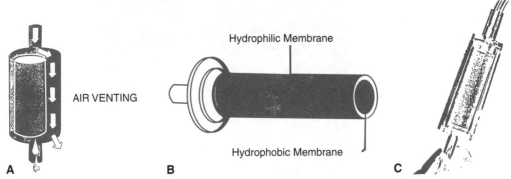

FIGURE 12-8 **A:** Air-eliminating properties of an IV filter. **B:** Hydrophilic/hydrophobic membrane properties of an IV filter. **C:** Optimal IV filter for add-on or in-line use. (Courtesy of Abbott Laboratories, Abbott Park, IL.)

absolute, bacteria-retentive, air-eliminating filter and decreases the complications of infection and the potential for air embolism.

The *United States Pharmacopeia* has established an acceptable limit of particles for single-dose infusion as not more than 50 particles/mL that are ≥ 10.0 μm and not more than 5 particles/mL that are ≥ 25.0 μm in effective linear dimension.

EFFECT OF PRESSURE AND AIR ON FILTERS

At a certain pressure, all filters allow air to pass from one side of the wetted hydrophilic membrane to the other. This pressure value is called the bubble point of that particular membrane. Distinguishing features that affect the bubble point are the different filter materials (e.g., hydrophobic, hydrophilic), depth, screen, different wetting (hydrophilic) or nonwetting (hydrophobic) characteristics, and the test liquid. Water or saline solution, for example, is the test liquid of choice when testing hydrophilic membranes for IV filters because fluids that are administered IV is primarily water. Water is inexpensive, can be filtered easily for control of particulates and microorganisms, and is readily available. There are other advantages to using water as a bubble point test fluid. Water tests the wetting characteristics of hydrophilic membrane filters. To define this point further, an explanation of bubble point tests in relation to membranes is required.

BUBBLE POINT TESTS

Bubble point testing is particularly important in infusion therapy because it is crucial that the filter in the IV line prevent air from passing through it at low pressures, such as those used in IV therapy.

Testing involves encapsulation of the membrane in an integral housing. Two different types of bubble point tests may be performed, open bubble and closed bubble point, depending on downstream flow and the ability to see the membrane (Figure 12-9). An open bubble point test can be performed only if the direction of normal flow is such that the bubbles produced can be seen as they form. This means that the housing of the filter must be transparent and the downstream side of the membrane can be observed. This test is performed by first flowing the test liquid through the device at low pressures until it is wetted out. Usually, this pressure is the same as that used in administering fluid by gravity feed

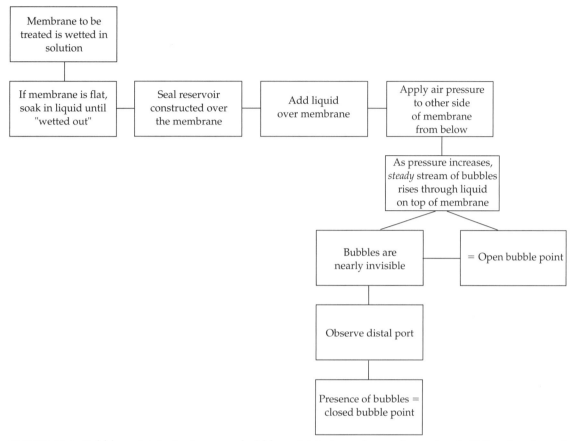

FIGURE 12-9 Bubble point tests. An open bubble point test can be performed only if the direction of normal flow permits bubbles to form.

pressures (36 to 39 inch of water). Then, after the membrane is wetted out, air pressure is applied as before. The bubble point has been reached when a steady stream of bubbles is seen on the downstream side of the membrane.

A closed bubble point test must be performed when the downstream side of the membrane cannot be visualized. Closed bubble points result in slightly higher values than open bubble points because the air pressure during the test is steadily increasing and it takes more time for the air bubbles to escape through the distal port. If the pressure is increased slowly, the test is more accurate.

Testing of IV membranes and filter devices with water is significant. Most hydrophilic membranes incorporate either external (applied after they are made) or internal (in the base formula) wetting agents to render them more wettable with water. It is particularly important in IV therapy because it is critical that the membrane should wet properly so that air does not pass the membrane at low pressures.

The 0.2-μm air-venting filters automatically vent air through a nonwettable (hydrophobic) membrane and permit uniform high gravity flow rates through large, wettable (hydrophilic) membranes. They prevent an air block, which could ultimately result in a plugged catheter.

Filters are also rated according to the pounds per square inch (**psi**) of pressure they withstand, an important consideration in selecting the proper filter. The filter should withstand the pressure exerted by the infusion pump or rupture may occur. If the psi rating of the housing is less than that of the membrane, excess force will break the housing, leaving the filter intact.

Optimal filters should (a) automatically vent air; (b) retain bacteria, fungi, and endotoxins; (c) not bind drugs; (d) allow high gravity flow rates; and (e) be able to withstand the pressure exerted by the infusion pump. The pressure rating of the housing, when less than that of the filter membrane, may provide added protection.

INFUSION ACCESSORIES

A plethora of accessories, such as injection caps, loops, latex ports, and needleless systems, is available today (Figure 12-10) and includes safety features. The injection port or catheter cap may be used to adapt any indwelling device to an intermittent infusion device. Available either as an individual unit or incorporated into the design of an ONC or winged infusion set, injection ports have simplified the administration of intermittent therapies using needleless systems.

Intermittent infusion devices may also be called *heparin locks*, *INTS*, or *PRN adapters* because heparin or saline is routinely instilled into the cap and its housing to maintain patency. Most health care organizations routinely instill saline rather than dilute heparin in such devices.

LATEX DEVICES AND SENSITIVITY

Latex sensitivity remains a challenge for health care workers and patients alike, with powdered latex gloves being the most common latex equipment to exacerbate allergies. In addition, many of the clinical supplies used to deliver IV fluids and fluids are made of latex.

The various types of latex reactions include irritant or contact dermatitis, allergic contact-type IV hypersensitivity, and type I hypersensitivity. Allergic reactions are potentially avoidable for both the patient and clinicians. The nurse delivering infusion therapy should be cognizant of the prevalence, symptoms, risk factors, diagnosis, and treatment of latex

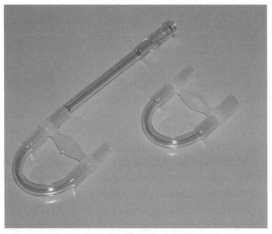

FIGURE 12-10 Accessories for IV therapy.

allergy. Standard precautions mandate that health care providers wear gloves for prolonged periods of patient care. Latex is a natural rubber product derived from the sap of the commercial rubber tree *Hevea brasiliensis*. The latex fluid is composed of carbohydrates, lipids, phospholipids, and *cis*-1,4 polyisoprene. Latex is a complex protein by-product of the rubber tree containing more than 28 antigenic peptide proteins and contributing to allergic reactions in people with hypersensitivity latex allergy (Table 12-4).

Exposure can occur through cutaneous, mucosal, parenteral, or aerosol routes. Parenteral exposure includes medications injected through latex IV injection sites or drawn through rubber stoppers of vials. Powder released into the air during the removal of a powdered latex glove may precipitate respiratory distress. Latex proteins may remain airborne for as long as 5 to 12 hours. Diagnosis is confirmed by detailed history, including risk factors and suspected reactions. Physical examination may reveal a lack of symptoms. A skin prick test is a reliable indicator of an antigen allergy. Radioallergosorbent testing (RAST) is an in vitro test for IgE antibodies to a specific antigen. The results of RAST may be inconclusive, however. Use, challenge, or patch tests may be performed, along with intradermal testing, basophil histamine release, and inhalation tests. Prevention is achieved by providing a latex-free environment. The National Institute for Occupational Safety and Health (NIOSH) recommends that if latex gloves are worn, they should be the low-antigen type and powderless. A part of the CDC, NIOSH is the federal agency responsible for conducting research and making recommendations for the prevention of work-related injury and illness.

FLOW CONTROL DEVICES: ELECTRONIC INFUSION DEVICES AND SMART TECHNOLOGIES

Complex infusions of medications are administered using EIDs that, although designed to be easy to use, have been associated with serious programming errors that can result in overdosing or underdosing. Smart computerized devices with comprehensive drug libraries, dosing limits, and best-practice guidelines have transformed the industry. Each hospital develops its own complete data set, including drug names, concentrations, dosing units, and dose limits, and loads the devices with this information. Some smart pumps include additional features such as drug information and weight, rate, and volume limits specific to the clinical area in which they are used. These devices add to a new level of safety in IV administration that was previously impossible (Schlotterbeck, Rickerson, Coffman, Vanderveen, & Lee, 2010).

The INS Standards of Practice address regulation of flow. EIDs should be used when warranted by the patient's age and condition, setting, and prescribed therapy. The nursing professional is responsible and accountable for the use of EIDs. Use of EIDs, their deployment, selection criteria, and classifications should be outlined in institutional policy and procedure

TABLE 12-4	TYPE I REACTIONS TO LATEX: FIVE STAGES
Stage	Clinical Manifestation
1	Local urticaria in the area of contact
2	Generalized urticaria with angioedema
3	Urticaria with asthma, eye or nose itching, and gastrointestinal symptoms
4	Urticaria with anaphylaxis
5	Chronic asthma and permanent lung damage

manuals. The nurse's knowledge base concerning EIDs should include, at the minimum, indications for use, mechanical operation, safe use and troubleshooting techniques, and the psi rating.

The psi rating is important because differential pressure is often a component of such devices. With a range of two or three levels, such equipment may sense a change in pressure, usually 5 psi over baseline, and some devices monitor and read out (display) line pressure. *Operating* or *line pressure* is the pressure generated by a pump that causes fluid to flow at a predetermined rate. *Maximum occlusion pressure* is the limit to operating pressure at which an occlusion alarm is triggered. Needle pressure is the same as venous pressure. During an infusion, pressure at the tip of the catheter is only slightly greater than the pressure in the vein or artery, regardless of the output pressure of the pump. The pressure at the needle tip needs to be slightly higher than vascular pressure for fluid to flow. An understanding of pressure and the psi rating is essential to safe use of EIDs, filters, and other components of the infusion system.

EIDs are invaluable in neonatal, pediatric, and adult intensive care units, where critical infusions of small volumes of fluid or doses of high-potency drugs are required. These devices have increased the level of safety in parenteral therapy. Today, the risk of air embolism is reduced by alarm systems and by the automatic interruption of the infusion when a container empties. A controlled rate of flow reduces the risk of circulatory overload.

AMBULATORY INFUSION DEVICES

Self-care is an important component of current health care delivery systems. The development of compact, battery-driven EIDs has simplified care in diverse ambulatory clinical settings, including home care. These products are small enough to be easily carried, allowing the patient freedom to return to work, school, and life. They employ a battery system that necessitates recharging and battery replacement.

The size, weight, and portability of the unit are important considerations in choosing a system. An active patient must be comfortable wearing the lightest pump possible; a sedentary patient may prefer the advantages of a larger device. Accessories and loading procedures vary with the manufacturer and the product selected. Infusion capacity may dictate the choice of the system. Pump-specific sets may be required, such as with the patient receiving nutritional support or pain medication. Integral safety features include

- Occlusion alarm
- Low-volume safety alarm
- Low-battery alarm

Competition in this exciting area of growth has stimulated many new companies to enter the electronic infusion market, resulting in greater availability of more sophisticated products.

ELASTOMERIC BALLOON DEVICES

An **elastomeric** device is made of a soft, rubberized material capable of inflating to a predetermined volume. The balloon deflates at a rate determined by the diameter of the restricting outlet located in the preattached tubing or in the neck of the container. The size of the tunnel controls the passage of fluid. The balloon, safely encapsulated inside a rigid, transparent container, becomes the reservoir for fluid. The shape of this device is manufacturer specific, and it may be round, disk shaped, or cylindrical. A tamper-proof port for injecting medication into the balloon is attached. Typically, the capacity is 50 to 100 mL, and the devices are for one-time use only.

SPRING-COIL PISTON SYRINGES

The volume of a spring-coil piston syringe ranges from 30 to 60 mL, and a spring powers the plunger in the absence of manual pressure. Like the elastomeric balloon, this device has limited applications and is for one-time use only. The syringe is filled by withdrawing the piston and overextending the spring. As the spring regains its shape, it forces the piston down, expelling its contents. The syringe has no incompatibilities associated with its use, making it ideal for the infusion of problematic drugs. Syringes may be prefilled and frozen until use.

SPRING-COIL CONTAINER

This container combines the principles of the spring-coil and a collapsible, flattened disk. An overextended spring in an enclosed space between two disks seeks to recover its original shape, pulling the top and bottom together and forcing the fluid contents out of the restricting orifice.

THERAPY-SPECIFIC DEVICES

EIDs are finding increasing use in keep-open arterial lines and infusion of drugs, blood, and viscous fluids such as parenteral nutrition fluids. Advances in technology have provided us with more sophisticated devices. Many types and models are available. In general, pumps are devices that generate flow under positive pressure. Such devices may be peristaltic, syringe, or pulsatile. Controllers are devices that generate flow by gravity and are capable of either drop counting or volumetric delivery.

CONTROLLERS

Controllers do not exert positive pressure greater than the head height of the infusion container, which is usually 2 psi. The controller is used to monitor the infusion for accuracy, to sound an alarm if flow is interrupted, and to provide even, consistent delivery of fluid. A controller uses drop-sensor technology. Manufacturers have developed variations on this theme, specific to patient populations and clinical needs.

PUMPS

By virtue of the name, a pump indicates that pressure is involved. The degree of pressure exerted must be sufficient to overcome resistance along the fluid pathway, including length of the administration set, kinked tubing, and accumulation of particulate matter in the tubing as well as the resistance caused by vascular pressure, presence of venous valves or fibrin/thrombus near the catheter tip, or positioning. A diversity of pump products is available, including syringe, positive pressure, and volumetric devices (Hadaway, 2010).

SYRINGE PUMPS

Many manufacturers have met the demand for syringe infusion systems. Syringe pumps are calibrated in milliliters per hour, are used with standard disposable syringes, and provide smooth and precise delivery of low volumes of fluid to specific patient populations. A variety of new products on the market may be configured to suit special clinical situations, with options such as auto bolus reduction to minimize the possibility of administering an accidental bolus of drug, preset upper bolus rates, maintenance notification, and downloading capability between instruments.

Negative Pressure Pumps

A negative pressure pump is composed of a double-sided chamber with one side serving as a vacuum or negative pressure and the other at atmospheric pressure. Filling the drug reservoir causes the creation of a vacuum. Pressure from a moveable wall is exerted against the drug reservoir as a result of differential pressure. Such devices are used to deliver pain medication when connected to a catheter immediately following surgical procedures.

Positive Pressure Infusion Pumps

A positive pressure device overcomes vascular resistance, tubing compromises such as excessive length, and the normal physical limitations that cause an IV to function improperly.

Pressure exerted by the unit is expressed in pounds per square inch (psi) or millimeters of mercury (mm Hg). One psi and 50 mm Hg exert the same amount of pressure. The psi rating of an EID is important because it may affect the type of filter being used or the ability of the unit to infuse fluids through arterial lines. The pressure exerted should not exceed the pressure the filter can withstand because otherwise a rupture may occur; when the pump is used for arterial infusion, the pressure must be high enough to overcome arterial pressure. Positive **pressure pumps** are used in most clinical settings.

Pole-mounted Volumetric Pumps

These devices lock onto a stationary or ambulatory IV pole and are applicable for use in all practice settings. Configurations abound with single, dual, and multiple channels.

Multichannel pumps may be two single-channel devices in one housing or two pump mechanisms with common controls and programming panels. The infusion nurse must be familiar with the type of device being used, potential for misuse, and possible interference from cellular telephones, portable radios, and electrosurgical equipment operating with high-frequency waves that could contribute to false alarms (Hadaway, 2010).

Computer-Generated Technology

The computer has become the focal point of the IV drug delivery system. Electronic flow is now the norm rather than the exception. EIDs today are available in diverse sizes and technologies for a broad range of purposes.

Accompanying these computerized systems is a whole new lexicon of terms with which the nurse must become familiar to use the equipment safely and properly. For example, commonly heard terms include *tapering* or **ramping**, which describe the progressive increase or decrease of infusion rate. Another common term is free flow. Free-flow alarms may be lifesaving if the administration set has no intrinsic valves or reservoirs that require motion of the pumping mechanism to propel the fluid. Many pumps incorporate free-flow alarms that are capable of detecting open flow of fluid to the patient. Others have internal clamps or devices that lock into place when tubing is removed from the pump, preventing free flow of fluid to the patient. Other safety features are available on a number of products.

Compared with a smart pump, an IV medication safety system offers a technology platform that can provide harm- and dose-error reduction software across multiple types of infusion devices. This type of system integrates infusion and patient monitoring modules using a common user interface. It may even be networked with a hospital's information technology system, providing immediate access to data and accelerating best practice and process improvements (Vanderveen, 2005; Schlotterbeck et al., 2010).

SAFETY SIGNALS

A "safety signal" is information that arises from one or more sources and suggests a new, potentially causal association or a new aspect of a known association, between a medical device and an event or set of related events. The aim of signal detection is to identify promptly possible unwanted or unexpected effects associated with a product. The decision whether a finding represents a "safety signal" and whether it warrants further investigation is a clinical challenge.

Factors that may influence the decision include the strength of the signal, whether or not the signal represents a new finding, the clinical importance and potential public health implications of the issue, and the potential for preventive measures to mitigate the adverse public health impact.

Alarms are intended to alert caregivers of potential problems but can compromise patient safety if they are not properly managed. Many patient care areas have numerous alarms, and the barrage of warning noises tend to desensitize caregivers and cause them to ignore alarms or even disable them. **Alarm fatigue** is a national problem and the number one medical device technology hazard today.

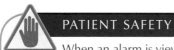

PATIENT SAFETY

When an alarm is viewed as a "nuisance," the caregiver may disable, silence, or ignore the warning that is intended to create a safer environment. This is a true safety issue!

Other issues associated with effective alarm management include too many medical devices with alarms or individual alarms that are difficult to hear. Preset or default settings also may cause problems because the device sounds a warning even when no action or decision by a caregiver is required. Rather than calling attention to a patient's needs, these settings may distract caregivers. The Joint Commission (TJC, 2013) recommends that health care organizations take actions, which correspond with recommendations made by both the American Association for Medical Instrumentation (AAMI) and the ECRI Institute (Box 12-7).

EQUIPMENT SAFETY AND USE

ECRI Institute (Plymouth Meeting, PA), an independent, nonprofit agency that tests equipment for safety and effectiveness and continually designs new criteria for evaluation of equipment, is dedicated to improving the safety, efficacy, and cost-effectiveness of health care technology, facilities, and procedures. Among the products assessed are EIDs from various manufacturers. The organization develops strict evaluation criteria aimed at helping care providers in the clinical setting perform with a high degree of safety and accuracy. ECRI Institute is a designated Evidence-Based Practice Center by the U.S. Agency for Healthcare Research and Quality (AHRQ) and listed as a federal Patient Safety Organization by the U.S. Department of Health and Human Services.

In relation to EIDs and infusion therapy, evaluation criteria are wide ranging to meet the needs of nursing staff in today's complex health care setting. The impact of downsizing and the integration of health care organizations have affected staffing patterns nationwide; therefore, nurses must be familiar with the literature and with the device to be used. They must take all precautions to ensure safe, efficient operation. One constant remains, however. The EID should never be used as a substitute for high-quality care and patient monitoring.

BOX 12-7   JOINT COMMISSION RECOMMENDATIONS FOR ALARMS/SIGNALS

- Ensure that there is a process for safe alarm management and response in areas identified by the organization as high risk.
- Prepare an inventory of alarm-equipped medical devices used in high-risk areas and for high-risk clinical conditions and identify the default alarm settings and the limits appropriate for each care area.
- Establish guidelines for alarm settings on alarm-equipped medical devices used in high-risk areas and for high-risk clinical conditions; include identification of situations when alarm signals are not clinically necessary.
- Establish guidelines for tailoring alarm settings and limits for individual patients. The guidelines should address situations when limits can be modified to minimize alarm signals and the extent to which alarms can be modified to minimize alarm signals.
- Inspect, check and maintain alarm-equipped medical devices to provide for accurate and appropriate alarm settings, proper operation, and detectability. Base the frequency of these activities on criteria such as manufacturers' recommendations, risk levels, and current experience.

Adapted from The Joint Commission. (2013). *Joint Commission Alert: Medical Device Alarm Safety in Hospitals [press release]*. April 8, 2013. http://www.marketwire.com/press-release/joint-commission-alert-medical-device-alarm-safety-in-hospitals-1776295.htm.

Product Selection and Evaluation

Selection of equipment is a complex task. Hospitalized patients now receive a multitude of therapies through their vascular systems. The type of device used to initiate flow depends on the complexity of care, the range of required flow, pressure, the insertion site, and the delivery rate.

Product selection should be a serious consideration and should be based on needs assessed in the clinical setting. The ability to deliver a specified dose in µg/kg/min, µg/kg/h, mg/kg/min, or mg/kg/h by entering the appropriate concentration, patient weight, bolus amount, and mass units is a feature often required in the critical care setting. Demands for features such as bolus capabilities, syringe size sensing, and delivery in body

EVIDENCE FOR PRACTICE

National attention to alarm hazards was created in 2010 by the death of a patient at Massachusetts General Hospital that was attributed to an alarm that had inadvertently been turned off. The federal report indicated that nurses working among constantly beeping monitors contributed to the death of the patient.

Wireless technologies may be viable alternatives to human monitor surveillance. Comparative studies are needed to identify the best approach to ensure positive patient outcomes. Potential study topics are as follows:

What strategies are effective in reducing alarm desensitization?

What is the effect of excessive alarms on staff?

weight, mass, continuous, or volume-over-time modes have challenged today's manufacturers to produce ever more advanced products.

Decision-Making Process

The product evaluation committee, regardless of the product being considered, is usually involved in the selection of products used in the clinical setting. Again, this group should be multidisciplinary and participate in the preliminary selection process and ongoing product evaluations as an end user. With all committee members working toward a common goal, an informed product choice can be made.

Considerations include identification of the need for a product change, technology, ease of use associated equipment, timing, features, and benefits—all with a focus on safety. This is certainly true of EIDs as well.

Patient Selection and Education

Patients should be carefully evaluated for their ability to comprehend and perform self-care procedures, especially when EIDs are to be used. The patient should be taught how to wear the pump, how to operate and care for the equipment (pump and line as well), and what troubleshooting steps to take in case of technical problems.

Complex infusion delivery systems enable us to ensure efficiencies in the delivery of care, regardless of the clinical setting. The infusion nurse plays a critical role in product selection, evaluation, and use. A dedicated, knowledgeable infusion specialist has a significant impact on patient safety. As technology continues to advance, the nurse's role will continue to escalate.

Review Questions   *Note: Questions below may have more than one right answer.*

1. Which of the following factors should be considered in selecting IV equipment?
   A. Latex-free components
   B. Safety design
   C. Performance
   D. All of the above

2. The porosity rating of an inline IV filter is what size in micrometers (μm)?
   A. 0.2
   B. 0.5
   C. 1.0
   D. 1.2

3. Which of the following factors may interfere with or inhibit fluid flow?
   A. Patient's vascular pressure
   B. Internal diameter of the tubing
   C. Neither of the above
   D. Both of the above

4. Which of the following is the aim of signal detection?
   A. Signal malfunction with other mechanical equipment
   B. Identify possible unwanted or unexpected effects
   C. Neither of the above
   D. Both of the above

5. Which of the following statements concerning hypovolemic patients is true?
   A. Plasma and blood must be delivered rapidly.
   B. Plasma and blood must be delivered slowly.
   C. Rate of infusion decreases with increased blood pressure.
   D. Rate of infusion increases with changes in blood pressure.

6. General infusion equipment includes which of the following?
   A. Durable medical equipment
   B. Single-use devices
   C. Reprocessed single-use devices
   D. All of the above

7. Latex fluid is composed of which of the following?
   A. Carbohydrates
   B. Lipids and phospholipids
   C. Neither of the above
   D. Both of the above

8. Which of the following systems may reduce the incidence of needlestick injuries?
   A. Needleless
   B. Filters
   C. Luer locks
   D. Universal connectors

9. Examples of sharps involved in IV practice include which of the following?
   A. Lancets
   B. Needles
   C. IV catheters
   D. B and C

10. Type I latex reactions manifested by the respiratory system include which of the following?
    A. Angioedema and respiratory arrest
    B. Shortness of breath and cyanosis
    C. Coughing and sneezing
    D. Rapid breathing

References and Selected Readings   *Asterisks indicate references cited in text.*

Alexander, M., Corrigan, A.M., Gorski, L.A., & Phillips, L. (2013). *Core curriculum for infusion nursing* (4th ed). Philadelphia, PA: Lippincott Williams & Wilkins.

Balkhy, H.H., El Beltagy, K.E., El-Saed, A., Sallah, M., & Jagger, J. (2011). Benchmarking of percutaneous injuries at a teaching tertiary care center in Saudi Arabia relative to United States hospitals participating in the Exposure Prevention Information Network. *American journal of infection control*, 39(7), 560–565.

Barnsteiner, J.H. (2005). Medication reconciliation: Transfer of medication information across settings—keeping it free from error. *Journal of Infusion Nursing*, 28(2 Suppl), 31–36.

Bolton L.B., Gassert, C.A., & Cipriano, P.F. (2008). Smart technology, enduring solutions. *Journal of Healthcare Information Management*, 22(4), 24–30.

*Burke, K.G. (2005). The state of the science on safe medication administration symposium. http://www.nursingcenter.com. *American Journal of Nursing*, 105(2 Suppl.), 4–9.

*Centers for Disease Control and Prevention. (2011). Guidelines for prevention of intravascular catheter-related infections. http://www.cdc.gov/hicpac/pdf/guidelines/bsi-guidelines-2011.pdf

Cohen, N.L. (2013). Using the ABCs of situational awareness for patient safety. *Nursing*, 43(4), 64–65.

*Cvach, M., (2012). Monitor alarm fatigue. *Biomedical Instrumentation and Technology*. 268–276

Djukic, M., Kovner, C.T., Brewer, C.S., Fatehi, F.K., & Cline, D.D. (2013). Work environment factors other than staffing associated with nurses' ratings of patient care quality. *Health Care Management Review*, 38(2), 105–114.

Dolan, S.A., Felizardo, G., Barnes, S., Cox, T.R., et al. (2010). APIC position paper: Safe injection, infusion and medication vial practices in health care. *American Journal of Infection Control*, 38(3), 167–712.

Dresser, S. (2012). The role of nursing surveillance in keeping patients safe. *Journal of Nursing Administration*, 42(7/8), 361–368.

ECRI Institute. (2011). Top 10 Health Technology Hazards for 2012. *Health Devices, 40*(11):358–373.

Groves, P.S., Meisenbach, R.J., & Scott-Cawiezell, J. (2011). Keeping patients safe in healthcare organizations: a structuration theory of safety culture. *Journal of advanced nursing, 67*(8), 1846–1855.

*Hadaway, L. (2010). In: Alexander M, Corrigan A. et al. (Eds.), *Infusion nursing: An evidence based approach* (391–393 and 213–214). St. Louis, MO: Saunders.

*Harding, A.D. (2013). Intravenous smart pumps. *Journal of Infusion Nursing 36*(3), 191–194

Hatcher, I., Sullivan, M., Hutchinson, J., et al. (2004). An intravenous medication safety system: Preventing high-risk medication errors at the point of care. *Journal of Nursing Administration, 34*(10), 437–439.

Henneman, E.A., Gawlinski, A., & Giuliano, K.K. (2012). Surveillance: A strategy for improving patient safety in acute and critical care units. *Critical Care Nurse, 32*(2), e9–e18.

*Hughes, R.G., & Ortiz, E. (2005). Medication errors. *Journal of Infusion Nursing, 28*(Suppl.), 14–23.

*Infusion Nurses Society. (2011). Infusion nursing standards of practice. *Journal of Infusion Nursing, 34*(1S), S1–S110.

*Institute of Medicine. (2004). *Keeping patients safe: Transforming the work environment of nurses.* Washington, DC: National Academies Press.

*Institute of Medicine. (2011). *Medical Devices and the Public's Health: The FDA 510(k) Clearance Process at 35 Years.* Washington, DC: National Academies Press.

Institute for Safe Medication Administration. (2004). ISMP list of high alert medications. Available at: www.ismp.org/MSAarticles/highalert.htm.

Institute for Safe Medication Practices. (2005). Safety issues with patient-controlled analgesia. *ISMP medication safety alert! 3:1–3.* Horsham, PA: ISMP Author.

Joint Commission on Accreditation of Healthcare Organizations. (2007). National patient safety goals. Available at: http://www.jointcommission.org/PatientSafety/NationalPatientSafetyGoals/07_npsgs.htm

*Ludeman, K. (2008). I.V. Essentials: Which vascular access device is right for your patient? *Nursing Made Incredibly Easy, 6*(4), 7–11.

*Metheny, N.M. (2012). *Fluid and electrolyte balance: Nursing considerations.* (5th ed.). Sudbury, MA: Jones & Bartlett Learning.

National Research Council. (2012). *Health IT and patient safety: Building safer systems for better care.* Washington, DC: National Academies Press.

*Nelson, R. (2006). AJN Reports: Reprocessed single-use devices—Safe or not? *American Journal of Nursing (106)* 25–26

*Nicholas, P.K., Agius, C.R. (2005). Toward safer IV medication administration. *Journal of Infusion Nursing, 28*(Suppl), 25–30.

Page, A. (Ed.); National Research Council. (2004). *Keeping patients safe: Transforming the work environment of nurses.* Washington, DC: National Academies Press.

*Prue-Owens, K.K. (2006). Use of peripheral venous access devices. *Critical Care Nurse, 28*(1), 30–38.

*Pugliese, G. (2013). http://www.healthleadersmedia.com/print/NRS-290704/Needlestick-Safety-Challenges-Continue.

Ring, L., & Fairchild, R.M. (2013). Leadership and patient safety: A review of the literature. *Journal of Nursing Regulation, 4*(1), 52–56.

Schneider, P.J. (Ed.). (2004). Addressing harm with high-risk drug administration. *Hospitals & Health Networks, 78* (Suppl), 18–20.

*Schlotterbeck, D.L., Rickerson, S.E., Coffman, D.J., Vanderveen, T.W., & Lee, B.A. (2010). *U.S. Patent No. 7,835,927.* Washington, DC: U.S. Patent and Trademark Office.

Siebig S., Kuhls S., Imhoff M., Gather U, Scholmerich J, and Wrede C. (2010). Intensive care unit alarms—How many do we need? *Critical Care Medicine, 3*(2): 451–56

Shively, M., Rutledge, T., Rose, B.A., Graham, P., Long, R., Stucky, E., & Dresselhaus, T. (2011). Real-Time Assessment of Nurse Work Environment and Stress. *Journal for Healthcare Quality, 33*(1), 39–48.

*Swenson, D. (2007). Best practices in action. *Patient Safety and Quality Healthcare* http://www.psqh.com/mayjun07/pointofcare.html.

*U.S. Food and Drug Administration. (2012a). National Medical Device Postmarket Surveillance Plan. http://www.fda.gov/AboutFDA/CentersOffices/OfficeofMedicalProductsandTobacco/CDRH/CDRHReports/ucm301912.htm

*U.S. Food and Drug Administration. (2012b). MedSun: Medical Product Safety Network. http://www.fda.gov/medicaldevices/safety/medsunmedicalproductsafetynetwork/default.htm.

*U.S. Food and Drug administration. (2013). There's no guarantee of 'latex free.' http://www.fda.gov/forconsumers/consumerupdates/ucm342641.htm.

Vanderveen, T. (2005) How IV safety systems have prevented medication errors. *Journal of Infusion Nursing, 28*(Suppl.), 40–41.

*Whittington, J., Cohen, H. (2004). OSF Healthcare's journey in patient safety. *Quality Management in Health Care, 13*(1), 53–59.

*Wilson, K., Sullivan, M. (2004). Preventing medication errors with smart infusion technology. *American Journal of Health-System Pharmacy, 61* (2), 177–183.

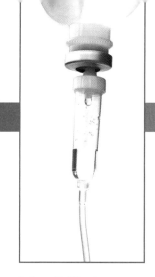

CHAPTER 13

Peripheral Venous Access

Mary E. Hagle
Martin Mikell

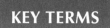

KEY TERMS	Alarm Reaction	Syncope
	Arteriospasm	Therapeutic
	Fear Cascade	Phlebotomy
	Midline Catheter	Vasovagal Reaction

INFUSION THERAPY WITH SHORT PERIPHERAL CATHETERS

Short peripherally placed catheters have long been the standard of care for time-limited infusion therapy and remain so today. The term short peripheral catheter denotes a product that is <3 inches long, usually about 1 inch in length; it is inserted into a peripheral vein, and the tip terminates in a peripheral vein. Still considered a peripheral catheter is the midline catheter; it is 3 to 8 inches in length and inserted in the upper arm or antecubital area. Short catheters are used for infusions, bolus drug administration, and phlebotomy for blood sampling. Midline catheters enable more concentrated solutions to be infused and may remain in place longer than does a short catheter.

In 2008, over 200 million short peripheral intravenous (PIV) catheters were used in the United States alone (Maki, 2008). Almost 70% of acute care inpatients receive a PIV at some point in their stay (Zingg & Pittet, 2009). Short PIV catheters encompass a variety of devices, including over-the-needle catheters (ONCs) with or without stabilizing features, winged infusion needles (butterfly needles), and blood collection needles.

Safety has become a priority in all health care settings. Considerations to promote safety with PIV catheters include minimizing blood exposure, clinician needlesticks, and leakage. Manufacturers tackle these issues through a variety of strategies, including closed systems and retractable needles. Needleless systems have been the standard of care for several years.

Devices and safety features are addressed in Chapter 12. Techniques associated with infusion therapy remain consistent regardless of the clinical settings in which care is delivered. Adherence to institutional guidelines and Standards of Practice (INS, 2011) ensures quality outcomes.

PATIENT PREPARATION FOR PERIPHERAL VENOUS ACCESS

The nurse's approach to the patient about to receive infusion therapy may have a direct bearing on that patient's response to treatment. Because an undesirable response can affect the patient's ability to accept treatment, the nurse's manner and attitude are significant factors. Although routine for the nurse, infusion therapy may be a new and frightening experience for any patient unfamiliar with the procedure and with the health care process in general.

Patient-centered care helps the nurse to focus on the patient's perspective of events. Being patient-centered means "providing care that is respectful of and responsive to individual patient preferences, needs, and values and ensuring that patient values guide all clinical decisions" (Institute of Medicine, 2001, p. 6). Components of patient-centered care include sharing with the patient relevant information and providing emotional support, such as relieving anxiety.

Prior experience with infusion therapy, good or bad, affects the patient's experience of, and agreement with, treatment. If the patient has had a positive and successful venipuncture by a clinician, he or she may feel more comfortable and relaxed. If the patient's history includes complications associated with intravenous (IV) therapy, venipuncture may be difficult. Other factors enter into the patient's perception of infusion care, including accounts in the mass media, rumors related to errors or fatalities, or simple miscommunications. By offering a careful explanation of the procedure and keeping the patient's privacy and comfort uppermost, the nurse can alleviate fear or anxiety and ensure patient compliance with the procedure and treatment.

Education is critical in allaying anxiety and preparing the patient for the procedure. Explain that an assessment is needed before a final decision on potential site and device can be made. Once a decision is made, in collaboration with the patient if possible, explain in lay terms what will happen and what the patient may feel and see. Education includes the necessity for infusion therapy, how long the catheter will remain in place, and signs and symptoms to report. Take time to explain the patient's role in the process, such as opening/closing the fist or remaining still. Repeating these instructions during the procedure keeps the patient involved and may distract him or her from the possible discomfort of the needle puncture.

Knowledge of the patient's past experiences with infusion therapy, as well as clinical condition, mental status, and other treatment modalities currently in place are important considerations in preparing the patient for venipuncture and successful infusion therapy.

Past Experience with Venipuncture and Infusion Therapy

A common reaction in health care situations is syncope. The patient may be feeling unwell, nauseous, or may have been standing and/or waiting an extended length of time. The patient may know they faint or become "light-headed" at the sight of blood. Alternatively, the patient may be experiencing emotional or physical strain. All of these situations can contribute to a **vasovagal reaction**, stimulated by the parasympathetic nervous system, part of the autonomic nervous system. The vasovagal reaction, which results in dilated blood vessels, slowed heart rate, and lowered blood pressure, manifests itself as syncope. It is important to assess the patient's current status and history so that venipuncture does not contribute to further anxiety or adverse events, such as a fall and possible injury. Precipitating and aggravating factors for vasovagal syncope are found in Table 13-1.

The critically ill patient is particularly susceptible to fears, triggering a fight or flight response, or an **alarm reaction**. This is an autonomic nervous system response, through the sympathetic nervous system, resulting in vasoconstriction, increased heart rate, increased blood pressure, and increased respiratory rate. Whether the fear is real or imagined, the patient experiences this physiologic response to a perceived threat. When there is an exaggerated reaction to fear, the **fear cascade** can result in decreased venous access and may constitute a real threat to the patient, particularly one with severe cardiac disease (Figure 13-1).

However, emotion and reason are difficult to separate, and researchers now believe that persons can regulate or adjust their own emotions to some extent (Kappas, 2011). In the concept of self-regulation, we do not live in an emotionally neutral state but seek out a desired state that is slightly positive. If past experiences with infusion therapy were unpleasant or painful or the patient anticipates this type of situation, it can trigger a negative feedback loop. This negative feedback loop can result in distress and anxiety for the patient, with the possible alarm reaction and attendant vasoconstriction, resulting in peripheral venous constriction and limited available veins for venipuncture. Repeated attempts at venipuncture can result in an experience so traumatic as to affect the further course of infusion therapy.

Several nursing interventions may reduce these experiences for the patient. The nurse needs to appear confident and reassuring. A skilled clinician will have a higher probability of initial venipuncture success with an anxious patient who has limited access and difficult veins. Helping the patient identify his or her commonly used coping strategies may also be effective. Or, the nurse can supplement these with other strategies such as distraction or emotional support. Establishing a relationship with the patient may assist the patient toward a more positive emotional state, as well as promote trust in the nurse's skill.

Clinical Condition and Mental Status

A patient's comorbidities and clinical history influence infusion therapy. A history of stroke, breast cancer, or renal dysfunction influences vein selection, as described later. If the clinician has minimal information about the patient, ask the patient if he or she has an implanted vascular device or tunneled catheter, using terms a patient would understand. A comprehensive assessment will avoid having a patient ask, "Why can't you use the port (or Hickman)

TABLE 13-1 PRECIPITATING AND AGGRAVATING FACTORS FOR VASOVAGAL SYNCOPE

Precipitated by	Aggravated by
• Sudden emotional stress (adaptogenicity)	• Fasting
• Pain or fear of anticipated harm	• Dehydration
• Sudden relief of anxiety	• Challenged physical condition
• Vascular cannulation	• Room temperature
• Arterial decannulation	• Fatigue

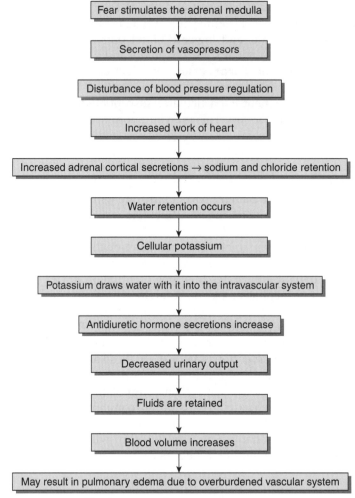

FIGURE 13-1 The fear cascade.

to draw blood?" This is an important assessment, particularly if the patient has a cancer or hematological diagnosis.

The ambulatory surgical patient has decidedly different needs than does the critically ill patient with multiple IV accesses. If the patient will be involved in self-care and self-administration of IV medications and solutions, the approach must encourage and support the patient's independence and confidence. Plans for promoting self-care and independence should begin at the time of admission to the hospital, treatment at the clinic, or with the patient's first encounter with infusion therapy.

Mental status influences the clinician's assessment. Is the patient able to provide an accurate history? Will mental status influence the patient's ability to comprehend instructions or follow directions? If a patient is confused, there may be a risk of inadvertent catheter removal. Last, is the patient able to give consent or assent to the procedure? Involving the family and/or caregiver may be key to the collection of this information.

Other Treatment Modalities

Use of multiple clinical modalities (i.e., nutritional support, antibiotics, or transfusions) has a significant effect on preparation for infusion therapy. In such cases, the clinician may consider using a multilumen catheter so that administration of subsequent medications can be timed to avoid interference with the line providing nutrition or the line providing transfusion therapy. Other concerns include non-IV therapies. For example, if the patient is also undergoing physical or occupational therapy, the nurse may find it difficult to use the dorsal aspect of the hand for an IV because such placement makes maintaining secure, dry connections and a tightly sealed dressing difficult.

CONSIDERATIONS FOR SHORT PERIPHERAL CATHETER INFUSION

There are several considerations in selecting peripheral venous access using a short catheter. Among these are patient preferences and values. Foremost is the patient's consent for treatment. Engaging the patient in the discussion, such as which type of device or which arm is more suitable for venipuncture, may promote a positive attitude and adherence to the plan. Other considerations are described below and outlined in Box 13-1.

Type of Therapy

Infusion therapy may involve isotonic solutions for hydration, solutions with high viscosity or high osmolarity, or vesicant or irritant medications, thus influencing the site for infusion and type of device selected. Additionally, the desired infusion rate needs to be considered. Larger veins have more blood flow volume, which provides rapid disbursement of fluid and rapid dilution. Thus, larger veins are recommended for infusions of

- Large quantities of solution with rapid administration
- Solutions using positive pressure
- Fluids with high viscosity, such as packed red blood cells (RBCs)
- Irritant or vesicant medications

A new peripheral venous access site is needed when vesicant medications are administered through a short catheter (INS, 2011, p. S88). Continuous infusions of vesicant medications should be administered only through a central vascular access device (CVAD), not a short peripheral catheter (INS, 2011, p. S88).

BOX 13-1 CONSIDERATIONS FOR SHORT CATHETER PIV INFUSION

- Patient preferences and values
- Type of therapy
- Duration of therapy
- Catheter gauge
- Vascular assessment

Parenteral nutrition administration is recommended through a CVAD. However, until a CVAD is placed, a short peripheral catheter or midline may be used for specific parenteral nutrition solutions. Only those solutions with a final concentration of 10% dextrose or lower, or with osmolarity not exceeding 600 mOsm, may be administered in this manner (INS, 2011, pp. S91–S92). However, peripheral administration of parenteral nutrition causes phlebitis; several strategies can minimize the inflammation and prolong the infusion until a CVAD is placed (INS, 2011, p. S92). More frequent site rotation can reduce the incidence of phlebitis; regular assessment and monitoring by the nurse will promote the most advantageous rotation for safety while reducing painful venipunctures for the patient.

If the solution's pH is <5 or >9, it must be administered through a CVAD (INS, 2011, S37). A final consideration is whether the medication is at risk for diversion. This would influence the type of device and the method of administration. All actions to prevent or reduce the risk of this scenario are necessary.

Duration of Therapy

A prolonged course of therapy requires multiple infusions and possibly multiple venipunctures, which makes preservation of the veins essential. Performing the venipuncture distally with each subsequent puncture proximal to the previous one and alternating arms contributes to venous preservation. Short peripheral catheters are usually indicated for infusion therapy of <1 week, and winged steel needles should be limited to single-dose administration or short-term therapy (INS, 2011, p. S37). Whether using and replacing a short peripheral catheter for 1 to several weeks or considering a midline, a peripherally inserted central catheter (PICC), or other CVAD, the health care team and patient need to discuss the options when infusion therapy is anticipated to be lengthy.

Patient comfort always needs to be considered, but especially when infusions are required over an extended period. For instance, performing venipunctures on veins located on the dorsal surface of the extremities provide more freedom and comfort for the patient.

Catheter Gauge

Selection of the gauge of the PIV catheter to be inserted is a nursing decision. The standard is to use the smallest gauge needed to accommodate the prescribed therapy (INS, 2011, p. S37). Short peripheral catheters come in sizes from 14- to 27-gauge. Small-gauge catheters are able to infuse solutions quite rapidly, almost 1 L/h for some sizes; for example, one 24-gauge peripheral catheter has the capacity to infuse 960 mL/h (BD Medical, 2013). Special populations, such as the elderly, neonates, and infants often require extremely small-gauge catheters. Otherwise, it is the type of therapy or procedure that drives the catheter gauge. If the catheter is to be used for a power injection, special catheters identified for this purpose are required to withstand the administration pressure. Patients having a surgical procedure may need a larger device, such as an 18 gauge; the gauge may be specified in preoperative orders. Transfusion of blood and blood products can generally be accommodated with short peripheral catheter gauges as small as 22 to 24 (INS, 2011, p. S37).

Vascular Assessment

The nurse responsible for venipuncture or team may make the vascular assessment. If findings confirm that limited vascular access precludes successful peripheral venipuncture or the treatment is long-term, consideration should be given to the use of alternative access devices, such as a midline, PICC, or other CVAD. If, after assessment of therapy type and duration, a PIV catheter is indicated, the nurse proceeds with vein selection and then the procedure for a PIV catheter insertion and infusion or locked catheter.

VEIN SELECTION

The selection of the vein may be a deciding factor in the success of the infusion and the preservation of veins for subsequent treatment (Table 13-2). The most prominent vein is not necessarily the most suitable for venipuncture. Prominence may result from a sclerosed condition, which occludes the lumen and interferes with the flow of solution, or the prominent vein may be located in an area impractical for infusion purposes. Scrutiny of the veins in both arms is desirable before a choice is made. Using the nondominant side is recommended to avoid restricting patient function. However, asking the patient which side is preferred or identifying benefits of using one side versus the other may elicit more cooperation from adult patients. Factors to be considered in selecting a vein include location and condition of the vein.

TABLE 13-	SITE SELECTION: SUPERFICIAL VEINS OF THE ARM		
Vein	**Location**	**Device**	**Considerations**
Cephalic	Radial aspect of lower arm along radial bone of the forearm	18- to 22-gauge cannula; usually ONC	Large vein, easily accessed Start distal and work upward Good for infusing blood or chemically irritating drugs
Basilic	Ulnar aspect of lower arm along the ulnar bone	18- to 22-gauge ONC	Difficult to access Large vein, easily palpated Stabilize during venipuncture
Accessory cephalic	Branches off cephalic vein along radial bone	18- to 22-gauge ONC	Medium–large vein, easily stabilized Valves at cephalic junction may inhibit catheterization Short length may require short (1-inch) catheter
Upper cephalic	Radial aspect of upper arm above elbow	16- to 20-gauge ONC	Difficult to visualize Good site for confused patients
Median antebrachial	Extends up front of forearm from median antecubital	18- to 22-gauge ONC	Nerve endings preclude cannulation Infiltration may occur
Median basilic	Ulnar aspect of forearm	18- to 22-gauge ONC	Appropriate site
Median cubital	Radial aspect of forearm	18- to 22-gauge ONC	Appropriate site
Veins in area of antecubital fossa	Bend of elbow	Any size; may be used for midline or PICC insertion	Best for emergency interventions

ONC, over-the-needle catheter.

Location

Most superficial veins are accessible for venipuncture (Figure 13-2), but some of these veins, because of their location, are not practical. For example, the antecubital veins are a poor choice for routine therapy because they are located over an area of joint flexion where any motion could dislodge the IV catheter and cause infiltration or result in mechanical phlebitis. If these large veins are impaired or damaged, phlebothrombosis may occur, which can limit access to the many available hand veins. The antecubital veins offer excellent sources for withdrawing blood and may be used many times without damage to the vein, provided good technique is used. However, one infusion of long duration may traumatize the vein, limiting the availability of vessels that most readily provide ample quantities of blood when needed.

Because of the proximity of the arteries to the veins in the antecubital fossa, special care must be taken to prevent intra-arterial injection when medications are introduced. Aberrant arteries in the antecubital area are present in 1 of 10 people. When a patient complains of

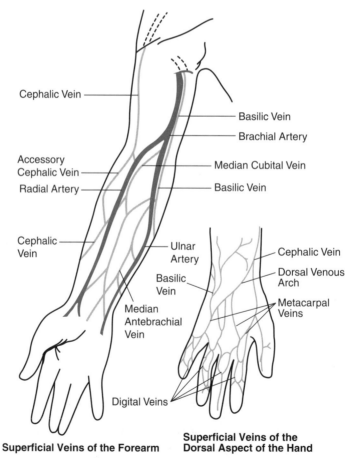

Superficial Veins of the Forearm

Superficial Veins of the Dorsal Aspect of the Hand

FIGURE 13-2 IV placement chart. (Courtesy of Becton Dickinson Vascular Access.)

severe pain in the hand or arm on infusion, an arteriospasm caused by an intra-arterial injection is to be suspected, and the infusion must be stopped immediately.

The ventral surface of the wrist should be avoided due to the pain on insertion and risk of damage to the radial nerve (INS, 2011, p. S41). Other potential venous sites to avoid would be areas of pain on palpation; compromised veins such as those that are bruised, infiltrated, inflamed, corded, or sclerosed; or areas of planned procedures (INS, 2011, p. S41).

Several factors influence which arm should be avoided, if possible. These include an upper extremity on the side with an axillary node dissection, radiation therapy, or lymphedema; these are conditions where circulation may be impaired, affecting the flow of the infusion and possibly increasing or causing edema. If a stroke has affected the functioning of an upper extremity, that side should be avoided. However, choices for venous access may be limited. In this case, a "collaborative discussion" between the patient and the physician/ licensed independent practitioner (LIP) and/or team is needed to review the risks and benefits of using a vein in the affected extremity (INS, 2011, p. S41).

For patients with renal dysfunction, several factors are identified. Avoid the use of an extremity with an arteriovenous fistula or graft inserted for dialysis. Additionally, for patients with chronic kidney disease stage 4 or 5, "avoid forearm and upper arm veins 'suitable for placement of vascular access'" (INS, 2011, p. S41). This protects vascular access for future use in the case of kidney failure and the need for hemodialysis or renal replacement therapy.

Surgery often dictates which extremity can be used and is often identified in the preoperative orders. When the patient is turned to the side-lying position during an operation, the upper arm is used for the infusion; increased venous pressure in the lower arm may interfere with free flow of the solution.

The use of veins in the lower extremities of adults is discouraged because of the risk of thrombophlebitis, tissue damage, and ulceration (CDC, 2011; INS, 2011, p. S41). There is also the danger of pulmonary embolism caused by a thrombus extending into the deep veins. Complications may arise from the stagnant blood in varicosities, which makes them susceptible to trauma. If a catheter is inserted into a lower extremity vein, replace the catheter into an upper extremity as soon as possible (CDC, 2011).

Condition of the Vein

Frequently, the dorsal metacarpal veins provide points of entry that may be used first to preserve the proximal veins for further therapy. The use of these veins depends on their condition. In some elderly patients, the dorsal metacarpal veins may be a poor choice; blood extravasation occurs more readily in small, thin veins, and it may be difficult to secure the catheter adequately because of thin skin and lack of supportive tissue. At times, these veins do not dilate sufficiently to allow for successful venipuncture; when hypovolemia occurs, the peripheral veins collapse more quickly than do larger, more proximal ones.

Palpation of the vein is an important step in determining the condition of the vein and in differentiating it from a pulsating artery. A thrombosed vein may be detected by its lack of resilience; its hard, cordlike feeling; and by the ease with which it rolls. Use of such traumatized veins results in repeated attempts at venipuncture, pain, and undue stress. Often, large veins may be detected by palpation and offer advantages over the smaller but more readily discernible veins. Because of the small blood volume, the more superficial veins may not be easily palpated and may not make a satisfactory choice for venipuncture.

Continual use by the nurse of the same fingers for palpation increases their sensitivity. The thumb should never be used because it is not as sensitive as the fingers; also, a pulse may be detected in the nurse's thumb, and this may be confused with an aberrant artery.

Although not apparent, edema may conceal an available vein; application of finger pressure for a few seconds may help to disperse the fluid and define the vein.

Large veins are used when hypertonic solutions or solutions containing irritating drugs are to be infused. Large vessels provide better hemodilution of the drug or solution, thereby minimizing the potential for developing phlebitis. Such solutions traumatize small veins; the supply of blood in these veins is not sufficient to dilute the infused fluid.

INITIATING PERIPHERAL VENOUS ACCESS WITH SHORT CATHETERS

Hand hygiene cannot be overemphasized. It "should be performed before and after palpating catheter insertion sites as well as before and after inserting, replacing, accessing, repairing, or dressing an intravascular catheter. Palpation of the insertion site should not be performed after the application of antiseptic, unless aseptic technique is maintained" (CDC, 2011, p. S3).

Environment

For patient privacy, close the door or the bedside curtains if the patient has a roommate. Ask the patient if they wish visitors to leave the room during the procedure. Clean an area on which to place the equipment and support the patient's arm. The patient should be in a comfortable position with the arm on a flat surface. If the patient is uncooperative or disoriented, determine the best method and/or strategy to prevent the patient from moving the arm during catheter insertion. A restraint may escalate the situation. Solicit the assistance of a family member or another caregiver to soothe or distract the patient and/or secure the arm. Last, the type of intervention is dependent on the urgency of the vascular access.

Proper lighting is very important and should not be overlooked. A few extra seconds spent in obtaining adequate light may actually save time and free the patient from unnecessary venipunctures. The ideal light is either ample daylight or a spotlight that does not shine directly on the vein but leaves enough shadow for clearly defining the vessel.

Solution, Administration Set, IV Pole, and Venipuncture Equipment

Venipuncture and initiation of an IV infusion or locked PIV are carried out upon the order of a physician/LIP. The solution, volume, any additives, rate, duration, and route (e.g., PIV, "Start IV") are specified in the order. Verify with the order that the solution obtained is that which is ordered.

Obtain all equipment and solution. A PIV kit is recommended to ensure that all supplies are easily available and to reduce time away from the patient by the nurse (Figure 13-3). Careful inspection is necessary to ensure that the fluid is clear and free of particulates and the container intact—with no cracks in the glass bottle or holes in the plastic bag. The label must be checked to verify that the correct solution is being used and that the container is not outdated. The nurse also needs to check the time and the date the container was opened. After 24 hours, the fluid is outdated and should not be used; expiration dates are specified in institutional policy.

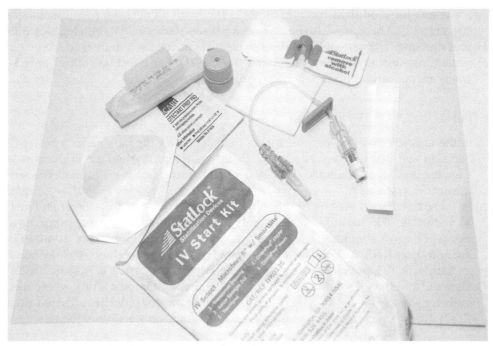

FIGURE 13-3 Peripheral intravenous catheter kit.

Open the IV administration set, close the roller clamp, remove the cap to the tubing insertion spike, and insert the spike into the container with a thrust, not a twisting motion. Hang the solution container on the pole. Squeeze the drip chamber so that it fills almost half full. Prime the tubing by slowly opening the roller clamp to fill the tubing fully. Close roller clamp. If extension tubing is needed, use sterile technique to attach it, and prime it as well. The fluid container is suspended approximately 3 feet above the injection site. The pressure from this height is adequate to ensure a maximum flow rate. The greater the height of the container, the greater the force with which the fluid flows into the vein should the flow-control clamp release. Many institutions have policies on which infusions require electronic control devices or pumps. Verify whether the ordered infusion requires a pump. Follow manufacturer's directions for priming the pump with device-specific tubing. Ensure that there is no air or air bubbles in the tubing; firm tapping will remove any air bubbles. Although air embolism is rare, air bubbles concern the nurse and alarm the patient (Cook, 2013; Wilkins & Unverdorben, 2012).

> ## PATIENT SAFETY
>
> To prevent air embolism, expel all air from IV tubing or pump cartridges before connecting to the patient's catheter. "Do not leave tubing attached to fluid but unprimed at the bedside if it is intended to be connected" (p. 32).
>
> Cook, L. S. (2013). Infusion-related air embolism. *Journal of Infusion Nursing*, 36, 26–36.

Many units or areas have an infusion tray with all necessary equipment and supplies to start a PIV. There may also be prepackaged sets with the PIV catheter, cleansing solution, and dressing. The patient's blood pressure cuff may be used to distend the vein or a single-patient use tourniquet may be applied (INS, 2011). For infection control purposes, tourniquets are not carried from patient to patient.

Vascular Access Site Preparation

If the area selected for venipuncture is hairy, clipping the hair permits better cleansing of the skin and makes removal of the catheter less painful when the infusion is terminated. Shaving is not recommended (INS, 2011, p. S44). If the area is visibly soiled, soap and water cleansing is necessary.

The designated venous site should be scrubbed with an antiseptic that remains in contact with the skin for at least 30 seconds before venipuncture. An appropriate single-dose antiseptic agent should be used. Site preparation with chlorhexidine solution is preferred for antisepsis (INS, 2011); other solutions that may be used include 70% alcohol, 2% tincture of iodine, or 10% povidone–iodine (CDC, 2011). It is important to note that a 2% chlorhexidine in 70% ethanol solution was used for site preparation in a study where the peripheral catheter was replaced only when signs and symptoms of phlebitis occurred (Rickard et al., 2012). Avoid aqueous benzalkonium-like compounds or hexachlorophene.

PATIENT SAFETY

Allow antiseptic agent to air dry. If using povidone–iodine as the primary antiseptic agent, do not apply alcohol, as it will negate povidone–iodine's antimicrobial effect. If using alcohol as a single agent, apply for a minimum of 30 seconds. If using tincture of iodine, allow it to dry, then remove with alcohol, and allow it to dry.

Local Anesthetic Considerations

It is important for the nurse to consider local anesthesia based on the patient's past experiences or current state. It is advised for all painful IV procedures in children and some adults (INS, 2011, p. S43). Using the least invasive method of local anesthesia will reduce the risk of infection.

A topical transdermal medication, such as EMLA™ (eutectic mixture of local anesthetics), is noninvasive. It is a cream mixture of two local anesthetics (lidocaine 2.5% and prilocaine 2.5%) and applied under an occlusive dressing for a specified time, from 30, 60, to 120 minutes (Table 13-3). The release of lidocaine and prilocaine into the epidermal and dermal layers of the skin provides anesthesia. The two agents stabilize neuronal membranes by inhibiting the conduction of impulses (Astra Zeneca). Use of this product is contraindicated in patients with a known history of sensitivity to local anesthetics of the amide type.

Intradermal injection of 1% buffered lidocaine is another method of local anesthesia before venipuncture. This is done with 0.1 to 0.2 mL of 1% buffered lidocaine and a tuberculin syringe. Lidocaine may, however, expose the patient to allergic reaction, anaphylaxis, inadvertent injection of the drug into the vascular system, or obliteration of the vein.

EVIDENCE FOR PRACTICE

Based on two robust studies, if the clinician wished to use an intradermal injection to reduce the pain of PIV insertion, the recommendation would be to use 1% buffered lidocaine. These studies are outlined in a commonly used method to summarize studies, an evidence table (Table 13-4).

Deguzman, Z. C., O'Mara, S. K., Sulo, S., Haines, T., Blackburn, L., & Corazza, J. (2012). Bacteriostatic normal saline compared with buffered 1% lidocaine when injected intradermally as a local anesthetic to reduce pain during intravenous catheter insertion. *Journal of Perianesthesia Nursing, 27*, 399–407.

Ganter-Ritz, V., Speroni, K. G., & Atherton, M. (2012). A randomized double-blind study comparing intradermal anesthetic tolerability, efficacy, and cost-effectiveness of lidocaine, buffered lidocaine, and bacteriostatic normal saline for peripheral intravenous insertion. *Journal of Infusion Nursing, 35*, 93–99.

Venous Distention

Special care must be taken to distend the vein adequately. To achieve this, a soft, preferably latex-free, tourniquet is applied with enough pressure to impede venous flow while maintaining arterial flow. If the radial pulse cannot be felt, the tourniquet is too tight. To fill the veins to capacity, apply pressure until radial pulsation ceases and then release pressure until pulsation begins. A blood pressure cuff may be used; inflate the cuff and then release it until the pressure drops to just below the diastolic pressure.

The tourniquet is applied to the midforearm if the selected vein is in the dorsum of the hand. If the selected vein is in the forearm, the tourniquet is applied to the upper arm.

TABLE 13-3	PROCEDURE FOR APPLYING EMLA CREAM

Equipment

Skin cleanser

Wipes or sponges

EMLA cream

Occlusive dressing

Action	Rationale
1. Cleanse skin.	
2. Use only over intact skin.	Prevents systemic absorption
3. Apply prescribed amount of EMLA cream thickly at intended site.	Ensures sufficient dermal analgesia
4. Place an occlusive dressing over the EMLA cream and smooth edges of the dressing. Keep dressing in place for 60 min for maximum effectiveness or until it is time for venipuncture, but not longer than 4 h.	Prevents spread of cream to unintended areas Prevents increased systemic absorption
5. Record application time.	Ensures appropriate absorption time and documentation of procedure

TABLE 13-4	EVIDENCE TABLE OF STUDIES COMPARING EFFECTIVENESS OF INTRADERMAL INJECTION SOLUTIONS TO REDUCE PAIN OF PIV CATHETER INSERTION				
Citation/ Country	Type of Evidence or Study Design	Research Question or Purpose	Sample/Setting *Did sample have adequate power?*	Intervention	Results or Findings
Deguzman et al. (2012) USA	Prospective, randomized, double-blind design	"…Determine whether there was a significant difference in patients' intradermal and IV pain levels when comparing the numbing effect of intradermally injected bacteriostatic normal saline with buffered 1% lidocaine before IV catheter insertion" (p. 400).	376 patients were included in the study; they were having same-day surgery, aged 18 y and older, able to communicate in English and rate and express pain, and had had no pain medication in the previous 4 h. Exclusions were known allergies to planned intervention or current condition/ history that may affect ability to provide pain ratings; an unsuccessful first IV attempt; or known needle phobia, anxiety, or panic attacks. Midwestern 638-bed community teaching hospital setting. Based on pilot data "…a minimum sample size of 300 was estimated to provide 80% statistical power to detect a 0.5 (± 1.5 standard deviation) difference" in pain ratings (p. 402).	Patients were randomized to one of two groups: Intradermal bacteriostatic normal saline with a benzyl alcohol preservative (184 subjects) or a control group of intradermal 1% buffered lidocaine (192 subjects). Very specific procedures were reported; a 0–10 numeric pain rating scale was used. Five study nurses were experienced in PIV insertion in study setting and conducted all study procedures.	Results demonstrated that patients who received the buffered lidocaine provided significantly lower pain ratings ($p =$ 0.025) during PIV insertion while intradermal pain was not different between the two groups. Average pain rating (standard deviation) during PIV insertion for each type of solution: • 1% buffered lidocaine: 1.19 (1.59) Bacteriostatic normal saline: 1.72 (1.58)

TABLE 13-4	**EVIDENCE TABLE OF STUDIES COMPARING EFFECTIVENESS OF INTRADERMAL INJECTION SOLUTIONS TO REDUCE PAIN OF PIV CATHETER INSERTION** *(Continued)*				
Citation/ Country	**Type of Evidence or Study Design**	**Research Question or Purpose**	**Sample/Setting** *Did sample have adequate power?*	**Intervention**	**Results or Findings**
Ganter-Ritz, Speroni, and Atherton (2012) USA	Prospective, randomized, double-blind, parallel design	"…Determine the tolerability, efficacy, and cost-effectiveness of three intradermal anesthetics for IV site preparation" (p. 94).	256 subjects were included in the study; preparing to have same-day surgery, age 18 y or older, visible or palpable veins in the hand or arm, consented to study; exclusions were inability to communicate in English, known allergies to planned intervention, or current condition/ history that may affect ability to provide pain ratings. Rural community hospital setting. Sample size was estimated using 0.95 level of confidence and 0.80 power for 252 completed subjects.	Patients were randomized to one of three groups: intradermal 1% lidocaine (84 subjects), intradermal 1% buffered lidocaine (85 subjects), or intradermal bacteriostatic normal saline with a benzyl alcohol preservative (83 subjects) prior to PIV catheter insertion. Very specific procedures were reported; a 0–10 numeric pain scale was used. Three IV nurse investigators conducted all study procedures.	Results demonstrated that both the lidocaine and buffered lidocaine provided significantly lower pain ratings ($p < 0.01$) during PIV insertion, although the discomfort (or tolerability) from the intradermal injection was lowest with the 1% buffered lidocaine ($p < 0.01$). Average pain rating (standard deviation) during PIV insertion for each type of solution: • 1% lidocaine: 0.8 (1.0) • 1% buffered lidocaine: 0.8 (1.1) • Bacteriostatic normal saline: 1.4 (2.1)

Quality of the body of evidence: II (Infusion Nurses Society. (2011). Infusion nursing: Standards of practice-strength of the body of evidence. *Journal of Infusion Nursing, 34*(Suppl.), S5.)

Very little pressure is applied when performing venipuncture on patients with sclerosed veins. If the pressure is too great or the tourniquet is left on for an extended time, the vein becomes hard and tortuous, causing added difficulty when the catheter is introduced. For some sclerosed veins, a tourniquet is unnecessary and only makes the phlebotomy more difficult.

If the pressure exerted by the tourniquet does not fill the veins sufficiently, the patient may be asked to open and close the fist. This action of the muscles forces the blood into the veins, causing them to distend considerably more. A light tapping usually fills the vein. It may be helpful, before applying the tourniquet, to lower the extremity below the heart level to increase the blood supply to the veins. On occasions when these methods are inadequate to fill the vein sufficiently, application of heat helps. To be effective, the heat must be applied to the entire extremity for 7 to 10 minutes and must be retained until the venipuncture is performed.

EVIDENCE FOR PRACTICE

Dry heat using warmed towels, wrapped around the entire arm for 7 minutes, was more effective than moist heat in decreasing the likelihood of multiple IV attempts and procedure time. Outpatient oncology patients found the procedure comfortable.

Fink, R. M., Hjort, E., Wenger, B., Cook, P.F., Cunningham, M., Orf, A., et al. (2009). The impact of dry versus moist heat on peripheral IV catheter insertion in a hematology-oncology outpatient population. *Oncology Nursing Forum, 36*(4), E198–E204.

Considerations for Venipuncture Procedure: Insertion

SITE ANTISEPSIS

Hand hygiene is imperative at all steps in the process. If a topical anesthetic was used, the injection site should be cleansed with the approved antiseptic and allowed to dry. Once the vascular site is antiseptically cleansed, the area for insertion may only be touched with a sterile, gloved finger or a gloved finger that has also been antiseptically cleansed. For short peripheral venipuncture, the clinician may use clean gloves if the cleansed insertion site is not touched (CDC, 2011).

VEIN VISUALIZATION

The vein is distended appropriately so that excessive pressure does not build up in the vein. If the vein has sustained a through puncture (evidenced by a developing hematoma) and the venipuncture is unsuccessful, the catheter should be removed immediately and pressure applied to the site. Consider the other extremity. Do not reapply a tourniquet to the extremity immediately after a venipuncture; a hematoma will occur, limiting veins and providing an excellent culture medium for bacteria.

An ongoing challenge, particularly for the less experienced nurse, is identifying available veins for venipuncture. Technologies are assisting with this task by providing non-invasive, direct, real-time visualization of vascular structures. Ultrasound imagery is available for identifying peripheral veins not visible on the surface. Commonly used for PICC insertion, it is also available for short peripheral catheter insertion, especially with difficult access. A narrative literature review summarizes the difficulties and recommends solutions for vascular access in individuals who are obese (Houston, 2013). For example, wiping a light-skinned arm with an alcohol swab or a dark-skinned arm with a Betadine swab to reflect light off a vein and provide shadowing may be helpful. Supporting evidence was reviewed and identified that ultrasound guidance is effective for successful PIV access in this population (Houston, 2013). Two researchers successfully implemented ultrasound-guided PIV catheter insertion for difficult to access sites with medical–surgical nurses; their findings demonstrated 71% success in placing difficult to access PIV catheters on the first attempt (Maiocco & Coole, 2012).

A more intuitive, and newer, technology is the near-infrared light for viewing veins. The device projects an image of the peripheral vascular system onto the skin (Figure 13-4). Much of the research around this device focused on usage with children, but it is applicable to adults with veins difficult to visualize, since the depth of visualization is up to 10 mm. Based on the evidence, for experienced clinicians, this technology was more effective in children with difficult to visualize veins (Hess, 2010; Kim et al., 2012; Perry et al., 2011).

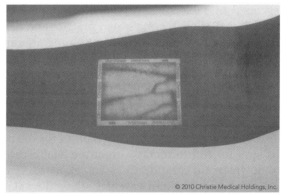

A

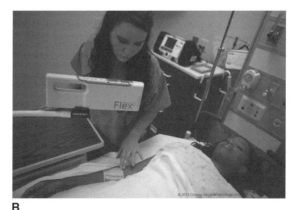

B

FIGURE 13-4 Near-infrared light imaging of peripheral vascular system for short peripheral catheter insertion. (Courtesy of Christie Holdings, Inc.)

INSERTION TECHNIQUES AND ISSUES

Variations in insertion techniques are common and depend on the clinician, the patient, the situation or context, and possibly the devices available. For example, three different short peripheral devices, all with safety features, could be used in the following situations with the nurse's clinical judgment and expertise considered:

- Single medication administration over a short period of time: a winged steel needle (if the medication is not a vesicant)
- Phlebotomy for blood sampling requiring several tubes: a winged blood collection set
- Infusion therapy for hydration, <6 days, in an older, frail person: 1-inch ONC with 24-gauge
- IV antibiotics for <6 days in an individual who is morbidly obese (body mass index more than 40): 2-inch ONC with 20-gauge

There are also variations in the method of device insertion. These direct and indirect methods are described in Table 13-5. A critical component to successful venipuncture is using the method that is feasible for one's own practice and developing expertise. Skill may be acquired initially through simulation with a training arm and then with patients having clearly visible veins and adequate subcutaneous tissue for anchoring. Some patient characteristics that can influence successful PIV catheter placement are obesity, chronic illness, sickle cell anemia, and IV drug use history (Brannam, Blaivas, Lyon, & Flake, 2004). Knowing some of the characteristics of difficult to place PIV catheters may assist in assignments of novice nurses, because solid competence is developed through repetition of successful venipuncture. Multiple unsuccessful attempts are painful for the patient, delay treatment, limit available venous sites for future therapy, frustrate health care professionals, and increase the likelihood of downstream complications and expense. "Patients with difficult vascular access require a careful assessment of vascular access device needs and collaboration with the health care team to discuss appropriate options" (INS, 2011, p. S44).

The number of venipuncture attempts can be viewed in two ways: attempts per nurse or clinician and attempts per patient. The standard of practice for attempts per nurse states, "No more than 2 attempts at vascular access placement should be made by any 1 nurse…" (INS, 2011, p. S44). This is commonly accepted practice as seen in many organizational policies and procedures.

TABLE 13-5 METHODS FOR VENIPUNCTURE

Direct (One Step)	Indirect (Two Complete Motions)
The nurse thrusts the catheter through the skin and into the vein with quick motion.	The nurse inserts the catheter through the skin below the point where vein is visible but above the vein.
The catheter enters directly over the vein.	This approach depresses the vein, obscuring its position.
Direct technique is not suitable for small veins because of potential for hematoma formation.	The catheter is adjacent to the vein but has not penetrated the vessel wall. Gently locate the vein, decrease catheter angle, and enter the vessel.

However, minimal attention is given to the number of attempts that the patient experiences in an episode of care requiring venous access for infusion therapy. Toward this end, a literature search using PubMed and CINAHL databases with subject headings and keywords: "Peripheral Catheterization," "Clinical Competence," and IV insertion attempts, was completed. From this search, 35 titles and abstracts were reviewed and 7 papers were retrieved and appraised. Reference lists were reviewed, and relevant articles were retrieved. Even though not all articles were reports of research findings, some articles were kept as contributing to the evidence. A total of 10 articles were reviewed, and 5 articles were summarized in an evidence table (Table 13-6). The evidence includes two articles of pediatric patients only, one article of adults only, and one article including both populations. The fifth article is a narrative literature review and addresses both pediatric and adult populations.

Based on the evidence, the success rate of PIV placement for children with one or two attempts ranges from 67% to 73% (Larsen et al., 2010; Lininger, 2003). For adults or adults and children, successful PIV placement is achieved with the first attempt between 60.8% and 64.6% of the time (Jacobson & Winslow, 2005; Witting, 2012); by the second attempt, there is an 86.4% success rate (Jacobson & Winslow, 2005). Thus, for a majority of the patients, often with difficult to access veins, successful PIV catheter insertion is possible on the first or second attempt. However, when is another resource called in?

From the summarized evidence, additional attempts by the same or different clinicians range from three to six attempts; in children, this is often higher. Mbamalu and Banerjee (1999) proposed an algorithm for difficult peripheral venous access. Based on this algorithm, it suggests that a maximum number of attempts per patient should be four, and then alternative sites or adjunctive measures should be considered. While emergent situations, or nursing staff experience, may result in one clinician making two or more PIV insertion attempts, the body of evidence is growing to support a practice that a patient receives no more than four PIV insertion attempts. One medical center has approved the nursing practice of limiting clinician insertion attempts to four per patient, "…And no more than four (4) peripheral IV insertion attempts for each patient by nurses or other staff" (Hagle, M., 2013, April, *personal communication*). Compliance with accepted Standards of Practice (INS, 2011) should be a guiding influence.

Considerations for Short Peripheral IV Catheter Maintenance

Catheter Patency

Maintaining **catheter patency** is critical to successful infusion therapy outcomes. Many PIV catheters remain in place far beyond the CDC (2011) recommendation of routine replacement every 4 days. Patency can be affected by several factors, but one under the clinician's control is the method of flushing and locking the PIV catheter. During flushing procedures, at the time of syringe disconnection from the injection cap/port, blood can be drawn back into the catheter lumen. This can lead to catheter occlusion and disruption of therapy. Clinicians have used a variety of techniques to prevent the reflux of blood back into the tip of the PIV catheter (Table 13-7). With the advent of needleless access systems to protect the health care worker from accidental needlesticks, innovations have occurred to also prevent blood reflux. Over the years, these needleless, Luer access products may have included internal mechanical valves that provide positive displacement, negative displacement, or neutral displacement of the internal fluid to prevent blood reflux (Hadaway & Richardson, 2010).

TABLE 13-6	EVIDENCE TABLE OF PIV CATHETER ATTEMPTS PER PATIENT			
Citation/ Country	Type of Evidence or Study Design	Research Question or Purpose	Sample/Setting/Method	Results or Findings
Jacobson and Winslow (2005) United States	Descriptive study	"…Determine what variables contribute to the difficulty of inserting IV catheters in hospitalized patients, what variables are associated with IV insertion failure and success, and what special techniques nurses use to facilitate IV catheter insertion" (p. 346).	34 nurses performed 339 PIV insertions (each nurse reported 10 insertions) Included inpatients/ outpatients, age range from 4–95 y Nurses: Female: 97% Certification: 35% Average age: 38 y (standard deviation, 9 y) Average experience as RN: 12 y (standard deviation, 11 y) Large urban hospital	64.6% (219/339) of PIV insertions were successful on the first attempt. 86.4% PIV insertions were successful on the second attempt. 13 insertions represented 3–6 previous attempts. "In two cases, the same nurse made three attempts in the same patient" (p. 348). Nurse-related variables associated with successful PIV insertion: age, years of experience as RN, years of experience with IV insertion, number of IV insertions per week, specialty certification, and self-rated skill. Methods used for vein distention: mechanical stimulation, vein stabilization, and good positioning of nurse and patient.
Larsen et al. (2010) United States	Prospective, observational study	"…Describe, with improved accuracy, the number of attempts and the amount of time required by general pediatric nurses to achieve successful PIV catheter placement in hospitalized children" (p. 227).	Convenience sample of *pediatric* inpatients 1,135 PIV attempts in 592 encounters Average age: 5.25 y Data obtained via independent direct observation Two pediatric hospitals: tertiary care teaching centers	73% of pediatric PIV insertions were successful after one or two venipuncture attempts Primary nurse may attempt two to three venipunctures; another nurse may then make an attempt. No IV teams

| TABLE 13-6 | | EVIDENCE TABLE OF PIV CATHETER ATTEMPTS PER PATIENT   *(Continued)* | | |

Citation/ Country	Type of Evidence or Study Design	Research Question or Purpose	Sample/Setting/Method	Results or Findings
Lininger (2003) United States	Prospective study; nonrandomized sample	Determine number of PIV attempts and success rates in a pediatric population	249 PIV placements *Pediatric* inpatients: ages ranged from 3 d–20 y 85% of PIVs placed by medical/surgical RN staff RN experience remained stable during three study periods at 5 y Data were collected at three time periods over 20 mo, self-reported data collection tool Children's hospital, inpatient medical/surgical RN staff and patients (self-reported data)	53% success on first attempt, 67% with 2 attempts, 91% with 4 attempts
Mbamalu and Banerjee (1999) England	Narrative literature review	Review of methods for obtaining PIVs under difficult situations	35 articles were reviewed	Proposed a sequential algorithmic approach for children and adults: for elective peripheral venous access, authors identified two attempts per arm. If unsuccessful, other steps are identified, such as alternative sites or adjunctive measures.
Witting (2012) United States	Prospective cohort study	"…Estimate the incidence of IV access difficulty in an urban tertiary care emergency setting" (p. 483).	107 patients with IV line placed Adult patients over 17 y of age likely to need a PIV; excluded if not able to give consent or PIV in place Setting was an ED, urban tertiary care university hospital with an annual census of 47,000	60.8% insertions successful on the first attempt Three or more punctures needed in 24 individuals (22%)

Quality of the body of evidence: IV (Infusion Nurses Society. (2011). Infusion nursing: Standards of practice-strength of the body of evidence. *Journal of Infusion Nursing, 34*(Suppl.), S5.) Other sources: Jacobson, A. F., & Winslow, E. H. (2005). Variables influencing intravenous catheter insertion difficulty and failure: An analysis of 339 intravenous catheter insertions. *Heart & Lung, 34*(5), 345–359; Larsen, P., Eldridge, D., Brinkley, J., Newton, D., Goff, D., Hartzog, T., et al. (2010). Pediatric peripheral intravenous access: Does nursing experience and competence really make a difference? *Journal of Infusion Nursing, 33*(4), 226–235; Lininger, R. A. (2003). Pediatric peripheral IV insertion success rates. *Pediatric Nursing, 29*(5), 351–354; Mbamalu, D., & Banerjee, A. (1999). Methods of obtaining peripheral venous access in difficult situations. *Postgraduate Medical Journal, 75*, 459–462; Witting, M. (2012). IV access difficulty: Incidence and delays in an urban emergency department. *Journal of Emergency Medicine, 42*(4), 483–487.

TABLE 13-7	CLINICIAN ACTIONS FOR POSITIVE DISPLACEMENT TO PREVENT BLOOD REFLUX
Practice	**Comments**
Applying pressure to the syringe plunger on needle withdrawal from the injection cap/port	This technique was very effective when using small-bore needles to flush through a rubber injection cap, not as effective with large-bore plastic cannula, and not effective with Luer-activated valves.
Withdrawing flush syringe/needle from the injection cap/port during the infusion of the last 1 mL of flush solution	Not effective with needleless Luer-activated valves.
Engaging the clamp on the catheter or extension set prior to syringe disconnection from the injection cap/port	This requires the presence of an extension set and clamp, and it is effective only as long as the clamp is left engaged.

And each of these devices requires different actions related to withdrawing the syringe or clamping the tubing. It is important to know what device your agency stocks and to be aware that clinician actions are clearly delineated in the procedures and accessible for ready reference. The earlier discussion of multiple venous access attempts and limiting vascular access is compounded when incorrect actions are taken that occlude the catheter.

Catheter patency is also affected by appropriate flushing and locking. The PIV catheter must be flushed prior to and after each medication administration or infusion (INS, 2011, p. S59). The PIV catheter is locked with preservative-free 0.9% sodium chloride after the completion of medication administration without an on-going infusion (INS, 2011, p. S60). If the PIV catheter is locked, it is flushed with 2 mL of preservative-free 0.9% sodium chloride at a frequency of every 12 hours (INS, 2008) or every 8, 12, or 24 hours (Camp-Sorrell, 2011), depending on institutional policy..

Catheter Stabilization, Dressing, and Anchoring

Once the catheter is in place, the nurse needs to make sure it stays securely in place, safe from dislodgment, and protected from the environment. This involves both a stabilization or securement device and a dressing (Hadaway, 2010). The stabilization device preserves the integrity of the device and minimizes catheter movement, which can cause mechanical phlebitis. With moderate support from the body of evidence (INS, 2011, p. S46) and a category II recommendation for practice (CDC, 2011), a stabilization device is recommended for use with vascular access devices. Stabilization devices may be separate from the vascular access catheter and attached once the catheter has been inserted (Figure 13-5) or may be integral with the PIV catheter (Figure 13-6).

The site dressing prevents infection. For a PIV catheter, a sterile, semipermeable, transparent dressing (e.g., Tegaderm™) is recommended since this dressing may remain in place up to 7 days. A gauze dressing may be needed if the patient is diaphoretic or unable to tolerate the semipermeable dressing. In general, a PIV catheter dressing does not need to be changed until the system is replaced or removed every 4 days (96 hours), unless the dressing is damp, loosened, or visibly soiled. The PIV catheter should be stabilized and covered with a dressing that does not interfere with assessment and monitoring or impede circulation (INS, 2011, p. S46) (Figure 13-7).

If a stabilization device is not available, the catheter needs to be secured; a dressing does not provide this type of stabilization (Hadaway, 2010). A traditional taping technique may

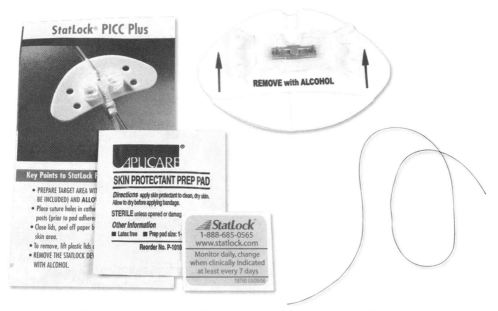

FIGURE 13-5 Vascular catheter stabilization device. (Courtesy of C.R. Bard.)

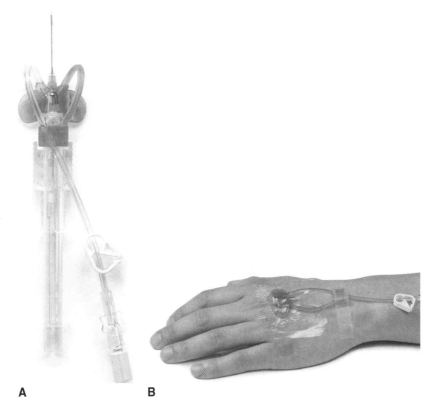

A   **B**

FIGURE 13-6 Vascular catheter stabilization device integral with catheter. (Courtesy of Tangent Medical.)

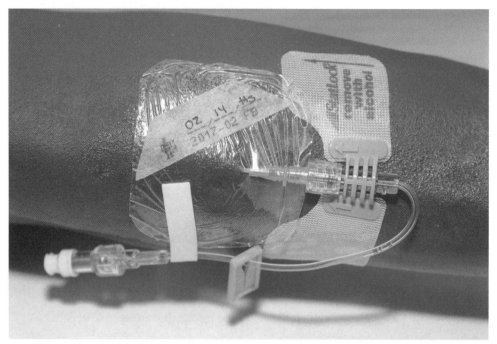

FIGURE 13-7 Short PIV catheter inserted into forearm with stabilization and sterile, semi-permeable, transparent dressing. (Courtesy of T.T. Smith, MS, RN-BC and A. Urrea; Clement J. Zablocki VA Medical Center.)

be used as illustrated in Figure 13-8. This method secures the catheter firmly and prevents any sideways movement. Tape should not be placed directly over the injection site. A dressing is put over the catheter insertion site.

After the catheter is secured by the dressing, the IV tubing is looped to relieve tension and anchored with tape independent of the catheter tape. This prevents dislodging the catheter by an accidental pull on the tubing.

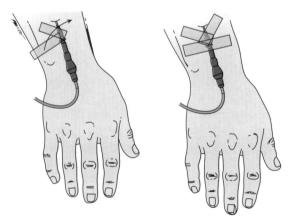

FIGURE 13-8 Chevron taping technique.

An arm board may be helpful for immobilizing the area, such as the hand, wrist, or elbow, when undue motion may cause catheter occlusion or movement. To preserve maximal function, the hand should rest in a functional position on the arm board. If an arm board or similar device is used, circulation must be maintained, and the insertion site remains visible; the arm board should be removed regularly, circulation assessed, and range of motion provided (INS, 2011, p. S48).

DOCUMENTATION

The dressing for a PIV catheter should be labeled with the insertion date and clinician's initials who initiated the procedure. The tradition of putting the time of insertion on the label is less critical with PIV catheters remaining in place every 4 days or until clinical signs and symptoms are evident. Additionally, unless there is another reason to wake the patient, a PIV catheter can be changed for routine replacement when the patient is normally awake.

In the patient's medical record, more information needs to be documented. This includes the catheter type, gauge, and length inserted; location; the date and time of insertion; number of attempts; any anesthetic used; patient response; and appropriate clinician signature per organizational policy for paper or electronic medical records (INS, 2011).

A step-by-step approach to basic venipuncture is provided in Table 13-8.

TABLE 13-8   A STEP-BY-STEP APPROACH TO BASIC VENIPUNCTURE

1. Obtain equipment and solution/medication. Identify the patient using two identifiers. Perform hand hygiene. Assess venous sites before applying tourniquet.
2. Select appropriate site that will best enhance venous distention.
3. Cleanse the skin using an approved antiseptic agent.
4. Prepare solution and administration set. Establish minimum rate of flow.
5. Apply tourniquet. Hold the patient's hand or arm with other hand using your thumb to keep skin taut. This helps to anchor the vein and prevent rolling.
6. Align steel introducer needle with the vein, approximately one-half inch from entry site. Keeping the needle in bevel-up position facilitates venipuncture and is atraumatic. (*Note: In some cases, the bevel-down approach may be used in small veins to avoid extravasation. Then, readjustment may be made before releasing the tourniquet to prevent puncturing the vein and producing a hematoma.*)
7. To ensure simultaneous entry through skin and tissue, insert the needle at a 45-degree angle.
8. Relocate the vein and decrease the angle slightly to minimize trauma.
9. Then, slowly (with a downward motion) pick up the vein. Doing this levels the introducer needle and catheter almost flush with the skin.
10. Watch for a flashback of blood, which may indicate successful entry. Also anticipate both a sense of increased resistance when the catheter meets the wall of the vein and a snap felt at the loss of resistance as the catheter enters the vein.
11. Release tourniquet, remove introducer needle, and activate the needleless cover. The catheter may then be advanced manually or with infusing fluid.
12. Connect administration set to hub and adjust flow.
13. Check the injection site for swelling.
14. Attach stabilization device. Apply dressing and label. Assess the patient's response. Document.

Assessment, Monitoring, and Removal or Replacement of Short Peripheral IV Catheters

Clinical assessment is more than collecting data. It is "an evaluation of a patient's physical condition and prognosis based on information gathered from physical and laboratory examinations and the patient's medical history" (Mosby's Medical Dictionary, 2012). This evaluation is considered in the context of the clinician's knowledge and expertise. The clinician needs to assess the PIV catheter site on a regular basis as well as the patient's response to the device and to the infusion therapy.

In an INS Position Paper (Gorski et al., 2012), the frequency of assessment and parameters of assessment, based on patient condition, are specified. The assessment includes any PIV, whether it is locked or has intermittent or continuous infusion therapy. The site should be assessed for "…Redness, tenderness, swelling, drainage, and/or the presence of paresthesias, numbness, or tingling…. Assessment should minimally include visual assessment, palpation, and subjective information from the patient. If there is tenderness at the site, the dressing may be removed to more carefully visualize the site" (p. 291–292). The frequency of assessment is highlighted in Box 13-2.

The frequency of routinely replacing PIV catheters to prevent infection has contradictory recommendations for adults. The CDC (2011) states that PIV catheters may be replaced every 72 to 96 hours in adults and only when clinically indicated in children (S6). Based on a Cochrane review and other evidence, INS (2011, p. S57) recommends that PIV catheters may be replaced when clinically indicated in adults, except if parenteral nutrition is infusing, and with a thorough assessment by the clinician. An updated Cochrane review (Webster, Osborne, Rickard, & New, 2013) supports this recommendation. However, the CDC (2011) states replacing PIV catheters only when clinically indicated as an unresolved issue. The PIV catheter must be removed if signs of infection, malfunctioning catheter, or phlebitis (warmth, tenderness, erythema, palpable venous cord) are present (CDC, 2011) or if the infusion has infiltrated. Last, "promptly remove any intravascular catheter that is no longer essential" (CDC, 2011, p. S3).

MIDLINE CATHETERS

Midline catheters were introduced in the 1950s and have undergone several transitions in technology and in placement. Currently, the design is 3 to 8 inches long and available as single or double lumen. The catheter may be placed in the basilic, cephalic, or median cubital veins of the upper arm or antecubital area, with the tip residing in the cephalic or basilic vein in the upper portion of the arm, at or below the axillary line.

The midline catheter is designed for peripheral infusion of general IV solutions and medications and for venous sampling. Indications for midline IV therapy include administration of antibiotics, hydration, pain medication, and selected antineoplastic agents (excluding continuous vesicant infusion). Solutions not appropriate for midline infusions include infusates with pH <5 or >9 and infusates with an osmolality >600 mOsm/L (INS, 2011). The midline is appropriate for infusion therapy of between 1 and 4 weeks, although the CDC (2011) states that the midline may remain in place until "there is a specific indication to remove it" (p. S6).

The procedure should be performed using sterile technique and a chlorhexidine solution for skin preparation. Only experienced nurses with excellent IV insertion skills should insert midline catheters, and then only after careful consideration of the possible risks,

BOX 13-2   FREQUENCY OF ASSESSMENT FOR PIV CATHETERS

Frequency	Patient Condition or Intermittent/Continuous Infusion
At least every 4 hours	• Patients who are receiving nonirritant/nonvesicant infusions *and* who are alert and oriented *and* who are able to notify the nurse of any signs of problems such as pain, swelling, or redness at the site
At least every 1 to 2 hours	• Critically ill patients • Adult patients who have cognitive/sensory deficits or who are receiving sedative-type medications and are unable to notify the nurse of any symptoms • Catheters placed in a high-risk location (e.g., external jugular, area of flexion)
At least every hour	• Neonatal and pediatric patients

More frequently: every 5 to 10 minutes	• Patients receiving intermittent infusions of vesicants.
	  ○ The peripheral infusion of vesicant agents should be limited to <30 to 60 minutes.
	  ○ In addition to visual assessment of the site, a blood return should be verified every 5 to 10 minutes during the infusion.
	• Patients receiving infusions of vasoconstrictor agents

With every home/outpatient visit	• For patients receiving peripheral infusions at home as overseen by home care or outpatient nurses
Frequency	**Locked PIV Catheter**
At a minimum of twice per day or with every catheter access/infusion	• For all patients who have a locked PIV catheter for intermittent infusions

Adapted from Gorski, L. A., Hallock, D., Kuehn, S. C., Morris, P., Russell, J. M., & Skala, L. C. (2012). INS Position Paper: Recommendations for frequency of assessment of the short peripheral catheter site. *Journal of Infusion Nursing, 35,* 291–292.

including thrombosis, phlebitis, air embolism, infection, vascular perforation, bleeding, and catheter transection (Perucca, 2010). As with any venipuncture, adequate assessment of the patient and the venous status is essential to ensure success. The basilic vein is the vein of choice for longer-line IV insertions because of its larger size, straighter course, and adequate hemodilution capability. Insertion technique is specific to the manufacturer's recommendations for the use of its product.

Catheter stabilization and dressing are similar to PIV catheter procedures. However, the dressing label also includes the external catheter length. Documentation is similar to that of the PIV catheter but also includes external catheter length and length of the catheter inserted (INS, 2011).

Midline catheter removal should be done with caution; apply digital pressure to the site until hemostasis is achieved. Use a petroleum-based ointment over the access site and a sterile dressing to "seal the skin-to-vein tract and decrease the risk of air embolus" (INS, 2011).

PHLEBOTOMY FOR THERAPEUTIC PURPOSES

The infusion nurse may perform phlebotomy for therapeutic purposes, as well as for blood sampling. Therapeutic phlebotomy, a bleeding of between 400 and 500 mL blood, is performed for polycythemia vera, hemochromatosis, and porphyria cutanea tarda. Therapeutic phlebotomy reduces the RBC mass, lowers the blood volume, reduces blood viscosity, and improves circulatory efficiency (Table 13-9). The practice requires a written order by the physician/LIP specifying the date, the amount of blood to be drawn, the frequency for performing the procedure, and the hemoglobin or hematocrit value at which the patient's blood should be drawn.

Polycythemia vera is characterized by a striking increase in the number of circulating RBCs; thus phlebotomy is a cornerstone of treatment (Tefferi, 2013). The number of and interval between phlebotomies should be specified by the physician/LIP and the hematocrit

---

TABLE 13-9 SUGGESTED THERAPEUTIC PHLEBOTOMY PROCEDURE

In therapeutic phlebotomies, collected blood must be discarded. The procedure itself is not adequate for recipient protection. Equipment needed includes a PIV insertion kit, phlebotomy pack, a counterbalance stand or small spring scale, blood pressure cuff or tourniquet, tincture of iodine (3% in 70% ethyl alcohol) swabs or iodophor (10% povidone–iodine) swabs, alcohol wipes, and sterile gauze.

The nurse proceeds as follows:
1. Put on gloves.
2. Select the most suitable vein. Apply a tourniquet or a blood pressure cuff inflated to 50–60 mm Hg. Have the patient open and close the fist to make the vein more prominent, if necessary. Remove the tourniquet.
3. Prepare the venipuncture site with cleansing swabs. Always start at the puncture site and move out in concentric spirals.
4. Begin blood collection by suspending bag from donor scale as far below patient's arm as possible. If counterbalance scales are used, adjust the balance for amount of blood to be drawn.
5. Make loose overhand knot in donor tube near needle.
6. Apply tourniquet (do not impair arterial circulation).
7. Do not touch or repalpate the vein.
8. Perform venipuncture.
9. Tape needle in place and cover with sterile sponge.
10. Pinch bead into bag from junction of donor tube and bag to open lumen and allow blood to flow.
11. Instruct the patient to open and close the fist slowly.
12. Collect blood until bag falls on scale. If spring scales are used, collect until prescribed amount has been withdrawn.
13. Pull knot tight.
14. Release tourniquet, withdraw needle, and apply pressure with gauze pad until bleeding has stopped. Do not flex arm. The arm may be elevated while applying pressure.
15. Dispose of blood and equipment as directed by hospital procedure.
16. Wipe site with alcohol to remove iodine solution and apply snug dressing.
17. Record procedure in clinical record.

value determined after the phlebotomy. Excessive body stores of iron characterize hemochromatosis. Weekly phlebotomy, as tolerated, is usually an outpatient procedure performed to reduce the total body iron concentration (Bacon, Adams, Kowdley, Powell, & Tavill, 2011). Because patients with hemochromatosis usually have a hematocrit value in the normal range, periodic checks on the hematocrit value are desirable. Therapeutic phlebotomy is often done for symptomatic porphyria cutanea tarda (Singal & Anderson, 2012). These patients may have a normal hematocrit reading; thus, they are likely to undergo phlebotomy too often. Hemoglobin or hematocrit is followed to prevent significant anemia.

Treatment of Adverse Reactions

Stop the phlebotomy at the first sign of reaction and call the physician/LIP. If the patient faints

- Elevate the patient's feet above head level.
- Loosen tight clothing.
- Ascertain that the patient has an adequate airway.
- Apply cold compresses to the forehead and back of the neck.
- Check and record blood pressure, pulse, and respiration periodically.

If the patient experiences nausea and vomiting, instruct the patient to breathe slowly. If the patient exhibits muscular twitching or tetanic spasms of hands or face, assist him or her to rebreathe into a paper bag. Do not give oxygen. If the patient has convulsions (rare), call for assistance. Then, prevent injury by turning the patient on the left side. Record the nature and treatment of all reactions on the patient's record.

Conclusion

The delivery of safe, quality infusion care is within the scope of practice of the professional nurse. A working knowledge of process, practice, and standards will help to ensure good outcomes.

Review Questions   *Note: Questions below may have more than one right answer.*

1. Which of the following is true of short peripheral catheter insertion?
   A. Techniques vary.
   B. Standards of practice should be followed.
   C. Skill is acquired with repeated successful attempts.
   D. All of the above

2. Polycythemia vera is characterized by which of the following?
   A. Decreased RBCs
   B. Increased RBCs
   C. Decreased eosinophils
   D. Increased eosinophils

3. Which of the following is true of blood obtained through therapeutic phlebotomy?
   A. It may be transfused.
   B. It should be stored at 4°C.
   C. It must be discarded.
   D. It does not require HIV testing.

4. A vasovagal reaction, an autonomic nervous system response, manifests itself as
   A. Stress
   B. Syncope
   C. Restlessness
   D. Fight or flight

5. Appropriate actions for the nurse to take if a patient's veins do not become prominent after application of a tourniquet include all of the following *except*
   A. Asking the patient to pump his or her hand
   B. Placing the extremity in a dependent position
   C. Tapping the vein gently
   D. Tightening the tourniquet to restrict arterial flow

6. Which of the following is true concerning the height of the fluid container?
   A. The greater the height, the lower the force
   B. The lower the height, the lower the force
   C. The greater the height, the greater the force
   D. The lower the height, the greater the force

7. The dorsal metacarpal veins may be a poor choice in which of the following patients?
   A. Elderly
   B. Home care
   C. Diabetic
   D. Renal patient

8. A thrombosed vein may be detected by which of the following factors?
   A. Resilience
   B. Lack of resilience
   C. Soft, pliable feel
   D. Cord-like feel

9. Before venipuncture, the injection site should be scrubbed with an antiseptic that is allowed to remain in contact with the skin for
   A. 15 seconds
   B. 30 seconds
   C. 45 seconds
   D. 60 seconds

10. Solutions with a pH of <5 or >9 may not be administered through a short PIV catheter.
    A. True
    B. False

References and Selected Readings   *Asterisks indicate references cited in text.*

Alekseyev, S., Byrne, M., Carpenter, A., Franker, C., Kidd, C., & Hulton, L. (2012). Prolonging the life of a patient's IV: An integrative review of intravenous securement devices. *Medsurg Nursing, 21*, 285–292.

Alexander, M., Corrigan, A., Gorski, L., Hankins, J., & Perucca, R. (2010). *Infusion nursing: An evidence based approach* (3rd ed.). St. Louis, MO: Mosby-Elsevier.

*Bacon, B.R., Adams, P.C., Kowdley, K.V., Powell, L.W., & Tavill, A.S. (2011). Diagnosis and management of hemochromatosis: 2011 Practice guideline by the American Association for the Study of Liver Diseases. *Hepatology, 54*, 328–343.

*BD Medical. (2013). *BD Nexiva Closed IV Catheter System-Single Port Resource: Flow Rates.* http://www.bd.com/resource.aspx?IDX=22133

*Brannam, L., Blaivas, M., Lyon, M., & Flake, M. (2004). Emergency nurses' utilization of ultrasound guidance for placement of peripheral intravenous lines in difficult-access patients. *Academy Emergency Medicine, 11*(12), 1361–1363.

*Camp-Sorrell, D. (Ed.). (2011). *Access Device Guidelines: Recommendations for nursing practice and education* (3rd ed.) (p. 8). Pittsburgh, PA: Oncology Nursing Society.

*Centers for Disease Control and Prevention (CDC). (2011). Guidelines for the prevention of intravascular catheter-related infections. http://www.cdc.gov/hicpac/pdf/guidelines/bsi-guidelines-2011.pdf

*Cook, L.S. (2013). Infusion-related air embolism. *Journal of Infusion Nursing, 36*, 26–36.

*Institute of Medicine: Committee on Quality of Health Care in America. (2001). *Crossing the quality chasm: A new health system for the 21st century* (p. 6). Washington, DC: National Academies Press.

*Deguzman, Z.C., O'Mara, S.K., Sulo, S., Haines, T., Blackburn, L., & Corazza, J. (2012). Bacteriostatic normal saline compared with buffered 1% lidocaine when injected intradermally as a local anesthetic to reduce pain during intravenous catheter insertion. *Journal of Perianesthesia Nursing, 27*, 399–407.

*Fink, R.M., Hjort, E., Wenger, B., Cook, P.F., Cunningham, M., Orf, A., et al. (2009). The impact of dry versus moist heat on peripheral IV catheter insertion in a hematology-oncology outpatient population. *Oncology Nursing Forum, 36*(4), E198–E204.

*Ganter-Ritz, V., Speroni, K.G., & Atherton, M. (2012). A randomized double-blind study comparing intradermal anesthetic tolerability, efficacy, and cost-effectiveness of lidocaine, buffered lidocaine, and bacteriostatic normal saline for peripheral intravenous insertion. *Journal of Infusion Nursing, 35*, 93–99.

Goode, C., Kleiber, C., Titler, M., Small, S., Rakel, B., Steelman, V.M., et al. (1993). Improving practice through research: The case of heparin vs. saline for peripheral intermittent infusion devices. *Medsurg Nursing, 2*, 23–27.

*Gorski, L.A., Hallock, D., Kuehn, S.C., Morris, P., Russell, J.M., & Skala, L.C. (2012). INS Position Paper: Recommendations for frequency of assessment of the short peripheral catheter site. *Journal of Infusion Nursing, 35*, 290–292.

*Hadaway, L. (2010). Infusion therapy equipment. In M. Alexander, A. Corrigan, L. Gorski, J. Hankins, & R. Perucca (Eds.), *Infusion Nurses Society Infusion Nursing: An evidence-based approach* (3rd ed., pp. 391–436). St. Louis, MO: Saunders Elsevier.

*Hadaway, L., & Richardson, D. (2010). Needleless connectors: A primer on terminology. *Journal of Infusion Nursing, 33*, 22–31.

*Hess, H. (2010). A biomedical device to improve pediatric vascular access success. *Pediatric Nursing, 36*, 259–263.

*Houston, P.A. (2013). Obtaining vascular access in the obese patient population. *Journal of Infusion Nursing, 36*, 52–56.

*Infusion Nurses Society. (2008). *Flushing protocols*. Norwood, MA: Author.

*Infusion Nurses Society. (2011). Infusion nursing: Standards of practice. *Journal of Infusion Nursing, 34*(Suppl.), S1–S110.

*Jacobson, A.F., & Winslow, E.H. (2005). Variables influencing intravenous catheter insertion difficulty and failure: An analysis of 339 intravenous catheter insertions. *Heart & Lung, 34*(5), 345–359.

*Kappas, A. (2011). Emotion and regulation are one! *Emotion Review, 3*(1), 17–25.

*Kim, M.J., Park, J.M., Rhee, N., Je, S.M., Hong, S.H., Lee, Y.M., et al. (2012). Efficacy of VeinViewer in pediatric peripheral intravenous access: A randomized controlled trial. *European Journal of Pediatrics, 171*, 1121–1125.

*Larsen, P., Eldridge, D., Brinkley, J., Newton, D., Goff, D., Hartzog, T., et al. (2010). Pediatric peripheral intravenous access: Does nursing experience and competence really make a difference? *Journal of Infusion Nursing, 33*(4), 226–235.

*Lininger, R.A. (2003). Pediatric peripheral IV insertion success rates. *Pediatric Nursing, 29*(5), 351–354.

*Maiocco, G., & Coole, C. (2012). Use of ultrasound guidance for peripheral intravenous placement in difficult-to-access patients: advancing practice with evidence. *Journal of Nursing Care Quality, 27*(1), 51–55.

*Maki, D.G. (2008). Improving the safety of peripheral intravenous catheters. *British Medical Journal, 337*, 122–123.

*Mbamalu, D., & Banerjee, A. (1999). Methods of obtaining peripheral venous access in difficult situations. *Postgraduate Medical Journal, 75*, 459–462.

*Mosby. (2012). *Mosby's medical dictionary* (9th ed.). St. Louis, MO: Mosby/Elsevier.

*Perry, A.M., Caviness, A.C., & Hsu, D.C. (2011). Efficacy of a near-infrared light device in pediatric intravenous cannulation: A randomized controlled trial. *Pediatric Emergency Care, 27*(1), 5–10.

*Perucca, R. (2010). Peripheral venous access devices. In M. Alexander, A. Corrigan, L. Gorski, J. Hankins, & R. Perucca (Eds.), *Infusion Nurses Society Infusion Nursing: An evidence-based approach* (3rd ed., pp. 456–479). St. Louis, MO: Saunders Elsevier.

Peterson, F.Y., & Kirchhoff, K.T. (1991). Analysis of the research about heparinized versus nonheparinized intravascular lines. *Heart & Lung, 20*(6), 631–640.

*Rickard, C.M., Webster, J., Wallis, M.C., Marsh, N., McGrail, M.R., French, V., et al. (2012). Routine versus clinically indicated replacement of peripheral intravenous catheters: A randomised equivalence trial. *Lancet 380*(9847), 1066–1074.

Sherwood, G., & Barnsteiner, J. (2012). *Quality and safety in nursing: A competency approach to improving outcomes.* Ames, IA: Wiley-Blackwell.

*Singal, A.K., & Anderson, K.E. (2012). Porphyria cutanea tarda and hepatoerythropoietic porphyria. *UpToDate.* http://www.uptodate.com/contents/porphyria-cutanea-tarda-and-hepatoerythropoietic-porphyria

*Tefferi, A. (2013). Prognosis and treatment of polycythemia vera. *UpToDate.* http://www.uptodate.com/contents/prognosis-and-treatment-of-polycythemia-vera

*Webster, J., Osborne, S., Rickard, C.M., & New, K. (2013). Clinically-indicated replacement versus routine replacement of peripheral venous catheters. *Cochrane Database of Systematic Reviews*, Issue 4. Art. No.: CD007798.

*Wilkins, R.G., & Unverdorben, M. (2012). Accidental intravenous infusion of air. *Journal of Infusion Nursing*, *35*, 404–408.

*Witting, M. (2012). IV access difficulty: Incidence and delays in an urban emergency department. *The Journal of Emergency Medicine*, *42*(4), 483–487.

Woody, G., & Davis, B. (2013). Increasing nurse competence in peripheral intravenous therapy. *Journal of Infusion Nursing*, *36*, 413–419.

*Zingg, W., & Pittet, D. (2009). Peripheral venous catheters: An under-evaluated problem. *International Journal of Antimicrobial Agents*, *34*(Suppl. 4), S38–S42.

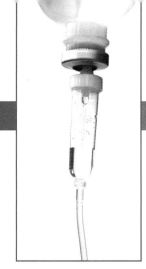

CHAPTER 14

Central Venous Access

Mary E. Hagle
Ann M. Cook

KEY TERMS

Add-on Device
Basilic Vein
Central Line Bundle
Central Venous
  Access Device
  (CVAD)
Central Venous
  Catheter (CVC)
Cephalic Vein
External Jugular Vein
Implanted Infusion
  Pump

Implanted Port
Nontunneled CVAD
Peripherally Inserted
  Central Catheter
  (PICC)
Pinch-Off Syndrome
Subclavian Vein
Superior Vena Cava
Thrombolytic
Tunneled CVAD
Valsalva Maneuver

CENTRAL VENOUS ACCESS

Definition

A central venous access device (CVAD) or central venous catheter (CVC), commonly referred to as a central line, is a catheter placed into the central venous vasculature. The CVAD tip is placed in the lower third of the superior vena cava or at the atriocaval junction. Central venous access permits rapid administration of solutions for replacing vascular volume, as well as administration of all other types of solutions, including highly concentrated or incompatible solutions. Another advantage of CVADs is that they may stay in place for weeks to years, depending on the type of CVAD.

Knowledge of the vascular system is essential for providing care to the patient with a CVAD. Vessels involved include the basilic, median cubital, brachial, cephalic, axillary, subclavian, external and internal jugular, and brachiocephalic veins as well as the superior vena cava (Figure 14-1).

Vascular Structures Used for Central Venous Access

Basilic Vein

The basilic vein is larger than the cephalic. It passes upward in a smooth path along the inner side of the biceps muscle and terminates in the axillary vein along with the brachial vein.

Median Cubital Vein

Distally from the basilic vein is the median cubital vein, located at the site of the antecubital space.

Brachial Vein

The *brachial vein* merges with the basilic vein and becomes the axillary vein.

Cephalic Vein

The cephalic vein ascends along the outer border of the biceps muscle to the upper third of the arm. It passes in the space between the pectoralis major and deltoid muscles. It terminates in the axillary vein, with a descending curve, just below the clavicle. The cephalic vein is occasionally connected with the external jugular or subclavian vein by a branch that passes from it upward in front of the clavicle.

Axillary Vein

The *axillary vein* starts upward as a continuation of the basilic vein, increasing in size as it ascends. It receives the cephalic vein and terminates immediately beneath the clavicle, at the outer border of the first rib, at which point it becomes the subclavian vein.

Subclavian Vein

The subclavian vein, a continuation of the axillary vein, extends from the outer edge of the first rib to the inner end of the clavicle, where it unites with the internal jugular to form the brachiocephalic vein. Valves are present in the venous system until approximately 1 inch before the formation of the brachiocephalic vein.

External Jugular Vein

The external jugular vein is easily recognized on the side of the neck. It follows a descending inward path to join the subclavian vein above the middle of the clavicle.

Internal Jugular Vein

The *internal jugular vein* descends first behind and then to the outer side of the internal and common carotid arteries. The carotid plexus is situated on the outer side of the internal carotid artery. The internal jugular vein joins the subclavian vein at the root of the neck.

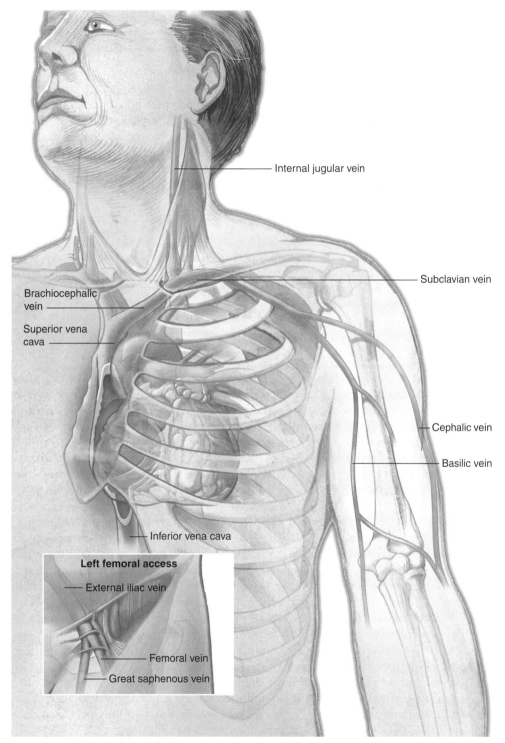

FIGURE 14-1 Central vascular structures.

At the angle of junction, the left subclavian receives the thoracic duct, whereas the right subclavian receives the right lymphatic duct.

BRACHIOCEPHALIC VEIN

The brachiocephalic vein is formed by the union of the right or left internal jugular vein and the corresponding subclavian vein. The *right brachiocephalic vein* is approximately 1 inch long. It passes almost vertically downward and joins the *left brachiocephalic vein* just below the cartilage of the first rib. The left brachiocephalic vein is approximately 2.5 inches long and larger than the right. It passes from left to right across the upper front chest in a downward slant. These vessels join to form the superior vena cava.

SUPERIOR VENA CAVA

The superior vena cava receives all blood from the upper half of the body. It is composed of a short trunk 2.5 to 3 inches long. It begins below the first rib close to the sternum on the right side, descends vertically slightly to the right, and empties into the right atrium of the heart.

INDICATIONS FOR CENTRAL VENOUS ACCESS DEVICES

CVADs are indicated when peripheral venous access is unavailable or not recommended. CVADs are used for rapid administration of large volumes of fluids in a short period of time. This is possible because the catheter tip is in a large vessel that can distribute the fluid rapidly. Other indications for a CVAD are for infusing highly concentrated fluids, such as parenteral nutrition (PN), or vesicant or irritating drugs, such as antineoplastic medications and some vasopressors. Because the CVAD tip rests in an area with a rapid flow of a large amount of blood, prompt dilution occurs of the infusing fluid. Rapid dilution reduces the risk of chemical phlebitis and venous sclerosis. A highly concentrated solution is one with an osmolarity >600 mOsm/L or a pH <5 or >9. These solutions would be irritating or damaging to a peripheral vein (INS, 2011). When this is the case, a CVAD must be used to administer the solution. CVADs may have one or several lumens, thus permitting concurrent administration of needed medications, even if they are incompatible solutions (Figure 14-2). Additionally, CVADs can be used to administer all other types of therapies, such as blood components and antibiotics. Again, a CVAD may remain in place, without being replaced, for several weeks up to several years, depending on the type of CVAD.

Candidates for a CVAD include most individuals. Trauma patients requiring massive fluid replacements or in surgery requiring rapid administration of fluids would need a CVAD. Hospitalized patients are candidates for a CVAD when they are in need of venous access with poor peripheral veins, have multiple therapies that may be incompatible, or have infusions that are irritating or damaging to peripheral veins. Patients in home care or receiving infusion therapy in an ambulatory care clinic or infusion center, who require administration of continuous or intermittent infusions over a long period of time, may also require a CVAD. Frequent blood sampling is less painful using a CVAD. Last, CVADs may be inserted without general anesthesia.

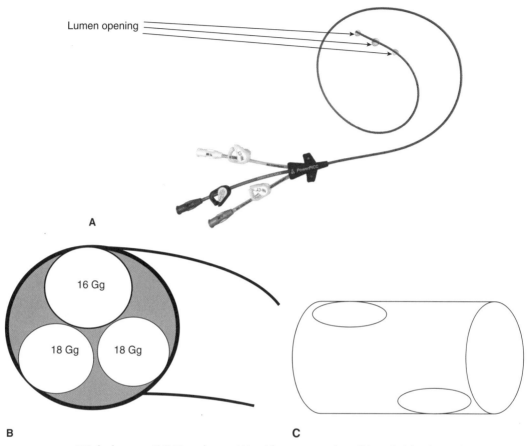

Lumen opening

16 Gg

18 Gg   18 Gg

A

B   C

FIGURE 14-2 Triple-lumen CVAD catheter **(A)** with cross-section **(B)** and side view **(C)**.

Another indication for a CVAD is to monitor central venous pressure (CVP). This is for detecting volume changes related to potential problems or to evaluate patient hemodynamic status, which is discussed in Chapter 15.

OVERVIEW OF CVAD TYPES

There are five main types of CVADs: **nontunneled CVADs, peripherally inserted central catheters (PICC) tunneled CVADs, implanted ports,** and **implanted infusion pumps** (Box 14-1). Their dwell time ranges from days to years, or indefinitely, until therapy is discontinued or a complication becomes evident. Improvements in catheter materials and properties, safety features, and device options have made this an ever-evolving field of technology. All CVADs are radiopaque, so tip placement may be verified and any adverse event may be detected, such as catheter embolism.

BOX 14-1 OVERVIEW OF CENTRAL VENOUS ACCESS DEVICES

Nontunneled CVAD
- Large-bore catheter inserted percutaneously into central venous structure and sutured into place
- Used for short-term therapy, days to weeks
- Most complications seen with these CVADs

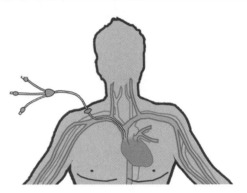

Nontunneled CVAD

PICC
- Very–small-gauge catheter inserted percutaneously into an upper extremity vein and then threaded into the superior vena cava
- Used for short- or long-term therapy, 7 days to months
- Variety of types available, including a rapid flow/power injectable PICC
- Fewer complications than nontunneled CVADs

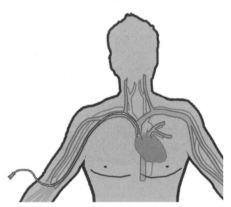

PICC

Tunneled CVADs
- Catheter inserted into a central venous structure; the distal end is pulled through subcutaneous tissue (tunneled) for a short distance before exiting the skin
- Has a cuff, usually Dacron
- Used for long-term therapy, 6 months or more
- Frequently used: Broviac, Groshong, Hickman
- Fewer complications than nontunneled CVADs

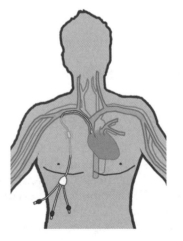

Tunneled CVAD

BOX 14-1 OVERVIEW OF CENTRAL VENOUS ACCESS DEVICES (*Continued*)

Implanted Port
- A tunneled catheter attached to a device with a hollow core, implanted into the subcutaneous tissue
- Used for long-term therapy
- Noncoring needle required to access port
- Variety of types:
  ○ May be a single or dual port
  ○ May be power injectable
- Fewest complications

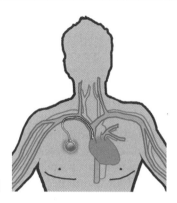

Implanted port

Implanted Infusion Pump
- A tunneled catheter attached to a device with a (a) refillable drug reservoir, (b) power source, and (c) septum/port for percutaneous access; implanted into the subcutaneous tissue around the lower abdomen or side
- Used for long-term therapy to artery, vein, or anatomical space
- Noncoring needle required to access port
- Variety of types based on energy source and number of ports
- Few complications

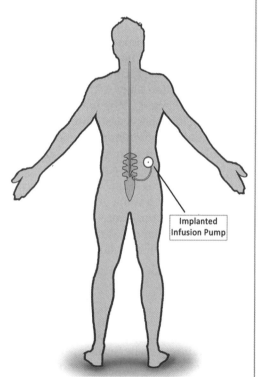

Implanted Infusion Pump

Implanted infusion pump

Illustrations courtesy of Elizabeth Hirschmann.

Catheter Materials

The ideal CVC would be composed of a material that inhibits thrombus formation, inserts easily, is chemically neutral, and is biocompatible. Catheters may be composed of polyurethane, silicone, elastomeric hydrogel, or Teflon®. Polyurethane is firm, allows for ease of insertion, softens after insertion, and is biocompatible so that tissues do not react to the material. It is less thrombogenic than materials used in the past. A thrombus forms as a result of intima irritation and reaction; softer materials are less irritating to the vein wall. The strength of the polyurethane allows for a thinner catheter wall and larger internal diameter when compared with same-sized silicone catheters. Silicone is more flexible, thus requiring special insertion techniques, and has increased biocompatibility. Elastomeric hydrogel catheters, primarily used in peripheral IVs, combine hydrogel and polyurethane to obtain the lowest coefficient of surface friction of the catheter, thus allowing for less thrombogenicity and decreased mechanical tissue trauma. The hydrogel allows the catheter to soften, whereas the polyurethane provides strength and prevents absorption of the infusate into the catheter.

Catheters and Thrombus Formation

Advancements in technology related to catheter materials and properties are aimed at reducing complications of catheter-related infections and thrombosis. Catheter-related bloodstream infection (CRBSI) occurs when microorganisms adhere to catheter materials and promote formation of a biofilm allowing cell proliferation, intercellular adhesion, and colonization. Polyurethane catheters have been associated with fewer CRBSIs than are silicone catheters along with decreased biofilm formation (CDC, 2011).

Thrombosis associated with CVCs has many contributing factors. Any foreign material in the bloodstream becomes coated with a protein and fibrin deposit as well as a biofilm. This in turn activates internal coagulation, causing platelet activation and platelet adherence to the catheter. Damage to endothelial cells at the puncture site also promotes platelet activation. Patients requiring CVCs often have activated coagulation systems because of trauma or severe disease, both of which promote the development of thrombosis. Thrombosis may be limited to a fibrin sheath formation or may be severe enough to occlude the vein. It may have no clinical significance or it may result in a fatal pulmonary embolism. Fibrin sheaths can lead to loss of function of the catheter and mediate bacterial adherence.

Antimicrobial and Antiseptic Catheters

Catheter properties aimed at reducing the complications of thrombosis and CRBSI include bonding with heparin or cefazolin; impregnating with silver sulfadiazine and chlorhexidine or small silver particles; and coating with minocycline and rifampin or silver. Multiple studies have demonstrated the effectiveness of these catheters at decreasing some CRBSIs in the short term due to the length of time the antimicrobial substance is released. Few studies have evaluated the use of heparin-coated catheters, but when examined, these catheters have demonstrated a decrease in CRBSIs.

Most of the literature has focused on chlorhexidine and silver sulfadiazine or minocycline and rifampicin. Studies have demonstrated decreased CRBSIs when compared with control catheters. Studies evaluating various silver technologies have been inconclusive. The Centers for Disease Control and Prevention (CDC) recommends use of antimicrobial or antiseptic-impregnated CVCs when the expected duration is for more than 5 days and a comprehensively implemented strategy to decrease rates of CRBSIs is ineffective (CDC, 2011). The strategy would need to include comprehensive education of those who insert and maintain the CVADs, use of maximum sterile barriers on insertion, and the use of a 0.5% chlorhexidine preparation for skin antisepsis. In such cases, use of these catheters may be cost-effective.

Anti-infective catheters may also be considered for patients who are neutropenic, have had a transplant, have severe burns, are on hemodialysis, or are critically ill. They should not be used if the patient has an allergy to silver, chlorhexidine, silver sulfadiazine, rifampin, or tetracycline (INS, 2011).

Catheter with Removable Introducer

Catheters with removable introducers are frequently made of polyurethane; a wide variety of products are available from today's manufacturers. These products have been developed with safety standards in mind in an effort to minimize the incidence of needlestick injury.

The unit consists of an introducer catheter or syringe and needle and a catheter with stylet. A catheter with a removable introducer is a single-lumen catheter with a fairly easy method of insertion. Because thrombus formation can be a problem with polyurethane, this may not be the catheter of choice for long-term therapy. However, minimal thrombus formation has been reported with hydromer-coated polyurethane and long-term use.

Insertion should be done using ultrasound technology to visualize the vein. The syringe is removed and the catheter threaded through the needle. The needle is withdrawn from the vein and removed from the catheter by splitting the needle into two parts.

Catheter with Introducer and Guidewire

A safety catheter with an introducer and guidewire allows for the insertion of a multiple-lumen silicone catheter. The unit consists of a syringe and needle or an over-the-needle catheter (ONC), a long central catheter, and a guidewire.

To insert the catheter, venipuncture is performed with the syringe and needle or safety-type ONC. The syringe or stylet is removed. The guidewire is threaded through the short catheter or needle, and the short catheter or needle is withdrawn (into a self-contained locking cover to avoid needlestick injury). The puncture site may be enlarged with a scalpel. The long catheter is threaded over the guidewire, which is then withdrawn, leaving the long catheter in the vein.

Tunneled Catheter Cuffs

Tunneled catheters are available with one or two small polyester fabric cuffs approximately 0.5 cm wide. These cuffs are made of the polymer Dacron and are commonly known as Dacron cuffs. Within weeks, the Dacron cuff becomes enmeshed in fibrous tissue securing the catheter in place. It lies within the subcutaneous tunnel 1 to 2 inches from the exit site. The cuff also inhibits migration of microorganisms into the tunnel. These measures reduce the risk of infection.

An antimicrobial cuff has been developed that provides stability while reducing the risk of infection. The cuff exhibits antimicrobial activity attributed to silver ions that are active for 4 to 6 weeks until they are absorbed (Bard). Another innovation to cuff design promotes tissue growth to help secure the catheter in place (Bard).

Catheter Tips and Valves

Catheters are available with open-ended or closed-ended tips. Open-ended catheters have a blunt tip. They require clamping when not in use. Most CVADs have this type of tip. Closed-ended catheters have a rounded closed tip with a side valve. The Groshong catheter has a rounded, closed tip and features a patented Groshong valve that opens inward for blood aspiration and outward for infusion but remains closed when not in use (Figure 14-3). Advantages of this type of catheter tip include the following:

- Decreased risk of bleeding or air emboli
- Elimination of catheter clamping
- Elimination of the use of heparin in the catheter
- Reduction of flushing between use; weekly flushing is all that is required

Catheters also are available with a pressure-activated safety valve (PASV) (Navilyst Medical). The valve is located in the catheter hub (Figure 14-4). The patented valve

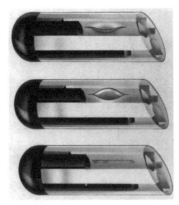

FIGURE 14-3 Groshong valve. (Courtesy of C. R. Bard.)

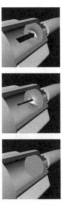

FIGURE 14-4 Pressure-activated safety valve. (Courtesy of Boston Scientific.)

opens with minimal positive pressure for infusion, yet requires four times as much negative pressure for aspiration. The PASV also reduces the reflux of blood into the end of the catheter during periods of increased CVP and decreases difficulties with poor blood return. Weekly saline-only flushing is needed, and the product is consistent with needleless systems. The valve may also be used with PICCs and midline catheters. It is important to note that changes in technique are needed when this type of catheter and valve are used. The catheter must not be clamped until after the syringe is removed or the valve will not function to prevent reflux. When the catheter is not in use, the catheter hub can be taped to the chest wall above heart level. This minimizes blood pressure at the catheter tip.

EDUCATION AND TRAINING FOR HEALTH CARE PERSONNEL

It is recommended that health care personal, including licensed independent practitioners (LIPs) and nurses, be trained with an organized training program regarding all aspects of infusion therapy. In relation to CVADs, this would include site selection, device selection, insertion, maintenance, removal, and appropriate infection control measures. A variety of methods should be used to validate competency on an ongoing basis. This is not limited to, but would include, written tests, clinical scenarios, observations in a skills laboratory, and observed performance of the skill in a clinical setting (CDC, 2011; INS, 2011). It is important for nurses to know the standards related to insertion and maintenance of CVADs and thus to understand the needs of individual patients. Competence in monitoring patients with CVADs and in maintaining CVADs is critical. Since its inception, Infusion Nurses Society' (INS) *Clinical Competency Validation Program* has been the ideal tool for clinicians seeking to validate their infusion skills in both acute care and alternate care settings (INS, 2013).

INFECTION PREVENTION AND CONTROL

In 1999, the often cited report by the Institute of Medicine (IOM), *To Err is Human: Building a Safer Health System*, sent a shock wave through the nation by reporting the unnecessary deaths occurring in health care settings to be as high as 98,000 annually (IOM, 1999). Since then, the IOM, the National Institutes of Health, The Joint Commission (TJC), the CDC, and others have focused on addressing the problems delineated in this report by improving processes and systems to affect change and improve patient outcomes. Preventing central line infections is one of the areas of focus as a result of this report.

Approximately 15 million CVAD days (the total number of days of exposure to CVADs by patients in a selected population) occur annually in intensive care units (ICUs) in the United States each year. Approximately 80,000 CRBSIs occur annually in ICUs with a total of 250,000 cases of bloodstream infections occurring in all areas of the hospital (CDC, 2011). Most CRBSIs originate from the catheter insertion site or the hub and increase the patient's stay in the hospital (Mermel et al., 2009).

Several recommendations have been made and are being implemented to decrease the incidence of CRBSIs. One recommendation is to have an effective education program for all health care providers and nurses inserting and maintaining CVADs as mentioned earlier (CDC, 2011; INS, 2011). Grouping key actions to prevent CRBSIs has been referred to as the **Central Line Bundle** (CDC, 2011; IHI, 2011; INS, 2011). These measures include optimal catheter and site selection (avoiding the femoral vein for a CVAD in an adult), appropriate hand hygiene (should be practiced before and after insertion site palpation, before and after insertion, and before and after donning and removing gloves), the use of chlorhexidine gluconate solution as a skin antiseptic, and maximal barrier precautions during insertion of the CVAD. This requires the use of a mask, cap, sterile gown, and sterile gloves for the health care provider and a sterile full body drape for the patient (CDC, 2011; IHI, 2011). Daily assessment of the need for the CVAD and prompt removal when indicated prevents infection (CDC, 2011). The Agency for Healthcare Research and Quality (AHRQ) developed a toolkit for preventing CRBSI; a daily audit form illustrates the best practices that should be followed (Figure 14-5). Reports of agencies implementing these actions and the reduction in adverse events, or the outcomes of monitoring adherence to procedures, all demonstrate the success of these interventions (Guerin, Wagner, Rains, & Bessesen, 2010; The Joint Commission, 2012; McMullan et al., 2013; Rupp et al., 2013).

CENTRAL VENOUS ACCESS DEVICE AND SITE SELECTION

CVAD selection requires a collaborative approach between health care team members and the patient. Considerations in access device selection include patient assessment, type of therapy, duration of therapy, type of CVAD, and patient's values and preferences.

Device selection is guided by the principles of the least invasive, fewest lumens, and smallest gauge catheter that are appropriate for the therapy and able to last for the duration of the therapy. The risk of adverse events decreases with less invasive insertion techniques, and reduced risk of infection may be associated with fewer CVAD lumens (CDC, 2011). A large external catheter diameter may cause damage to the intima, impede venous flow around the catheter, and interfere with appropriate dilution of medications. The internal diameter of the catheter may affect flow rate and ability to draw blood samples.

The types of prescribed medication and nutrition therapy influence device selection as well. Multiple therapies that are incompatible require multiple lumens. Therapies that are irritants or of high osmolarity, acidity, or alkalinity can cause endothelial damage and increase risk of phlebitis and thrombosis. An algorithm assists with matching the appropriate device to the specific criteria (Figure 14-6).

Nontunneled CVADs are used for short-term therapy, are often placed when there is an emergent need for central venous access, and account for the majority of CRBSIs. The subclavian vein is the preferred site for nontunneled CVADs as it poses the least risk for complications (CDC, 2011).

PICC lines are used for therapies of 7 days or more and up to approximately 1 year. Recommended veins include the basilic, median cubital, cephalic, and brachial veins. Veins in the upper extremity should be avoided in patients with stage 4 or 5 chronic kidney disease. The extremity should be avoided on the same side where there has been breast surgery with axillary node dissection, radiation therapy, lymphedema, or in the affected extremity from a stroke (INS, 2011).

Central Venous Catheter Maintenance Audit Form

Audit Date: ____/____/20____   Addressograph Here

1. **Was the need for a central line for this patient discussed on patient rounds?**
    [ ] Yes   [ ] Yes, as part of Daily Goals   [ ] No

2. **Was proper hand hygiene used by all personnel involved in line care for this patient (i.e., hand washing with soap and water or with alcohol-based hand sanitizer)?**
    [ ] Yes   [ ] No, not during: _Dressing change _Accessing the line _Port/clave change _Other

3. **If the line was percutaneously placed, was this line placed in a recommended site?**
    [ ] Yes (IJ, SC)   [ ] No (femoral)

4. **Was the dressing changed during this shift?**

    [ ] Yes, changed because:
       [ ] Dressing soiled, damp or non-occlusive
       [ ] Due to be changed (7 days for transparent
          OR 1 day for gauze)
       [ ] Changed by specific team (e.g., PICC,
          TNA)
       [ ] Dressing was overdue to be changed?
       ____ days for transparent
       ____ days for gauze

    [ ] No, not changed because:
       [ ] It was intact and not due
       [ ] It was due but could not be completed.
       Explain:

5. **Was Chloraprep© or 2% chlorhexidine in 70% Isopropyl alcohol used for skin antisepsis?**

    [ ] Yes:
    Was it used appropriately?
    [ ] Scrub vigorously back and forth for 30
       seconds
    [ ] Groin sites 2 minutes
    [ ] Air dry up to 2 minutes
    [ ] No – Explain:

    [ ] No, Povidone iodine used
    Secondary to allergy?
    [ ] Yes   [ ] No – Explain:

    Did scrub comply with recommendations?
      1. Clean with soap and water or alcohol, air
         dry
      2. Povidone iodine air dry 2 minutes
        [ ] Yes   [ ] No – Explain:

6. **Were central line tubing and all additions (secondary tubing, etc.) changed during this shift?**

    [ ] Yes, completed because:
       [ ] Tubing due to be changed
       [ ] 72 hours since last change
       [ ] 24 hours for intralipids
       [ ] Medication tubing expired

    [ ] No, not completed because
       [ ] Not due to be changed
       [ ] Due but could not be completed – Explain:

7. **Was there blood return from each lumen?**   [ ] Yes [ ] No [ ] Unable to assess
                                          (infusion can't be stopped)

    Please specify lumen: _____

USE OF ADVANCED TECHNOLOGY

8. **Was a chlorhexidine impregnated BioPatch used?**   [ ] Yes   [ ] No

9. **Was a chlorhexidine impregnated occlusive dressing used?**   [ ] Yes   [ ] No

10. **Was an antibiotic coated catheter used at insertion?**   [ ] Yes   [ ] No

11. **What will you change to improve line maintenance practices?**

FIGURE 14-5 AHRQ CVC Maintenance Audit Form. (From Agency for Healthcare Research and Quality. [2013].)

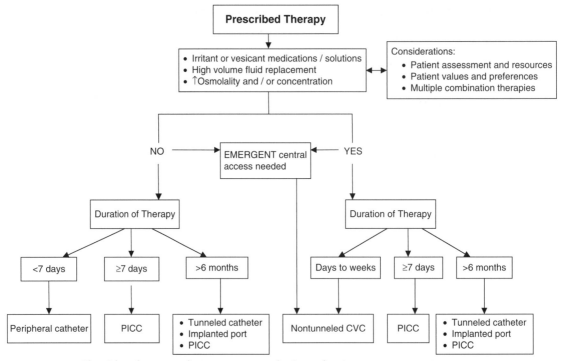

FIGURE 14-6 Algorithm for central venous access device selection.

Tunneled CVADs (Hickman, Groshong, and Broviac are common trade names), implanted ports, and implanted infusion pumps are recommended when therapy is expected to be longer than 6 months.

For all types of CVADs in adults, the femoral vein should be avoided as it has high colonization rates of bacterial flora. Additionally, catheters should be placed as far as possible from any open wounds to decrease the risk of infection (CDC, 2011).

Patient Assessment and Informed Consent

Patient assessment includes health history and physical assessment. Medical conditions of concern, besides allergy status, include coagulation status, diabetes, renal disease, trauma, and previous CVCs. Other conditions to note are previous arm, neck, or chest trauma; surgery; or radiation. Physical assessment is needed for circulatory status, lymphedema, and skin integrity. For long-term CVADs, patient activity level and lifestyle must be considered. Any limitations of patient activity the device may create should be thoroughly discussed. Additionally, mental and emotional status, physical dexterity, and financial capacity to manage long-term care of the device must be assessed from the patient and/or family perspective.

Consent should be obtained by the health care provider performing the procedure, and confirmation of informed consent should be obtained by the nurse based on institutional policies and procedures (INS, 2011).

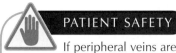

PATIENT SAFETY

If peripheral veins are adequate and can be used for the prescribed therapy, a CVAD should not be inserted.

PREPARATION FOR CVAD INSERTION

Patient Education

Some of the information about the CVAD insertion technique will be explained to the patient during device selection. However, once the type of device is selected, specific education about the device and insertion is necessary. Explaining the reasons for the CVAD and the procedure for inserting it will allay fears and help the patient participate as much as possible. Engaging the patient and the family in all aspects of care, particularly infection prevention and control measures and maintenance of the CVAD, will help to improve patient outcomes (National Quality Forum, 2009).

Patient education should include a description of the procedure, expected postprocedure discomfort, and the need for comfort measures. It may be necessary to use some form of premedication sedation for the procedure depending on the type of device, insertion site, and individual patient needs (Box 14-2). If a tunneled catheter, implanted port, or implanted

---

BOX 14-2 PATIENT TEACHING FOR CVAD INSERTION AND MAINTENANCE

- Assessment of patient's readiness for learning, potential barriers to learning-health literacy, and preferred learning style(s)
- Rationale for CVAD placement and device options including length of therapy and impact on patient's lifestyle
- Discussion of the insertion procedure and maintenance of the CVAD: Include patient and health care provider responsibilities for the maintenance of the CVAD once inserted
- Explanation of possible risks and complications of CVAD insertion and continued CVAD utilization
- Emergency information includes what to do and whom to call if the external catheter is cut, breaks, cracks, or is accidently removed
- When to return for follow-up appointments for assessment and maintenance of the CVAD
- Use of multiple methods of instruction including written materials, multimedia presentations, hands-on opportunities, and interactive learning whenever possible

Follow-up evaluation of teaching includes

- Assessment of patient and/or caregiver comprehension through discussion and return demonstration
- Opportunities for patient and caregiver questions and/or concerns

infusion pump is being inserted, offer the patient the opportunity to see and/or handle a sample of the CVAD that will be placed. This often helps to reassure many patients. Explain to the patient that he or she will be covered with a sterile drape, and the health care providers will wear gowns, caps, masks, and gloves.

Patient Positioning

If the catheter will be inserted by a subclavian approach, explain to the patient that he or she is positioned flat in bed with the head lowered and knees bent (Trendelenburg position). This position facilitates entry to the vein by distending the vein and increasing CVP and the venous blood supply. A rolled towel is placed under the back along the spinal cord and between the shoulders to hyperextend the neck and elevate the clavicle. For the jugular approach, the head is turned to the opposite direction and extended. This stretches and stabilizes the vein and accentuates the muscular landmarks. During a cephalic or brachial approach, abduction of the arm may be required to pass the catheter past the shoulder area. Explaining this to the patient before the procedure promotes patient cooperation when the uncomfortable position must be maintained.

Valsalva Maneuver

Practicing the Valsalva maneuver before the insertion also promotes cooperation when the patient is asked to hold her or his breath and bear down when the catheter is open to the air (INS, 2011).

Laboratory Tests

Prior to CVAD insertion, several laboratory tests for assessment may be needed. These include platelet count and international normalized ratio/prothrombin time (INR/PT). Any abnormal findings may require correction with vitamin K, fresh frozen plasma, or platelet concentrates before catheter insertion is attempted. This should be explained to the patient. Contraindications for a CVAD include

- Abnormal coagulation studies
- Septicemia
- Anomalies of the central venous vascular structures
- Thrombosis of the subclavian or brachiocephalic veins or the superior vena cava

INSERTION OF THE CENTRAL VENOUS CATHETER

CVAD insertion is a medical act. CVAD insertion and infusion therapy need to be initiated, changed, or discontinued with an order by a physician/LIP (INS, 2011). Insertion of some types of catheters, such as PICCs, may be delegated to specially trained RNs according to each state's Nurse Practice Act. Additionally, the CDC (2011) made a strong recommendation to use ultrasound guidance for placing CVCs (if this technology is available) to reduce the number of cannulation attempts and mechanical complications. Of course, ultrasound guidance should only be used by those with validated competency.

There are three basic approaches for CVC insertions. The veins used for entry are the subclavian vein and the internal or external jugular veins for most CVAD insertions; for PICCs, access to the vascular system is through the cephalic, basilic, brachial, or median cubital vein.

Subclavian Approach

The subclavian vein is the entry site of choice for nontunneled centrally inserted catheters and is recommended, if not contraindicated, to minimize risk of infection (CDC, 2011). This approach requires the shortest catheter length because it is closest to the superior vena cava. However, subclavian entry can foster major complications both during and after insertion.

The subclavian entry may be performed using the infraclavicular or supraclavicular approach. In both approaches, the catheter is inserted under the clavicle, aiming for the jugular notch. For the infraclavicular approach, the catheter is inserted at approximately the midpoint of the clavicle. For the supraclavicular approach, the catheter is frequently inserted at the base of the triangle formed by the sternal and clavicular heads of the sternocleidomastoid muscle. Contraindications to the subclavian approach may include the following:

- Radiation skin damage at intended insertion site
- Fractured clavicle
- Hyperinflated lungs
- Malignant lesion at the base of the neck or apex of the lungs

Internal Jugular Vein Approach

The internal jugular vein is preferred by many practitioners as the site of first choice for inserting a CVC. The constant anatomic location of the internal jugular vein makes it easier to catheterize than is the subclavian vein. The right internal jugular vein is usually chosen because it forms a straighter, shorter line to the superior vena cava. It also avoids the higher left pleura and thoracic duct.

External Jugular Vein Approach

The external jugular vein is observable and easily entered. Insertion complications are rare. The external jugular vein varies in size, and its junction with the subclavian vein is acutely angulated. It contains two pairs of valves: the uppermost pair is 4 cm above the clavicle and the lower pair is located at the vein's entrance to the subclavian vein. Because of these factors, central catheterization can be difficult. Because a short catheter may be inserted easily, central catheterization may be achieved by using an introducer with a guidewire. Entry into the superficial vein is performed by directing the catheter toward the ipsilateral nipple.

The main objections to any jugular catheterization are the following:

- Catheter occlusion, resulting from the patient's head movement, is a persistent problem.
- Vein irritation also results from head movement, with a shorter catheter life as a consequence.
- Maintaining an intact dressing on the area is difficult.
- The idea of having a catheter in the neck may be aesthetically and psychologically disturbing to many patients and families.

CVAD Insertion Complications and Tip Placement Verification

Prevention is the best intervention for CVAD insertion complications. Patient safety initiatives include using two identifiers to ensure having the right patient, doing a preprocedure verification, and having systems in place for high-alert medications. A CVAD insertion checklist has been found to be effective and several examples are available (The Joint Commission, 2012). However, there are several potential complications that result from CVC insertion. Nursing surveillance during and after the procedure with prompt recognition of signs and symptoms of a complication and rapid response to the complication can keep patients safe. Table 14-1 outlines the major potential complications of CVC insertion with appropriate interventions.

PATIENT SAFETY

The risk of air embolism is always present during catheter insertion because CVP can be negative. Placing the patient in the Trendelenburg position increases CVP. If possible, the patient should perform the Valsalva maneuver whenever the catheter is opened to the air. If the catheter stylet has been removed, the hub should be occluded either with a syringe or a sterile gloved finger to prevent air entry.

Verifying the CVAD tip placement also prevents potential complications from mechanical trauma of the catheter against the cardiac wall or infusion of fluids, medications, or nutrition into nonvasculature or inappropriate vasculature. The preferred tip placement for all CVADs is at the junction of the superior vena cava and the right atrium. If the tip lies in the right atrium, atrial arrhythmias may occur as a result of the catheter irritating the chamber. Proper placement also decreases the incidence of dislodgment, vessel wall erosion and stenosis, and device dysfunction.

A chest radiograph or fluoroscopy is used to confirm tip placement. Fluoroscopy can be used to verify tip placement if this method is being used to insert the catheter. The chest radiograph, if used, is always obtained immediately after catheter insertion to rule out pneumothorax and to document tip placement. The catheter should not be used until tip placement is confirmed. The site should be observed for any signs of excess bleeding

TABLE 14- POTENTIAL COMPLICATIONS OF CVC INSERTION OR CVADs

Complications	Signs/Symptoms	Treatment
Embolus of Catheter, Thrombus, or Air An embolus can be caused by catheter shearing, dislodgment of a thrombus, or air drawn into the central venous circulation during tubing disconnection.	Dyspnea, tachypnea, hypoxia, cyanosis, tachycardia, hypotension, precordial murmur, chest pain	Emergency situation • For a catheter embolus, apply tourniquet to upper arm. • For thrombus, anticoagulants and thrombolytic agents are ordered. • For air embolus, position the patient on left side in Trendelenburg position and give the patient oxygen (may require air aspiration from right atrium). *Notify physician/LIP immediately.*
Catheter Occlusion • Catheter tip positioned against vein wall or valve • Mechanical: clamped or kinked catheter; tight sutures • Precipitate or lipid buildup • Thrombotic: fibrin tail, fibrin sheath, intraluminal occlusion, mural thrombus—may be due to inadequate flushing	Inability to infuse and/or aspirate; sluggish infusion or aspiration	• Have the patient cough, raise arm, and change position. • Alleviate mechanical cause. • Flush catheter with normal saline using 10-mL syringe. • Consider flow study or other radiologic exam to determine source and site of occlusion. • Consider instillation of precipitate-clearing agent or instillation of thrombolytic agent for clot after discussion with physician/LIP and pharmacist, and with order.
Pinch-off Syndrome Mechanical compression of a CVC catheter by the clavicle and first rib at the costoclavicular space; results in catheter compression or possibly catheter fracture with resultant catheter embolism. Catheter fracture may occur as the catheter weakens owing to the scissoring action of the clavicle and first rib on the catheter (Gorski, 2003a, 2003b).	Difficulty infusing or withdrawing fluids until the patient repositions shoulder or lies supine. Symptoms of catheter fracture and embolism may include chest pain, palpitations, swelling, or pain with flushing.	Chest radiography with the patient upright and arms at side; confirmation is luminal narrowing Catheter may be removed and reinserted carefully to stay within vein.
Thrombosis Related to CVC Compromising Blood Flow Through Superior Vena Cava (Also Known as SVCS) May be caused by malposition of catheter, intima damaged on insertion, irritating drugs, venous stasis, increased blood viscosity, or hypercoagulability	Edema of the entire extremity, upper chest, and neck; tenderness or pain in affected extremity; inability to aspirate blood and/or infuse through the catheter; discoloration of extremity	Venogram to establish diagnosis; thrombolytics, anticoagulants, and elevate extremity CVC may have to be removed.
Catheter-Related Infections May result from contamination during insertion and/or maintenance; seeding from another site; migration of microorganisms along catheter	Local: erythema, induration, tenderness, purulent drainage from site Systemic: fever, chills.	Blood culture from catheter and a peripheral site; remove catheter if indicated; warm moist compresses Appropriate antibiotic therapy may be ordered.

(Continued)

Complications	Signs/Symptoms	Treatment
Damaged Catheter May occur owing to small syringe used with excessive force; use of pins or scissors near catheter; needle puncture; hemostat with teeth used on catheter	Fluid leak from catheter; ruptured catheter; popping sound heard while flushing; burning or pain with flush or infusion	Notify physician/LIP if internally ruptured. Remove catheter. If damage is external, clamp catheter proximal to tear and apply sterile dressing over tear. Repair if possible.
Catheter Tip Migration May happen because of coughing, vomiting, or excessive activity	Referred pain in jaw, ear, or teeth, distended veins on side of malposition; flushing or sense of fullness in head during rapid infusions	Radiograph or flow study to verify tip placement. Consult with physician/LIP to determine next steps.
Mechanical Phlebitis For PICCs, phlebitis at the insertion site is common during the 1st week after insertion. Redness at the IV site usually appears within the first 48 h after insertion and may last the 1st week. The incidence is 12.5%–23%.	Redness along the catheter line without induration, warmth, tenderness, or inflammation. The clinical signs will occur anywhere between the insertion site and the catheter tip location. Other complications (infection, infiltration, or loss of catheter integrity) should be ruled out.	• Warm moist compresses for 60 min three times daily to the affected area for 72 h • Rest and elevation of the extremity • Physician/LIP prescription for PO anti-inflammatory drugs, unless contraindicated For mechanical phlebitis, the catheter may continue to be used for IV therapy. *Observe for improvement within the first 24 h.* Continue heat application until complete resolution occurs, usually within 72 h. • Restrict movements to mild arm activity.
Extravasation From Implanted Port or Pump During Infusion or Cracked Catheter Occurs if noncoring needle not completely inserted into reservoir or it becomes loose or dislodged during infusion of vesicant or irritant drugs; CVC may have cracked owing to excessive flush pressure or scissors/pins used near catheter	May have pain or burning in area, depending on the infusate May have redness, edema, swelling, or difficulty infusing solution	• Prevention is the best intervention: use external catheter for vesicant solutions, infuse only if blood return present or correct needle placement is verified. • Stabilize needle during infusion; check infusion frequently. • Teach the patient signs and symptoms of extravasation with instructions to call nurse if a problem. • If extravasation is suspected: Stop infusion. Aspirate residual drug. Give appropriate antidote. Apply heat or cold as indicated. Notify physician/LIP. Follow up with the patient for observation of site, measure, and photograph site for evaluation.

Adapted from Andris et al. (1997); Arrants, Awillis, Stevens, et al. (1999); Bagnall-Reed (1998); Camp-Sorrell (2011); CDC (2011); Cook (2013); Forauer & Alonzo (2000); Gorski (2003a,2003b).

or swelling, and the patient's breathing should be monitored for any signs of respiratory distress. Abnormal assessments or changes in patient condition should be reported immediately to the physician/LIP who inserted the CVAD, as should complications associated with central line placement.

CVAD DESCRIPTIONS

An extensive description of nontunneled CVADs, PICCs, tunneled CVADs, and implanted ports is presented in Table 14-2. The table also includes insertion technique descriptions and considerations for uses, replacement, and recommendations. Since many nurses insert PICCS, a more complete description is included below, as well as more information on implanted ports and pumps. Once a CVAD is inserted, accurate documentation is critical to ensure communication of the insertion, patient tolerance of the procedure, and a record of the actual device specifications (Box 14-3).

Peripherally Inserted Central Catheters

A CVAD that offers a good choice between a short-term CVC and a long-term CVAD requiring a surgical procedure is a PICC. A PICC is a very small outer diameter catheter but as large as 18 gauge; it can have one to three lumens and is 55 cm long for adults. The length is necessary since it must reach from the area of the antecubital fossa to the superior vena cava. With an increasing need to use one catheter for multiple purposes, including injections for radiologic imaging, certain PICC types can accommodate power injections of up to 300 psi (pounds per square inch) at 5 mL/s (Hadaway, 2010). The power injectable catheters need to be adequately labeled for this purpose. Most catheters are capable of withstanding up to 40 psi. When a power scan is required, a power or pressure injection catheter must be used for the scan.

PICC Advantages and Considerations

The PICC has many advantages for patients and health care providers. These include the following:

- May be inserted at the bedside or in radiology under fluoroscopy by either RNs or physicians/LIPs
- Decreased risk of insertion-related complications compared with other CVADs
- Lower infection rates than other CVADs
- Better suited for young children or the elderly because of the small gauge
- Cost-effective when compared with surgically placed CVADs

A PICC does require patient-related and therapy-related cautions. It is not suitable for rapid, high-volume infusions, and blood sampling may be difficult. A PICC may restrict arm movement as well as the patient's lifestyle and activities. Also, blood pressures and

TABLE 14-2 CVAD DESCRIPTIONS, INSERTION TECHNIQUES, AND CONSIDERATIONS

CVAD	Insertion Techniques	Considerations

Nontunneled CVAD
Large-bore catheter percutaneously inserted directly into the subclavian, internal jugular, or femoral vein
• Length ≥8 cm
• Size: 14–22 gauge
• Single to multiple lumens
• Silicone, polyurethane
• Distal tip openings are open ended
• Options: radiopaque, antimicrobial, or heparin impregnated
	• Inserted by physician/LIP with validated competency
	• Inserted using ultrasound technology for correct placement
	• 15-degree Trendelenburg position assists with vein distension and prevention of air emboli
		• Recommended for short-term use (usually ≤6 wk)
		• Appropriate for multiple therapies:
		  ○ Continuous or intermittent infusions including antibiotics, blood products, vesicants
		  ○ Multiple infusions as well as incompatible infusions
		  ○ CVP monitoring
		  ○ Emergency or critical situations—this catheter can accept rapid and high-volume fluid or medication infusions
		• Subclavian site preferred
		• Routine replacement not recommended
		• Accounts for majority of CRBSIs

PICC Nontunneled CVAD inserted through peripheral arm vein into superior vena cava • Length: ≥20 cm • Size: 16–28 gauge • Single and double lumen • Silicone, polyurethane, or elastomeric hydrogel • Distal openings may be open or closed ended • Options: radiopaque, peripheral port, power injection	• Inserted by physician/LIP or RN with validated competency • Inserted into basilic, cephalic, or median cubital veins • Inserted using ultrasound technology for correct placement	• Recommended for therapy >7 d • Can remain in place for up to a year • Appropriate for multiple therapies: antibiotics, blood products, vesicants • Often the CVAD of choice for home care patients receiving intermittent therapies and frequent blood draws • Adequate flushing is necessary to maintain catheter patency • Lower rate of infections than nontunneled CVADs • If a power PICC is placed, may be used for rapid infusions for diagnostic studies • Gravity flow rates will vary based on the gauge and the PICC material, with flow rates through a silicone catheter being slower than through one made of polyurethane.
Tunneled CVAD Flexible catheter inserted into the subclavian or internal jugular vein with tip in the superior vena cava and then tunneled under the skin exiting distally from insertion site. • Length: 35–100 cm • Size: 2.7–12.5 French • Single to triple lumen • Polyurethane, silicone, or combination • Dacron cuff may have antimicrobial cuff • Distal tip openings are open or closed ended • Three-way safety valve (PASV) available Options: Broviac, Hickman, Groshong, power injection	• Inserted by physician/LIP with validated competency • Inserted using ultrasound technology for correct placemen • Cut down or percutaneous puncture is used to access the vasculature. • From central vasculature, the catheter is tunneled 3–5 cm through subcutaneous tissue to an exit site on the chest. A catheter cuff lies within the subcutaneous tunnel securing the catheter. • Catheter is secured with absorbable sutures at the exit site	• Recommended for frequent or continuous therapy lasting 6 mo or longer • Appropriate for all types of infusion therapies • Fibrous tissue forms around the Dacron cuff, anchors the catheter, and inhibits migration of microorganisms • Lower rate of infections than nontunneled CVADs • Open-ended catheters require clamping; closed-ended or valved catheters do not.

TABLE 14- **CVAD DESCRIPTIONS, INSERTION TECHNIQUES, AND CONSIDERATIONS**   (*Continued*)

CVAD	Insertion Techniques	Considerations
Implanted Ports Tunneled CVAD is attached to an implanted port with a self-sealing septum. The port is implanted into the subcutaneous tissue. • Length: ≥8 cm • Gauge: 4–12 French • Single or dual lumen • Silicone or polyurethane • Port is made of plastic, titanium, polysulfone, stainless steel, or a combination. • The port houses a self-sealing silicone septum. • Diameter of the port body is 16.5–40 mm	• Insertion is similar to tunneled catheter insertion with the additional step of creating a pocket through blunt dissection to accommodate the port. • The port is sutured in the pocket to prevent port movement or from flipping over.	• Septum can withstand 1,000–3,600 punctures, depending on the product. • Port is accessed with special noncoring needle (often a Huber needle) as a sterile procedure. • Access with the smallest needle gauge and length. • Vascular access ports may be side entry or top entry. In a side-entry port, the needle is inserted almost parallel to the reservoir. In a top-entry port, the needle is inserted perpendicular to the reservoir. • Lowest risk for CRBSI • The port does not need site care when not in use. • Flushed monthly when not in use • Port device can cause artifact on diagnostic imaging studies.

Implanted Pumps
Infusion device with a power source, refillable drug reservoir, and catheter that allows drug delivery to an artery, vein, or anatomical space
• Length: 76–114 cm
• Size: 6.5 French
• Single-lumen silicone catheter; may have separate port for direct access to the CVAD. Port is attached to the pump housing.
• Titanium pump and reservoir.
• Pump powered via pressurized gas or lithium battery
• Reservoir volume: 10–60 mL
• Flow rate preset or programmable
• Flow rate: 0.3–21.6 mL/d
• Silicone septum to refill reservoir
• Dose titration: reprogrammable or remove drug and replace with new concentration
• Designed for continuous, low-volume, long-term therapy
• Some uses: intra-arterial infusion to the liver, intrathecal morphine, intrathecal baclofen
	• The pump is implanted surgically under anesthesia, usually in the abdomen, in a subcutaneous pocket just above or below the beltline. The catheter is connected to the pump and tunneled under the skin to the intended delivery site in the body.
	• Pump preparation in the surgical suite is dependent on the type of pump and planned infusate.
		• The patient is evaluated at regular intervals depending on his or her therapy protocol for pump refills and response to therapy.
		• Factors that influence flow rate:
		  ○ Viscosity of solution
		  ○ Arterial pressure on the catheter tip
		• Several factors influence gas-powered pumps:
		  ○ Body temperature
		  ○ Pump reservoir volume
		• MRI should not be done with implanted pumps.
		• Patient education: Importance of returning for refill as scheduled, pump alarms, avoid traumatic physical activity around pump site, symptoms of pump malfunction (symptoms related to type of drug, such as withdrawal symptoms, excessive sedation, increase in underlying symptoms of the disorder, delivery of medication into the pump pocket, increased pain)
		• Use strict aseptic technique when accessing pump.
		• Use only access and refill kits designed for the pump with noncoring needles.
		• Refill procedures are specific to pump.
		• Know the pump model, reservoir size, and flow rate.

Adapted from Camp-Sorrell (2011); CDC (2011); Gorski and Czaplewski (2004).

BOX 14-3   DOCUMENTATION OF CVAD INSERTION AND PROCEDURE OUTCOMES

Documentation supports the continuity of care within and among caregivers and organizations or institutions and on discharge to continuing care or home care. Document the following information as appropriate for each type of device:

- Patient's informed consent (consent obtained prior to insertion)
- Date and time of catheter or device insertion, number and location of attempts, specific vein used, insertion methodology, use of ultrasonography, sedatives, or local anesthetic
- Catheter or device information (as appropriate): type, lumens, manufacturer, lot number, size/original length, actual length inserted, external length
- Function of catheter—ease of flush and quality of blood return
- Fluid currently infusing: type, flow rate, and method of administration or locking solution used and amount
- Appearance of catheter site, site care, and dressing applied
- Method of verifying catheter tip location
- Patient's response to placement
- Patient/caregiver teaching, verification of his or her understanding, and materials given
- A manufacturer's registration card or a hospital information card should be completed for the patient to carry at all times. This card should contain all information about the CVAD or device, such as name of device, serial and model number, type of catheter material, gauge, tip position, frequency of maintenance procedures (flushing, locking, dressing change, or refills), and phone number for concerns or questions

---

blood sampling should not be taken from the arm with a PICC insertion. The presence of any of the following conditions may be a contraindication for a PICC in that extremity:

- Arm contractures, injury, or other musculoskeletal or vascular condition.
- Axillary lymph node dissection, such as in breast cancer surgery, is considered a lifetime precaution for avoiding vascular access in that extremity.
- Affected arm from a stroke or lymphedema
- Vein preservation for possible future arteriovenous fistula for patients with chronic renal insufficiency should be considered.

PICCs Inserted by RNs: Training

Most state boards of nursing permit nurses with specialized training and demonstrated competency to insert PICCs with a physician/LIP's or authorized prescriber's order as a delegated medical act. Many training programs are available; these programs should include

- 4- to 8-hour class with didactic content
- Observation of insertion with three PICC insertion demonstrations by the learner
- Supervision as requested by the learner until ease of insertion and comfort are present

Content should include anatomy and physiology of pertinent structures and vasculature, patient assessment, insertion technique, contraindications to the PICC, possible complications and appropriate interventions, and PICC product information. Last, a thorough understanding of the state Nurse Practice Act is required. A skills competency checklist should be used to determine competencies of nurses who have completed the PICC training program. An annual supervised demonstration of competency ensures ongoing quality and safety for both patient and nurse. Providing patients with information on what to do when at home or in the community empowers patients to participate in their own care (Box 14-4).

BOX 14-4   PATIENT AND CAREGIVERS' GUIDE TO MANAGING PICC PROBLEMS

Problem	Signs and Symptoms	Action
Air enters bloodstream	Shortness of breath, coughing, chest pain	Clamp catheter. Patient should lie on left side with head down. Call Emergency Medical Services (EMS) for assistance.
Catheter breaks or is accidentally cut	Noticeable damage or leakage	Clamp catheter. Notify nurse or physician/LIP.
Access cap disconnects	Blood inside cap or leakage	Clamp catheter and notify nurse. Apply new sterile access cap. Flush catheter as directed.
Evidence of infection	Pain, redness, swelling, fever, drainage at site	Notify health care provider. Keep dressing dry and intact. Avoid infection by using sterile technique as instructed.
Occluded catheter	Resistance is met when infusing medications or when flushing	Stop infusion immediately; do not force it. Call health care provider.
Central vein thrombosis	Swelling around hand, arm, or neck	Call health care provider.
Phlebitis	Small area of redness 7 cm in diameter surrounding insertion site; evidence of tenderness or swelling	Call health care provider; early treatment is necessary (may include warm, moist compresses for 20 minutes four times daily). If no improvement within 24 hours, contact health care provider.

PICC Insertion Techniques

VEIN SELECTION

Veins considered for use for PICC placement are the basilic, median cubital, cephalic, and brachial veins (INS, 2011). The basilic vein is usually the first choice for the peripheral insertion of a CVC. It ascends obliquely in the groove between the biceps brachii and pronator teres and perforates the deep fascia slightly distal to the middle of the upper arm. With the arm held at a 90-degree angle, it forms the straightest, most direct route into the central venous system.

The median cubital vein is the second choice. Ascending on the ulnar side of the forearm, the vein may be divided into two vessels, one joining the basilic vein and the other the cephalic vein. This vein varies substantially, and the proper branch must be ascertained before venipuncture for PICC placement. The median antecubital basilic is preferred.

The cephalic vein runs proximally along the lateral side of the antecubital fossa in the groove between the brachioradialis and the biceps brachii. It becomes a deep vein at the clavipectoral fascia, ending in the axillary vein immediately caudal to the clavicle. It is much more tortuous than the basilic vein and presents a greater potential for catheter tip malposition. It is not preferred because it may also be difficult to thread.

KEY STEPS FOR PICC INSERTIONS

There are several key steps for PICC insertions. Anatomical measurements are taken to determine the length of the catheter required to ensure catheter tip placement in the superior vena cava. Maximal sterile barrier precautions are used. For patients older than 2 months of age, the preferred site preparation is with a 2% chlorhexidine preparation, 3 mL, applied vigorously with friction for 30 seconds and then allowed to air dry completely before insertion.

BREAKAWAY NEEDLE TECHNIQUE

Use of a breakaway needle facilitates venipuncture with an introducer needle. The catheter, with or without a guidewire, is threaded through the introducer. The introducer is removed from the venipuncture site, broken in half, and peeled away. Catheterization technique involves using an introducer needle to place a plastic catheter (peel-away sheath) into the vein. The catheter is then threaded through this sheath. The sheath is removed from the insertion site and peeled away from the catheter.

MICROINTRODUCER ALTERNATIVE TECHNIQUE

As with the guidewire, a modified Seldinger technique is used for inserting a central catheter with the microintroducer. A hydrophilic coating facilitates vascular access device exchanges. Disadvantages include the need for specialized training and additional components compared with standard PICC placement. Potential complications associated with this technique include venous rupture or perforation, arterial puncture, hematoma, and embolization. The clinician should consult product literature and institutional guidelines before using any PICC product.

Ultrasonography

The use of ultrasound for placing peripheral IV catheters has increased the success of PICC insertion and is recommended for insertion use (CDC, 2011). With ultrasonography, the nurse may identify arterial vessels by applying pressure with the probe against the patient's arm and noting the relative ease of vein compression compared with artery compression. The ultrasound device also facilitates visualization of solid material in the lumen of the vessel, such as catheters or thrombus formations. Thus, a comprehensive assessment of cannulated and uncannulated veins is ensured.

Catheter Securement

The PICC must be secured to stabilize the catheter, thus preventing inadvertent dislodgment and catheter migration. Sutureless securement devices are the recommended choice to help reduce the risk of infections (CDC, 2011). Sutures are no longer a preferred option, as they can be a source of infection, cause inflammation and discomfort, and may cause catheter occlusion if they are too tight. Sterile tape secures the catheter well but can be difficult to remove. The adhesive can make the catheter sticky and may harbor microorganisms that could contaminate if used on the catheter itself. Securement devices are specifically designed to stabilize catheters and are safe and effective. A sterile, transparent semipermeable dressing occludes the site. In the initial 24 hours, a gauze dressing under the transparent dressing may be needed for drainage and would be replaced in 24 hours if blood or drainage is present.

Use of a standardized checklist is recommended for placement of a peripherally inserted central, nontunneled catheter (Box 14-5).

Verification of Tip Placement When Inserting PICCs

PICC tip location is verified before initial use. Tip location may be needed in the following clinical situations: difficulty with catheter advancement, pain or discomfort after catheter advancement, inability to obtain positive aspiration of blood, inability to flush the catheter easily, and difficulty in removing guidewire or guidewire is bent on removal.

IMPLANTED PORTS

Components and Features

An implanted port allows access to the central venous system without a catheter exiting the skin. It is the least visible and intrusive device for the patient. Maintenance is monthly, and minimal surveillance is necessary.

The implanted port may have one or two portals with a separate self-sealing septum for each portal, accessed with a noncoring needle. Ports are used for medication administration into the vascular system as well as into specific body cavities. The port is connected to a catheter; the tip may be placed into the superior vena cava as a CVC, or it may be placed into other structures, such as the peritoneum or pleural cavity. When the port is connected to a CVC, the same potential for complications exists as for other CVADs.

BOX 14-5 STANDARDIZED CHECKLIST FOR PLACEMENT OF A NONTUNNELED PICC

1. Perform hand hygiene with antiseptic soap.
2. Identify known patient allergies.
3. Explain the procedure and rationale to the patient.
4. Obtain consent.
5. Assess the patient.
6. Assemble equipment and use maximal sterile barrier precautions with insertion (CDC, 2011).
7. Observe standard precautions throughout the procedure.
8. Position the patient.
9. Remove excess hair from the intended insertion site with clippers or scissors.
10. Cleanse the intended insertion site with a chlorhexidine preparation (CDC, 2011); if an allergy to chlorhexidine is present, alternative antiseptic solutions include tincture of iodine, an iodophor, or 70% alcohol (CDC, 2011).
11. Stabilize catheter after placement and attach securement device.
12. Dress the access site with sterile gauze if drainage is present and cover with sterile, transparent, semipermeable dressing.
13. Secure connection junctions.
14. Before initiating therapy, radiographically confirm catheter placement in the superior vena cava.
15. Initiate prescribed therapy.
16. Discard used equipment in appropriate receptacles.
17. Document the procedure.

Ports can come as a power injectable device allowing for the injection of contrast media for contrast-enhanced computed tomography (CECT). CECT scans allow for better visualization in tracking tumor markers or visualizing pulmonary embolisms. They also allow for better visualization of soft tissues. Injecting the contrast media at a high rate improves the result of the scan. This process or technique is referred to as power injection.

The implanted port comes with preattached or separate catheters. It is important that surgical staff know that special noncoring needles should be used to verify patency of the port (Figures 14-7 and 14-8). Additionally, a needle guard covers the area where the catheter connects to the port, protecting the catheter from inadvertent puncture during access. Implanted ports may be made with titanium or a plastic body. Magnetic resonance imaging (MRI) should not be done with titanium-implanted ports. Implanted ports with a plastic body were designed to be compatible with MRI and to eliminate interference caused by metal ports. When a port is implanted, the patient is given a card stating the type of port that was implanted, the placement of the catheter tip, and any precautions that must be observed.

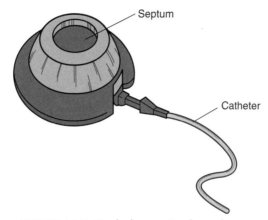

FIGURE 14-7 Single-lumen implanted port.

Implanted Peripheral Port

An implanted peripheral port is an option when continuous infusions are not required, but frequent venous access is needed. The device consists of a small, flat port with a self-sealing septum, accessible by percutaneous needle puncture, and a catheter for the parenteral delivery of medications and fluids. The catheter tip ending in the superior vena cava is considered a CVC. These ports are accessed in the same manner as other implanted vascular access

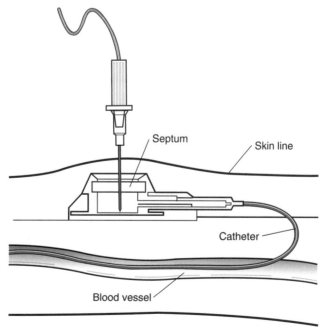

FIGURE 14-8 Cross-section of implanted port with noncoring needle inserted.

devices located on the chest wall. Depending on the material of the implanted peripheral port, plastic or titanium, it may be MRI compatible.

Noncoring Needles

Implanted ports or implanted pumps must be accessed only by noncoring needles. These needles are often referred to as Huber needles as this is a common brand name for this type of needle. A noncoring needle has an angled or deflected point that slices the septum on entry. When removed, the septum reseals itself. Noncoring needles are available in straight and 90-degree angle configurations, with or without extension sets.

Noncoring needles at a 90-degree angle are used for continuous or frequent intermittent infusions. Noncoring needles are also available with a permanently attached extension tubing and clamp and are preferred. A needleless connector cap should be attached to the end of the tubing of the noncoring needle. The port can then be accessed with any Luer lock syringe or tubing for saline flushes, heparin flushes, bolus injection, or blood drawing.

Needles are available with metal or plastic hubs, in gauges 24 to 19, and in lengths from 0.5 to 2.5 inches. The required needle length depends on how superficially or deeply the septum lies. The needle gauge depends on the type and rate of infusate to be given. Packed red blood cells may require a 20-gauge needle, whereas a 24-gauge needle may be adequate for flushing. The needle must meet safety specifications.

Accessing and Deaccessing Implanted Ports

Access an implanted port with the smallest needle gauge appropriate for therapy and length sufficient to touch the backstop of the implanted port body. Needles that are too short can become dislodged and may lead to infiltration and extravasations when the needle is infusing into tissue.

Prior to accessing an implanted port, it is important for the nurse to explain the procedure to the patient. Some patients have anxiety related to the accessing procedure due to the insertion of the noncoring needle and may want something to help decrease the discomfort. Although most patients do not require anything, some patients would prefer the use of a topical anesthetic cream prior to the procedure. If this is used, it is important to leave the cream on for the recommended amount of time to obtain the greatest effect from the anesthetic. A cold pack can also be used to numb the area before insertion.

Accessing an implanted port is a sterile procedure and requires sterile gloves, a sterile noncoring needle, extension set if used, a needleless connector or access cap, a 0.9% normal saline flush, a chlorhexidine swab or sponge, and sterile 2 × 2 or 4 × 4 gauze, tape, or a sterile, transparent, semipermeable dressing if the needle is to remain in place.

Inserting a noncoring needle into an implanted port is a common procedure. Follow the steps in Box 14-6. If the needle is to remain in place, dress the insertion site with a sterile, transparent, semipermeable dressing. The noncoring needle may stay in the implanted port for up to 7 days.

If the implanted port will be deaccessed and not used, the nurse will flush with 0.9% normal saline followed by a heparin lock (100 unit/mL). If the heparin flush is performed without extension tubing, 3 mL of heparin solution is used. If extension tubing is used, 5 mL of heparin solution may be required.

The implanted port is deaccessed by first removing the dressing, and gauze if present, with clean gloves. Stabilize the implanted port with the nondominant hand; grasp the

BOX 14-6 PROCEDURE TO ACCESS AN IMPLANTED PORT

1. Perform hand hygiene.
2. Explain the procedure and rationale to the patient.
3. Palpate the implanted port to identify the septum for needle insertion.
4. Cleanse the insertion site and surrounding skin with a chlorhexidine solution swab or pad with friction for 30 seconds; allow to dry completely.
5. Put on sterile gloves, attach the extension set and needleless connector to the non-coring needle and flush with 0.9% normal saline to prime the tubing and the non-coring needle while maintaining sterility.
6. Stabilize the implanted port with the nondominant hand; holding the noncoring needle in the dominant hand, push the noncoring needle into the implanted port with one smooth, steady motion (accessing the port). The noncoring needle will have wings similar to a butterfly needle to hold on to. An angular motion or twist of the needle must be avoided once the needle is seated in the septum to prevent cutting the septum and creating a path for medication leakage.
7. The nurse will feel the noncoring needle touch the back stop of the implanted port.
8. Aspirate for blood return; if blood is seen, then vigorously flush the implanted port with the normal saline.
9. Gauze may be place under the wings of the noncoring needle as a cushion. It is important not to block visibility of the insertion site with the gauze.

wings of the noncoring needle with the dominant hand and pull back in a straight, smooth motion until the noncoring needle is removed. The safety mechanism may be activated upon removal based on the manufacturer's design or it may need to be activated by the nurse and then placed in a sharps container. The nurse needs to be aware of the manufacturer's recommendations in terms of how the products are used; these recommendations can assist in developing institutional policy.

IMPLANTED INFUSION PUMP

Over the years, various models of implanted pumps have been developed and tested. They have been used to infuse opioids, anesthetics, antineoplastic agents, and insulin. Additionally, the catheter tip may end in the vascular system, venous or arterial, or other body spaces. Technology is ever-evolving; thus, it is important that the nurse who is called upon to care for a patient with such a pump, and safely manage this device, understand the particular pump that is implanted, where the tip terminates, and the infusate that is being administered.

Components and Features

The implanted infusion pump contains a power source and refillable drug reservoir; many times, there is a programmable mechanism as well. The infusion pump is powered by a replaceable battery. The battery life extends for 5 to 7 years, depending on the volume of infusion, frequency of reprogramming, and other factors.

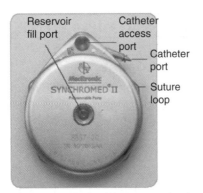
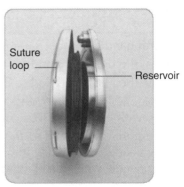

FIGURE 14-9 Exterior front and side view of Synchromed II implantable pump. (Reprinted with the permission of Medtronic, Inc. © 2012.)

The implanted pump may have a direct-access side port that bypasses the reservoir for administering bolus injections as well as the drug reservoir administering medication (Figure 14-9). The silicone catheter results in a low incidence of thrombus formation. Delivering medications by pump is an excellent method for continuous long-term administration of low-volume infusates, such as analgesics or antineoplastic agents. The pump must have some solution infusing to prevent occlusion; otherwise, it requires no care between refills. Accurate fill and refill records are essential to ensure that the pump is refilled at the required intervals; these records also document appropriate pump functioning.

Contraindications

Contraindications to the implanted pump include body size that cannot support the size and weight of the pump. In addition, an implanted pump can deliver only small volumes of drugs, so the device is unsuitable for patients needing large volumes of medication.

MAINTENANCE OF CENTRAL VENOUS ACCESS DEVICES

Site Assessment

The catheter–skin junction (insertion) site should be inspected, assessed, and palpated for tenderness daily through the intact dressing (CDC, 2011). Regular site inspection and standardized dressing changes should minimize the incidence of CRBSI. If there is tenderness at the site, fever without known source, drainage, or symptoms of local or systemic infection, the dressing should be removed and the site inspected directly. Signs of CVAD-related complications include pain, redness, swelling, induration, tenderness, drainage, fever, chills, and inability to infuse or withdraw. Documentation should reflect routine assessment. Patient/caregiver education on assessment parameters can be provided as assessment is being performed.

Site Care

Organizations should have established policies and procedures regarding the maintenance of CVADs. Maintaining a clean, dry, and occlusive dressing is one of the most important mechanisms to prevent infection in CVADs. There are four possible routes of contamination of a CVAD. The most common routes are migration of organisms from the skin at the insertion site to the catheter and then into the vascular system and direct contamination of the catheter or catheter hub by contaminated hands, fluids, or devices. Less common routes include infections spread hematogenously from another area of infection, and contaminated infusates (CDC, 2011). CVADs are associated with a higher rate of CRBSIs than other catheters, and most of the organisms appear to originate from the patient's skin (Gillies et al., 2005).

Thus, the use of an antiseptic solution for cleansing and a sterile dressing is necessary in the maintenance of CVADs. A 2% chlorhexidine with 70% isopropyl alcohol preparation is recommended for cleansing with a 30-second scrub time over the insertion site and area under the dressing. If the patient has allergies or sensitivity to this solution, 1% to 2% tincture of iodine, povidone–iodine, or 70% alcohol may be used (CDC, 2011; INS, 2011).

Dressings

A sterile dressing is applied following cleansing with an appropriate solution. Sterile gauze, with edges secured with occlusive material, or sterile, transparent semipermeable membrane dressings are recommended. Evidence is inconsistent to support a recommendation of one dressing over the other (INS, 2011).

Gauze dressings are recommended if the site is bleeding or oozing; they should be changed every 48 hours. There is often bleeding at the insertion site (or exit site for a tunneled catheter) within the first 24 hours of insertion, so a gauze dressing is often put under the transparent dressing. If this is the case, it is considered a gauze dressing and must be changed within 48 hours or sooner. With bleeding and oozing, it is critical to visually inspect the site and change the dressing if needed. After this first dressing change, it may not be necessary to use gauze. The patient may be able to have only the transparent dressing.

Transparent dressings allow for better assessment of the insertion site. They should be changed every 7 days. The dressing should be changed immediately if the integrity of the dressing is compromised (it is wet, soiled, or loose). The routine use of antimicrobial ointment at the insertion or catheter exit site is not recommended (CDC, 2011).

The dressing change procedure may be modified for the tunneled catheter. If the patient is immunosuppressed or if site healing is not complete, the same care given to the nontunneled catheter may be used for this catheter. If the patient is not immunosuppressed and site healing is complete, site care may be limited to daily inspection and cleansing with soap and water while bathing (CDC, 2011). Site preparation prior to accessing the port includes 2% chlorhexidine for a 30-second friction rub and aseptic technique. If the access needle is left in place, a sterile transparent dressing is used to cover the port/pump access site.

The dressing protects the CVAD site, but it can also be a source of skin damage, up to 20% incidence for the older population (Thayer, 2012). Two common types of skin damage are skin stripping and tension blisters. Skin stripping occurs with the removal of adhesive dressings, from careless removal, extra adhesion skin barriers, or due to fragile skin. Tension blisters are a result of a pressure dressing; in the case of CVAD dressing, it could be to stop drainage or bleeding. In either case, on the removal of the dressing, the adhesive tears away the top layer of skin or dermis (Thayer, 2012). The nurse is in an excellent position to prevent skin damage and monitor its occurrence to detect any trends due to a possibly new product or procedure.

CHLORHEXIDINE-IMPREGNATED SPONGES

A chlorhexidine-impregnated sponge may be used at the insertion site under the transparent dressing after cleansing. They are recommended for use in patients where the rate of CRBSIs is not decreasing and a comprehensively implemented strategy to decrease rates of CRBSIs is ineffective. Evidence does not recommend the routine use of these sponges (CDC, 2011).

Biopatch (Ethicon 360) is an example of this sponge. It is a quarter-sized disk and placed around a central line insertion site. It contains polyurethane, absorptive foam, and chlorhexidine gluconate, a well-known antiseptic agent with antimicrobial and antifungal properties. Highly absorbent, this disk stays in place and inhibits growth of bacteria for up to 7 days. When applied to a CVAD site, the sponge may help to reduce catheter tip colonization and bloodstream infection. As with all products, follow the manufacturer's directions for application and removal. The most common maintenance procedures for CVADs are summarized in Table 14-3.

Needleless Connectors and Access Caps

Over the last several years, many products related to the maintenance of infusion therapy have entered the market. Different health care organizations use different products, and the variety has caused some confusion in terms of what to call the products and how they are used. It has been proposed that the term *needleless connector* be used for any add-on device that allows connection to a catheter with potential for blood contact. Because of the possibility of blood contact, needleless devices are required to be used (Hadaway & Richardson, 2010). **Add-on devices** are any device added to the catheter or to the tubing in relation to the patient's therapy. These were formerly known as injection caps. Some examples of add-on devices would be extension sets, in-line filters, extension loops, and stopcocks.

It is recommended that all CVADs have a Luer lock needleless connector or access cap in place. The Luer lock design allows for leak free fitting between the "female" hub of the catheter and the "male" end of a cap, which screw together. Luer lock products are recommended for any device that is attached to the cap, tubing, or other add-on device used with a CVAD (CDC, 2011; INS, 2011). This prevents accidental detachment of any item attached to the CVAD or tubing. The hubs of a CVAD should not be directly hooked to any IV tubing without a needleless connector, or access cap, in place. It is not recommended to tape catheter connections. Health care personnel need to be responsible for knowing their organization's policies and procedures related to CVAD maintenance, and they must also know the manufacturer's recommendation with the products they are using.

Access caps or needleless connectors can be simple or complex. The simple caps have no internal mechanisms. They may require a blunt tip on the end of a syringe or tubing to access the cap. Complex access caps have an internal mechanical valve. Needleless connectors can also be described by how they function in relation to fluid displacement. There are currently three different types of access caps related to function: they are negative fluid displacement caps, positive fluid displacement caps, and neutral caps (Table 14-4).

Negative fluid displacement access caps allow for blood to be pulled back into the end of the catheter with removal of a syringe or tubing. The flushing technique of maintaining pressure upon the syringe during removal is needed to keep blood from refluxing back into the catheter and causing a possible occlusion. Positive fluid displacement access caps work

TABLE 14-3	CVAD MAINTENANCE PROCEDURES: DRESSING AND CAP CHANGE, FLUSHING, LOCKING			
CVAD	Dressing/Access Cap Change	Flushing	Locking	Special Instructions for Blood Sampling and Accessing
Nontunneled CVAD	**Dressing:** Change every 7 d if a sterile transparent, semipermeable membrane (e.g., Tegaderm®) is used Change every 48 h if gauze is used. Maintain aseptic technique, use "either clean or sterile gloves" (CDC, 2011, p. S4) Change securement device with dressing **Access Cap:** Change with administration set or every 7 d and prn (no more frequently than every 72 h)	5 mL of 0.9% NaCl before and after infusions If not used: Nonvalved catheter: flush every 24 h Valved catheter: flush weekly	2 mL of 10 units/mL heparin per lumen per day (Camp-Sorrell, 2011) Heparin not required for valved CVAD	Flush with 5 mL of 0.9% NaCl predraw; discard a minimum of 4–5 mL of blood to clear infusate (do not reinfuse blood (INS, 2011, p. S79)). Flush 10 mL of 0.9% NaCl postdraw. Follow with lock solution if catheter is not used.
Tunneled CVAD Nonvalved: Broviac, Hickman Valved: Groshong	**Dressing:** Change every 7 d if transparent dressing is used Change every 48 h if gauze is used. Maintain aseptic technique, use "either clean or sterile gloves" (CDC, 2011, p. S4) Change securement device with dressing **Access Cap:** Change with administration set or every 7 d and prn (no more frequently than every 72 h)	5 mL of 0.9% NaCl Before and after infusions If not used: Nonvalved: one to two times per week Valved: weekly	5 mL of 10 units/mL heparin three times per week (Camp-Sorrell, 2011) Heparin not required for valved CVAD	Flush with 5 mL of 0.9% NaCl predraw; discard a minimum of 4–5 mL of blood to clear infusate (do not reinfuse blood (INS, 2011, p. S79)). Flush 10 mL of 0.9% NaCl postdraw. Follow with lock solution if catheter is not used.

(Continued)

| TABLE 14-3 | CVAD MAINTENANCE PROCEDURES: DRESSING AND CAP CHANGE, FLUSHING, LOCKING *(Continued)* | | | |

CVAD	Dressing/Access Cap Change	Flushing	Locking	Special Instructions for Blood Sampling and Accessing
PICC May be nonvalved or valved (Groshong PICC)	**Dressing:** Change every 7 d if transparent dressing is used Change every 48 h if gauze is used. Maintain aseptic technique; use "either clean or sterile gloves" (CDC, 2011, p. S4) Change securement device with dressing **Access Cap:** Change with administration set or every 7 d and prn (no more frequently than every 72 h)	5 mL of 0.9% NaCl before and after infusions If not used: Nonvalved: every 24 h Valved: weekly	3 mL of 10 units/mL heparin three times per week (Camp-Sorrell, 2011) Heparin not required for valved PICC	Flush with 5 mL of 0.9% NaCl predraw; discard a minimum of 4–5 mL of blood to clear infusate (do not reinfuse blood (INS, 2011, p. S79)). Flush 10 mL of 0.9% NaCl postdraw. Follow with lock solution if catheter is not used. Vacutainer may collapse catheter; follow institutional policy for use.
Implanted Ports	**Dressing:** For an accessed port: Change the dressing and noncoring needle every 7 d if a transparent dressing is used and if a gauze dressing is used with a visible access site. Maintain aseptic technique (mask, sterile gloves). **Access Cap:** Change with a new noncoring needle and tubing (no more frequently than every 72 h).	Accessed port: 5 mL 0.9% NaCl before and after infusions Accessed but not used: Nonvalved: 1–2 times per week Valved: weekly Deaccessed: monthly	5 mL of 100 units/mL heparin monthly Heparin not required for valved port Deaccessed: monthly after NaCl flush	Flush with 5 mL of 0.9% NaCl predraw; discard a minimum of 4–5 mL of blood to clear infusate (do not reinfuse blood (INS, 2011, p. S79)). Flush 10 mL of 0.9% NaCl postdraw. Follow with lock solution if port is not used. Change noncoring needle every 7 d.

Note for all CVADs:
Change any dressing that is damp, loosened, soiled.
Disinfect access cap with alcohol *using vigorous scrub for 15 seconds* prior to access (Alexander et al., 2010, p. 503; Guerin et al., 2010).
Adapted from Alexander et al. (2010); Camp-Sorrell (2011); CDC (2011); INS (2011).

TABLE 14- NEEDLELESS CONNECTORS OR ACCESS CAPS

Type of Cap	Cap Description	Flushing Applications
Neutral Caps • Luer-activated valve Examples: InVision-Plus (RyMed Technologies), MicroClave (ICU Medical), One-Link (Baxter)	Prevents fluid from moving into or out of the catheter when a syringe or tubing is disconnected; there is no flow or a "neutral" flow • Luer activated • Some types have directions for saline only flushes, thus eliminating the need for a heparin lock. • Disinfect prior to use.	Function of the valve is *NOT* dependent on the flushing technique.
Negative Displacement *Caps*: **Two types**	Blood can move into the catheter end when syringe or tubing is disconnected and the catheter is NOT clamped, causing negative fluid displacement.	For both types: • Requires positive-pressure flushing technique Clamp tubing *after* flushing and *before* removing syringe.
• Split Septum Example: Interlink (Baxter)	• Requires blunt adapter tip attached to tubing or syringe in order to access split septum negative displacement cap • Accepts needles • Disinfect prior to use	
• Mechanical Valve Examples: Antimicrobial Clave (ICU Medical), Clearlink (Baxter), SmartSite (CareFusion)	• Luer-activated mechanism • Does not accept needles • Disinfect prior to use	
Positive Displacement Caps • Luer-activated valve Examples: CLC2000 (ICU Medical), Flolink (Baxter), MaxPlus (Maximus), Posiflow (BD Medical), SmartSite (CareFusion)	Has a fluid reservoir, within cap, that releases fluid into the catheter when a syringe or tubing is disconnected, causing positive fluid displacement • Some types have directions for saline only flushes, thus eliminating the need for a heparin lock. • Disinfect prior to use	• *DO NOT* use positive-pressure flushing technique. This will override the fluid reservoir and permit blood to move back into the catheter. • Clamp catheter *after* flushing AND *after* removal of tubing or syringe.

Needleless connectors should be changed with the administration set or weekly (no more than every 72 h).
Adapted from Alexander et al. (2010); CDC (2011); Hadaway (2006); Hadaway and Richardson (2010).

by producing positive fluid displacement when a syringe or tubing is removed from the access cap thus preventing blood from backing up into the catheter. Therefore, it is important to wait to clamp the tubing until after the syringe or tubing is removed, otherwise blood will reflux into the catheter and possibly cause an occlusion. Neutral displacement caps prevent blood reflux into the catheter during connection and disconnection through use of positive pressure (Hadaway & Richardson, 2010).

The needleless connector must be changed at routine intervals but no more frequently than every 72 hours. They are often changed with the tubing (CDC, 2011). It is generally recommended that needleless connectors on CVADs be changed at least as frequently as the administration set changes, usually every 96 hours (CDC, 2011). These devices should also be changed when residual blood remains within the connector or cap before blood cultures are drawn or when contaminated (INS, 2011).

If the catheter has more than one lumen, the nurse needs to change the needleless connectors on all unused lumens. If the catheter is made of a material that cannot be clamped without catheter damage, the patient needs to lie flat in bed and perform the Valsalva maneuver whenever the cap is changed to prevent an air embolism.

PATIENT SAFETY

It is important for the nurse to know what type of access cap is on the CVAD since it will impact how the nurse flushes and locks the CVAD. This reduces the risk of occlusion and infection.

Alcohol Wipes and Caps

All access ports and caps should be disinfected prior to use. Friction should be used while disinfecting the port or cap. The preferred type of disinfecting agent (70% isopropyl alcohol, chlorhexidine, povidone–iodine, or an iodophor) and preferred technique in using them are also unresolved issues (CDC, 2011; INS, 2011). The most common product used is an alcohol pad (70% isopropyl alcohol). A new pad should be used to cleanse each port if more than one port or cap is accessed.

The preferred length of time used to disinfect a cap or port is an unresolved issue based on the current available research, but evidence is accumulating that swabbing for <10 seconds is not adequate (Menyhay & Maki, 2006; Smith et al., 2012). Currently, the phrase "scrub the hub" has been used in clinical and educational settings with a recommendation of scrubbing the hub of a port or access cap for 15 seconds prior to each access of the cap or port (Alexander, Corrigan, Gorski, Hankins, & Perucca, 2010, p. 503; Guerin et al., 2010). Although this evidence has been communicated, an observational and qualitative study reported nurses' challenges to adhere to best practices. One quote from the study may not be an isolated belief, "I don't scrub the hub for 15 seconds, and I know of no nurse that would do that" (Morrison, 2012, p. 325). The agency in this study implemented best practices to prevent central line–associated bloodstream infection (CLABSI), including "underscoring the nurses' individual role and accountability" in preventing CVAD infections (p. 327). The steps in the infection program were listed, and CLABSI was reduced, and the reduction was sustained.

A newer category of disinfecting products on the market are disinfecting caps. The single-use caps are permeated with 70% isopropyl alcohol. The caps are used to disinfect the ports or access cap rather than an alcohol pad. A cap is put on each access cap and port when not in use. When the cap or port is accessed, it is simply removed without the need to cleanse the cap again. After the cap or port is used, a new cap is put in place and left on until it is used again. It is thought that keeping the cap in place will protect the cap or port from touch or airborne contamination. The orange SwabCap by Excelsior Medical Corporation and the green Curos Port Protector by Ivera Medical are two examples of disinfecting caps. The Site-Scrub IPA device by Bard is a single blue cap meant to be used in place of an alcohol pad and does not stay on the access cap or port (Figure 14-10). Further research is needed to determine if these products are superior to the traditional alcohol prep pad.

Catheter Stabilization

Catheter securement by the use of tape is no longer recommended. The use of stabilization devices for all CVADs is recommended as their use helps to prevent infection and irritation at the catheter exit site (CDC, 2011; INS, 2011). Various products are on the market for non-tunneled, PICC, tunneled, and port CVAD securement.

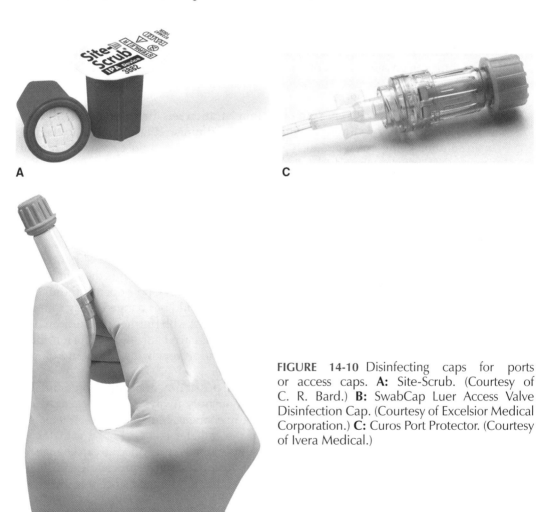

FIGURE 14-10 Disinfecting caps for ports or access caps. **A:** Site-Scrub. (Courtesy of C. R. Bard.) **B:** SwabCap Luer Access Valve Disinfection Cap. (Courtesy of Excelsior Medical Corporation.) **C:** Curos Port Protector. (Courtesy of Ivera Medical.)

Catheter Clamps

Smooth-jaw clamps are used when tunneled silicone catheters are placed to prevent damage to the catheter material. Ideally, the clamp is applied to the distal two thirds portion of the external catheter. If clamp damage should occur, catheter repair is easily facilitated in this area. Clamp sites should be alternated to prevent weakening an area on the catheter itself. Second-generation silastic catheters use integral, soft-jaw clamps.

Administration Sets and Add-On Devices

When using IV administration sets or tubing and any add-on devices, the nurse needs to make sure items are compatible with the administration system they are using. There is a risk of contamination whenever a new device is added or when tubing or caps are changed. It is also important to trace all catheters, administration sets, and add-on devices from the patient to the point of origin before adding any new devices. The system should be opened as few times as possible. Ports on the tubing or access caps need to be disinfected with 70% alcohol before each access. The access port or access cap should only be accessed with a sterile device (INS, 2011).

Recommendations for changing IV administration sets are based on whether the tubing is used continuously or intermittently. Primary administration set refers to the primary or main solution being infused, which is usually a hydration fluid. Secondary administration sets are shorter in length and are usually used for medications; they are often attached to one of the hubs of the primary set.

Primary and secondary continuous administration sets that are used to administer fluids other than blood products or lipids should be changed no more frequently than every 96 hours (4 days) (CDC, 2011). If the secondary administration set is detached at all from the primary set, it is an intermittent set and should be changed every 24 hours. Primary and secondary intermittent administration sets should be changed every 24 hours (INS, 2011). A new sterile, compatible cover needs to be attached to the end of the administration set after each intermittent use. It cannot be left to hang on the IV pole open to the air (INS, 2011).

Administration sets used to administer lipids should be changed every 24 hours (CDC, 2011). The standards and other publications from the AABB (formerly, American Association of Blood Banks) (2009, 2010, 2011) should be referenced for all transfusion information, administration set and filter change frequency, and in reviewing blood and blood component administration.

The IV nurse must always keep in mind the possibility of negative pressure with a central catheter. Therefore, the risk of an air embolism is always present when the catheter is open to the air during needleless connector cap changes. Make sure the catheter is clamped prior to cap changes or tubing changes. If the catheter is a Groshong catheter without a clamp, the patient should perform the Valsalva maneuver during the cap change.

Many times the extension set is attached during the sterile procedure of CVC insertion. If this is the case, the extension set may not need to be changed since it is integral with the

PATIENT SAFETY

Do not leave unprimed administration sets or tubing attached to the container at the bedside (Cook, 2013).

CVC. Between changes of components, the system should be maintained as a closed system. All entries into the system should be made through access caps that have been disinfected immediately before use.

Looping the tubing and taping it to the chest wall prevents any related stress to the connection or insertion site when the tubing is pulled or inadvertently stretched. Tape used for CVADs should be designated for each patient to decrease the spread of infection. All connections should use Luer-locking connections, consistent with INS Standards of Practice and CDC guidelines. The procedure for CVAD dressing change is outlined in Table 14-5.

Infusion Containers and Admixtures

All recommendations for peripheral containers or admixtures should be strictly adhered to for CVAD usage. To prevent risks of contamination, all manipulations for admixture and container changes must be performed with strict adherence to aseptic technique. Single-dose use is recommended for all medications and flushes pertaining to IV infusion.

Catheter Flushing and Locking

Adequate flushing is the most important factor in preventing blood, fibrin, and drug precipitates from building up and causing occlusions. Prior to use, a CVAD will be assessed by aspirating for a blood return and flushing with preservative-free 0.9% normal saline. After

---

TABLE 14-5   DRESSING CHANGE AND SITE CARE FOR CVADs

---

1. Obtain dressing materials or prepackaged kit and prepare a clean table for a work area.
2. Position the patient comfortably.
3. Perform hand hygiene; have the patient turn head away from CVAD side or have the patient wear a mask if he or she is unable to move the head away from the site of the CVAD dressing area. Put on clean gloves. There are no recommendations from the CDC (2011) to use a mask during the dressing change.
4. Carefully remove the old dressing. Gently lifting the tape from the outside edges inward toward the center prevents stress at the insertion site. Discard dressing and gloves. Do not touch the insertion site.
5. Inspect the catheter insertion site for signs of discharge or leakage. Inspect the catheter to ensure that the sutures are intact (if there are sutures), that the length of the external portion has not increased, and that the catheter and hub are intact.
6. Perform hand hygiene.
7. Open the kit. The overlay provides a sterile field.
8. Don sterile gloves. Arrange your items for the dressing.
9. Clean all debris from the insertion site and from the portion of the catheter close to the site with an alcohol swab if required by the agency. Clean the site with 2% chlorhexidine in back-and-forth fashion with friction scrub for 30 s; allow the skin to dry completely. (Do not create a breeze with your hand or other item.)
10. Apply transparent dressing or a gauze dressing with a transparent dressing over it. Maintain aseptic technique throughout the procedure.
11. Inspect the catheter hub–tubing connection to ensure that it is clamped. You may loop the tubing and tape it to the chest wall to prevent stress at the connection or insertion site when the tubing is pulled or stretched. Use tape that is designated for that patient.
12. Initial and date the dressing change label and apply it to the dressing. Do not cover the insertion site.

Remember to review institutional or agency policy and procedure before performing site care.

each infusion, the CVAD will be flushed again with preservative-free 0.9% normal saline to clear the medication from the lumen to prevent contact between incompatible solutions. After the final flush, the CVAD should be "locked" (formally known as capped) to decrease the risk of occlusion (INS, 2011).

The push/pause or pulsing flushing technique, rather than even syringe pressure, is recommended to create a turbulent flow. Using a positive-end pressure technique while flushing, such as clamping catheter while continuing pressure on syringe, minimizes blood reflux into the lumen that may result in catheter clotting (INS, 2011). This technique involves injecting the flush solution and clamping the catheter before the syringe is completely empty. Then, the syringe and needle are removed while pressure is applied on the plunger. Of course, this technique changes when a positive-pressure access valve is in place.

Care must be taken when administering solutions and flushing through a CVC because excessive pressure can be generated from a small syringe. The manufacturer of the specific device outlines the maximum recommended pressure in psi. The smaller the size of the syringe used to flush the catheter, the greater the pressure in psi exerted on the catheter. Pressure in excess of 40 psi may cause catheter rupture with possible embolization. A wide-barrel syringe (diameter of 10 mL), which exerts <10 psi, is recommended for use with all CVCs to avoid excessive pressure when administering medication and flushing the catheter.

PATENCY AND LOCKING SOLUTIONS FOR CVCS

CVC locking solutions and frequencies depend on the devices' characteristics, uses, and institutional policy. Heparin sodium is a protein that inhibits the conversion of prothrombin to thrombin and fibrinogen to fibrin, thus inhibiting coagulation. A recent study indicates that preservative-free 0.9% sodium chloride as a locking solution is as effective as heparin (Schallom, Prentice, Sona, Micek, & Skrupky, 2012). Preservative-free 0.9% sodium chloride (normal saline) has approximately the same osmotic pressure and composition as extracellular fluid and is thus an ideal solution for flushing blood and infusate from catheters. Preservative-free 0.9% sodium chloride is the only flush solution used for Groshong catheters that have the specialized closed-tip three-way valve. With potential adverse effects from heparin, normal saline may be recommended for short-term CVADs, although many authors still recommend heparin (Camp-Sorrell, 2011; Gorski, Perucca, & Hunter, 2010; INS, 2008).

Flush solutions should be at least two times the internal volume of the catheter (INS, 2011). For almost all CVCs, 3 mL is an adequate amount to use as a flush solution. Using a prefilled syringe reduces the risk of touch contamination during preparation but should not be used to dilute medications (INS, 2011). Use one syringe for initial flushing and another syringe for the final flush or lock, preventing risk of contamination from re-use.

Implanted ports require heparin flushing after each use and monthly when not in use. This recommended dose is 5 mL of 100 unit/mL of heparin. Positive pressure must be maintained when withdrawing the needle to avoid reflux of blood into the catheter.

A potential problem of overheparinization exists when devices are locked frequently with heparin solution, ranging from one to six times per day. The nurse needs to recognize this increased risk. It is recommended to lock the device with normal saline when the device is accessed frequently during a 24-hour period. INR/PT may need to be monitored for these patients. Special note should be made on the plan of care to revert to the usual locking order when the frequency matches the order. See Table 14-3 for regular maintenance and flushing procedures.

ADDITIONAL RECOMMENDATIONS

The CDC does not recommend routine use of antibiotics as a prophylactic measure to prevent infection or the use of antibiotic lock solutions. The CDC recommends the following: *Use prophylactic antimicrobial lock solution in patients with long-term catheters who have a history of multiple CRBSI despite optimal maximal adherence to aseptic technique.* The CDC (2011) also does not recommend the use of anticoagulation therapy as a prophylactic measure to prevent CVAD occlusion.

Venous Sampling

Many CVADs are placed in patients who do not have peripheral veins available or who need multiple venipunctures for blood sampling. Therefore, drawing blood specimens through CVADs is common practice. Because each catheter is different, the nurse must follow the manufacturer's instructions for use and adhere to institutional policy that should be evidence based. The withdrawal of blood through a CVAD can contribute to thrombotic catheter occlusion when the catheter is not flushed adequately.

To withdraw a blood sample, the syringe can be attached directly to the needleless connector. Check with the manufacturer's directions to see if the needleless connector needs to be changed after blood withdrawal. An evacuated tube (e.g., Vacutainer) can be used to draw blood samples with most catheters. The specific catheter's specifications should be checked to confirm that it can withstand the pressure without collapsing.

The first aspirate of blood is discarded to reduce the risk of drug concentration or a diluted specimen. Reinfusion of this aspirate is not recommended owing to the risk of introducing clots into the system. The following key steps should be part of each agency's policy and procedure:

- If IV fluids are infusing, stop the infusion in *all* lumens while samples are drawn.
- Flush the catheter with normal saline prior to blood withdrawal.
- Withdraw an aspirate of 4 to 5 mL (or approximately three times catheter volume) of blood to discard before drawing laboratory sample.
- Withdraw laboratory sample.

Flush catheter vigorously with a sufficient amount (10 to 20 mL) of preservative-free 0.9% normal saline to adequately clear blood from the catheter. Use a push/pause or pulsing technique to create turbulent flow to better clear catheter.

CVADs that have been locked with heparin or that have heparin as a solution additive should be a secondary source for drawing blood samples for INR/PT or partial thromboplastin time. Because heparin adheres to the catheter, falsely elevated test values may result. Coagulation studies should be drawn peripherally when possible. If the patient has no peripheral venous access, some institutions have procedures that allow for withdrawal of coagulation studies after a larger amount of blood has been withdrawn. The laboratory results should be evaluated for the possibility of false results.

Electronic Infusion Devices and Power Injection of Contrast Media

Electronic infusion pumps should be used to maintain flow accuracy and catheter patency. The diversity of electronic infusion devices today ensures availability for patients with CVADs. When a positive-pressure instrument is used, the pressure must not exceed that recommended for the type of catheter or electronic infusion device in use.

The question is often raised as to whether a tunneled catheter can be used for power injection of contrast media for computerized tomography examinations. The primary concern with power injection is catheter rupture. Manufacturers specify the psi that a catheter should be able to tolerate. Variables that affect or increase the psi are internal diameter, outer diameter, partial or complete occlusion, catheter material, and catheter length. Power injectors should not be used on VADs that are difficult to flush (Camp-Sorrell, 2011). Power injectors should be used cautiously with tunneled catheters and only by health care professionals who understand power injection and the properties of the specific catheter.

COMPLICATIONS OF CENTRAL VENOUS CATHETERS OR DEVICES

Excellent care of patients with CVCs and devices requires skilled staff who is knowledgeable about the devices, their care, and the potential complications. Ongoing monitoring will assist in identifying problems or undesirable trends before an adverse event occurs. Complications associated with CVADs are reduced when the nurse is part of a health care team that monitors related quality indicators, such as infection rates or adherence to appropriate CVAD maintenance procedures, and implements solutions when needed (CDC, 2011; INS, 2011; McMullan et al., 2013). Astute nursing assessment and a comprehensive understanding of the vascular access device in place may avert complications such as dislodgment, migration, pinch-off syndrome, and occlusion. Potential complications and their definition, signs and symptoms, and treatment are outlined in Table 14-1. As needed, more specific information is provided below for some complications.

Catheter Occlusion

Catheter-related obstructions are categorized as nonthrombotic and thrombotic. Nonthrombotic catheter occlusions include clamped or kinked tubing, pinch-off syndrome, catheter fracture, catheter migration, and precipitation of drug. Thrombotic occlusions occur with the initiation of the coagulation process. Contributing factors include vessel wall trauma, venous stasis, enhanced coagulation, and improper flushing and locking. Risk factors for these conditions include dehydration, hypotension, atrial fibrillation, disease states (chronic renal failure, sepsis, and malignancy), medications, traumatic insertion, large diameter catheters, and catheter malposition (Gorski, 2003a, 2003b; Mayo, 2001; McKnight, 2004). It is estimated that thrombotic catheter occlusions account for about 60% of occlusions. Four categories of thrombotic catheter occlusions are commonly described in the literature:

- *Fibrin tail* is a layer of fibrin encasing the CVC at its tip. Flushing is easy, but withdrawal of blood is not possible as the "tail" acts as a one-way valve as it closes over the CVC tip.

- *Fibrin sheath* is a layer of fibrin that forms around the external surface of the catheter and can potentially extend to the entire exterior wall of the vessel. It is as if a sock were pulled over the CVC from the tip toward the hub. Any infusate administered may travel in a retrograde fashion along the fibrin sheath and could cause tissue irritation or necrosis depending on the nature of the infusate.
- *Intraluminal occlusion* occurs when the fibrin accumulates within the lumen of the CVC. Flow becomes sluggish and may progress to a complete occlusion. Causes include insufficient flushing, frequent blood withdrawal, or reflux of blood into the catheter.
- *Mural thrombus* is caused by catheter tip irritation against the inner lining of the vein. An accumulation of fibrin from the injury attaches to the fibrin buildup on the catheter surface causing the CVC to adhere to the vessel wall.

Symptoms of catheter occlusions include sluggish infusion, resistance to flushing, inability to aspirate blood, inability to infuse, or ability to infuse or aspirate dependent on patient positioning. Adherence to proper insertion, flushing, and locking technique according to institutional policy and guidelines decreases the incidence of catheter occlusion. Catheter occlusions can interfere with therapy and lead to CRBSI, pulmonary emboli, vein thrombosis, or superior vena cava syndrome (SVCS). Symptoms of serious complications include edema in the neck, chest, or upper extremities, jugular vein distension, or difficulty breathing. Descriptions of radiologic testing for possible catheter occlusions are given in Box 14-7.

Catheter Declotting

Clots develop when thrombin, an enzyme made from prothrombin, converts fibrinogen to fibrin, a collagen. The fibrin forms the clot. Activated plasminogen forms plasmin, an enzyme that dissolves the clot and keeps fibrinogen from reforming fibrin; this process is known as *fibrinolysis*. Within the lumen of a CVC, a clot or fibrin sheath occludes the line, and fibrinolytic agents are often used to restore patency. Thrombolytic agents dissolve clots by stimulating the conversion of plasminogen to plasmin, thereby triggering

BOX 14-7   RADIOLOGIC CONFIRMATION OF CATHETER OCCLUSION

Test	Evaluation	Indication for Test
Chest radiograph	Catheter placement	Suspected malposition—pinch-off syndrome, which may result from the patient's position whereby the pressure of the clavicle against the first rib pinches the catheter closed
Contrast study	Flow at distal tip of catheter	Suspected fibrin sheath formation
Venogram	Vessel patency	Suspected superior vena cava thrombosis

fibrinolysis. When alteplase (tPA), for example, is used as directed for CVC clearance, therapeutic serum levels are not observed, because only minute amounts of the drug enter the bloodstream.

INTRALUMINAL PRECIPITATES OR LIPID BUILDUP

Precipitate may form from the mixing of incompatible drugs or solutions within the catheter or port and lead to occlusion of the catheter. Crystallization or drug-to-drug or drug-to-solution incompatibilities may exist, or an alteration in pH may cause precipitation. Precipitates may build up gradually or occur suddenly. A registered pharmacist should be consulted on issues of compatibility. Examples of solutions causing intraluminal precipitates are as follows:

- low-pH drugs (e.g., vancomycin)
- high-pH drugs (e.g., phenytoin)
- PN formula with a high amount calcium or lipids (e.g., in 3-in-1 PN)
  (Adapted from Gorski (2003a, 2003b))

In assessing occlusion, other more common causes such as mechanical obstruction and patient's position should be ruled out first. The infusate and other IV solutions are evaluated for compatibility and potential for precipitate. Intervention is initiated only after careful assessment of these factors. Depending on the nature of the precipitate, treatment may be possible with the use of a precipitate-clearing agent specifically indicated for dissolving medication and/or solution precipitate.

Measures to restore patency from nonthrombotic occlusions are considered investigational. The instilled volume of the precipitate-clearing agent solution is no greater than the internal volume of the catheter. It is allowed to dwell in the lumen of a catheter for a designated period of time, and the contents of the catheter are then aspirated. The nurse using a precipitate clearance agent should have knowledge of dosage, contraindications, side effects, and mechanism of instillation. Occlusions resulting from precipitates may result in catheter removal. Recommendations for declotting technique are found in Table 14-6.

Infection

The use of CVCs is indispensable, especially in critical care settings but also in acute care setting and in the clinic or home environment. However, it puts patients at risk for local and systemic infections. These infectious complications include local site infections, catheter-related bloodstream infections, septic thrombophlebitis, endocarditis, and other infections such as osteomyelitis. The CDC (2013) monitors CVC infections and practices through the National Healthcare Safety Network (NHSN): (a) CLABSI and (b) central line insertion practices adherence. Reporting these data regularly to the health care team has demonstrated effectiveness at reducing CRBSIs (CDC, 2011).

LOCAL SITE INFECTION

Infection at the CVC insertion or exit site is often called a local site infection and is diagnosed based on the absence of a catheter infection. There is erythema localized around the site, no purulence, and no fever (CDC, 2011). There may also be tenderness at the site. Neutropenic

TABLE 14--	DECLOTTING A CENTRAL VENOUS CATHETER

EQUIPMENT:

Gloves, alcohol wipe

Alteplase (r-tPa) 1 mg/mL drawn up into a 3-mL syringe

Sterile needle

Blue plastic catheter clamp (for use with silicone plastic type catheters)

10-mL syringe (empty; 2)

10-mL syringe containing 10 mL sterile normal saline

Needleless connector

1. Disconnect IV tubing or cap from catheter. Swab catheter hub with alcohol.
2. Attach empty 10-mL syringe to hub of catheter.
3. Draw back gently on plunger to aspirate blood from catheter. If no blood is obtained, the catheter is occluded; proceed to step 5.
4. Reattach IV tubing to catheter or attach injection cap and flush central line.
5. Notify physician/LIP that catheter is occluded and obtain order for use of alteplase to declot the catheter.
6. Obtain alteplase from pharmacy (1 mg/mL). Only the specified amount of drug is to be used to surround and dissolve the clot. If required, follow the alteplase with 0.9% sodium chloride to fill the remaining volume of the catheter.
7. Disconnect the IV tubing or cap at the catheter hub. *Remember*: any time the catheter hub is open to air, the line must be clamped. If clamping is not possible, instruct the patient to exhale and then hold breath during the time that the catheter is open.
8. Attach the 3-mL syringe filled with 0.5 mL of alteplase (r-tPa; 1 mg/mL). Inject the drug *slowly* and gently into the catheter. If required, follow the alteplase with 0.9% sodium chloride to fill the remaining volume of the catheter. *Never* forcefully push on the syringe. Excessive pressure should be avoided when injecting a fibrinolytic drug into the catheter because such force could cause rupture of the catheter or expulsion of the clot into circulation. When the drug is injected slowly, the catheter can expand, allowing the drug to surround the clot.
9. Attach a needleless connector to the catheter and wait 60 min.
10. Remove connector; attach and draw back *gently* with an empty 10-mL syringe to attempt to aspirate the drug and residual clot with the attached syringe.
11. If blood is not aspirated: Attempt to aspirate the first alteplase (r-tPa) dose, discard it, and instill 1 mL of alteplase 1 mg/mL. If required, follow alteplase with 0.9% sodium chloride to fill the remaining volume of the catheter. Attach a needleless connector to the catheter and wait an additional *60 min*.
12. Remove connector. Attach empty 10-mL syringe. Draw back gently on an empty 10-mL syringe to attempt to aspirate the drug and residual clot with the attached syringe.
13. Notify the physician/LIP if catheter remains occluded.
14. When the blood can be aspirated, aspirate clot into 10-mL syringe.
15. Disconnect 10-mL syringe. Attach an empty 10-mL syringe and withdraw 5–10 mL of blood. *Do not reinfuse this blood; it contains the thrombolytic.*
16. Remove blood-filled syringe and discard.
17. Connect syringe containing 10 mL normal saline. Flush catheter gently with 10 mL normal saline. Remove syringe from catheter. Reconnect IV tubing or lock with appropriate solution and attach needleless connector.
18. Assess patient's tolerance to the procedure; document patient's response and outcome of intervention.

Sample internal volume for one CVAD: 11-French Hickman = 0.8–0.9 mL.

patients may not produce a typical inflammatory response. These infections may be treated with local wound care and oral antibiotics. If signs of bacteremia are present, additional treatment may be necessary and if necessary, the catheter removed.

SYSTEMIC OR CENTRAL LINE–ASSOCIATED BLOODSTREAM INFECTIONS

The incidence of CRBSI varies by type of catheter, frequency of catheter access, and patient-related factors such as severity of illness and medical condition. Most serious catheter-related infections are associated with CVC, especially those that are placed in critical care units. The most common type of organism that causes hospital-acquired CRBSIs remains coagulase-negative staphylococci, *Staphylococcus aureus*, enterococci, and *Candida*. Antimicrobial resistance continues to be a problem. The incidence of MRSA CRBSI has decreased, and this may be due to prevention techniques. These infections are costly in terms of patient morbidity and in financial resources (CDC, 2011). A checklist for prevention of CLABSI may be found in Box 14-8.

Laboratory confirmation and specific signs/symptoms are used to classify CLABSI. This is defined as "a laboratory-confirmed bloodstream infection (LCBI) where central line (CL) or umbilical catheter (UC) was in place for greater than 2 calendar days when all elements of the LCBI infection criterion were first present together, with day of device placement being Day 1, *and* a CL or UC was in place on the date of event or the day before. If the patient is admitted or transferred into a facility with a central line in place (e.g., tunneled or implanted central line), day of first access is considered Day 1" (CDC, 2013). Because of public reporting and identifying where infections initiated so that agencies may make any needed changes in procedures, definitions are very specific as to when an infection is identified.

Whenever a patient with a CVC has an unexpected high fever, CVC-related sepsis must be suspected. The insertion site should be inspected for signs of infection. A blood specimen may need to be drawn through the catheter and cultured. To rule out all sources of contamination, all tubings, add-on devices, and containers should be changed immediately and sent promptly for bacteriologic culturing. A complete fever workup must be performed to rule out any other obvious source of infection. If the fever remains and no other possible source can be established, catheter removal may be necessary.

Some practitioners perform a catheter exchange with a guidewire. Guidewire exchange should not be performed in the presence of bacteremia due to the usual source of the infection being skin colonization. However, in some patients with a tunneled hemodialysis catheter, the catheter may be replaced over a guidewire along with antibiotic treatment if they have limited venous access (CDC, 2011).

If the blood culture is positive or the semiquantitative culture of the catheter tip yields 15 or more colonies, the new catheter is removed and the patient is considered to have catheter sepsis. If both culture results are negative, then the catheter can be used despite the fever. In cases of septic shock, shaking chills, recent positive blood cultures for *Staphylococcus* or *Candida*, or local infection of the catheter entry site, the catheter must be removed immediately. In some facilities, in situ treatment of catheter-related sepsis with a combination of systemic antibiotics and local thrombolytic agents has been reported.

Of primary importance in preventing CVC-related infection is maintaining strict aseptic technique during insertion, admixture, and CVC manipulations. The nurse must also perform recommended site dressing and tubing and cap changes, using aseptic technique.

BOX 14-8   CENTERS FOR DISEASE CONTROL AND PREVENTION CHECKLIST FOR PREVENTION OF CLABSI

For Clinicians:

Promptly remove unnecessary central lines
- Perform daily audits to assess whether each central line is still needed

Follow proper insertion practices
- Perform hand hygiene before insertion
- Adhere to aseptic technique
- Use maximal sterile barrier precautions (i.e., mask, cap, gown, sterile gloves, and sterile full-body drape)
- Perform skin antisepsis with >0.5% chlorhexidine with alcohol
- Choose the best site to minimize infections and mechanical complications
  - Avoid femoral site in adult patients
- Cover the site with sterile gauze or sterile, transparent, semipermeable dressings

Handle and maintain central lines appropriately
- Comply with hand hygiene requirements
- Scrub the access port or hub immediately prior to each use with an appropriate antiseptic (e.g., chlorhexidine, povidone–iodine, an iodophor, or 70% alcohol)
- Access catheters only with sterile devices
- Replace dressings that are wet, soiled, or dislodged
- Perform dressing changes under aseptic technique using clean or sterile gloves

For Facilities:

- Empower staff to stop non-emergent insertion if proper procedures are not followed
- "Bundle" supplies (e.g., in a kit) to ensure items are readily available for use
- Provide the checklist above to clinicians, to ensure all insertion practices are followed
- Ensure efficient access to hand hygiene
- Monitor and provide prompt feedback for adherence to hand hygiene http://www.cdc.gov/handhygiene/Measurement.html
- Provide recurring education sessions on central line insertion, handling and maintenance

Supplemental Strategies for Consideration:

- 2% Chlorhexidine bathing
- Antimicrobial/antiseptic-impregnated catheters
- Chlorhexidine-impregnated dressings

Based on 2011 CDC guideline for prevention of intravascular catheter-associated bloodstream infections: http://www.cdc.gov/hicpac/pdf/guidelines/bsi-guidelines-2011.pdf

SINGLE-LUMEN VERSUS MULTILUMEN CATHETERS

The minimal number of lumens necessary for treatment is recommended to prevent infec-

PATIENT SAFETY

• National and professional association guidelines, evidence-based practice, and health care–related agencies provide best practices that must be considered and adopted in agencies and institutions.

• Caregiver skill demonstration, policies, technology, and outcomes need to be reviewed regularly and on an appropriate basis that addresses the rapid changes in evidence and technology and helps maintain competent practitioners.

• Patients need to be involved in their own care, knowledgeable about care-related decisions and expected outcomes (Institute of Medicine, 2004).

tion (CDC, 2011). However, in many patient circumstances, especially in critical care, the advantages of using a multilumen catheter outweigh the slight increase in infectious risk.

OTHER STRATEGIES TO PREVENT INFECTION

Overall, the CDC (2011, p. S2) identified that "the goal of an effective prevention program should be the elimination of CRBSI from all patient care areas." Although a challenge, it is imperative for patient safety. A number of "strongly recommended" (categories IA and IB) strategies, not already presented, were identified as being effective in preventing infection (CDC, 2011):

- Specific and ongoing staff education with regular demonstrations of adherence to protocols
- Designated "trained" staff for insertion and maintenance of CVCs
- Appropriate levels and type of nursing staff in critical care
- Removing the CVC within 48 hours if adherence to aseptic technique cannot be ensured
- Daily review of line necessity and prompt removal of any unnecessary lines
- Not routinely replacing CVCs to prevent infection
- Use quality improvement initiatives to implement bundled strategies to prevent infections and monitor adherence as well as clinical outcomes

Catheter Damage and Repair

Catheters can be damaged by excessive pressure with flushing, accidental cutting by scissors or clamps, or dislodgment of the catheter from an implanted portal body. Implanted ports need to be removed or replaced in the event of catheter damage. Nontunneled catheters can be replaced with guidewire exchange. Emergency information for the patient includes being able to identify a leak and knowing how to clamp or fold over the catheter until the patient can be seen. A decision will need to be made whether to replace or repair the catheter. Factors to consider include risk of infection, expected duration of the catheter, cost, and risk of infection during the procedure (Alexander et al., 2010).

Catheter repair kits are available for tunneled catheters and PICC lines from individual manufacturers. Select a repair specific to the manufacturer and size of the catheter. Repair kits are sterile and include at least the replacement catheter, syringe, and Luer-lock cap. They are also available to repair double- and triple-lumen catheters. It is important to follow manufacturer instructions when repairing a catheter. Because catheter repairs are extremely rare, it is often helpful to have two people do the procedure: one to do the repair and one to assess the patient and read the directions. The following are general guidelines:

- Provide a sterile field: Assemble supplies including a sterile scissors.
- The catheter should already be clamped proximal to the rupture.
- Prep the site.
- Cut the damaged catheter to remove the damaged portion and provide a clean edge.
- Apply the repair sleeve, blunt connector, and adhesive as directed by the manufacturer.
- Secure the repaired area per manufacturer's directions.

A sterile repair kit, specific to the individual type of catheter, should be readily available. Repairing the external portion of a tunneled catheter is a sterile procedure requiring surgical gloves, gown, mask, and cap. (Note that some manufacturers provide generic catheter repair kits that may be used for most catheters.)

Once the catheter repair is achieved, attaching a Luer-lock 0.2-μm air-eliminating filter directly to the catheter hub reduces the risk of connection separation and air infusion that could result in a fatal embolism. If a separation occurs distal to the filter, this device prevents air infusion and an inadvertent bleed. The 0.2-μm filter can also prevent any particulate matter, fungi, bacteria, and endotoxins from entering the system through the filter.

Removal of PICCs and Nontunneled CVADs

Removal of PICCS and nontunneled CVADs requires a physician/LIP order. RNs with training are able to remove nontunneled CVADs and PICC lines. There is much research-based information related to the insertion and maintenance of CVADs, but there is minimal research regarding removal of CVADs. While removal is a common procedure with a low incidence of complications, when a complication does occur, there is an overall mortality rate of 57% (Drewett, 2000).

It is imperative for the nurse to be aware of possible complications during CVAD removal; this includes air embolism, catheter fracture with embolism, thrombus dislodgement, bleeding and arterial complications, and compression of the brachial plexis (Drewett, 2000).

PICC Removal

PICCs may be removed by an RN with training. Being aware of possible complications and the reason for catheter removal is necessary before removing the CVAD. Catheters are removed when therapy is complete, the device has exceeded its recommended use or dwell time, when there is a confirmed thrombosis, an unresolved occlusion, an unresolved infection, or an unresolvable phlebitis or thrombophlebitis (Drewett, 2000).

The procedure for removing a PICC involves turning off any infusions and flushing with 0.9% bacteriostatic normal saline. Position the patient comfortably with the arm outstretched. The next step would be to perform hand hygiene and put on clean gloves to remove the old dressing and securement device. Inspect and cleanse the catheter/skin junction (Alexander et al., 2010). Then, don sterile gloves and gently pull the catheter out while placing traction at the skin exit site. Do not remove the catheter quickly, and use a moderate rate of removal to reduce the possibility of venous spasm (Drewett, 2000).

Take precautions to prevent air embolism by instructing the patient to take a deep breath and hold it as you gently pull the catheter out, 2 to 5 cm at a time. Pressure is held over the site with sterile gauze and a gloved finger for 1 to 5 minutes until hemostasis is achieved. A petroleum-based ointment and a sterile occlusive dressing should be applied to the site. Application of ointment may occlude the skin-to-vein tract and prevent air embolism (INS, 2011). If you suspect that the catheter has broken, have the patient lie still on the left side and notify the physician/LIP *immediately*.

If resistance occurs during removal, *do not force removal*. Wait 30 minutes and try again. Vasospasm is the most common problem when removing a PICC. Apply heat to the upper arm, axilla, and hand; warming the extremity may decrease vasospasm and allow catheter removal. Try relaxation techniques or have the patient drink warm liquids. Flush the catheter gently with 10 mL 0.9% NaCl. If all of the above fail, notify the physician/LIP, who may consult an interventional radiologist. After 24 hours, if the PICC is unable to be removed, the surgeon may need to do a surgical cut down procedure to remove it.

After PICC removal, the dressing should be changed and the access site assessed every 24 hours until the site is epithelialized. Documentation of discontinuation of therapy includes catheter length and integrity, site appearance, dressing applied, and patient tolerance.

Nontunneled CVAD Removal

A nurse may remove nontunneled CVADs after training and a physician/LIP order. Similar complications to PICC removal may occur. An arterial hemorrhage may occur after a nontunneled CVAD is removed if there was an arterial tear during the insertion and the catheter had plugged the hole. Ensure that the patient is well hydrated. A dehydrated patient will have a low CVP, which allows air to be aspirated into circulation more easily (Drewett, 2000).

Explain to the patient what will happen and risks of removal; this will enable the patient to understand why it is important to adhere to specific instructions. Assist the patient to a supine position. Have the patient lie in the Trendelenburg position (10- to 30-degree head down tilt) if dehydrated (Drewett, 2000). Follow the same steps for PICC removal. Remove sutures if present. Instruct the patient to take a deep breath and then hold it while withdrawing the catheter. If the patient is on a ventilator, withdraw the catheter during the expiratory cycle. Grasp the catheter with the dominant hand and steadily withdraw the catheter in one continuous motion while stabilizing the site with gauze in the other hand. Note that the distal end of a multilumen catheter should be removed quickly, since the exposed proximal and medial openings could permit air entry. Apply pressure with sterile gauze over the insertion point for a minimum of 1 to 5 minutes or until bleeding has stopped. Apply a petroleum-based ointment and a sterile occlusive dressing to the site; it should remain in place for 24 hours. Application of ointment may occlude the skin-to-vein tract and prevent air embolism (Cook, 2013; INS, 2011). Have the patient lie still for 30 minutes if possible. Instruct the patient to notify the nurse if any bleeding is noted. If you suspect that the catheter has broken, have the patient lie still on the left side and notify the physician/LIP *immediately*. Document removal of catheter and any significant findings. The dressing should be changed and the access site assessed every 24 hours until the site is epithelialized.

NURSING PRACTICE: SKILLED, KNOWLEDGEABLE, AND SAFE

A focus on system safe practices and a nonpunitive environment for safe reporting is paramount for continually improving practice. Evidence-based practices, policies and procedures based on the best evidence, continuing education, and annual skill demonstrations will provide practitioners with the tools to care for patients with these technologies. Competency checklists ensure thorough training and accurate return demonstrations. A documentation record that lists all the steps for accessing and maintaining long-term venous access assists family members and skilled technicians in consistently following safe practices and records their actions if follow-up is necessary.

Nursing can impact patient-centered care by developing a multidisciplinary team to systematically select products and benchmark patient outcomes. Products should be reviewed annually and updated based on a body of sound research.

Nurse-sensitive and health care team outcomes for CVADs have been identified by the American Nurses Association, National Quality Forum, and Institute for Healthcare Improvement (IHI, 2005). Outcomes for these indicators need to be measured, collected, and reported regularly to key stakeholders, including the Infection Control and Prevention Committee, LIPs, and the IV team, and to nursing staff and other clinicians on ICU and medical/surgical units (TJC, 2012). Data need to be reported so that improvements may be tracked and communicated. Generating knowledge to improve nursing practices and using data to improve care and system processes advances quality care for all patients.

Review Questions   *Note: Questions below may have more than one right answer.*

1. Which vein should be avoided for CVAD use in adults?

   A. Subclavian vein

   B. Internal jugular vein

   C. Median cubital vein

   D. Femoral vein

2. Which of the following is *true* of a valved (Groshong) catheter?

   A. It must be clamped when not in use.

   B. Heparin (10 unit/mL) is the preferred lock solution.

   C. You must aspirate a blood return from the catheter before infusing fluids or medications.

   D. You must increase the number of times flushing is required between use.

3. An air embolism may be avoided by using which of the following techniques?

   A. Place the patient in high Fowler position during CVAD removal.

   B. Have the patient use the Valsalva maneuver during CVAD insertion and removal.

   C. Have the patient use deep breathing techniques to reduce anxiety during CVAD insertion.

   D. Use a dry 2 × 2 gauze and tape as a dressing after CVAD removal.

4. Radiologic testing for catheter occlusion includes all of the following tests *except*

   A. Chest radiograph

   B. Contrast study

   C. Venogram

   D. MRI scan

5. Which of the following statements concerning CVC patency are correct? *Select all that apply.*
   A. Patency includes the ability to infuse through and aspirate blood from the catheter.
   B. Risk for occlusion increases with dehydration and atrial fibrillation.
   C. It is not possible for catheter occlusion to lead to CRBSI or SVCS.
   D. Catheter occlusion and decreased catheter patency may be caused by pinch-off syndrome.

6. The most common cause of catheter occlusion is
   A. Catheter malposition
   B. Catheter material defects
   C. Catheter-related bloodstream infections
   D. Thrombotic occlusions

7. What are some of the components of the central line bundle? *Select all that apply.*
   A. Weekly CVAD assessment to assess for the need of a CVAD
   B. The use of maximum sterile barriers during CVAD insertion
   C. Adequate hand hygiene after vein palpation
   D. The use of chlorhexidine gluconate as a skin antiseptic

8. The CVAD with the least risk for CRBSI is a (an)
   A. Implanted port
   B. PICC
   C. Tunneled catheter
   D. Nontunneled catheter

9. Catheters can be made of all of the following materials *except*
   A. Silicone
   B. Polyurethane
   C. Elastomeric hydrogel
   D. Polyethylene glycol

10. Which type of access cap or needleless connector requires the nurse to clamp the CVAD after the final flush or lock is done and the syringe is removed?
    A. Positive displacement access cap
    B. Negative displacement access cap
    C. Interlink access cap
    D. Neutral access cap

References and Selected Readings   *Asterisks indicate references cited in text.*

*AABB. (2010). *Primer of blood administration.* Bethesda, MD: Author.

*AABB. (2011). *Standards for blood banks and transfusion services* (27th ed.). Bethesda, MD: Author.

*AABB, the American Red Cross, America's Blood Centers, & the Armed Services Blood Program. (2009). *Circular of information for the use of human blood and blood components.* Bethesda, MD: Author. http://www.aabb.org/resources/bct/Documents/coi0809r.pdf

*AHRQ (Agency for Healthcare Research and Quality). (2013). *Tools for reducing central line-associated blood stream infections: Appendix 6: Central Line Maintenance Audit Form.* Rockville, MD: Author. http://www.ahrq.gov/professionals/education/curriculum-tools/clabsitools/clabsitoolsap6.html

*Alexander, M., Corrigan, A., Gorski, L., Hankins, J., & Perucca, R. (2010). *Infusion Nursing: An evidence based approach* (3rd ed.). St. Louis, MO: Mosby-Elsevier.

Bartock, L. (2010). An evidence-based systematic review of literature for the reduction of PICC line occlusions. *Journal of the Association for Vascular Access, 15*(2), 58–63.

*Camp-Sorrell, D. (Ed.). (2011). *Access Device Guidelines: Recommendations for nursing practice and education* (3rd ed.). Pittsburgh, PA: Oncology Nursing Society.

*Centers for Disease Control and Prevention (CDC). (2011). Guidelines for the prevention of intravascular catheter-related infections. http://www.cdc.gov/hicpac/pdf/guidelines/bsi-guidelines-2011.pdf

*Centers for Disease Control and Prevention (CDC). (2013). National Healthcare Safety Network (NHSN). http://www.cdc.gov/nhsn/PDFs/pscManual/1PSC_OverviewCurrent.pdf

*Cook, L.S. (2013). Infusion-related air embolism. *Journal of Infusion Nursing, 36,* 26–36.

*Drewett, S. (2000). Central venous catheter removal procedures and rationale. *British Journal of Nursing, 9,* 2304–2315.

Earhart, A. (2013). Recognizing, preventing, and trouble-shooting central-line complications. *American Nurse Today, 8*(11), 18–23.

Frey, A. (2003). Drawing blood samples from vascular access devices: Evidence-based practice. *Journal of Infusion Nurses, 26*(5), 285–293.

Galloway, M. (2002). Using benchmarking data to determine vascular access device selection. *Journal of Intravenous Nursing, 25*(5), 320–325.

*Gillies, D., O'Riordan, L., Carr, D., Frost, J., Gunning, R., & O'Brien, I. (2005). Gauze and tape and transparent polyurethane dressings for central venous catheters. *Cochrane Database of Systematic Reviews, 1.*

*Gorski, L.A. (2003a). Central venous access device occlusions, pt. 1: Thrombotic causes and treatment. *Home Healthcare Nurse, 21*(2), 115–121.

*Gorski, L.A. (2003b). Central venous access device occlusions, pt. 2: Non-thrombotic causes and treatment. *Home Healthcare Nurse, 21*(3), 168–171.

Gorski, L.A. (2004). Central venous access device outcomes in a homecare agency: A 7-year study. *Journal of Infusion Nursing, 27*(2), 104–111.

*Gorski, L.A., Perucca, R., & Hunter, M.R. (2010). Central venous access devices: Care, maintenance, and potential complications. In M. Alexander, A. Corrigan, L. Gorski, J. Hankins, & R. Perucca, (Eds.), *Infusion Nurses Society Infusion Nursing: An evidence-based approach* (3rd ed., pp. 495–515). St. Louis, MO: Saunders Elsevier.

*Guerin, K., Wagner, J., Rains, K., & Bessesen, M. (2010). Reduction in central line-associated bloodstream infections by implementation of a postinsertion care bundle. *American Journal of Infection Control, 38,* 430–433.

*Hadaway, L. (2006). Technology of flushing vascular access devices. *Journal of Infusion Nursing, 29*(3), 137–145.

*Hadaway, L. (2010). Infusion therapy equipment. In M. Alexander, A. Corrigan, L. Gorski, J. Hankins, & R. Perucca (Eds.), *Infusion Nurses Society Infusion Nursing: An evidence-based approach* (3rd ed., pp. 391–436). St. Louis, MO: Saunders Elsevier.

*Hadaway, L., & Richardson, D. (2010). Needleless connectors: A primer on terminology. *Journal of Infusion Nursing, 33,* 22–31.

Holmes, K.R. (1998). Comparison of push-pull versus discard method from central venous catheters for blood testing. *Journal of Intravenous Nursing, 21*(5), 282–285.

Hornsby, S., Matter, K., Beets, B., Casey, S., & Kokotis, K. (2005). Cost losses associated with the 'PICC, stick, and run team' concept. *Journal of Infusion Nursing, 28*(1), 45–53.

*Infusion Nurses Society. (2008). *Flushing protocols.* Norwood, MA: Author.

*Infusion Nurses Society. (2011). Infusion Nursing: Standards of practice. *Journal of Infusion Nursing, 34*(Suppl.), S1–S110.

*Infusion Nurses Society. (2013). Clinical Competency Validation Program. Author http://www.ins1.org/i4a/ams/amsstore/category.cfm?product_id=216

*Institute for Healthcare Improvement (IHI). (2005). 100k Lives Campaign at http://www.ihi.org/IHI/Programs/Campaign/Campaign.htm

*Institute for Healthcare Improvement (IHI). (2011). Implement the IHI Central Line Bundle at http://www.ihi.org/knowledge/Pages/Changes/ImplementtheCentralLineBundle.aspx

*Institute of Medicine. (1999). *To err is human: Building a safer health system.* Washington, DC: National Academies Press.

*Institute of Medicine. (2004). *Keeping patients safe: Transforming the work environment of nurses.* Washington, DC: National Academies Press.

Jackson, D. (2001). Infection control principles and practices in the care and management of vascular access devices in the alternate care setting. *Journal of Intravenous Nursing, 24*(Suppl. 3), S28–S34.

*The Joint Commission. (2012). *Preventing central line–associated bloodstream infections: A global challenge, a global perspective.* Oak Brook, IL: Joint Commission Resources. http://www.jointcommission.org/CLABSIToolkit

*Mayo, D.J. (2001). Catheter-related thrombosis. *Journal of Intravenous Nursing, 24*(3), S13–S22.

Mayo, D., Dimond, E., Kramer, W., & Horne, M. (1996). Discard volumes necessary for clinically useful coagulation studies from heparinized Hickman catheters. *Oncology Nursing Forum, 23*(4), 671–675.

*McKnight, S. (2004). Nurse's guide to understanding and treating thrombotic occlusion of central venous access devices. *Medsurg Nursing, 13*(6), 377–382.

*McMullan, C., Propper, G., Schuhmacher, C., Sokoloff, L., Harris, D., Murphy, P., et al. (2013). A multidisciplinary approach to reduce central line-associated bloodstream infections. *Joint Commission Journal on Quality and Patient Safety, 39*(2), 61–69.

Mehall, J.R., Saltzman, D.A., Jackson, R.J., & Smith, S.D. (2002). Fibrin sheath enhances central venous catheter infection. *Critical Care Medicine, 30*(4), 908–912.

*Menyhay, S.Z., & Maki, D.G. (2006). Disinfection of needleless catheter connectors and access ports with alcohol may not prevent microbial entry: The promise of a novel antiseptic-barrier cap. *Infection Control and Hospital Epidemiology, 27*, 23–27.

*Mermel, L.A., Allon, M., Bouza, E., Craven, D.E., Flynn, P., O'Grady, N.P., et al. (2009). Clinical practice guidelines for the diagnosis and management of intravascular catheter-related infection: 2009 Update by the Infectious Diseases Society of America. *Clinical Infectious Diseases, 49*, 1–45.

*Morrison, T. (2012). Qualitative analysis of central and midline care in the medical/surgical setting. *Clinical Nurse Specialist, 26*, 323–328.

*National Quality Forum (NQF). (2009). Safe Practice 21: Central line-associated bloodstream infection prevention. *Safe practices for better healthcare–2009 update: A consensus report.* Washington, DC: Author.

Penney-Timmons, E., & Sevedge, S. (2004). Outcome data for peripherally inserted central catheters used in an acute care setting. *Journal of Infusion Nursing, 27*(6), 431–436.

*Pronovost, P., Needham, D., Berenholtz, S., Sinopoli, D., Chu, H., Cosgrove, S., et al. (2006). An intervention to decrease catheter-related bloodstream infections in the ICU. *New England Journal of Medicine, 355*(26), 2725–2732.

Ruesch, S., Walder, B., & Tramer, M. (2002). Complications of central venous catheters: Internal jugular versus subclavian access—A systematic review. *Critical Care Medicine, 30*(2), 454–460.

*Rupp, M.E., Cassling, K., Faber, H., Lyden, E., Tyner, K., & Van Schooneveld, T. (2013). Hospital-wide assessment of compliance with central venous catheter dressing recommendations. *American Journal of Infection Control, 41*, 89–91.

Saxena, A.K., Panhotra, B.R., Sundaram, D.S., Al-Hafiz, A., Naguib, M., Venkateshappa, C.K., et al. (2006). Tunneled catheters' outcome optimization among diabetics on dialysis through antibiotic-lock placement. *Kidney International, 70*(9), 1629–1635.

*Schallom, M.E., Prentice, D., Sona, C., Micek, S.T., & Skrupky, L.P. (2012). Heparin or 0.9% sodium chloride to maintain central venous catheter patency: A randomized trial. *Critical Care Medicine, 40*, 1820–1826.

Sherwood, G., & Barnsteiner, J. (2012). *Quality and safety in nursing: A competency approach to improving outcomes.* Ames, IA: Wiley-Blackwell.

Simmons, S., Bryson, C., & Porter, S. (2011). "Scrub the hub": Cleaning duration and reduction in bacterial load on central venous catheters. *Critical Care Nursing Quarterly, 34*(1), 31–35.

*Smith, J.S., Irwin, G., Viney, M., Watkins, L., Morris, S.P., Kirksey, K.M., et al. (2012). Optimal disinfection times for needleless intravenous connectors. *Journal of the Association for Vascular Access, 17*, 137–143.

*Thayer, D. (2012). Skin damage associated with intravenous therapy. *Journal of Infusion Nursing, 6*, 391–401.

*The Joint Commission. (2012). Hospital National Patient Safety Goals. http://www.jointcommission.org/assets/1/18/NPSG_Chapter_Jan2013_HAP.pdf

Von Eiff, C., Jansen, B., Kohnen, W., & Becker, K. (2005). Infections associated with medical devices: Pathogenesis, management, and prophylaxis. *Drugs, 65*(2), 179–214.

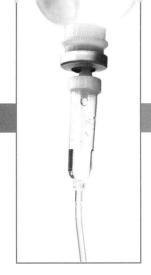

CHAPTER 15

Expanded Approaches to Access and Monitoring

Maureen T. Greene

KEY TERMS		
	Acid–base Balance	Hypodermoclysis
	Alveolar PaO_2	Intraosseous Infusion
	Arterial Blood Gas	Metabolic Acidosis
	(ABG) Analysis	Metabolic Alkalosis
	Arterial Pressure	Oxyhemoglobin
	Monitoring	Dissociation
	Base Bicarbonate	pH Value
	Bicarbonate Excess	Pseudoaneurysms
	Hemodynamic	Renal Replacement
	Monitoring	Therapy
	Hemoglobin	Ventricular Reservoir
	Desaturation	
	Hypercapnia	

SIGNIFICANCE OF EXPANDED ACCESS

Having alternatives to intravenous (IV) access provides patients with lifesaving options. Expanded access includes vascular infusions via the intraosseous route, unique access for hemodialysis, and medication and fluid administration via the subcutaneous route. Intra-arterial access for critically ill patients provides the ability to monitor pressures and sample blood. These modalities are featured in this chapter; also included are detailed explanations of arterial and venous pressure monitoring as well as interpretation of relevant laboratory values.

One of the most common procedures carried out in acute care hospitals and a high priority for the care of a critically ill and unstable patient is establishing vascular access. The patient's condition plays a role in the likelihood of attaining vascular access; conditions associated with difficult vascular access include obesity, sepsis, chronic illness, hypovolemia, IV drug abuse, and vasculopathy (Miles, Salcedo, & Spear, 2011; Nafiu et al., 2010).

Central venous catheterization is a common approach to cannulation in patients with difficult venous access. The central venous catheter (CVC) provides vascular access for fluid resuscitation, and additionally allows for hemodynamic monitoring, but not without risk to the patient. Common complications are pneumothorax, venous thrombosis, arterial puncture, and central line–associated bloodstream infection.

Given the time required to establish central venous access, the increased risk to the patient, and the skill required of the provider, alternatives for vascular access are desirable. Another method for monitoring a patient's hemodynamic status includes arterial pressure monitoring through vascular access lines and the use of sophisticated monitoring equipment.

ARTERIAL BLOOD SAMPLING AND PRESSURE MONITORING

Invasive hemodynamic monitoring allows direct measurement of arterial blood pressure (BP), central venous pressure (CVP), intracardiac pressures, and pulmonary artery (PA) pressures. Hemodynamic monitoring contributes to the diagnosis of a patient's underlying condition and can be useful in predicting prognosis. Arterial pressure monitoring via an indwelling peripheral catheter is the most common mode of invasive hemodynamic monitoring. It is used to draw blood samples, to monitor arterial BP when rapid fluctuations are anticipated, to maximize drug therapy, and when vasopressor therapy is in use. Complications of continuous arterial pressure monitoring include ecchymosis, hematoma, and soreness at the insertion site. Arterial laceration, arteriovenous (AV) fistulas, and aneurysms are rare.

Arterial Puncture Sites and One-Time Blood Sampling

The radial artery is the most common access site for placement of a peripheral arterial catheter. It has the least discomfort, allows freedom of motion, and usually does not require joint immobilization. Radial arterial lines are associated with a low risk of ischemic injury to the hand as there is usually adequate collateral circulation via the ulnar artery. Other sites for monitoring arterial pressure include the femoral, brachial, and dorsalis pedis arteries (Table 15-1).

The femoral artery, the preferred site for emergency cannulation, is easily cannulated. The femoral artery, located midway between the anterior superior spine of the ilium and the symphysis pubis (Figure 15-1), is the largest accessible artery and is easily palpated, stabilized, and entered. However, focused digital pressure is required for postpuncture pressure. If postpuncture thrombosis should occur, though this is considered low risk in the femoral artery, a limb- or life-threatening condition may result.

TABLE 15-	SITES FOR ARTERIAL BLOOD SAMPLING OR CANNULATION	
Site	Advantages	Disadvantages
Radial artery	Close to the surface Easily palpable Easy to check site	Pulsation is difficult to palpate on obese patients with short arms
Brachial artery	Largest artery in upper arm Close to surface Extension of the arm stretches the artery Easily accessed Easily observed after puncture	May lie deep in muscular or obese patients Traumatic puncture may damage adjacent nerve and ligaments
Ulnar artery	Fairly close to surface and therefore accessible Good alternative to radial artery	Palpation difficult if artery is small or deep Difficult to stabilize Difficulty in extending wrist if patient is uncooperative
Femoral artery	Relatively large artery Easily palpated Allows direct, perpendicular approach Incidence of arterial spasm is rare	Risk of contamination at site (groin) Possible to puncture femoral vein accidentally during procedure

Brachial artery access is the least preferred as it limits mobility of the patient and interferes with nursing care. The ulnar artery is usually much deeper and more difficult to stabilize than is the radial artery, so, although it may be larger, it is usually not the first choice as an entry site. The dorsalis pedis artery of the foot can be used for arterial monitoring but may be the least favorable site due to distal ischemic blood flow issues. This vessel is supported by collateral circulation over the arch of the foot but with comorbid conditions, such as peripheral vascular disease and vascular changes associated with diabetes, this site should be avoided.

Arterial blood is obtained for an arterial blood gas (ABG). Single stick blood sampling can be used for ABG sampling using a rigid needle sampling method. A cannulated arterial line can also be used for continuous arterial monitoring for hemodynamic pressure monitoring and frequent blood sampling using a flexible catheter.

PATIENT PREPARATION

Initially, the nurse reviews the physician/licensed independent practitioner's (LIP) order. Unless a postexercise blood sample is ordered, the patient also should be at rest for 15 to 20 minutes before the blood sample is drawn. The most comfortable position for the patient should be used for all blood sampling procedures.

The laboratory requisition form should have all identifying patient information plus the oxygenation status of the patient, time of day (important when drawing serial samples), and, if the patient is on a ventilator, all pertinent ventilator settings (i.e., FIO_2). In some institutions, the patient's temperature and hemoglobin count are also required. In any institution, the nurse follows recommended institutional policy.

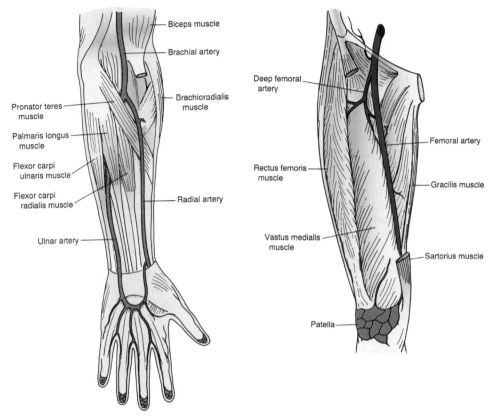

FIGURE 15-1 Location of radial, ulnar, and brachial arteries **(left)** and location of the femoral artery in the leg **(right)**.

 PATIENT SAFETY

While positioning the patient, the nurse fully explains the procedure to alleviate anxiety and fear, which can cause hyperventilation in the patient and hence an alteration of the blood analysis findings.

EQUIPMENT

Arterial blood samples are drawn with a syringe and needle from available stock, or a prepackaged kit may be used. An ABG kit is inexpensive and contains all equipment needed to perform a one-time arterial puncture, except for the ice and tape. If the kit contains a heparinized prefilled syringe, the nurse removes the syringe cap, places and secures the appropriate-size needle, wets the inner walls of the syringe with heparin (to prevent blood clotting), and expels excess heparin and air with the same method used for a syringe that is not prefilled. Most ABG kits contain a plastic bag for the iced blood sample and for lab transport of specimens.

To heparinize a syringe, the nurse attaches a needle (other than the one to be used for the arterial puncture) to the syringe, cleanses the top of the heparin vial with an alcohol swab, and opens the vial. One milliliter of heparin is withdrawn into the syringe. The nurse then moves the plunger back and forth several times to coat the plunger with heparin and rotates the plunger to eliminate dry spots. To eliminate air bubbles, the nurse holds the syringe with the needle bevel upright and gently taps the sides of the syringe or turns the syringe with the needle pointed downward and slowly inverts the syringe upright. The needle used for heparin withdrawal is discarded.

The nurse replaces the needle used for heparinization with a sterile, tightly secured needle selected for arterial puncture. Then with the syringe pointing skyward, the plunger is pushed up and all excess heparin expelled. The only heparin remaining should be in the dead space of the needle and on the walls of the syringe. Excess heparin or air bubbles alter the results of the ABG analysis.

Radial Puncture

The site is palpated for a pulse, and the condition of the skin and surrounding tissues is inspected particularly for previous arterial puncture marks. Allen test is performed to ensure the adequacy of collateral circulation (Figure 15-2). Local anesthesia prior to the arterial puncture should be considered, since it appears to prevent pain without adversely impacting the success of the procedure (Hudson, Dukes, & Reilly, 2006).

The radial artery is best palpated between the distal radius and the tendon of the flexor carpi radialis when the wrist is flexed. A rolled towel may be placed under the wrist, promoting hyperextension of the hand to stretch and stabilize the artery. Taping the forearm and the palm to the insertion field or via an armboard can help maintain the position. The planned puncture site should be sterilely draped. The skin is prepared with chlorhexidine or other agency-specific product by wiping the area in a back and forth friction motion and allowing at least a 30-second drying time at the intended puncture site. Hand hygiene is used, gloves are required, and Occupational Safety and Health Administration standards should be met.

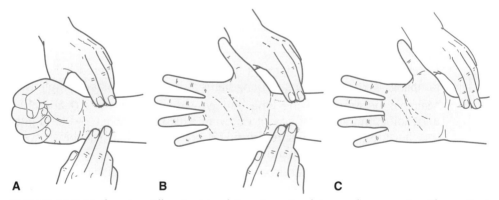

A   **B**   **C**

FIGURE 15-2 Performing Allen test to determine circulatory adequacy. **A:** The patient clenches the fist while nurse applies pressure to both the radial and ulnar artery. **B:** The patient opens the hand and nurse noting the pallor of the palm surface, releases the ulnar pressure releases pressure while watching to see how long it takes for the hand to color (signifying circulation and patency of vessels). **C:** Evaluating pulse and blood return.

To perform a radial puncture, the nurse uses one gloved hand to palpate the artery and aligns two or three fingertips along the direction the artery follows. A small needle (e.g., 22- to 25-gauge) should then be attached to the syringe. The plunger should be withdrawn 1 to 2 mL before the stick, for two reasons: if the sample is indeed arterial and not venous, the patient's pressure causes a brisk and often pulsatile reflux of blood into the syringe (unless the patient is severely hypotensive), and it prevents complications such as arterial spasm and blood hemolysis.

Holding the syringe and the needle in a bevel up position at an angle no higher than 30 degrees directly toward the artery, the nurse enters the skin and artery smoothly in one quick motion. Arterial pressure usually causes the blood to pulsate spontaneously back into the syringe. If BP is low or the syringe not free flowing, however, the nurse may need to pull back gently on the plunger or reposition the needle to achieve intralumen artery access. The blood return stops when the blood reaches the automatic shutoff level. If the equipment does not have a shutoff feature, a volume of 1 to 2 mL blood is a sufficient quantity for the blood gas analyzer.

Immediately after quickly withdrawing the needle and blood-filled syringe, the nurse applies digital pressure to the puncture site with a 2 × 2-inch sterile sponge folded to form a pressure point. Then, taking precautions not to encircle the entire wrist, a secure dressing is firmly secured with tape. Additional postprocedure interventions are listed in Box 15-1.

If the syringe will be capped, the nurse resheaths the needle using a quick-cover cap. The nurse rolls the syringe back and forth between the hands for 5 to 10 seconds to ensure that the blood mixes with the heparin lining the syringe. The unit is then placed in an iced container and taken to the laboratory immediately for analysis. A small amount of cold water added to the ice provides for even cold distribution and facilitates placement of the sample so that all the blood in the barrel is chilled by iced water. Ice bathing ABG blood draws is not needed for transport of samples when using a fast, pneumatic tube system. Lab personnel will process all STAT lab requisitions within the guidelines established by the facility.

BOX 15-1   POSTPROCEDURAL PATIENT INTERVENTIONS

- Determine if the oxygen status of the patient has been altered only for the blood sampling. If so, resume presampling status as soon as the blood sample is drawn.
- Maintain pressure dressing long enough—usually between 10 and 20 minutes depending on the access site—to prevent excessive seepage of blood into the tissue. Be sure that the pressure dressing is not so tight that blanching occurs or that venous blood flow in the hand is severely restricted.
- If the patient is receiving anticoagulation therapy, apply digital pressure. Digital pressure is also preferable to the use of a C-clamp at the femoral site because significant occult bleeding into the retroperitoneal space can occur rapidly and may result in unnecessary blood loss and discomfort for the patient.
- Remove pressure dressing after bleeding stops.

FEMORAL PUNCTURE

For femoral artery access, palpate the vessel below the midpoint of the inguinal ligament, when the lower extremity is extended. The needle should be inserted at a 90-degree angle just below the inguinal ligament. The femoral artery is usually easily palpated with the patient in the supine position. If the patient is obese, assistance may be needed to hold the abdomen away or the patient's buttocks may be placed on an inverted bedpan. A pendulous abdomen may be taped up and away to provide easier access and maintain sterility. Procedures for wearing gloves and preparing the skin are the same as for a radial artery puncture.

The following two techniques may be used for a femoral arterial puncture:

- The artery is located and kept between two fingers held in a "V" pattern, allowing pulsation to be felt on both fingers laterally but at the same time allowing enough room between them for the needle entry. The syringe and needle are held almost straight down. When the puncture is made in this manner, care must be taken not to pierce through the other wall of the artery. The acronym "NAV" (nerve, artery, vein) can assist the practitioner in focusing on the right femoral puncture location by remembering the *n*erve innervating the leg is to the left of the stick, the *a*rtery is central, and the *v*ein is in the direction of the pubis symphysis.
- Vessel entry may be performed with the same techniques used for a radial artery puncture. Two or three fingertips are placed along the direction of the femoral artery to the left over the ilium, and the syringe and needle are held at an angle no higher than 90 degrees. This method must be used for femoral artery catheter placement due to the need to manipulate more equipment; if used for a one-time needle and syringe sample, there is less chance of artery perforation using this approach.

Regardless of the method used, when pulsation is strong, it is relayed up through the needle and syringe as the needle touches and penetrates the artery. The walls of the femoral artery are usually thick and resistant to puncture, so feeling pulsations can be a good guide to needle tip placement. When the artery is entered, the blood usually pulsates back into and fills the syringe without any traction being applied on the plunger. See Box 15-1 for postprocedure interventions and nursing responsibilities.

Other Arterial Access Sites

Variations in arterial puncture for the brachial access site include palpation of the vessel medial to the biceps tendon in the antecubital fossa, when the arm is extended in the palm up fashion. The dorsalis pedis artery is best palpated lateral to the extensor hallucis longus tendon. It receives collateral flow from the lateral plantar artery through the arch similar to that of the hand. The needle should be inserted just above the elbow crease or at the level of the dorsal arch, respectively.

> **EVIDENCE FOR PRACTICE**
>
> An ABG sample that is not placed immediately on ice can produce faulty results on analysis because leukocytes increase oxygen consumption at higher temperatures (leukocyte larceny) causing fictitiously low PaO_2 (Hess et al., 1979). Ice retards the process.

PERIPHERAL ARTERIAL CATHETERS AND MONITORING

Catheter Insertion and Blood Sampling

Most arterial access devices use a guidewire and hollow needle for insertion using the Seldinger technique, defined as a method of percutaneous insertion of a vascular access catheter (VAC) into a blood vessel. The vessel is accessed with a needle, and a guidewire is placed through the needle. The needle is removed, and a catheter is placed over the guidewire and advanced into the desired position. The guidewire is removed, leaving the catheter in place (Bullock-Corkhill, 2010).

To obtain a blood sample for ABG analysis from a catheter with a heparin lock device, the nurse puts on gloves and prepares three syringes. A needleless access cap should be used to access the line and prevent open system contamination:

- A heparinized syringe
- A plain syringe for withdrawal of dilute heparin from the injection port
- A syringe with dilute heparin solution for flushing the catheter after drawing the blood sample

Next, the nurse cleanses the capping port of the catheter with antiseptic, securely anchors the catheter hub with the free hand to prevent excessive pressure at the insertion site, and inserts a plain syringe. Approximately 0.5 mL of blood of the heparin-capped line is withdrawn from the catheter and is discarded.

The cap is recleansed, the heparinized syringe inserted, the syringe allowed to fill with enough blood for the ABG analysis, and the syringe is removed and closed with the proper transport cap. Finally, the injection port is recleansed, and the nurse, still securely anchoring the catheter hub, inserts the syringe containing dilute heparin, flushes the catheter, and removes the syringe leaving the catheter with a heparinized cap. The blood sample is treated in the same manner as the sample obtained for a one-time analysis. Key interventions may be found in Table 15-2.

Continuous Arterial Pressure Monitoring

Arterial pressure monitoring via an indwelling peripheral catheter is the most common mode of invasive hemodynamic monitoring. Continuous arterial pressure monitoring requires inserting an indwelling arterial catheter, which permits the infusion nurse and other health care personnel to obtain continuous systolic, diastolic, and mean arterial pressure readings; to assess the cardiovascular effects of vasopressor or vasodilator drugs during the treatment

TABLE 15-2	KEY INTERVENTIONS: POSTARTERIAL CATHETER INSERTION CARE

1. Observe the catheter site for signs of arterial thrombosis, hematoma formation, arterial perforation, and catheter kinking or dislodgment.
2. Check the patient's extremity for adequate blood supply by noting color and temperature.
3. Maintain secure, clean, and intact dressings.
4. Avoid placing undue stress at the insertion site by using the unaffected arm for BP monitoring and venipunctures.
5. Femoral arterial lines may hamper patient mobility and a physician/licensed independent practitioner's order is required for out of bed activity. Patients with femoral lines can be positioned in a side-lying position, but hemodynamic measures should be taken in a neutral, re-zeroed position for best accuracy.

of shock; and, at the same time, to draw arterial blood for ABG measurement and other sampling.

EQUIPMENT

Following insertion into the artery, the catheter is connected to a flush bag with pressurized saline solution, a three-way stopcock, flush valve, and transducer with tubing connected both to the patient and to the monitor through cabling. A cardiac monitor with a module for measuring arterial pressure is required. The monitor is connected by cable and a transducer to a special IV setup (Figure 15-3). The IV system consists of a 500-mL bag of normal saline solution connected to IV tubing and placed inside a pressure infuser bag with a gauge and inflation bulb. This pressure infuser bag is the same type used to pump blood transfusions. The pressure is set at 300 mm Hg. Most pressure infusion systems deliver 3 to 5 mL of solution under pressure.

The monitoring system transforms the electrical impulses into an arterial pressure waveform. The nurse calibrates the equipment to assure accurate measurement. The entire system is flushed with saline to remove excess air. Air bubbles and blood clots in the tubing or transducer can dampen the waveform and skew hemodynamic values. The transducer can be attached to an IV pole at the level of the patient's right atrium. Alternately, the transducer can be secured to the patient's limb on the side of insertion close to the right atrium. The goal is to achieve a sufficient arterial waveform for interpretation on the monitor. Each manufacturer provides detailed instructions for this setup.

OBTAINING BLOOD FOR ABG ANALYSIS

When an ABG sample is needed, a sampling port using a three-way stopcock provides an easy arterial access. The nurse removes the cap when sampling and attaches an appropriate syringe. The stopcock is turned off to pressure and open to the sampling site, and the nurse gently withdraws the sample and handles it consistent with institutional policy. The port is then flushed using the transducer fast-flush valve and the stopcock turned back to its original position. Many arterial blood drawing systems are prepared with a blood-sparing in-line syringe device whereby a waste sample is drawn into the syringe and the stopcock is turned off to the waste and on to a sampling syringe. The lab sample is withdrawn, and the waste syringe volume is reintroduced to the patient by turning the stopcock open to the patient. This reduces the extrinsic blood loss associated with frequent lab tests.

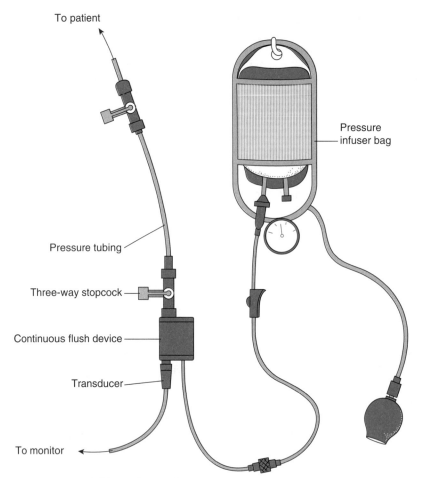

To patient

Pressure
infuser bag

Pressure tubing

Three-way stopcock

Continuous flush device

Transducer

To monitor

FIGURE 15-3 Cable and transducer setup.

Malfunctions and Complications

Common malfunctions occurring in arterial pressure lines are listed in Table 15-3. Common complications related to arterial pressure lines include thromboses, hematomas, **pseudoaneurysms**, and prolonged arterial spasms. These problems may be reduced by clinical expertise during catheter insertion and by careful monitoring of insertion sites.

Infection is a serious complication as well. Evidence including a randomized controlled trial (Marik, Flemmer, & Harrison, 2012), Cochrane review (Ge et al., 2012), and practice guideline (CDC, 2011) has indicated that centrally placed lines, like arterial, subclavian, internal jugular, and femoral, should be selected for the least risk of injury and infection. No difference in infection rate was found between internal jugular and subclavian lines; however, subclavian CVC was preferable to femoral lines for short-term catheter use because of the lower risk for hospital-acquired bacterial colonization.

As with any invasive line, consideration of the need for the arterial catheter should be determined on a daily basis. Agency-specific IV tubing changes and invasive line change

TABLE 15-	MALFUNCTIONS OCCURRING IN ARTERIAL PRESSURE MONITORING	
Malfunction	**Intervention**
• Air bubbles may distort wave patterns.	• Eliminate air from system during setup; avoid entry of air in manipulation.
• Near-exsanguination has been reported.	• Secure all connections.
• Damped pressure tracing (almost flat) may occur if tip lies against artery wall.	• Secure catheter hub; ensure use of intact dressings.
• Catheter clotting can occur if pressure is <300 mm Hg.	• Check pressure bag to ensure that it is maintained.
• Abnormally high or low reading may occur if height of transducer is at zero reference point or is the type placed with a plate on an IV pole.	• Monitor cable malfunctions to the bedside computer.

practices should be used to reduce nosocomial infection rates. Thorough hand hygiene before catheter insertion and maintenance of aseptic technique during setup of the system, during insertion, and during all manipulations of the line are mandatory. Use of observation monitoring and checklist compliance to sterile technique and practitioner insertion methods have been incorporated into line insertion practices in hospital settings to enhance sterile insertion and reduce infection rates of invasive lines.

PURPOSE AND USE OF ARTERIAL BLOOD GAS ANALYSIS

Arterial blood with all its nourishing elements supplies all body tissues; thus, arterial blood is used routinely for diagnosing abnormalities and assessing patients' conditions. Intra-arterial therapy may involve one-time or daily blood sampling to analyze the concentration of gases, such as oxygen, and other components, or it may involve inserting an indwelling catheter to obtain serial or daily samples for arterial blood gas (ABG) analysis and continuous arterial pressure monitoring.

Although venous, arterial, and capillary blood all contain comparable levels of carbon dioxide and base bicarbonate, the levels of oxygen in venous and capillary blood vary significantly from the level of oxygen in arterial blood.

Oxygen in Plasma

Oxygen moves through the circulatory system in plasma and hemoglobin; because the small amount of oxygen dissolved in plasma cannot be measured directly, its presence is expressed as the tension or partial pressure it exerts on plasma (PaO_2—the letter P symbolizes the pressure value; the letter a signifies that the partial pressure of oxygen measured is that in arterial blood).

Oxygen in Hemoglobin

Oxygen level determination is the most common reason for taking blood gas readings. The major portion of blood oxygen is bound to hemoglobin and measured as a percentage of the hemoglobin saturated with oxygen (SaO_2). Tissue is adequately oxygenated when the partial pressure of oxygen in arterial blood (PaO_2) is in the normal range between 80 and 100 mm Hg and when SaO_2 ranges from 93% to 100% (Horne & Derrico, 1999; Tortora & Grabowski, 2003). Under normal resting conditions, blood contains 20 mL oxygen per 100 mL blood. Of that, 97% (19.4 mL) is attached to hemoglobin of the red blood cells, and 3% (0.6 mL) is dissolved in the plasma (Margereson, 2001). If the PaO_2 is high, more oxygen is able to bind with hemoglobin; the converse is also true. It is important to interpret SaO_2 and PaO_2 values in relation to the amount of supplemented oxygen the patient is receiving. The alveolar–arterial gap is the difference between the mean alveolar PaO_2 and the measured arterial PaO_2. The alveolar PaO_2 is always higher than the arterial PaO_2. Elevations in the gap indicate a ventilation perfusion imbalance in the lungs and inadequate diffusion of oxygen to carbon dioxide at the pulmonary blood supply.

Under normal circumstances, when the PaO_2 value decreases slightly, there is an incremental drop in the SaO_2 value. However, when PaO_2 falls below 60 mm Hg, the association is disturbed and subtle decreases in partial pressure cause significant drops in SaO_2, known as hemoglobin desaturation. The oxyhemoglobin dissociation curve is illustrated in Figure 15-4.

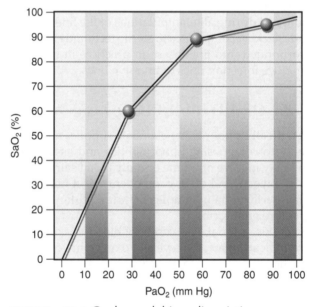

FIGURE 15-4 Oxyhemoglobin dissociation curve. Normally, PaO_2 and SaO_2 values are closely related. When PaO_2 decreases slightly, so does SaO_2. However, when PaO_2 drops below 60 mm Hg, the close association is disrupted. The disruption is represented graphically as the oxyhemoglobin dissociation curve, which illustrates the relationship between PaO_2 and SaO_2 values known as the 30–60–90 rule. When PaO_2 measures 30 mm Hg, SaO_2 is usually 60%, and when PaO_2 is 60 mm Hg, SaO_2 is usually 90%. (Adapted from Horne, C., & Derrico, D. (1999). Mastering ABGs: The art of arterial blood gas measurement. *American Journal of Nursing*, 99(8), 26–33.)

BOX 15-2   NORMAL ARTERIAL BLOOD GAS VALUES*

pH: 7.35–7.45
$PaCO_2$: 38–42 mm Hg
PaO_2: 75–100 mm Hg
PCO_2: 35–45 mm Hg
PO_2: 80–100 mm Hg
SaO_2: 94%–100%
HCO_3^-: 22–26 mEq/L
Base excess: ± 2 mEq/L

*At sea level for adults (Fischbach & Dunning, 2009).

ABG Parameters and Interpretation

ABG measurements are used to detect and address respiratory imbalances. Specific uses include diagnosing and regulating oxygen therapy and evaluating all other therapy and metabolic imbalances. In particular, ABG measurements assess the effectiveness of the therapy. To interpret ABG values, the nurse must understand the physiologic, chemical, and physical processes that influence each parameter. Normal ABG values are outlined in Box 15-2.

pH

The **pH value** refers to the degree of acidity or alkalinity of the blood. It is not an absolute measurement but gives an approximation of hydrogen ion concentration. The pH scale is as follows (*numbers are inversely related to the degree of acidity*): the range compatible with life is roughly 6.8 to 7.8, and the normal range lies between 7.35 and 7.45. A pH increase represents a decrease in acidity, and a pH decrease represents an increase in acidity. A pH decrease of 0.3 shows a doubling of hydrogen concentration (e.g., blood pH of 7.10 has twice the hydrogen concentration of blood pH 7.40) (Woodrow, 2010).

The ABG analyzers measure:

- pH
- Respiratory function
- Metabolic function
- Electrolytes + metabolites

Thus, analysis by the nurse should follow a systematic sequence:

1. pH
2. Respiratory function—three core measurements ($PaCO_2$, PaO_2, and SaO_2)
3. Metabolism function—two core measurements (bicarbonate, HCO_3^- and base excess, BE) noting whether each aspect of one to three as normal, low, or high to baseline ranges

4. Is compensation occurring (compare pH with respiratory and metabolic function)? If so, which direction is the change?
5. Note electrolytes + metabolites

HYDROGEN

Cell metabolism produces hydrogen, which combines with bicarbonate to form carbonic acid. This breaks down into water, which is excreted by the kidneys, and carbon dioxide, which is excreted by the lungs. Acid–base balance is the maintenance of hydrogen ion (H^+) concentration in the blood at a level that enables normal cell function. The normal pH of the arterial blood is 7.35 to 7.45, and normal H^+ concentration is 36 to 44 nmol/L (Kindlen, 2003). H^+ and pH have an inverse relationship, that is, as one increases, the other decreases.

Acid–base balance is achieved through (1) cellular processing of hydrogen with no appreciable change in blood concentration by elimination of volatile acid as carbon dioxide by the lungs, (2) by excretion and reabsorption of fixed acid and bicarbonate by the kidneys, and (3) by chemical buffering. When the pH is below 7.0 or above 8.0, survival is unlikely (Woodrow, 2010). Three mechanisms help to maintain acid–base balance in the blood:

- Buffer systems
- Exhalation of carbon dioxide
- Excretion of H^+ by the kidneys

BUFFERS

A buffer is a solute that resists pH change when acids or bases are added. The buffer base consists of bicarbonate and all nonbicarbonate buffers. The bicarbonate buffer system cannot buffer volatile acids but does buffer approximately 75% of all the fixed acid generated by the body. The nonbicarbonate buffer system consists primarily of proteins, hemoglobin, and phosphate. Nonbicarbonate buffers volatile nonfixed acids.

BICARBONATE

The primary metabolic parameter, bicarbonate, may be reported as carbon dioxide content, carbon dioxide combining power, carbon dioxide, or standard bicarbonate, any of which refers to the same factor. Bicarbonate is measured by concentration and reported as milliequivalent per liter (mEq/L). It is universally related to the quantity of fixed acid excess and therefore is more a controlled than a controlling factor.

Sources of fixed acids include organic and inorganic dietary acids, lactic acid as a by-product of cell metabolism without oxygen, and ketoacids as by-products of cell metabolism without glucose or insulin. The normal excretion rate of fixed acid by the kidneys is 50 mEq/d. However, the excretion and reabsorption of both hydrogen and bicarbonate can be greatly increased or decreased by body demands. The normal bicarbonate range is 24 ± 3 mEq/L. The minimum level compatible with life is 1 mEq/L; the maximum level is 48 mEq/L.

BASE EXCESS

The BE parameter is the sum total in concentration of all the buffer anions (bicarbonate and nonbicarbonate) in a sample of whole blood, equilibrated with a normal partial pressure carbon dioxide PCO_2 (40 mm Hg). Because BE is equilibrated with a normal PCO_2, it is not affected by primary respiratory imbalances.

Normal BE is 48 ± 3 mm/L but is reported as plus or minus zero. In metabolic acidosis, BE is minus; in metabolic alkalosis, BE is plus.

Physics of Gas

The parameters discussed so far are measured by concentration. The two respiratory parameters measured by pressure (intensity) warrant a brief review of the physics of gas.

Gas has volume, which refers to the space the gas occupies, and is measured in milliliters (mL). Gas has pressure, which is measured mathematically as force per unit area by noting the height to which the force can support a column of mercury. This measurement is expressed in millimeters of mercury (mm Hg). Gas has temperature, which is generated by gas molecules in constant motion and is measured in degrees Celsius (°C) or Fahrenheit (°F). Dalton's law regarding the behavior of gas in a mixture, as applied to oxygen in the atmosphere (room air), indicates the following:

- The total pressure of the gas mixture equals the sum of the partial pressures of each gas or total pressure of atmosphere (P_{atm}) = partial pressure oxygen (PO_2) + partial pressure nitrogen (PN_2) + partial pressure carbon dioxide (PCO_2).
- Each gas acts independently, as if it alone occupied the total space.
- Each gas contribution to the total pressure depends solely on the percentage of the total gas it occupies. The contribution of oxygen to the total atmospheric pressure is 21%. (Other variables not discussed here can exist.)
- The partial pressure of each gas depends on the number of molecules existing in the fixed space. At high elevations, the number of oxygen molecules is decreased; therefore, PO_2 is decreased.
- Each gas is unaffected by any changes in other gas molecules. The PO_2 does not increase or decrease in relation to changes of PCO_2.

PARTIAL PRESSURE OF CARBON DIOXIDE

The PCO_2 value reflects the adequacy of alveolar ventilation. It is the primary respiratory parameter. Carbon dioxide is eliminated by the lungs at the same rate it is formed by the tissues and at the same time maintains constant blood levels.

Arterial PCO_2 is inversely related to the level of ventilation. With hypoventilation, carbon dioxide is retained and the PCO_2 elevates; with hyperventilation, carbon dioxide is blown off and the PCO_2 decreases. The normal range for PCO_2 is 40 ± 4 mm Hg. The minimum value compatible with life is 9 mm Hg; the maximum value is 158 mm Hg.

The carbonic acid–bicarbonate buffer system is the most important regulator of extracellular fluid. It is able to control two constituents: CO_2 via the lungs and HCO_3^- via the kidneys (Kindlen, 2003). Buffers are only a temporary means of acid–base balance as they are unable to excrete acid actively like the lungs and kidneys.

LUNGS

Retention of arterial CO_2 produces an increase in extracellular H^+ and a subsequent decrease in pH (**hypercapnia** and acidosis); the opposite is also true. An increase in respirations permits the exhalation of more CO_2, H^+ concentration falls, and pH rises. Changes in respiratory rate and depth of breathing can alter body pH within minutes (Woodrow, 2010).

KIDNEYS

The renal system is slower and can take several hours or days to compensate for a change in H^+. The kidneys alter H^+ concentrations in the following ways:

- Adjusting the amount of bases secreted in the urine
- Altering the amount of hydrogen secreted in the urine
- Generating new bicarbonate to raise plasma levels

Bases are gained through diet or during metabolism. The control of pH is also dependent on the secretion of H^+ in the urine by renal tubular absorption. H^+ is secreted into the tubular fluid in competition with sodium in the potassium–sodium pump. This explains why patients with acidosis are often hyperkalemic. Lastly, the renal system uses hydrogen phosphate (HPO_4^{2-}) and ammonia (NH_3) to bind with H^+ and excrete them in the form of dihydrogen phosphate ($H_2PO_4^-$) and ammonia (NH_4^-) (Kindlen, 2003).

PARTIAL PRESSURE OF OXYGEN

The PO_2 value is also an intensity factor, measured in millimeters of mercury. It tells how fast and for how long oxygen passes from blood into tissue. The PO_2 is usually not a direct influence in acid–base balance.

Normal PO_2 values are oxygen and age dependent. When the fraction of inspired oxygen (FiO_2) is 21% (room air) and the patient is 60 years of age or younger, the PO_2 should be at least 80 mm Hg. With each 10-year advance in age, the normal PO_2 decreases by 10 mm Hg. If the PO_2 is 50 mm Hg or lower in a patient younger than 60 years of age, respiratory failure is present. A PO_2 between 50 and 75 mm Hg reflects moderate hypoxemia.

HYPOXEMIA

Hypoxemia is insufficient oxygenation of the blood and can be measured directly by the PO_2. Hypoxia—insufficient oxygenation of the tissues—cannot be directly measured but is presumed if the partial pressure of oxygen in venous blood $(P\bar{v}o_2)$ is 30 mm Hg or lower. To avoid hypoxia when hypoxemia is present, the cardiovascular system must increase the rate of tissue perfusion or the hemoglobin content must be elevated.

Shunting is a common cause of hypoxemia. *Shunting* is any impediment in the blood transport system that results in blood not coming in contact with oxygen. This can be seen in vascular lung tumors, a right-to-left intracardiac shunt, or capillary shunting in which pulmonary capillary blood comes in contact with totally unventilated alveoli (dead space).

OXYGEN SATURATION

Oxygen saturation (SaO_2) is the parameter that reflects the amount of oxygen taken up by hemoglobin when fully saturated. It is a quantity factor and is measured in percentage. It may also be called $PO_2\%$. The normal adult values are 96% to 97% before 65 years of age and 95% to 96% in older patients. Oxygen saturation

- depends on PO_2. When the pressure exceeds a certain value, the amount of oxygen taken in no longer increases.
- is altered by pH. If PO_2 remains constant, oxygen saturation decreases when the pH decreases and increases when the pH increases.
- is altered by temperature. If the PO_2 is constant, oxygen saturation decreases when the temperature increases and increases when the temperature decreases.

This indicates that hyperthermia causes metabolic acidosis and hypothermia causes metabolic alkalosis. In hypothermia, the oxygen need is decreased, but the oxygen is bound so tightly to the hemoglobin that the ability to deliver it is greatly decreased. Inhalation of carbon dioxide may be used to cause acidosis and release the bound oxygen.

Chemoreceptors and Primary Acid–Base Imbalances

Chemoreceptors located peripherally in aortic and carotid vessels and centrally in the brain play a role in body responses to abnormal PCO_2 and PO_2 values. Chemoreceptors signal the brain to stimulate or depress ventilation, according to body needs. The response to an elevated PCO_2 is greater than to a decreased PO_2 because PCO_2 elevation is a danger signal of respiratory failure. At high altitudes where oxygen supply is decreased, oxygen need is greater than PCO_2 constancy; the chemoreceptors stimulate hyperventilation to obtain more oxygen; thus this hyperventilation results in a decreased PCO_2.

METABOLIC ACIDOSIS

Metabolic acidosis results from an excess of fixed acids or a primary bicarbonate deficit. The primary causes are as follows:

- Increased production of fixed acids, including ketoacids, which are evident in diabetic acidosis or starvation when glucose and insulin are unavailable for cell metabolism, and lactic acid, which is evident in cardiopulmonary failure when oxygen is unavailable for cell metabolism
- Failure of kidneys to excrete fixed acid
- Primary bicarbonate deficit—severe diarrhea or bowel or biliary fistula

This is a metabolic imbalance because bicarbonate is the parameter primarily affected. Acidosis is present because the carbon dioxide level has not changed, but the decrease in bicarbonate has caused the ratio to go closer than 1 part acid to 20 parts base. It can be between 1:16 and 1:5, depending on the degree of bicarbonate deficit. Because pH depends on the acid–base ratio, and this ratio has now narrowed, acidosis is present. BE is minus because there is not enough bicarbonate to buffer the fixed acid.

ABG values in metabolic acidosis:

- pH: <7.35
- HCO_3^-: <22 mEq/L
- PCO_2: normal (40 ± 4 mm Hg)
- BE: <– 3

If the metabolic acidosis is of renal origin, the kidneys cannot respond. If it is of nonrenal origin, the kidneys increase the excretion of hydrogen and the reabsorption of bicarbonate. This response is slow, but once started, can be maintained for weeks or months.

The chemoreceptors are sensitive to the increase in hydrogen and stimulate compensatory hyperventilation to blow off carbon dioxide, decreasing the PCO_2 < 40 mm Hg to obtain an acid–base ratio closer to normal (1:20) needed for a normal pH. This compensatory respiratory response is prompt and predictable; it occurs within minutes but becomes less effective with time. The limit of compensatory hyperventilation occurs when the PCO_2 reaches 12 mm Hg.

After the kidneys and lungs respond, bicarbonate increases to a level closer to normal. PCO_2 decreases and the acid–base ratio moves closer to 1:20 with a resultant pH closer to normal. Compensation thus occurs.

With bicarbonate administration, the bicarbonate level reverts to normal and the lungs stop hyperventilation. Therefore, PCO_2 reverts to normal, resulting in a 1:20 acid–base ratio and allowing a normal pH (7.35 to 7.45). Correction thereby is achieved.

METABOLIC ALKALOSIS

Metabolic alkalosis results from a decrease in body content of fixed acids or a primary bicarbonate excess. The primary causes are as follows:

- Excessive loss of fixed acids resulting, for example, from prolonged vomiting, gastric suctioning, potassium deficit
- Primary bicarbonate excess resulting, for example, from excessive administration of sodium bicarbonate, sodium citrate, or chloride deficit, whereby bicarbonate increases to maintain cation–anion balance or sodium deficit, with bicarbonate excretion dependent on sodium

This is a metabolic imbalance because the primary parameter affected is bicarbonate. Alkalosis occurs because the acid–base ratio has widened to 1 part acid to 25 to 50 parts base. This ratio results in a pH elevation. Because there is an excess of bicarbonate, the BE is plus.

ABG values in metabolic alkalosis:

- pH: >7.45
- HCO_3^-: >26 mEq/L
- PCO_2: normal (40 ± 4 mm Hg)
- BE: > +3

Whether the kidneys respond to metabolic alkalosis depends on several factors. An increase in bicarbonate causes bicarbonate excretion to increase, provided there is no deficit of chloride or potassium. If a chloride depletion is present, bicarbonate is reabsorbed as the accompanying anion for sodium. Because a bicarbonate increase is usually accompanied by an increase in sodium, a decrease in chloride, and a potassium deficit, bicarbonate is not excreted but reabsorbed.

Compensatory respiratory response to metabolic alkalosis is variable. The degree of hypoventilation that occurs depends on the causative factors. Regardless of the cause, hypoventilation as a compensatory response is rarely sufficient to bring the PCO_2 > 55 mm Hg because an elevated PCO_2 causes the chemoreceptors to stimulate breathing to prevent respiratory failure.

When the lungs and kidneys do respond, some compensation occurs: bicarbonate falls, PCO_2 rises, and the acid–base ratio comes closer to 1:20. The pH thus decreases to a level closer to normal.

Correction occurs with the administration of solutions containing chloride and potassium. In assessing and treating respiratory imbalances, ABG measurements are an absolute clinical necessity because ventilation is reflected in PCO_2 and oxygenation in PO_2. Furthermore, acute respiratory failure may occur with slight changes in pulse, BP, or alertness until cardiopulmonary collapse occurs.

RESPIRATORY ACIDOSIS

Respiratory acidosis is always caused by carbon dioxide retention from hypoventilation. This is rarely seen without hypoxemia (PO_2 < 60 mm Hg). The causes of hypoventilation include

- Anesthesia, narcotics, sedation
- Central nervous system disease such as polio, spinal cord lesions
- Severe hypokalemia
- Intrathoracic collection of blood, fluid, or air
- Pulmonary diseases, both restrictive (heart failure, tumors, atelectasis) and obstructive (bronchitis, emphysema, asthma, or foreign body)

The acidosis process is respiratory because the PCO_2 is the primary parameter involved. Nonfixed, volatile acid (PCO_2) is in excess, but the base (bicarbonate) is normal. The acid–base ratio is closer than 1:20; it is between 1:5 and 1:20, resulting in acidosis.

ABG values in respiratory acidosis:

- pH: <7.35
- PCO_2: >44 mm Hg
- HCO_3^-: normal (24 ± 2 mEq/L)

Because the lungs are always the primary cause of respiratory acidosis, they cannot play a role in compensation. Renal compensation is always slow in onset but effective once started: generation and reabsorption of bicarbonate increases, excretion of hydrogen increases, and the excretion of chloride increases, resulting in a chloride deficit.

With renal response, bicarbonate rises above normal and PCO_2 remains unchanged. The acid ratio comes closer to 1:20, allowing for some compensation, with a pH closer to normal.

Correction of respiratory acidosis is possible only by correction of the pulmonary cause. Chloride solutions are usually given to treat the chloride deficit.

RESPIRATORY ALKALOSIS

Respiratory alkalosis is always caused by a carbon dioxide deficit owing to hyperventilation.

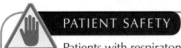

PATIENT SAFETY

Patients with respiratory alkalosis are at risk for hypokalemia and hypocalcemia.

Factors causing hyperventilation include the following:

- Chemoreceptor response to hypoxemia. The chemoreceptors sense the decrease in oxygen and send a message to the brain to stimulate ventilation. This hyperventilation results in carbon dioxide being blown off thus decreasing PCO_2. This is normal at high altitudes.
- Respiratory response to metabolic acidosis. This response can persist for several hours or days after the metabolic acidosis is corrected because of higher levels of hydrogen excess in cerebrospinal fluid (CSF) and the fact that chemoreceptors are more responsive to CSF than to blood.
- Central nervous system malfunctions (trauma, infection, brain lesions)
- Anxiety, pain, fever, shock
- Anemia, carbon monoxide poisoning
- Epinephrine, salicylates, and progesterone
- Improper mechanical ventilation. Any patient with chronic obstructive pulmonary disease who is overcorrected by mechanical ventilation so that the PCO_2 decreases faster than 10 mm Hg/h will have respiratory alkalosis.

This hyperventilation process is respiratory because PCO_2 is the primary parameter affected. Alkalosis is present because carbon dioxide is decreased and the bicarbonate value is normal, resulting in an acid–base ratio between 1:25 and 1:50. This ratio results in a pH above 7.45.

ABG values in respiratory alkalosis:

- pH: >7.45
- PCO_2: <36 mm Hg
- HCO_3^-: normal (24 ± 2 mEq/L)

Because the lungs are the primary cause of respiratory alkalosis, they cannot respond for compensation. Renal response occurs after several hours or days. The kidneys decrease excretion of hydrogen and increase excretion of bicarbonate. The urine cannot become more alkaline than pH 7.0. This renal response creates some compensation. The bicarbonate value drops < 24 mEq/L. The acid–base ratio comes closer to 1:20, allowing the pH to come closer to normal.

Respiratory alkalosis can be corrected by administering chloride solutions to replace the bicarbonate ion load. However, the buffering capacity of the plasma has been compromised as a result of the alkalosis, and any additional insult to the balance is poorly tolerated.

MIXED ACID–BASE IMBALANCES

In the hospital setting, two or more primary imbalances may coexist in the same patient. The following combinations sometimes occur:

- Metabolic acidosis and metabolic alkalosis in a patient who has diabetic acidosis and who is vomiting
- Metabolic acidosis and respiratory acidosis in a patient with severe pulmonary edema, followed by cardiogenic shock
- Metabolic acidosis and respiratory alkalosis in a patient with both kidney and liver failure
- Respiratory acidosis and metabolic alkalosis in a patient who has chronic respiratory insufficiency and who is on a salt-poor diet and taking diuretics
- Respiratory alkalosis and metabolic alkalosis are usually seen as a result of mechanical overventilation.

Respiratory acidosis and respiratory alkalosis cannot coexist because a person cannot hypoventilate and hyperventilate at the same time.

Hemodynamic Monitoring

Critically ill patients require continuous assessment of their cardiopulmonary system to diagnose and manage complex medical conditions. This is most commonly achieved by using direct pressure monitoring systems. Pulmonary artery pressure (PA), central venous pressure (CVP), and intra-arterial blood pressure (BP) monitoring are the most common forms of hemodynamic monitoring. These invasive monitoring techniques are being replaced by noninvasive impedance methods of dynamic monitoring (Corley, Barnett, Mullany, & Fraser, 2009; McCoy et al., 2009).

Hemodynamic instability is defined as a global or regional perfusion that is inadequate to support normal organ function. The two variables that most directly reflect organ perfusion are BP and cardiac output. Because of the limits on coronary and cerebral autoregulation, hypotension may compromise adequate perfusion of the brain and heart.

The basic tenet of hemodynamic monitoring is the control of adequate oxygen delivery to tissues. The primary physiologic response to an increased demand in tissue oxygen or to a reduced content in arterial oxygen is to increase cardiac output. However, most cardiovascular disorders limit the heart's ability to respond to these needs. As a result, tissues rely on a second compensatory mechanism by drawing on the venous oxygen reserve. When the tissue oxygen supply becomes inadequate, even for brief periods, lactic acidosis and tissue damage may arise. The primary objective is to prevent tissue hypoxia through critical care interventions.

CENTRAL VENOUS PRESSURE

CVP reflects the pressure of blood in the right atrium or vena cava and relates to an adequate circulatory blood supply. CVP is affected by a myriad of intrinsic and extrinsic factors including IV fluids, positioning, intrathoracic pressures, blood volume, heart rate, contractility, and myocardial and venous compliance, among others. Further confusing the issue is discrepancy between normal physiology and disease state pathology.

BLOOD VOLUME

Changes in blood volume alter the tone of the blood vessels and the ability of the heart to circulate the blood. Reduced blood volume results in less pressure at the right atrium, indicated by a drop in CVP; an increased blood volume produces more pressure at the atrium, with a rise in CVP.

In managing inadequate circulation, the clinician must first establish a normal blood volume. If the inadequate circulation results from deficient blood volume, pressure may be manipulated by administering blood volume expanders. In instances of increased volume, phlebotomy may be used to reduce volume. If circulation is still insufficient, the clinician needs to evaluate the remaining two essential components: cardiac contractility (myocardial status) and vascular tone.

CARDIAC CONTRACTILITY

Cardiac contractility may be affected by disease, drugs, fluids, or anesthetics. Because the CVP is a measure of the capacity of the myocardium as well as the blood volume, it is invaluable in monitoring the effects of anesthesia and surgery on elderly patients with arteriosclerosis or patients with myocardial insufficiency. Normally, the right atrial pressure is 0 mm Hg, approximately equal to atmospheric pressure around the body. The right atrial pressure, reflected in CVP readings, can vary to 30 mm Hg in a variety of clinical conditions and as low as −5 mm Hg during hemorrhage (Hadaway, 2010). The CVP rises if the heart muscle is impaired. The pressure of the volume of blood at the heart increases because the heart muscle can no longer pump an adequate flow of blood out of the right atrium. A high CVP may suggest cardiac failure, which is one of the most common causes of elevated CVP in shock. Drugs or chemicals are administered to improve myocardial response, thus increasing cardiac output and lowering the CVP.

VASCULAR TONE

The third essential component, vascular tone, depends on the arterial pressure and on external and internal pressures on the veins. The arterial pressure arises from the contractile force of the left ventricle and is transmitted through the capillaries to the veins.

Compensatory external pressures on the veins usually result from muscular and fascia tissue pumping action in the extremities, intra-abdominal pressure from straining and distention, and the intrathoracic pressure from contraction of the diaphragm and chest wall. CVP of patients on positive-pressure respirators is usually increased by 4 cm H_2O; patients on negative pressure show a decreased CVP.

The blood volume, myocardial response, and sympathomimetic amines (epinephrine, norepinephrine) produce internal pressure on the veins. By stimulating contraction of the venous wall, vasopressors decrease the capacity of the venous system and improve vascular tone. Various methods are used to detect change in a patient's blood volume, including hematocrit, changes in patient weight, and blood volume computations. CVP is a parameter used to assess blood volume.

Central Venous Pressure Monitoring

The CVP catheter is used to measure the filling pressures of the right side of the heart. During diastole, when the tricuspid valve is open and the blood is flowing from the right atrium to the right ventricle, the CVP accurately reflects fluid volume pressures in the right ventricle (Urden, Stacy, & Lough, 2004). The CVP waveform reflects the contraction of the atria and the concurrent effect of the ventricles and surrounding major vessels. Normal parameters vary with the patient's clinical condition and the measurement methodology; as discussed previously, values are affected by circulating volume, cardiac contractility, and vascular tone.

CVP monitoring may be accomplished by using a water manometer (rarely used today), which records pressure in units of centimeters of water (between 4 and 12 cm H_2O), or more commonly by transducer and monitor, which records pressure in units of millimeters of mercury (between 0 and 15 mm Hg). CVP readings indicate changes in preload (filling pressure in the right ventricle). Abnormal readings may indicate inadequate or increased preload, decreased contractility, or increased afterload (pressure against which the left ventricle contracts). Abnormal pressures may appear in many patients. The procedure for using a transducer is seen in Box 15-3.

Assessing and Documenting Central Venous Pressure

CVP is usually read at intervals directed by the patients' condition and/or therapy. When obtaining a CVP reading, the patient must be quiet, not coughing or straining, and in a supine position with the zero point on the manometer at the mid-atrial level. The procedure involves turning the stopcock open to the patient and reading either through the vacillations on the water manometer until the meniscus settles to the appropriate reading or by transducing a pressurized bag to the CVP component of a bedside monitor. In this instance, the computer system is zeroed to atmospheric air by opening the stopcock to air and pressing the system's zero button. The stopcock is then readjusted to permit equilibration between the pressure bag and the patient vascular flow. The CVP waveform should appear on the

---

BOX 15-3   MEASURING CVP WITH A TRANSDUCER

1. Complete hand hygiene
2. Place the patient in supine position and explain the procedure
3. Identify the phlebostatic axis at the intersection of the midaxillary line and the fourth intercostal space
4. Temporarily stop any IV solution in progress to avoid artifacts
5. Adjust the three-way stopcock off to the patient and remove the protective cap from the port to open the system to air
6. Press zero on the monitor and look for the display indicative of zero level
7. Replace cap on stopcock and turn stopcock on to the patient
8. Observe and record the waveform and reading as well as the patient's position
9. Resume the infusion as indicated

monitor and be interpreted along with the resulting CVP value on the monitor. Figure 15-5 shows how the CVP waveform corresponds to the electrocardiogram (ECG).

Pulmonary Artery Pressure

Since the mid-1950s, the concept of a balloon-assisted arterial catheter has been explored. Two physicians, H.J.C. Swan and William Ganz, further developed intracardiopulmonary monitoring and a cardiac output thermodilution method. These developments of the 1970s introduced the balloon-tipped, flow directed, PA catheter, also known as the Swan-Ganz catheter.

The PA catheter as a diagnostic tool may be used for the following diagnostic needs or indicators in complex patient situations: shock states, differentiation of high- and low-pulmonary edema, primary pulmonary hypertension, valvular disease, intracardiac shunt, cardiac tamponade, pulmonary embolus, monitoring and management of complicated acute myocardial infarction, assessing hemodynamic response to therapies, management of multiorgan failure, severe burns, and hemodynamic instability after cardiac surgery. The therapeutic indications for use of a PA catheter are aspiration of air emboli and direct infusions of medication for pulmonary hypertension. PA catheters are contraindicated in patients with tricuspid or pulmonary valve mechanical prosthesis, right heart mass (thrombus or tumor), and tricuspid or pulmonary valve endocarditis (Manoach, Weingart, & Charchaflieh, 2012; Mathews, 2007).

The PA catheter is inserted into a large vein and threaded into the pulmonary outflow track distal to the right ventricle transiting the pulmonary tricuspid valve. PA systolic and diastolic pressures are transferred through a transducer to an amplifier or monitor, which converts the electrical signals to waveform displays on the bedside monitor. Computer algorithms and programs can be used by the experienced practitioner to gain additional physiologic parameters for hemodynamic interpretation of systemic circulation, oxygen perfusion and delivery, and patient response to vasoactive medication.

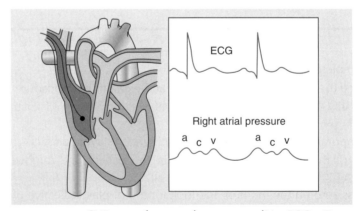

FIGURE 15-5 CVP waveform and corresponding ECG. (From Burchell, P. L., & Powers, K. A. (2011). Focus on central venous pressure monitoring in an acute care setting. *Nursing, 41*(12), 38–43.)

PA CATHETER SYSTEM AND INSERTION

Catheters are approximately 110 cm long and come in sizes 5, 6, 7, and 7.5 French. The lines may be color-coded blue to differentiate them from arterial lines, which may be color-coded red. Basic PA catheters have multiple lumens. This multilumen catheter contains a clear port used as an infusion and medication port. The blue, distal port is used for CVP monitoring, which is connected to an IV system and a transducer to measure the right atrial pressure CVP. A yellow port is transduced to monitor hemodynamic pressures. A red specialized smaller port is manufactured with a two-way stopcock for inflation and deflation of the balloon that is inflated with 0.8 to 1.5 mL air, depending on the size and manufacturer. The infusion system contains an IV bag, pressure infuser bag, pressure tubing with stopcocks, and transducer with cable connected to a monitor.

The PA catheter may be inserted either percutaneously or by a cut down procedure in any accessible vein large enough to allow passage of the catheter. The right subclavian or internal jugular positions are the preferred location, but left-sided access is possible. As the catheter is threaded and the tip passes the superior vena cava, the balloon is inflated. Normal blood flow then assists catheter advancement. The tip enters the right atrium and passes through the tricuspid valve, entering the right ventricle. It then passes through the pulmonic valve into the PA. Use of a cardiac monitor is essential during insertion because the waveform pattern defines changes with each advancement, thereby providing a guide for tip location, and simultaneously monitoring the patient's condition throughout the procedure. The catheter tip placement must be confirmed by radiography.

Pulmonary capillary wedge pressure, which reflects left heart pressure, is measured intermittently by inflating the balloon to its recommended level (Figure 15-6). Care should be taken not to overinflate the balloon and not to inflate it too frequently. Typically, the balloon is inflated every 4 hours, with the inflation pressure maintained no longer than 1 to 2 minutes. The measurement achieved when a PA catheter floats to the wedged position in the pulmonary outflow tract is the pulmonary artery wedge pressure (PAWP) or also called the pulmonary artery occlusive pressure (PAOP). The PAWP is calculated as left-sided heart entering pressure as the blood ceases when the balloon is wedged in the PA and provides indirect measures of pulmonary venous pressure and the left ventricle heart pressure.

Indications for proper placement include a decline in pressure as the catheter moves from the PA into the wedged position, ability to aspirate blood from the distal port, and a decline in end-tidal CO_2 concentration with the inflation of the balloon (produces a rise in alveolar dead space).

COMPLICATIONS

Possible complications include the following:

- Catheter migration backward to the right ventricle as evidenced by a change in the waveform on the monitor to an RV waveform. Prompt removal or advancement by a trained practitioner should be completed to thwart the risk of a lethal catheter-induced ventricular rhythm

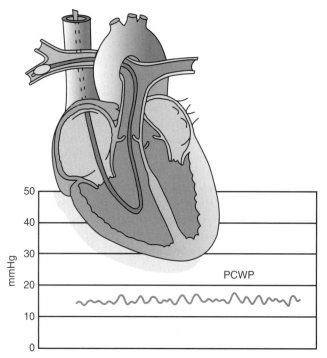

FIGURE 15-6 Balloon inflation in pulmonary capillary wedge pressure.

- Cardiac arrhythmias, which may occur during insertion. Lidocaine hydrochloride and defibrillation equipment must be readily available. Serious dysrhythmias during insertion are rare
- Catheter knotting
- Balloon rupture, which is possible in a patient without intracardiac shunting of blood
- Pulmonary damage, which may result from obstructed PA blood flow caused by peripheral migration of the catheter to a wedged position. This is avoidable with constant monitoring and by following recommendations regarding balloon inflation
- Infection, which is always a threat. The use of disposable equipment has minimized the occurrence of infection. Strict adherence to aseptic technique is mandatory.

PA CATHETER HEMODYNAMIC MONITORING PARAMETERS

The PA catheter monitoring parameters that are transduced to the bedside monitor include PA systolic and diastolic pressure with a calculated mean and PAWP with the balloon inflated when the practitioner uses a synchronized method of ECG monitoring with PA catheter balloon inflation. Using the thermodilutional or continuous cardiac output method, additional intracardiac and systemic hemodynamic parameters can be obtained. See Table 15-4 for select parameters, definitions, and values for PA monitoring interpretations.

TABLE 15-4	SELECT PA MONITORING PARAMETERS

The following definitions and values represent a standard range of hemodynamic parameters.

RAP/CVP:
RAP is the right atrial pressure or central venous pressure. The normal range is 2–6 mm Hg.

RVP:
RVP is the right ventricular pressure. The normal systolic range is 20–30 mm Hg. The normal diastolic range is 0–5 mm Hg.

PAP:
PAP is the pulmonary artery pressure. The normal systolic range is 20–30 mm Hg. The normal diastolic range is 8–12 mm Hg. The normal mean range is 10–20 mm Hg.

PAWP:
PAWP (also known as PAOP) is the pressure generated by the left ventricle in the PA. This is performed by inflating a balloon in the PA catheter. The normal range is 4–12 mm Hg.

PAWP, pulmonary artery wedge pressure; PAOP, pulmonary artery occlusive pressure.

Use of PA Catheters

One important factor regarding PA catheters is that there is widespread controversy and debate regarding the use of PA catheters in the critically ill. The debate was seriously raised by Connors et al. (1996). The group indicated that an increase in mortality, cost, and length of hospital stay was related to PA catheter utilization. A recent Cochrane review (Rajaram et al., 2013) concluded that PA catheters did not decrease mortality, length of stay, or cost for ICU patients. They recommended that additional research is needed to support the efficacy of PA catheter use; for example, its effect on vasopressor use in specific patient populations.

The efficacy of PA catheter use may be related to the fact that physicians and nurses are often inadequately trained in its use and thus incorrectly measure and/or misinterpret the data obtained from the PA catheter. This subsequently leads to making inappropriate clinical decisions. Ultimately, the outcome of the patient is based on the proper use of the technology and accurate clinical interpretation of data provided, not on the technology that is providing the information (Murphy & Vender, 2007).

HEMODIALYSIS/RENAL REPLACEMENT THERAPY

Hemodialysis Catheters

Hemodialysis, also called renal replacement therapy, may be needed to correct acute renal failure, for patients with acute drug intoxication, or for patients with chronic renal failure needing maintenance therapy. Requirements for assuring adequate therapy include (1) well-trained nursing staff, (2) an appropriate prescription, (3) an efficiently operating dialysis machine, (4) satisfactory access, (5) an informed patient or designated surrogate, and (6) ongoing data review. Vascular access is needed to perform hemodialysis and can be provided with a double-lumen VAC, an external AV shunt, or a surgically created AV anastomosis (e.g., fistula or graft). For needle access, the common sites for VAC include the internal jugular or subclavian vein. Common sites for the external shunt include the forearm (radial artery to the cephalic vein) or the leg (posterior tibial artery to saphenous vein). The subclavian vein is not recommended for temporary access because of the increased risk for vascular stenosis. When this complication occurs, the use of the opposite side of the subclavian system for chronic dialysis is precluded (Tolwani, 2013). The internal jugular is the most common access site; however, the femoral vein for venovenous dialysis has been reported.

The double-lumen dialysis catheter is inserted into the prepped site under sterile procedure using ultrasound-guided equipment to reduce the risk of arterial or venous vascular damage. The hemodialysis catheter is made of polymers (usually polyurethane or silicone) that ensures adequate resistance combined with softness and hemocompatibility. Semirigid catheters are preferred over rigid catheters. The right jugular vein typically requires a 15- to 16-cm catheter, and the subclavian vein requires a 19- to 20-cm catheter; a 24-cm catheter is used for femoral access (Vijayan, 2009). A triple-lumen temporary hemodialysis catheter is available with a midcentral port for administration of medication and IV fluids. Complications related to dialysis catheter use are the same as for other central vascular access devices. Differences in performance during dialysis have been reported to be similar between the jugular and femoral sites (Parienti et al., 2010). Authors have cautioned about the use of invasive lines for patients who are better candidates for longer-term hemodialysis access devices. Proper patient selection by knowledgeable and skilled practitioners is necessary to curtail the growing incidents of patients on dialysis (Hakim & Himmelfarb, 2009).

Hypodermoclysis and Subcutaneous Infusions

Hypodermoclysis is an infusion method that should be considered in patients with limited vascular access. It is ideal for elderly patients in long-term care facilities when dehydration poses a serious problem and in hospice clients for palliative care. Hypodermoclysis should not be confused with the subcutaneous administration of medication. Although many medications can be given subcutaneously, the volume of fluids necessary for hydration is much larger than the small amounts given subcutaneously. The most common problems with subcutaneous infusion of opioids are local irritation at the needle insertion site and subcutaneous scarring. Frequent site changes (every other day) and reducing the infusion volume can minimize these complications.

Continuous subcutaneous therapies fall into two categories: (1) continuous subcutaneous infusion (CSI) of medication and (2) hypodermoclysis or clysis. The aim of administering medication through the subcutaneous route is to attain appropriate medication blood levels for desired symptom control or disease management.

There are numerous advantages and disadvantages to administering medication through the CSI route are as follows: (1) medications are absorbed avoiding the "first pass" of liver metabolism seen in oral administration; (2) titration of opioid medication can be achieved rapidly similar to IV administration; (3) the burden of numerous oral pill administration is relieved; (4) generally less expensive and less time consuming than IV access and administration; (5) the insertion procedure is easy to learn; and (6) it can be used easily in diverse settings, including the home. The disadvantages and contraindications of this route of administration are (1) local site discomfort and edema; (2) limited application in certain patient conditions such as a contraindication in patient with pulmonary congestion (heart failure) and in patients with skin disorders due to excessive bleeding; (3) hypodermoclysis is contraindicated in the emergency resuscitation of patients; and (4) it should not be used when hypertonic or electrolyte-free infusions are being used (Walsh, 2005). Medications commonly administered via CSI may be found in Box 15-4.

BOX 15-4   MEDICATIONS ADMINISTERED VIA CSI

Opioids
Insulin
Terbutaline
Deferoxamine mesylate
Antiemetics
Steroids
Midazolam
Haloperidol
Hyoscine

When performing hypodermoclysis, the subcutaneous route is used as a vehicle for absorption of IV isotonic hydration fluids. Fluid selection is tantamount to success, and solutions containing sodium chloride, with or without glucose, are most commonly used. Electrolyte solutions, including Ringer solution, lactated Ringer solution, and Normosol-R, may also be used. Additives, such as the enzyme hyaluronidase, are used to enhance absorption within the tissues (Walsh, 2005).

Sites for using hypodermoclysis include posterior upper arm, upper chest avoiding breast tissue, anterior and lateral thighs, abdomen at least 2 inches from the navel, infraclavicular area, and the flank in some patients (Figure 15-7). Be sure to avoid areas of ecchymosis, erythema, or impaired skin integrity.

The hypodermoclysis technique is uncomplicated. Fluid is infused into the subcutaneous space, below the epidermis and dermis. The adipose tissue in this space is rich in blood vessels. Fluid is disbursed into the circulation though the subcutaneous space by diffusion and perfusion. When the infusion is given at a rate of 1 mL/min, the fluid can be absorbed without significant edema (Walsh, 2005).

Hypodermoclysis is ideal for preventing dehydration in those with mild to moderate dehydration and in patients who are confused or dysphasic. Patients with limited IV access or frequent IV reinsertions are ideal for this therapy. Drip infusion rates of 50 mL/h achieving 1.2 L/24 h, or with two needle access sites, running subcutaneously for a total of 100 mL/h, 2.4 L/24 h can be infused comfortably. Less than 3 L of fluid in a day are well tolerated by this method (Thomas et al., 2008).

Advantages of this method include ease of administration and maintenance by nurses, fewer complications, less cost, less pain reported by patients, and less time invested by nurses. Contraindications for this method include rapid need for fluid hydration in shock, electrolyte-free solutions, or hypertonic solutions require an alternate method of vascular administration. Hypodermoclysis may not be appropriate in emaciated patients or in hypoalbuminemic states as diffusion may be impaired in the subcutaneous space.

Insertion

Currently, there are three devices for accessing subcutaneous tissue for infusion of medication and isotonic fluids: (1) stainless steel winged needles, (2) over-the-needle catheters, and (3) subcutaneous infusion sets (Parker & Henderson, 2010). Placement of the 1-inch subcutaneous needle, 22 to 24 gauge, via a straight or butterfly hub, should be inserted after

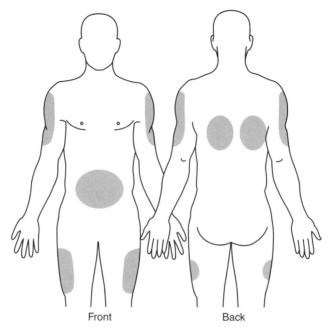

Front Back

FIGURE 15-7 Sites for hypodermoclysis medication and fluid administration.(From Cadogan, M., Brown, A. F. T., & Celenza, T. (2011). *Marshall & Ruedy's on call: Principles & protocols* (2nd ed.). © 2011, Sydney, Elsevier Australia.)

cleansing the skin per institutional policy and Infusion Nurses Society (INS) standards, at a 45- to 60-degree angle. Assure no blood return, as aspirating blood would suggest capillary or vascular breach. It is imperative that the needle be placed in the subcutaneous tissue such that the muscle and the tissue move freely around the needle. Painful infusions are reported when the needle is placed too high in the subcutaneous tissue, and muscle irritation will occur if the need is misplaced in the deeper muscle tissue. The tubing and infusion pump are the same as for an IV infusion method. Monitoring of the site is mandatory as with venous access devices. The needle is secured with tape, and a transparent dressing completes the insertion (Parker & Henderson, 2010).

INTRAOSSEOUS INFUSION DEVICES

Intraosseous access was first considered by Drinker, Drinker, and Ludd (1922) who proposed the sternum as a potential site for infusion. Intraosseous infusion of IV fluids was initiated in 1934, particularly for shock, pediatric emergencies, adults with mutilated skin, and transport of uncooperative patients. The technique has endured, despite dwindling interest after the advent of disposable needles and catheters for vascular access. Commonly administered fluids were colloids, crystalline solutions, plasma, blood products, antibiotics, epinephrine, morphine, and glucose. A renewed acceptance and interest in the technique as a viable alternative to peripheral or central venous access has grown since the 1970s. Military conflicts led to enhancements of the devices and expanded use of this modality. Research by Von Hoff, Kuhn, Burris, and Miller (2008) provided additional evidence for using this vast and noncollapsible venous matrix for infusion therapy. Intraosseous infusion may be considered during venous collapse in shock, when there is an anatomic scarcity of veins, and if thrombosis of venous sites preclude the ability to establish peripheral venous access.

Current indications for intraosseous infusion are anaphylaxis, burns, cardiac arrest, coma, dehydration, drowning, respiratory arrest, septic shock, hypovolemia, diabetic acidosis, status epilepticus, status asthmaticus, trauma, and sudden infant death syndrome. Standard protocol calls for establishing an intraosseous line in children if percutaneous peripheral venous access cannot be established within 60 to 120 seconds. It may be the route of choice in event of cardiac arrest or hypotension.

Bones are vascular structures with dynamic circulation capable of accepting large volumes of fluid and rapidly transporting fluids or drugs to the central circulation. Long bones consist of a shaft called the *diaphysis* with a very dense cortex, the *epiphysis* (or the rounded ends of the bone), and the *metaphysis* (the transitional zone). The epiphysis and the metaphysis have a much thinner cortex and contain cancellous, or spongy, porous bone. It structurally resembles honeycomb and accounts for about 20% of bone matter in the human body. The iliac crest is made of a thin cortex and is filled with cancellous bone. The hollow core of the shaft of long bones and the spaces within the cancellous bone are referred to as the *medullary space*, which contains the marrow.

The bone marrow cavity has an extensive virtually noncollapsible vascular network directly communicating with the systemic circulation. Comprising a highly interconnected network of venous sinusoids, analogous to a sponge, the intramedullary space is an integral part of the vascular system. Nutrient arteries that penetrate the cortex of the bone supply the marrow. Many bone sites have been used for intraosseous infusions, including the sternum, the tibia (Figure 15-8), the femur, and the iliac crest. In children younger than 5 years of age, the site of choice is the flat anterior medial surface of the proximal tibia just below the tibial tubercle or the distal tibia, followed by the distal femur. In adults, the iliac crest or sternum is the bone of choice. Strict asepsis is essential, and the skin preparation should be consistent with INS standards of practice (INS, 2011).

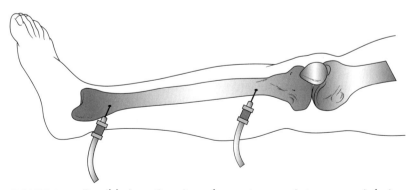

FIGURE 15-8 Possible insertion sites of percutaneous intraosseous infusion device in the lower extremity.

Intraosseous Needles

Intraosseous needles are categorized with steel needles. The marrow space of the human bone, especially in children, is capable of providing an infusion route for any IV drug or solution. The tip end of the intraosseous needle is very sharp and may have circular screwing threads that help penetrate the bone. The hub end is secured by a manual or battery-operated handle that fits into the operator's hand so that positioning and pressure may be exerted at an appropriate angle for stable insertion.

The needle size for a child is 18 gauge, and the 15- to 16-gauge needle is for adults. The long bones of the leg or the iliac crest are usually the point of insertion (Hadaway, 2010). The needle must be able to stand without support once the stylet is removed, and it must facilitate aspiration of blood and marrow. A needle with a short shaft prevents dislodgment.

Insertion Technique

After the patient receives a local or general anesthetic, the intraosseous needle is quickly advanced through the skin to the bony cortex. With firm pressure and a rotary motion in the hand device or by trigger activation with the battery-operated device, the needle is advanced into the marrow cavity. Insertion resistance decreases as the needle penetrates the cortex (known as the "trap-door effect"). The stylet is removed, and the correct position is verified by observing the needle standing without support and the ability to aspirate blood and marrow contents. Once the insertion is complete, the device is ready for use and a continuous infusion can begin.

If the attempt at implantation is unsuccessful, further attempts must be undertaken in other bones. If an infusion was established in the same bone, the infused fluid would leak from the original abandoned hole in the cortex.

VENTRICULAR RESERVOIRS

The use and benefit of an implanted ventricular reservoir has been documented as an early intervention in the management of posthemorrhagic hydrocephalus in neonates (Gaskill, Martin, & Rivera, 1988; Shooman, Portess, & Sparrow, 2009). The implanted **ventricular reservoir** provides direct access to the CSF without performing a spinal tap. The reservoir is also used to measure CSF pressure, obtain CSF specimens, and instill medication. Implanted surgically, it is positioned in the right frontal region's lateral ventricle, sutured to the pericranium, and covered with a skin flap (Figure 15-9).

Major complications associated with ventricular reservoirs include infection, malfunction, and displacement. Infection is characterized by tenderness, redness, drainage, fever, neck stiffness, and headache with or without vomiting. Malfunction typically results when the catheter is obstructed by the distal subarachnoid blockage of CSF. This is characterized by the inability to aspirate or inject the port and slow refilling of the reservoir after manual expression of fluid.

Catheter displacement or migration is also characterized by slow or absent refilling of the reservoir after manual expression of fluid. The complication is confirmed by computed tomography and change in neurologic status.

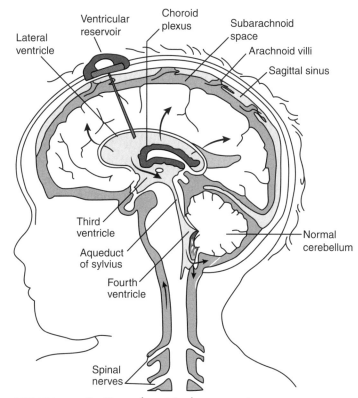

Ventricular reservoir

Lateral ventricle

Choroid plexus

Subarachnoid space

Arachnoid villi

Sagittal sinus

Third ventricle

Aqueduct of sylvius

Fourth ventricle

Normal cerebellum

Spinal nerves

FIGURE 15-9 Position of ventricular reservoir.

As clinicians, we are fortunate to have methods of expanded access to ensure safe delivery of infusions and medications for specific patient populations.

Review Questions   *Note: Questions below may have more than one right answer.*

1. Which of the following tests should be performed before insertion of an indwelling catheter in the radial artery?
   A. Allen's
   B. PA
   C. Serial
   D. Dalton's

2. Oxygen dissolved in plasma is expressed as
   A. PaO_2
   B. PO_2
   C. PCO_2
   D. pH

3. ABG values may be altered by
   A. Bicarbonate
   B. Air bubbles
   C. Excess heparin
   D. Dry spots

4. Which of the following is true of the ulnar artery?
   A. It is deep.
   B. It is difficult to stabilize.
   C. It lies close to nerves.
   D. A and B only

5. Mixed acid–base imbalances may coexist in the same patient. Which of the following are examples?
   A. Metabolic acidosis and metabolic alkalosis in a patient who has diabetic acidosis and who is vomiting
   B. Metabolic acidosis and respiratory acidosis in a patient with severe pulmonary edema
   C. A only
   D. A and B

6. Continuous arterial monitoring is used for
   A. Systolic, diastolic, and mean arterial pressure readings
   B. Assessment of cardiovascular effects of vasopressor or vasodilator drugs during shock
   C. Simultaneous ABG sampling
   D. All of the above

7. The relationship of blood pH to acidity, or hydrogen ion concentration, is
   A. Direct: as acidity increases, pH increases
   B. Indirect: as acidity increases, pH decreases
   C. Inverse: as acidity decreases, pH increases
   D. Nonexistent

8. In metabolic acidosis, BE is
   A. Plus
   B. Minus
   C. Zero
   D. Minimal

9. Which of the following is *not* an advantage of intraosseous infusion?
   A. Fluids are rapidly absorbed.
   B. It is a long-term infusion option.
   C. It is an option during circulatory collapse.
   D. Clotting and lung puncture problems are eliminated.

10. A ventricular reservoir may be used for which of the following?
    A. Access to CSF
    B. Measurement of CSF pressure
    C. Instillation of medication
    D. All of the above

References and Selected Readings   *Asterisks indicate references cited in text.*

Alexander, M., Corrigan N., Gorski, L., Hankins, J., & Perucca, R. (2010). *Infusion nursing: An evidence-based practice approach* (3rd ed.). St. Louis, MO: Saunders Elsevier.

*Bullock-Corkhill, M. (2010). Central venous access devices: Access and insertion. In M. Alexander., A. Corrigan., L. Gorski., J. Hankins., & R. Perucca (Eds.), *Infusion Nurses Society Infusion Nursing: An evidence-based approach* (3rd ed., pp. 480–494). St. Louis, MO: Saunders Elsevier.

*Centers for Disease Control and Prevention (CDC). (2011). *Guidelines for the prevention of intravascular catheter-related infections.* http://www.cdc.gov/hicpac/pdf/guidelines/bsi-guidelines-2011.pdf

*Connors, A.F. Jr., Speroff, T., Dawson, N.V., Thomas, C., Harrell, F.E., Wagner, D., et al. (1996). The effectiveness of right heart catheterization in the initial care of critically ill patients. SUPPORT Investigators. *JAMA, 276*, 889–897.

*Corley, A., Barnett, A.G., Mullany, D., & Fraser, J.F. (2009). Nurse-determined assessment of cardiac output: Comparing non-invasive cardiac output device and pulmonary artery catheter: A prospective observational study. *International Journal of Nursing Studies, 46*, 1291–1297.

Dalal, B.I., & Brigden, M.L. (2009). Factitious biochemical measurements resulting from hematologic conditions. *American Journal of Clinical Pathology, 131*, 195–204.

Day, M.W. (2011). Intraosseous devices for intravascular access in adult trauma patients. *Critical Care Nurse, 31*, 76–90.

*Drinker, C.K., Drinker, K.R., & Ludd, C.C. (1922). The circulation of the mammalian bone marrow. *American Journal of Physiology, 62*, 1–92.

*Fischbach, F.T., & Dunning, M.B. (2009). *A manual of laboratory and diagnostic tests* (8th ed., pp. 944–1015). Philadelphia, PA: Wolters Kluwer/Lippincott Williams & Wilkins.

*Gaskill, M.J., Martin, A.E., & Rivera, S. (1988). The subcutaneous ventricular reservoir: An effective treatment for posthemorrhagic hydrocephalus. *Childs Nervous System*, 4(5), 291–295.

*Ge, X., Cavallazzi, R., Li, C., Pan, S.M., Wang, Y.W., & Wang, F.L. (2012). Central venous access sites for the prevention of venous thrombosis, stenosis and infection. *Cochrane Database of Systematic Reviews*, Issue 3, CD004084. http://onlinelibrary.wiley.com/doi/10.1002/14651858.CD004084.pub3/pdf

*Hadaway, L. (2010). Infusion therapy equipment. In M. Alexander, A. Corrigan, L. Gorski, J. Hankins, & R. Perucca. (Eds.), *Infusion Nurses Society Infusion Nursing: An evidence-based approach* (3rd ed., pp. 391–436). St. Louis, MO: Saunders Elsevier.

*Hakim, R.M., & Himmelfarb, J. (2009). Hemodialysis access failure: A call to action-revisited. *Kidney International*, 76, 1040–1048.

Harvey, S., Harrison, D.A., Singer, M., Ashcroft, J., Jones, C.M., Elbourne, D., et al. (2005). Assessment of the clinical effectiveness of pulmonary artery catheters in management of patients in intensive care (PAC-MAN): A randomized control trial. *The Lancet*, 366, 472–477.

Hess, D., Nichols, A.B., Hunt, W.B., & Suratt, P.M. (1979). Pseudohypoxemia secondary to leukemia and thrombocytosis. *New England Journal of Medicine*, 301, 361.

Hind, D., Calvert, N., McWilliams, R., Davidson, A., Paisley, S., Beverly, C., et al. (2003). Ultrasonic locating devices for central venous cannulation: Meta-analysis. *British Medical Journal*, 327, 361. http://www.ncbi.nlm.nih.gov/pmc/articles/PMC175809/pdf/el-ppr361.pdf

*Horne, C., & Derrico, D. (1999). Mastering ABGs: The art of arterial blood gas measurement. *American Journal of Nursing*, 99(8), 26–33.

*Hudson, T.L., Dukes, S.F., & Reilly, K. (2006). Use of local anesthesia for arterial punctures. *American Journal of Critical Care*, 15, 595–599.

*Infusion Nurses Society. (2011). Infusion nursing standards of practice. *Journal of Infusion Nursing*, 34, S1–S100.

*Kindlen, S. (2003). *Physiology for health care and nursing* (2nd ed). London, UK: Churchill Livingstone.

Klabunde, R.E. (2012). *Cardiovascular physiology concepts* (2nd ed.). Philadelphia, PA: Wolters Kluwer/Lippincott Williams & Wilkins.

Levy, F.I., Schiffrin, E.L.O., Mourad, J., Agostini, D., Vicaut, E., Safar, M.E., et al. (2008). Impaired tissue perfusion: A pathology common to hypertension, obesity, and diabetes mellitus. *Circulation*, 118, 968–976.

Loiacono, L.A., & Shapiro, D.S. (2010). Detection of hypoxia at the cellular level. *Critical Care Medicine*, 26, 409–421.

Luck, R.P., Haines, C., & Mull, C.C. (2010). Intraosseous access. *Journal of Emergency Medicine*, 39(4), 468–475.

*Manoach, S., Weingart, S.D., & Charchaflieh, J.C. (2012). The evolution and current use of invasive hemodynamic monitoring for predicting volume responsiveness during resuscitation, perioperative, and critical care. *Journal of Clinical Anesthesia*, 24, 242–250.

Margereson, C. (2001). Anatomy and physiology. In G. Esmond (Ed.), *Respiratory nursing* (pp. 1–19). London, UK: Bailliere Tindall.

*Marik, P.E., Flemmer, M., & Harrison, W. (2012). The risk of catheter-related blood infections with femoral venous catheters as compared to subclavian and internal jugular venous catheters: A systematic review of the literature and meta-analysis. *Critical Care Medicine*, 40, 2479–2485.

*Mathews, L. (2007). Paradigm shift in hemodynamic monitoring. *Internet Journal of Anesthesiology*, 11(2), 33. http://archive.ispub.com/journal/the-internet-journal-of-anesthesiology/volume-11-number-2/paradigm-shift-in-hemodynamic-monitoring.html#sthash.QgFvKcXN.dpbs

*McCoy, J.V., Hollenberg, S.M., Dellinger, R.P., Arnold, R.C., Ruoss, L., Lotano, V., et al. (2009). Continuous cardiac index monitoring: A prospective observational study of agreement between a pulmonary artery catheter and a calibrated minimally invasive technique. *Resuscitation*, 80, 893–897.

*Miles, G., Salcedo, A., & Spear, D. (2011). Implementation of a successful registered nurse peripheral ultrasound-guided intravenous catheter program in an emergency department. *Journal of Emergency Nursing*, 38, 353–356.

Mosteller, R.D. (1987). Simplified calculation of body-surface area. *The New England Journal of Medicine, 317,* 1098.

*Murphy, G.S., & Vender, J.S. (2007). Con: Is the pulmonary catheter dead? *Journal of Cardiothoracic and Vascular Anesthesia, 21,* 147–149.

*Nafiu, O.O., Burke, L., Cowan, A., Tutuo, N., Maclean, S., & Tremper, K.K. (2010). Comparing peripheral venous access between obese and normal weight children. *Paediatric Anaesthesia, 20,* 172–176.

*Parienti, J., Megarbane, B., Fischer, M., Lautrette, A., Gazui, N., Marin, N., et al. (2010). Catheter dysfunction and dialysis performance according to vascular access among 736 critically ill adults requiring renal replacement therapy: A randomized controlled study. *Critical Care Medicine, 38,* 1118–1125.

*Parker, M., & Henderson, K. (2010). Alternative infusion access devices. In M Alexander, A Corrigan, L Gorski, J Hankins, & R Perucca. (Eds.), *Infusion Nurses Society Infusion Nursing: An evidence-based approach* (3rd ed., pp. 516–524). St Louis, MO: Saunders Elsevier.

Peters, S.G., Afessa, B., Decker, P.A., Schroeder, D.R., Offord, K.P., & Scott, J.P. (2003). Increased risk associated with pulmonary artery catheterization in the medical intensive care unit. *Journal of Critical Care, 18,* 166–171.

Phillips, L., Proehl, J., Brown, L., Miller, J., Campbell, T., & Youngberg, B. (2010). Recommendations for the use of intraosseous vascular access for emergent and non-emergent situations in various health care settings: A consensus paper. *Journal of Infusion Nursing, 33,* 346–351.

*Rajaram, S.S., Desai, N.K., Kalra, A., Gajera, M., Cavanaugh, S.K., Brampton, W., et al. (2013). Pulmonary artery catheters for adult patients in intensive care. *Cochrane Database of Systematic Reviews,* Issue 2, CD003408. http://onlinelibrary.wiley.com/doi/10.1002/14651858.CD003408.pub3/pdf

Richard, C., Warszawski, J., Anguel, N., Deye, N., Combes, A., Barnoud, D., et al. (2003). Early use of the pulmonary artery catheter and outcomes in patients with shock and acute respiratory distress syndrome: A randomized control trial. *JAMA, 290,* 2713–2720.

Royal College of Nursing. (2010). *Standards for infusion therapy* (3rd ed.). London, UK: Author.

*Shooman, D., Portess, H., & Sparrow, O. (2009). A review of the current treatment methods for posthaemorrhagic hydrocephalus of infants. *Cerebral Spinal Research, 6*(1), 1–15. http://creativecommons,org/licenses/by/2.0

Simpson, H. (2004). Interpretation of arterial blood gases. *British Journal of Nursing, 13*(9), 522–524.

Swan, H.E., Ganz, W., Forrester, J., Marcus, H., Diamond, G., & Chonette, D. (1970). Catheterization of the heart in man with use of a flow-directed balloon-tipped catheter. *The New England Journal of Medicine, 283,* 447–451.

*Thomas, D.R., Cote, T.R., Lawhorne, L., Leverson, S.A., Rubenstein, L.Z., Smith, D.A..; Dehydration Society. (2008). Understanding clinical dehydration and its treatment. *Journal of the American Medical Directors Association, 9,* 292–301.

*Tolwani, A. (2013). Continuous renal-replacement therapy for acute kidney injury. *The New England Journal of Medicine, 367,* 2505–2514.

*Tortora, G.L., & Grabowski, S.R. (2003). *Principles of anatomy and physiology* (10th ed.). New York: John Wiley & Sons.

*Urden, L., Stacy, K., & Lough, M. (2004). *Priorities in critical care nursing.* St Louis, MO: Mosby.

*Vijayan, A. (2009). Vascular access for continuous renal replacement therapy. *Seminars in Dialysis, 22,* 133–136.

*Von Hoff, D.D., Kuhn, J.G., Burris, H.A., & Miller, L.J. (2008). Does intraosseous equal intravenous? A pharmacokinetic study. *American Journal of Emergency Medicine, 26,* 31–38.

*Walsh, G. (2005). Hypodermoclysis: Alternative for hydration in long term care. *Journal of Infusion Nursing, 28*(2), 123–129.

West, J.B. (2012). *Respiratory physiology: The essentials* (9th ed.). Philadelphia, PA: Wolters Kluwer/Lippincott Williams & Wilkins.

*Woodrow, P. (2010). Essential principles: Blood gas analysis. *British Association of Critical Care Nurses: Nursing in Critical Care, 15,* 152–156.

PART 4

PATIENT-SPECIFIC THERAPIES

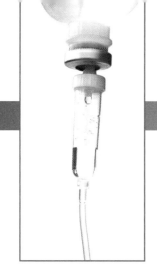

CHAPTER 16

Parenteral Nutrition

Mary E. Hagle
Sharon M. Weinstein

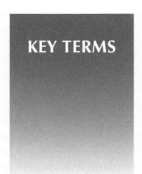

KEY TERMS	Drug–Nutrient Interaction	Nutritional Screening
	Enteral Nutrition	Nutritional Support
	Kwashiorkor	Parenteral Nutrition
	Malnutrition	Protein Malnutrition
	Marasmus	Total Nutrient Admixture
	Nutrients	

HISTORY OF PARENTERAL NUTRITION

The term parenteral hyperalimentation was coined by Dr. Jonathan E. Rhoads and Dr. Stanley J. Dudrick over four decades ago. In a classic citation from the literature, they defined it as "the intravenous administration of nitrogen, calories, and other nutrients sufficient to achieve tissue synthesis and anabolism in patients with normal or excessive nutritional needs" (Wilmore & Dudrick, 1968). These accomplishments led to further research and application as other clinicians and researchers realized the potential of this approach to feeding. Hyperalimentation soon became a recognized specialty resulting in nutritional support teams being formed. Nutritional support provides specially formulated or delivered parenteral or enteral nutrients to maintain or restore optimal nutrition status.

In 1976, a multidisciplinary group of professionals (physicians/licensed independent practitioners [LIPs], nurses, dietitians, and pharmacists) was organized, and the American Society for Parenteral and Enteral Nutrition (A.S.P.E.N.) held its first clinical congress in Chicago.

Hyperalimentation evolved as a science in the 1980s and became more commonly known as total parenteral nutrition, and eventually as parenteral nutrition (PN), the term used throughout this chapter. Disease-specific formulas were developed to address the particular needs of patients with renal, cardiac, or hepatic disease and became commercially available. Multiple organizations, such as the Oley Foundation and hospital-based support groups, grew out of need for the rehabilitation of patients surviving catastrophic illnesses by maintenance on home parenteral nutrition (HPN). PN has evolved into a sophisticated field of therapeutic intervention that has its own multidisciplinary specialists and a large body of established knowledge.

With the changing health care environment, including the emergence of care management, accountable care organizations, changing practice settings, and more, the field continues to change.

Practice Guidelines

Practice guidelines are just that—a guideline. The use of practice guidelines does not project or guarantee outcome or survival. The judgment of the health care professional based on individual circumstances of the patient must always take precedence over the recommendations in any guidelines.

In general, guidelines offer basic recommendations that are supported by review and analysis of the pertinent available current literature, by other national and international guidelines, and by the blend of expert opinion and clinical practicality (McClave et al., 2009).

EVIDENCE FOR PRACTICE

Current research addresses the following key issues:

- Reduced morbidity and mortality with enteral versus parenteral nutrition in critical care units
- Use of practice guidelines for nutritional support in different care settings
- Usage of glutamine (an amino acid)
- Trials of designer lipid emulsions, for example, soybean oil (SO), medium-chain triglycerides (MCTs), olive oil (OL), and fish oil (FO)
- Infusion-related support for PN: administration set changes, dressing guidelines, prevention of infection and extravasation, rate of infusion, and thrombosis prevention

OVERVIEW OF PARENTERAL NUTRITION

Parenteral nutrition is the intravenous (IV) provision of nutrients in patients without a functional or accessible gastrointestinal (GI) tract. PN provides protein in the form of amino acids, carbohydrates as dextrose, fats, vitamins, minerals, and trace elements to sustain life. The goals of PN are to ease the metabolic response to stress, prevent oxidative cellular injury, and to modify the immune response in a positive way (McClave et al., 2009). In many cases, PN is lifesaving.

PN is administered via a short peripheral IV catheter or central venous access device (CVAD). *Peripheral parenteral nutrition* (PPN) is used when CVAD placement cannot be achieved. PPN has a lower concentration of nutrients in a dilute solution and may not meet the protein and caloric needs of the patient. The osmolarity of the PPN solution must be

<600 mOsm and the final concentration of dextrose 10% or lower. Solutions with an osmolarity >600 mOsm are known to cause phlebitis. Typically, PPN is given for 7 days or less. It is not intended for prolonged nutrition support. It is also not appropriate for patients who cannot tolerate large volumes of fluid. Risk versus benefit must be weighed before the decision to treat with PPN is made. Strategies to reduce the risk of phlebitis should be implemented if PPN is selected as a course of treatment:

- Addition of a steroid such as hydrocortisone to the solution
- Addition of heparin
- Concomitant administration of fat emulsion
- Infusing the solution using a cyclic schedule such as infusing over 12 hours per day (INS, 2011)

Parenteral nutrition is a formula that contains complete nutrition and can only be given via a CVAD with catheter tip location in the cavoatrial junction due to its high osmolarity.

Nutrients in greater concentrations with smaller fluid volumes are administered. PN can be given for a short period of time such as days to weeks. Some patients with chronic conditions may require therapy for years to a lifetime.

Home parenteral nutrition (HPN) is the term used for PN administered in the home care or alternative care setting such as a long-term care setting. Indications for HPN are chronic diseases such as Crohn's disease where therapy may continue from months to years or a lifetime.

Enteral nutrition (*tube feeding*) is the administration of liquid nutrients through a tube, catheter, or stoma directly into a functional GI tract (A.S.P.E.N., 2009a, 2009b). It is the preferred method of nutrition when feasible and safe in a patient because it has the advantages over PN of decreased risk of metabolic complications, infection, reduced cost, and shorter hospital stays.

INDICATIONS FOR TREATMENT

Malnutrition is the primary indication for PN. It is defined by A.S.P.E.N. as "an acute, subacute, or chronic state of nutrition, in which varying degrees of overnutrition or undernutrition with or without inflammatory activity have led to a change in body composition and diminished function" (A.S.P.E.N., 2009a, 2009b). Up to 62% of hospitalized patients are malnourished (Somanchi, Tao, & Mullin, 2011). Effects of malnutrition affecting patient and facility are found in Table 16-1. In malnutrition, there is an increased loss of lean body mass, higher rates of infection and other complications, impaired wound healing, and increase in length of hospital stays and in readmissions (Barker, Gout, & Crowe, 2011).

TABLE 16-1 EFFECTS OF MALNUTRITION	
Patient	Institutional
Impaired immune response	Possible increased length of stay
Impaired wound healing	
Increased risk of infection	Possible increase in complications
Loss of muscle mass	
Atrophy of visceral organs	

In contrast to malnutrition resulting from famine, the pathophysiology of malnutrition in disease is associated with acute or chronic inflammation. This inflammation can lead to loss of lean body mass and protein and altered body function. Overall, malnutrition leads to an increase in morbidity and mortality. Types of malnutrition have been categorized based on the causes

- *Starvation-related malnutrition* where there exists a chronic state of malnutrition without inflammation. Anorexia nervosa is an example of this type.
- *Chronic disease–related malnutrition* exists when there is a chronic state of mild to moderate inflammation. Examples of this type are pancreatic cancer, rheumatoid arthritis, chronic renal failure, and in obesity with loss of muscle mass.
- *Acute disease– or injury-related malnutrition* that occurs with acute, severe inflammation. This type of malnutrition occurs in conditions such as trauma, burns, sepsis, head injuries, and acute inflammatory bowel disease (Jensen et al., 2010).

In the acute care setting, PN is used to support patients in the critical care arena as well as on the medical/surgical units. See Table 16-2 outlining potential indications for PN in the intensive care unit (ICU). Many of these patients are immobile and are on complete bed rest. Immobility over an extended period of time can cause progressive muscle loss. Ventilated patients experience insulin resistance, increased energy requirements, and increased protein catabolism (Jeejeebhoy, 2012). In general, if the gut can be used, enteral nutrition (EN) is preferred; PN may also be used to supplement EN. Conditions that may impact the need for PN include

- Major trauma
- Radiation enteritis

TABLE 16-2 POTENTIAL INDICATIONS FOR PN FOR PATIENTS IN THE ICU

If the patient in the ICU was healthy and nourished prior to ICU admission, PN is initiated after the first 7 d of hospitalization when EN is not available.
Evidence from Casaer et al. (2011); McClave et al. (2009)

If the patient is protein–calorie malnourished on ICU admission and EN is not feasible, PN is initiated as soon as possible following admission and adequate resuscitation.
Evidence from McClave et al. (2009)

"If a patient is expected to undergo major upper GI surgery and EN is not feasible, PN should be provided under very specific conditions" which accounts for the ICU patient's nutritional status (malnourished), when surgery is anticipated (5 d are available to start PN), and how long the PN therapy is expected to last (more than 7 d).
Evidence from McClave et al. (2009)

If the patient intake is unable to meet energy requirements (100% of target goal calories) after 7–10 d by the EN, initiate supplemental PN.
Evidence from McClave et al. (2009)

- Severe diarrhea
- Pancreatitis when EN is not tolerated
- Extensive burns
- Acute abdomen or ileus
- GI hemorrhage
- Ischemic bowel disease
- Bowel obstruction
- Severe short bowel syndrome
- Inflammatory bowel disease
- Enterocutaneous fistula
- Intractable nausea/vomiting
- Daily surgeries planned
- Severe mucositis
- Aggressive attempt at EN failed

Contraindications

When the GI tract is functional, EN is preferred over PN. If central vascular access cannot be achieved, then peripheral vascular access may be a short-term suboptimal alternative.

NUTRITIONAL ASSESSMENT

Nutritional assessment is necessary because inadequate nutrition increases the complications of disease, especially infection; decreases the ability to heal wounds; prolongs the length of the hospital stay; and contributes to anorexia and weakness. Malnutrition is determined through a nutritional assessment reviewing body weight, body composition, somatic and visceral protein stores, and laboratory values. Early nutritional intervention is recommended to avoid additional complications of malnutrition, including impaired respiratory muscle function, renal failure, and nonhealing wounds.

Two common types of protein–energy malnutrition include marasmus and kwashiorkor. Marasmus is characterized by catabolism of fat and muscle tissue, lethargy, generalized weakness, and weight loss. Visceral proteins are relatively preserved with serum albumin >3 g/dL. Patients are generally <80% of standard weight for height (Hammond, 2004). Kwashiorkor is characterized by edema, catabolism of muscle tissue, weakness, neurologic changes, secondary infections, stunted growth in children, and changes in hair. Visceral proteins are depressed with serum albumin <3 g/dL. Patients are generally >90% of standard weight for height (Hammond, 2004).

Another type of protein–energy malnutrition is characterized by a combination of marasmus and kwashiorkor symptoms. Patients are generally <60% of standard weight for height and have depressed visceral proteins with serum albumin <3 g/dL. This type of malnutrition usually occurs when a patient with marasmus is exposed to stress.

Nutritional Screening and Assessment Standards

Nutrition screening, assessment, and intervention in patients with malnutrition are key components of nutrition care. A.S.P.E.N. defines nutrition screening as *a process to identify an individual who is malnourished or who is at risk for malnutrition to determine if a detailed nutrition assessment is indicated.* In the United States, The Joint Commission (TJC) identifies a standard to screen nutrition within 24 hours of admission to an acute care center. The goal of nutrition assessment is to identify any specific nutrition risk(s) or clear existence of malnutrition. Nutrition assessments may identify recommendations for improving nutrition status (e.g., an intervention such as change in diet, enteral or parenteral nutrition, or further medical assessment) or a recommendation for rescreening (Mueller, Compher, Druyan, & American Society for Parenteral and Enteral Nutrition (A.S.P.E.N.) Board of Directors, 2011). Nutrition assessment has been defined by A.S.P.E.N. as "a comprehensive approach to diagnosing nutrition problems that uses a combination of the following: medical, nutrition, and medication histories; physical examination; anthropometric measurements; and laboratory data" (Mueller et al., 2011). A nutrition assessment provides the basis for a nutrition intervention. A focus on mandatory screening and nutritional assessment as part of the specific nutritional care standards began with TJC in 1995. The standards emphasize an interdisciplinary approach. In many settings, the nutritional screen is completed by a health professional other than the dietitian. The goal of nutritional screening is to identify individuals who are at nutrition risk, as well as to identify those who need further assessment.

Many hospitals have established formal nutritional screening programs for all hospital admissions to identify those patients most at risk or already malnourished. An algorithm for nutritional screening is presented in Figure 16-1. Once a nutritional screen is completed, patients who are at nutritional risk are usually referred to a dietitian.

A nutritional assessment should be included in the overall assessment of patients, particularly on admission to the hospital and periodically throughout the hospital stay. It should also be a component of nursing assessment in all health care settings, with reassessment at appropriate intervals, depending on the patient's status. Studies indicate that when admitted to acute care facilities, between 33% and 65% of all patients have some degree of malnutrition, and nutritional status deteriorates when patients are hospitalized >2 weeks (Hammond, 2004). Primary care, outpatient management, and the new standards have moved the role of nutritional assessment into the physician/LIP's office and home care setting as well. Mechanisms for documenting nutritional screening and assessment should be established and monitored. Suggested goals of nutritional assessment include the following:

- To identify individuals who require aggressive nutritional support
- To restore or maintain an individual's nutritional status
- To identify appropriate medical nutrition therapies
- To monitor the efficacy of these interventions (Hammond, 2004)

A nutritional assessment traditionally begins with a complete history, which includes a diet history, anthropometric measurements, physical assessment, and complete medical history, including drug–nutrient interactions and biochemical evaluation.

HEALTH, WEIGHT, AND DIETARY HISTORY

The patient's usual and current dietary intake is helpful in identifying the adequacy of nutrients (i.e., protein, carbohydrate, lipid, vitamins, minerals, trace elements, and water) and possible nutritional deficiencies. Nutrients in the medical history should include any acute or chronic diseases that may have an impact on nutrient intake or utilization and conditions that increase metabolic needs or fluid and electrolyte losses. Surgical history,

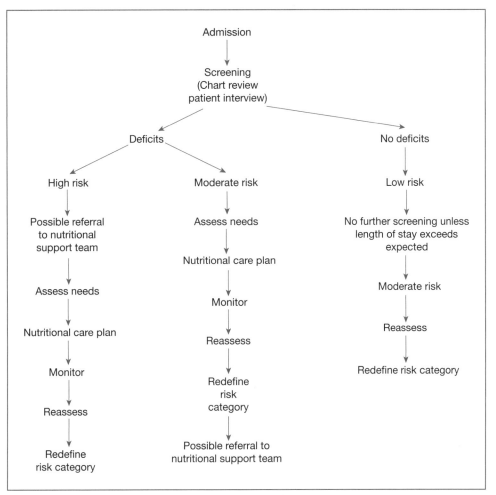

FIGURE 16-1 Nutritional screening. (Courtesy of Grant, A., & DeHoog, S. (1999). *Nutritional assessment, support and management* (5th ed). Seattle, WA: Authors.)

certain medications, and social factors also have an impact on nutritional status and should be evaluated. Multiple computerized programs for dietary assessment are available, each providing different end points of data (Probst & Tapsell, 2005). Benefits of a computerized assessment include standardized questioning, immediate micronutrient information, and possible recommendations; additionally, these programs may be used for practice or research. Specific factors that may alter nutritional status are listed in Box 16-1.

PHYSICAL ASSESSMENT

A thorough physical assessment by an experienced clinician can detect signs and symptoms suggesting nutritional deficiencies. These include but are not limited to changes in hair, eyes, skin, nails, and all organ systems (Table 16-3). Anthropometric measurements consist of simple, noninvasive, inexpensive techniques for obtaining body measurements useful

---

BOX 16-1 FACTORS INFLUENCING FOOD INTAKE

Diet

Food allergies, aversions, and intolerance
Fad diets
Diet modifications (low sodium, low fat)
Ethnic and cultural factors
Poor dentition or ill-fitting dentures
Mucositis or ulcerative lesions of the oral cavity
Alteration in taste or smell
Breathing difficulty
Inability to prepare food or feed self
Frequent fasting (NPO) status, clear liquid diet

Health Factors

Chewing or swallowing difficulty
Neurologic impairment
Malabsorption
Inflammatory bowel disease
Chronic illness (i.e., chronic obstructive pulmonary disease, human immunodeficiency virus infection, liver disease, end-stage renal disease, cancer)
Eating disorder (e.g., anorexia nervosa, bulimia nervosa, binge-eating disorder)
Increased losses from draining wounds, ostomies, fistulas, effusions, diarrhea

Surgical History

Small or large bowel obstruction
Surgical reconstruction (i.e., gastrectomy, gastrojejunostomy, esophagogastrectomy, small intestine resection)
Head and neck surgery
Surgical procedure for morbid obesity

Medications (may alter dietary intake or nutrient utilization):

Analgesics
Antacids
Antibiotics
Anticonvulsants
Antineoplastic agents
Diuretics
Laxatives
Oral contraceptives

BOX 16-1   FACTORS INFLUENCING FOOD INTAKE   *(Continued)*

Psychosocial and Psychological Factors

Alcohol or substance abuse

Depressive disorders

Income

Institutionalization

Mental illness

Religion

---

in evaluating for overnutrition or undernutrition. The patient's actual height and weight should be obtained and used to help determine nutritional status.

Body weight can by assessed by several methods including (a) body mass index (BMI), (b) comparison with usual body weight (UBW), and (c) comparison with ideal body weight (IBW). BMI is a tool for judging body weight in relation to height and risks for weight-related health problems such as heart disease, diabetes, and certain types of cancer (Box 16-2). Electronic medical record (EMR) systems often provide BMI once height and

---

TABLE 16   PHYSICAL ASSESSMENT FINDINGS IN NUTRITIONAL DEFICIENCIES

Physical Changes	Deficiency
Hair	
Lackluster, thin, sparse; pigmentation changes	Protein, calorie, zinc, linoleic acid
Mouth	
Angular stomatitis: cracks, redness at one or both corners of the mouth	Vitamin B
Cheilosis—vertical cracks in the lips	Riboflavin and niacin
Varicose veins under the tongue	Vitamin C
Tongue	
May become purplish, red, or beefy red or may appear smooth and pale; one or more fissures, atrophy of taste buds	Vitamin B
Skin	
Dryness, flakiness	Vitamin A, essential fatty acids
Petechiae or easy bruising; hemorrhagic spots on skin at pressure points; may occur in the presence of liver disease or during anticoagulation	Vitamins C and K
Musculoskeletal	
Muscle wasting (especially quadriceps, deltoids, and temporalis)	Protein, calorie
Kyphosis, osteoporosis	Calcium and vitamin D
Neurologic	
Confusion, listlessness	Protein malnutrition
Sensory motor, vibratory	Thiamine and vitamin B_{12}

BOX 16-2 INTERPRETING BODY MASS INDEX

Formula

Metric formula: BMI = Weight (kg)/Height (m²)

Recommended Classification

Underweight	<18.5
Normal	18.5–24.9
Obesity, grade I	25–29.9
Obesity, grade II	30–40
Obesity, grade III	>40

---

weight are entered. This information may be part of the clinical decision support system and provide an automatic consultation to the dietitian for specific BMI parameters indicating that a patient is at nutritional risk. The Centers for Disease Control and Prevention (CDC) also provides a Web site for calculating BMI for adults and children: http://www.cdc.gov/healthyweight/assessing/bmi.

UBW is obtained from past medical records or subjectively from the patient or family member. Actual weight as a percentage of UBW is usually the most accurate determinant of weight loss. Minimum weight for survival is 48% to 55% of UBW (Hammond, 2004). UBW can be calculated as follows:

$$\text{Percent weight change} = \frac{\text{Usual weight} - \text{actual weight}}{\text{Usual weight}} \times 100$$

Percentage of IBW may also be used and can be determined with the preceding formula by substituting IBW for usual weight. This method is not as effective when assessing the nutrition risk of a critically ill patient. A normally thin person, with stable weight, may be incorrectly identified as malnourished if weight is less than IBW; the obese patient with significant recent weight loss may be overlooked if weight is still above IBW (Grant & DeHoog, 2008).

Many of the nutrition screens examine BMI, weight loss, and weight history (Mueller et al., 2011). Recording actual weight and weight history carefully will inform the team and enable appropriate interventions. Additionally, weight will be used to assess for fluid overload, along with other parameters, as well as to track progress of nutrition support. The significance for weight loss over specific time periods is outlined in Table 16-4.

Other anthropometric measurements include triceps skinfold thickness, which estimates subcutaneous fat stores, and mid–arm muscle circumference, which estimates somatic protein stores (skeletal muscle mass). These measurements can be helpful in assessing individuals over time but not in the critical and acute care settings because changes in body fluid and composition may influence the results (Hammond, 2004). Reproducibility of accurate measurements requires strict adherence to protocol and may vary widely in the same individual with different examiners.

For the patient in the ICU, the A.S.P.E.N. guideline directs an "evaluation of weight loss and previous nutrient intake prior to admission, level of disease severity, comorbid

TABLE 16- ESTIMATING BODY WEIGHT AND PERCENTAGE LOSS IN PN		
Duration of Therapy	Considerable Weight Loss	Serious Weight Loss
10 d	1%–2%	>2%
1 mo	5%	>5%
3 mo	7.5%	>7.5%

Common anthropometric measurements include weight, height, and weight/height and their comparisons to standard values. To calculate the percent weight change (PWC) in the patient receiving parental nutrition, follow this formula:

$$PWC = \text{usual body weight}\,(UBW) - \frac{\text{actual body weight}}{UBW} \times 100 = \%UBW$$

conditions, and function of the GI tract" (McClave et al., 2009). Traditional anthropometric measures are not validated in critical care (McClave et al., 2009).

LABORATORY ANALYSIS (BIOCHEMICAL ASSESSMENT)

A variety of biochemical tests are used to assess nutritional status, with a broad range of sensitivity. The most commonly used, and most readily available, are visceral proteins and tests to evaluate immune function.

VISCERAL PROTEINS

Depletion of visceral proteins is characteristic of protein malnutrition, which occurs acutely in the hospitalized patient (hypoalbuminemia). An estimate of visceral protein status can be obtained from measurements of specific serum transport proteins that are synthesized in the liver. These include albumin, transferrin, prealbumin, and retinol-binding protein (Table 16-5). Serum albumin is useful for helping to determine nutritional status but has limited value in assessing acute changes in nutritional status related to its long half-life (Carney & Meguid, 2002). It is recommended that serum albumin measurements be included in the initial chemical profile when screening for malnutrition. An albumin concentration of <3.5 g/dL is associated with increased morbidity in hospitalized patients (Carney & Meguid, 2002). However, in the critically ill patient, these traditional measures (albumin and prealbumin) are not validated in the ICU (McClave et al., 2009).

Transferrin has a shorter half-life than albumin but does not respond rapidly enough to protein–energy status to be useful in acute care settings (Litchford, 2012). Retinol-binding protein also has a shorter half-life but does not accurately reflect protein–energy status in acutely stressed patients. It is also not useful for patients with vitamin A deficiency or renal failure (Litchford, 2012). Prealbumin, with a shorter half-life, seems to be a more sensitive and specific indicator for monitoring the effectiveness of nutritional support. It is more expensive and may be limited in smaller hospitals. Consideration should also be given to assessing non-nutritional factors, such as inflammation, that may affect these visceral proteins. Even though these tests are useful, new nutritional markers are needed that better identify malnourished patients and precisely monitor the effectiveness of nutritional intervention on nutritional status. Other proteins are being investigated to determine their efficacy in nutritional assessment.

TABLE 16-5 VISCERAL PROTEINS

Visceral Protein	Half-Life	Normal Range	Causes of Decrease	Causes of Increase
Albumin Maintains plasma oncotic pressure Carrier protein (zinc, calcium, magnesium, fatty acids)	18–21 d	Normal: >3.5 g/dL Mild depletion: 2.8–3.5 g/dL Moderate depletion: 2.1–2.7 g/dL Severe depletion: <2.1 g/dL Reflects *chronic*, not acute change	Metabolic stress Infection, inflammation Liver disease ↑ Losses (wounds, burns, fistulas) Inadequate protein intake Fluid imbalance (ascites, edema, overhydration) Malabsorptive states	Dehydration may falsely ↑ levels Salt-poor albumin infusion
Transferrin Carrier protein for iron	8–10 d	Normal: >200 mg/dL Mild depletion: 150–200 mg/dL Moderate depletion: 100–150 mg/dL Severe depletion: <100 mg/dL	Chronic infection Inflammatory state Acute catabolic states ↑ Iron stores Liver damage Overhydration	Pregnancy Hepatitis Iron deficiency anemia Dehydration Chronic blood loss
Thyroxine-binding prealbumin (transthyretin) Carrier protein for retinol-binding protein Transport protein for thyroxine	2–3 d	Normal: >20 mg/dL Mild depletion: 10–15 mg/dL Moderate depletion: 5–10 mg/dL Severe depletion: 5 mg/dL Sensitive to acute changes in protein status Limited use in situation in which there is a sudden demand for protein synthesis	Infection Acute catabolic state Postsurgery (5–10 mg/dL drop 1st week) Liver disease Altered energy and protein balance Hyperthyroid	Chronic renal failure Corticosteroids
Retinol-binding protein Transport retinol (alcohol of vitamin A)	10–18 h	Normal: 3–5 mEq/dL Reflects acute change	Vitamin A deficiency Acute catabolic states Postsurgery Liver disease Hyperthyroid	Renal disease

Immune Function Tests

Alterations in the immune system may be influenced by stress, specific disease states, and malnutrition. The total lymphocyte count (TLC) is indicative of a patient's ability to fight infection and is known to decrease with malnutrition, especially inadequate calories and protein. TLC may be calculated using the complete blood count with differential: TLC = white blood cell (WBC) count × lymphocytes. Normal levels range from 1,500 to 1,800 mm^3. However, TLC is affected by many medical disease states and varies widely; thus, it is of limited value.

Cell-mediated immunity is most frequently evaluated with delayed cutaneous hypersensitivity skin tests. Intradermal injections of specific recall antigens, such as *Candida*, mumps, or tuberculin, are used. Patients who are immunocompetent will exhibit a positive response within 24 to 48 hours; this response consists of a small, reddened area (5 mm) around the test site. Patients who are malnourished and possibly immunosuppressed may exhibit a delayed response, a response to only one of the antigens, or no reaction. These results are classified as normal or reactive if there is a response to two or more antigens, relatively anergic if only one response occurs, and anergic if there is no response to any of the antigens. These results must be weighed with other findings in the nutritional assessment because non-nutritional factors, such as infection, sepsis, cancer, liver disease, renal failure, immunosuppressive diseases, and immunosuppressive drugs, may also affect immunocompetence.

DECISION FOR NUTRITIONAL SUPPORT

Many nutritional assessments are available for different health care providers (Brogden, 2004; Rodriguez, 2004), as well as technologies that provide information on the individual's metabolic analyses (Stanberry et al., 2013). There is no single indicator of nutritional status. A global assessment of many indices, and the patient's clinical status, is necessary to determine the degree of nutritional deficiency. Based on the nutrition assessment, the guideline recommendation states that nutrition support is recommended for patients identified as at risk for malnutrition or who are malnourished (Mueller et al., 2011). A small body of sound evidence identifies quality outcomes for patients who receive nutrition support when they are malnourished; outcomes include improved nutrition status, nutrient intake, physical functioning, as well as fewer hospital readmissions (Mueller et al., 2011).

Reassessment is individualized whenever the clinical status changes and periodically throughout the course of nutritional therapy. Once the nutritional assessment data have been collected and evaluated, the optimal method for nutritional support must be selected. This decision process is depicted in Figure 16-2.

A growing body of evidence supports the use of EN, rather than PN, for the critically ill patient in the ICU (Casaer et al., 2011; Jeejeebhoy, 2012; McClave et al., 2009). However, specific guidelines outline when PN is appropriate for the patient in the ICU (McClave et al., 2009).

NUTRITIONAL REQUIREMENTS

The practical outcome of the nutritional assessment is to determine the caloric and protein needs of the patient. These requirements change in acute, catabolic illness, and in some chronic conditions.

Energy Requirements

Nutrient energy requirements are usually expressed in kilocalories (kcal). Numerous methods for determining a person's nutritional requirements are available, with varying degrees of sophistication. Indirect calorimetry is one of the most accurate ways of determining a patient's energy needs. In the clinical setting, metabolic charts are often used to determine

A. Diagnosis
  If the patient has at least ONE of the following diagnoses, circle and proceed to section E to consider the patient
      AT NUTRITIONAL RISK and stop here.
  Anorexia nervosa/bulimia nervosa
  Malabsorption (celiac sprue, ulcerative colitis, Crohn disease, short bowel syndrome)
  Multiple trauma (closed-head injury, penetrating trauma, multiple fractures)
  Decubitus ulcers
  Major gastrointestinal surgery within the past year
  Cachexia (temporal wasting, muscle wasting, cancer, cardiac)
  Coma
  Diabetes
  End-stage liver disease
  End-stage renal disease
  Nonhealing wounds
B. Nutrition intake history
  If the patient has at least ONE of the following symptoms, circle and proceed to section E to consider the patient
      AT NUTRITIONAL RISK and stop here.
  Diarrhea (>500 mL × 2 days)
  Vomiting (>5 days)
  Reduced intake (<1/2 normal intake for >5 days)
C. Ideal body weight standards
  Compare the patient's current weight for height to the ideal body weight chart on the back of this form. If at
      <80% of ideal body weight, proceed to section E to consider the patient AT NUTRITIONAL RISK and stop
      here.
D. Weight history
  Any recent unplanned weight loss? No_____ Yes _____ Amount (lb or kg)_____
  If yes, within the past _____ weeks or _____ months
  Current weight (lb or kg) _____
  Usual weight (lb or kg)_____
  Height (feet, inch, or cm)_____
  Find percentage of weight lost: usual wt − current wt × 100 = _____ % wt loss
                                    usual wt
  Compare the % wt loss with the chart values and circle appropriate value

Length of time	Significant (%)	Severe (%)
1 week	1–2	>2
2–3 weeks	2–3	>3
1 month	4–5	>5
3 months	7–8	>8
5+ months	10	>10

  If the patient has experienced a significant or severe weight loss, proceed to section E and consider the patient
      AT NUTRITIONAL RISK
E. Nurse assessment
  Using the above criteria, what is this patient's nutritional risk? (circle one)
      _____ LOW NUTRITIONAL RISK
      _____ AT NUTRITIONAL RISK

FIGURE 16-2 Decision-making process for nutritional support. (Adapted from Grant, J., & DeHoog, S. (1999). *Nutritional assessment, support, and management* (2nd ed.). Seattle, WA: Authors; and Livingston, A., Seamons, C., & Dalton, T. (2000). If the gut works, use it. *Nursing Management, 31*(5), 39–42.)

the oxygen consumption and carbon dioxide production of the body over a period of time. This helps to determine actual energy expenditure. Indirect calorimetry requires expensive equipment and therefore is not available at all institutions (Hammond, 2004).

A classic equation used to estimate energy expenditure is the Harris-Benedict Equation, which was derived from healthy individuals. It estimates basal energy expenditure (BEE) in kilocalories, using weight, height, age, and sex with the following equations:

$$BEE(male) = (66 + 13.8W + 5H) - 6.8A$$

$$BEE(female) = (655 + 9.6W + 1.8H) - 4.7A$$

where W is weight in kilograms, H is height in centimeters, and A is age in years.

UBW is most commonly used, although an adjusted body weight is often recommended if the patient is obese (BMI > 30). Stress and activity factors are often added to predict energy expenditures of critically ill or injured patients, which can range from an addition of 30% to 50% above resting energy expenditure (Ireton-Jones, 2002). Actual energy requirements are then estimated by multiplying BEE × AF × IF. Correction factors (for activity [AF] and stress/injury [IF]) to estimate nonprotein energy requirements of hospitalized patients are listed in Table 16-6.

Another common method to estimate energy needs is by calculating energy per kilogram. It has been estimated that 25 to 35 kcal/kg body weight is needed for total energy

TABLE 16-6   CORRECTION FACTORS FOR ESTIMATING NONPROTEIN ENERGY REQUIREMENTS OF HOSPITALIZED PATIENTS

Activity Description	Activity Factor
Chair or bed bound	1.2
Out of bed	1.3
Little movement and little or no leisure activity	1.4–1.5
Seated work with requirement to move but little strenuous leisure activity	1.6–1.7
Clinical Status	**Stress Factor**
Elective surgery	1–1.1
Peritonitis	1.05–1.25
Multiple/long bone fractures	1.1–1.3
Cancer	1.1–1.45
Severe infection	1.2–1.6
Closed head injury	1.
Infection with trauma	1.3–1.55
Multiple trauma	1.4
Burns	1.5–2.1

Actual energy requirements = basal energy expenditure (BEE) × activity factor (AF) × injury factor (IF).
Adapted from Rychlec, G., Edel, J., Murray, M., Schurer, D., & Tomko, M. M., (2000). Nutrition assessment of adults. In B. Hornick. (Ed.), *Manual of clinical dietetics* (6th ed., pp. 3–33). Chicago, IL: American Dietetic Association.

expenditure in the nonobese population, whereas only 21 kcal/kg body weight is needed in the obese critically ill population (Rychlec, Edel, Murray, Schurer, & Tomko, 2000).

Regardless of the method chosen, it is important to avoid overfeeding. The early adage of nutritional support "the more, the better" is no longer advocated. Overfeeding, which causes hyperglycemia and has deleterious effects on respiratory and hepatic function, should be avoided, especially in the acutely ill patient. Additional calories for desired weight gain should be held until the patient recovers.

Protein Requirements

Protein requirements for healthy people are based on the amount needed to maintain nitrogen equilibrium, assuming energy needs are being met by nonprotein kilocalories. The recommended daily allowance for healthy adults is 0.8 g/kg/d. Protein requirements are increased during illness to meet stress needs for wound healing, promote immune competence, and replace losses. Critically ill patients require an increased protein intake of 1.5 to 2.0 g/kg/d (Cresci, 2002).

CALORIE–NITROGEN RATIO

A nonstressed patient can achieve nitrogen balance with adequate calorie intake and protein accounting for 8% of calories. When a patient becomes stressed, both calorie and protein requirements increase. Protein should contribute 15% to 20% of energy in a stressed patient. The optimal calorie:nitrogen ratio for critically ill patients is 150:1.

NITROGEN BALANCE

Nitrogen balance is an objective method of evaluating the efficacy of the patient's nutritional regimen. For a patient to be in a positive nitrogen balance or anabolic state, the amount of nitrogen taken in by the patient (IV and orally) needs to be more than that excreted. A 24-hour urine collection is needed to measure the amount of urinary urea excreted. A factor of 4 g is added (2 g for fecal losses and 2 g for integumentary losses) to measure total nitrogen excretion. A nitrogen balance of 2 to 4 g of nitrogen per day indicates that the patient is in an anabolic state. It is nearly impossible to achieve positive nitrogen balance immediately after a metabolic insult. Nitrogen balance studies are not accurate for patients with impaired creatinine clearance, severe hepatic failure, massive diuresis, or abnormal nitrogen losses through diarrhea or large draining wounds (Cresci, 2002). The nitrogen balance formula and measures that reflect the severity of the catabolic state can be found in Box 16-3.

Fluid Requirements

Individual fluid requirements vary greatly and can fluctuate on a daily basis. Fluid needs should be carefully assessed when designing the PN formula. The minimum daily requirement for healthy adults is 1 mL/kcal. Factors that may increase fluid needs include fever and increased losses from diuresis, diarrhea, vomiting, and drainage from wounds and fistulas.

BOX 16-3   NITROGEN BALANCE

Formula

Nitrogen balance is calculated by subtracting the amount of nitrogen lost from the amount of nitrogen given or taken by the patient, as follows:

$$\text{Nitrogen balance} = \frac{\text{Protein intake}}{6.25} - \left(\text{urine urea nitrogen} + 4\right)$$

Interpretation

Normally at equilibrium, the following measures reflect the severity of the catabolic state:

Equilibrium	0 g/d
Mild	−5 to −10 g/d
Moderate	−10 to −15 g/d
Severe	>−15 g/d

Usual goal during nutritional support = +2/–4 g nitrogen/24 h

---

Environmental factors such as specialized high–air-loss beds, ultraviolet light therapy, and radiant warmers also increase fluid requirements. Humidified air reduces insensible fluid loss and results in lower fluid requirements. Preexisting excess or deficiency states and cardiac and renal function must also be evaluated.

Fluids may be required in addition to the fluids provided by PN. Because fluid requirements shift rapidly with changes in clinical status in hospitalized patients, this is best done by giving additional crystalloid IV fluids, such as dextrose 5% in water (D_5W) or dextrose 5% in 0.45% sodium chloride solution by a separate lumen or route. These can be frequently adjusted as necessary without affecting nutrient delivery. They can also be used as additional vehicles for electrolyte corrections, avoiding possible wastage of the PN solution. The PN solution can be formulated using concentrated nutrients (70% dextrose, 15% amino acids, 15% lipids) to provide adequate nutrients when fluid restriction is needed.

PARENTERAL NUTRITION SOLUTIONS

The complex solutions used in PN can provide all the necessary nutrients to meet requirements for growth, weight gain, anabolism, and wound healing.

Components

Total nutrient admixtures (TNA) are formulations consisting of carbohydrates, amino acids, lipids, vitamins, minerals, trace elements, water, and other additives in a single container. The proportion of each component is individualized based on the patient's clinical status, chronic diseases, fluid and electrolyte balance, and specific goals of PN.

CARBOHYDRATES

Glucose is the primary energy source in most PN solutions. Concentrations from 10% to 70% glucose may be used with a final solution concentration of no more than 10% to 12% for peripheral infusion and no more than 35% for central venous infusion. A carbohydrate, parenteral glucose is hydrolyzed and provides 3.4 kcal/g. Consistent with a classic study by Galica, at least 150 to 200 g of glucose is needed to meet the obligate needs for glucose by the brain, central nervous system, red blood cells, WBCs, active fibroblasts, and certain phagocytes, which normally require glucose as the sole or major energy source (Galica, 1997). No more than 5 to 7 mg/kg/min (equals a maximum of 5 to 7 g/kg/d, which is easier to calculate) should be given, which is the maximum rate of glucose oxidation. Less is given to the diabetic, hyperglycemic, or critically ill patient—usually no more than 4 g/kg/d. The incidence of hyperglycemia seems to increase if excess quantities are administered. Overfeeding carbohydrates may result in conversion of excess glucose to fat, which requires energy (increased oxygen consumption and carbon dioxide production), and leads to fatty liver changes with prolonged use. From 50% to 70% of the daily nonprotein kilocalories usually are given as glucose.

LIPIDS

Lipids (fats) provide the second source of nonprotein calories for PN solutions. IV lipid emulsions are given to prevent essential fatty acid deficiency (EFAD) and as a concentrated source of energy (each gram of fat provides 9 kcal). The only recommendation regarding specific fatty acids is that 1% to 2% of daily energy requirements should be derived from linoleic acid and about 0.5% of energy from α-linoleic acid to prevent EFAD (Kris-Etherton, Taylor, Yu-Poth, et al., 2000). EFAD has been detected as early as 3 to 7 days after initiation of fat-free PN, although clinical signs of dietary inadequacy may take 3 to 4 weeks to become evident. Clinical signs include dry or scaly skin, thinning hair, thrombocytopenia, and liver function abnormalities. Prevention of this deficiency state is desirable because EFAD is associated with decreased ability to heal wounds, adverse effects on red blood cell membranes, and a defect in prostaglandin synthesis.

PATIENT SAFETY

When administering lipid emulsions, prevent adverse events due to excess amounts administered too rapidly.

Lipids provide an energy-dense source of calories and, when used, may decrease the fluid volume of PN required to achieve the caloric intake desired. Thus, use of IV lipids with glucose in a daily PN solution decreases the glucose calories and minimizes insulin requirements. Lipids should provide 30% to 50% of the nonprotein calories in PN solutions but should not exceed 60% or 2.5 g/kg or an infusion rate of 1.7 mg/kg/min (Galica, 1997). Some data support the use of a maximum of lipid of 1 mg/kg/d intravenously, especially in critically ill patients (Cresci, 2005).

Because early administration of intravenous fat emulsions (IVFEs) has been linked to infectious complications in trauma patients, Gerlach et al. (2011) examined the effect of withholding IVFE for the first 7 to 10 days of PN in all surgical intensive care unit (SICU) patients. Prior to this, IVFE had been infused from the start of PN. Sixty-four patients received IVFE; 30 at initiation of PN and 34 starting after 7 to 10 days. The two groups had similar demographics, severity of illness, transfusion requirements, and duration of PN. Infectious complications occurred in 65.6% of patients (63.3% having immediate IVFE vs. 67.6% having delayed IVFE; $p = 0.79$). Equal numbers of patients developed bloodstream infection (BSI) or catheter-related bloodstream infection (CRBSI), and mortality rates were similar. Outcomes of interest were not clinically or statistically different. Thus, delaying IVFE did not reduce infections, mortality, or average hospital length of stay (Gerlach et al., 2011) in the SICU patient population; this may not be generalizable to all critically ill patients.

A position paper from A.S.P.E.N. (Vanek et al., 2012) encourages further research on the use of alternative, oil-based, IVFEs. Currently available standard SO-based IVFEs meet the needs of most PN patients. However, alternatives are available and have been extensively used in Europe; these include MCTs, OOs, and FOs. They seem to have an equivalent safety profile to SO. Alternatives, widely accepted in the European communities, are not available for wide distribution within the United States. Table 16-7 highlights the plethora of commercially available fat emulsion solutions in the United States and in Europe. The A.S.P.E.N. position paper recognized that "… Alternative oil-based IVFEs may have less proinflammatory effects, less immune suppression, and more antioxidant effects than the standard SO IVFEs and may potentially be a better alternative energy source" (Vanek, Seidner, et al., 2012).

IV lipids are available in 10% (1.1 kcal/mL), 20% (2 kcal/mL), and 30% (3 kcal/mL) formulations. They provide fatty acids solely as long-chain triglycerides and contain egg phospholipid as an emulsifier. They should not be used in patients with severe egg allergies. In general, 20% and 30% solutions are used because less volume is needed. Adverse reactions may occur, although the incidence is <1%. Symptoms include dyspnea, cyanosis, nausea, vomiting, headache, dizziness, increased temperature, sweating,

TABLE 16-7   TYPES OF COMMERCIALLY AVAILABLE LIPID EMULSION

Product Name	Manufacturer/ Distributor	Lipid Source	Concentrations of Selected FA, % by Weight				n–6:n–3 Ratio	α-Tocopherol, mg/L	Phytosterols, mg/L
			Linoleic	α-Linolenic	EPA	DHA			
IVFE Available in United States									
Intralipid®	Fresenius Kabi/Baxter	100% soybean oil	44–62	4–11	0	0	7:1	38	348 ± 33
Liposyn® III	Hospira	100% soybean oil	54.5	8.3	0	0	7:1	NA	NA
IVFL Available Only Outside of the United States									
Intralipid®	Fresenius Kabi	100% soybean oil	44–62	4–11	0	0	7:1	38	348 ± 33
Ivelip®	Baxter Teva	100% soybean oil	52	8.5	0	0	7:1	NA	NA

(Continued)

TABLE 16-7	TYPES OF COMMERCIALLY AVAILABLE LIPID EMULSION		(Continued)						
Product Name	Manufacturer/ Distributor	Lipid Source	Concentrations of Selected FA, % by Weight				n–6:n–3 Ratio	α-Tocopherol, mg/L	Phytosterols, mg/L
			Linoleic	α-Linolenic	EPA	DHA			
Lipovenoes®	Fresenius Kabi	100% soybean oil	54	8	0	0	7:1	NA	NA
Lipovenoes® 10% PLR	Fresenius Kabi	100% soybean oil	54	8	0	0	7:1	NA	NA
Intralipos® 10%	Mitsubishi Pharma Guangzhou/ Tempo Green Cross Otsuka Pharmaceutical Group	100% soybean oil	53	5	0	0	7:1	NA	NA
Lipofundin-N®	B. Braun	100% soybean oil	50	7	0	0	7:1	180 ± 40	NA
Soyacal	Grifols Alpha Therapeuticas	100% soybean oil	46.4	8.8	0	0	7:1	NA	NA
Intrafat	Nihon	100% soybean oil	NA	NA	0	0	7:1	NA	NA
Structolipid® 20%[a]	Fresenius Kabi	64% soybean oil 36% MCT	35	5	0	0	7:1	6.9	NA
Lipofundin® MCT/LCT	B. Braun	50% soybean oil 50% MCT oil	27	4	0	0	7:1	85 ± 20	NA
Lipovenoes® MCT	Fresenius Kabi	50% soybean oil 50% MCT oil	25.9	3.9	0	0	7:1	NA	NA
ClinOleic® 20%	Baxter	20% soybean oil 80% olive oil	18.5	2	0	0	9:1	32	327 ± 8
Lipoplus®	B. Braun	40% soybean oil, 50% MCT, 10% fish oil	25.7	3.4	3.7	2.5	2.7:1	190 ± 30	NA
SMOFlipid®	Fresenius Kabi	30% soybean oil, 30% MCT, 25% olive oil, 15% fish oil	21.4	2.5	3.0	2.0	2.5:1	200	47.6
Omegaven®	Fresenius Kabi	100% fish oil	4.4	1.8	19.2	12.1	1:8	150–296	0

[a]Fat source uses structured lipids.

DHA, docosahexaenoic acid; EPA, eicosapentaenoic acid; FA, fatty acid; IVFE, intravenous fat emulsion; MCT, medium-chain triglyceride; n-6:n-3 ratio, ratio of ω-6 fatty acids to ω-3 fatty acids; NA, not available.

From Vanek, V. W., Seidner, D. L., Allen, P., Bistrian, B., Collier, S., Gura, K., et al. (2012). A.S.P.E.N. position paper: Clinical role for alternative intravenous fat emulsions. *Nutrition in Clinical Practice, 27*, 150–192.

chest or back pain, pressure over eyes, and hyperlipidemia. Administration of IV fat emulsions is contraindicated in patients with disturbances in normal fat metabolism such as pathologic hyperlipidemia, lipoid nephrosis, or acute pancreatitis if accompanied by hyperlipidemia.

Because lipids are isotonic (300 mOsmol/L), up to 50% of nonprotein calories may be supplied as lipids in peripheral PN to decrease the incidence of phlebitis. Lipids are better tolerated and utilized if they are infused slowly, not to exceed 1.7 mg/kg/min. Fast infusion rates have been associated with deleterious effects on pulmonary function and impairment of the reticuloendothelial system function, potentiating the inflammatory response by altering the ability of this defense system to respond to bacterial invasion.

PROTEIN

Protein is used in PN solutions to maintain lean body mass and maintain nitrogen balance. In the absence of an adequate energy source, protein is used for energy. The protein or nitrogen source is provided by synthetic crystalline amino acid solutions. Essential amino acid makes up about 40% to 50% of standard amino acid solutions while 50% to 60% of these solutions are nonessential amino acids. Protein requirements are determined by metabolic demands and underlying organ function. For the unstressed patient with adequate organ function, 0.8 g/kg/d may be adequate, but requirements may rise with metabolic demands to 2 g/kg/d.

ELECTROLYTES

Electrolytes are essential to maintain normal metabolic function. They include sodium, potassium, chloride, calcium, magnesium, phosphorus, and acetate. A variety of standard electrolyte solutions are available, as well as individual electrolytes. The requirements of individual patients may vary depending on their nutritional status and underlying disease process. Table 16-8 provides standard ranges for electrolyte additions to PN solutions. The activity of electrolytes in the body is usually characterized by interrelated patterns; no one

TABLE 16-8 ELECTROLYTE MANAGEMENT—DAILY PARENTERAL NUTRITION	
Electrolyte	Standard Daily Requirement
Sodium (Na)	1–2 mEq/kg
Potassium (K)	1–2 mEq/kg
Calcium (Ca)	10–15 mEq
Magnesium (Mg)	8–20 mEq
Phosphorus (P)	20–40 mmol
Acetate	PRN to maintain balance
Chloride	PRN to maintain balance

electrolyte can function, be deficient, or be overabundant in the body without affecting other electrolytes.

VITAMINS

Vitamins are organic compounds essential for maintenance and growth that are not synthesized by the body. There are two main groups: fat soluble (A, D, E, and K) and water soluble (B complex and C). Vitamins are sensitive to or become inactive with temperature changes and exposure to light. Therefore, they are added before administration and protected from direct light. Parenteral multivitamins are available to meet the daily requirements as recommended by A.S.P.E.N. guidelines (Vanek, Borum, et al., 2012). Vitamin K, a fat-soluble vitamin necessary for clotting, is included in new formulations of parenteral multivitamins.

TRACE ELEMENTS

Trace elements are required in small amounts and are referred to as *micronutrients*. They are essential components of metabolic pathways. Those commonly added to PN solutions include zinc, copper, chromium, manganese, and selenium. They are available individually or as multitrace solutions.

DRUGS AND MEDICATIONS

A variety of drugs and medications have been found to be compatible with PN solutions, although compatibility studies are lacking for many. Compatibility studies that have been done used specific PN or TNA solutions and specific concentrations of drugs tested. Compatibility results may be different if a different solution or medication dose or concentration is used. Compatibilities also differ depending on whether the medication is being added to a traditional dextrose and amino acid solution or to a TNA.

PATIENT SAFETY

Preserve the integrity of the line.
Attach new primed TNA tubing to dedicated lumen of CVAD. If multilumen CVAD, designate a lumen for TNA and label that lumen. If single lumen, label lumen as TNA. Ensures safety in that the same lumen is always used for TNA and not used alternately for medications or other fluids; additionally, blood sampling for some lab work is not recommended from lumens used for PN.

The most commonly added medications are heparin, regular insulin, and histamine-2 blockers. It is preferable not to add multiple drugs to the solution. For current information about drug compatibility with PN solutions and drug–nutrient interactions, the infusion nurse is referred to their pharmacist specializing in PN. A certification for pharmacists is available in nutrition support, demonstrating knowledge in this complex area of patient care. An excellent resource is the *Handbook on Injectable Drugs* (Trissel, 2013), which is updated and published yearly and available in hospital pharmacies.

PATIENT SAFETY

The feasibility of mixing drugs with PN solutions depends on various factors, including the physical compatibility of the admixed components, the chemical stability of the drug, the retention of drug concentration over time, and the bioactivity of the components after admixture. For safety, the nurse should check with the pharmacist when the compatibility of drugs and PN solutions is a concern.

Preparation of Total Nutrient Admixtures Solution

Safe preparation of solutions requires that trained personnel mix the solution under a laminar-flow hood using strict aseptic technique. Specific protocols covering all aspects of preparation, storage, and quality assurance should be established. Guidelines may vary from institution to institution but should meet established standards. Practice guidelines for labeling, formulation and nutrient ranges, nutrient prescription, compounding, quality assurance, stability and compatibility, and in-line filtration are included (INS, 2011; Kochevar et al., 2007). Adoption of these standards should ensure patient safety and also serve as a catalyst for future research.

Solutions may be prepared as traditional dextrose–amino acid solutions or as TNAs. If dextrose–amino acid solutions are used, the IV lipid emulsions are usually piggybacked to the PN or administered by a separate route. TNAs consist of all components, including lipids, mixed together in one large bag. These solutions are used almost exclusively by home care companies and increasingly in many hospitals.

All additives should be added to the PN solution in the pharmacy under sterile conditions. Additives should not be added on the nursing unit or after the PN container has been spiked and hung. If additional additives are needed after the container is hanging, alternate methods or routes should be considered.

PATIENT SAFETY

Medications cannot be added to TNA solutions on the nursing unit; they must be added in the pharmacy.

TNA solutions offer a significant advantage in the ability to provide cost-effective, patient-specific nutrition support. Having only one solution container to hang each day saves nursing time. Pharmacy admixing is simplified by the use of computerized automixing systems, which also allow for more patient-specific formulations. Potential bacterial contamination of either the solution or the line is decreased because of decreased accessing of the line. The increased use of TNA reflects the trend toward the daily use of lipid emulsions as a daily calorie source.

The stability of TNA is affected by many factors, including admixture contents, storage time and conditions, addition of non-nutrient drugs, pH of the solution, and variability in temperature. A TNA solution is normally milky white and opaque, although a faint yellow

TABLE 16-9	VISIBLE PHENOMENA IN TOTAL NUTRIENT ADMIXTURE SOLUTIONS	
Phenomena	Characteristics	Considerations
Physical phenomena		
Aggregation (stratification)	Rare white streaks (early stages of creaming)	Readily reverses with *gentle* agitation Not harmful
Creaming	Dense white color at top of solution ("cream" layer) Aggregates migrate to top of the solution	Reverses with *gentle* agitation If creaming reappears in 1–2 h or decreases after agitation, it may indicate an unstable emulsion If left undistributed, may begin to coalesce (see below)
Chemical phenomena		
Coalescence/cracking (breaking/oiling out)	Oil globules on the surface of creamed emulsion coalesce or fuse to form larger oil droplets May appear as an oil layer on top of the solution, as large oil globules, or streaks of oil throughout the solution	Irreversible Cannot be dispersed Do not hang the container If coalescence appears during infusion, take container down and return it to pharmacy immediately

hue may be evident with the addition of vitamins. The nurse should examine the solution for any signs of instability before hanging and periodically thereafter. Particulate matter is hard to detect because of the opacity of the solution. Other physical or chemical phenomena may occur and are outlined in Table 16-9. Nurses should be aware of these phenomena and be able to recognize a stable lipid emulsion or TNA solution. A TNA solution is usually stable for 24 hours after admixing with the addition of vitamins, and for up to 7 days if vitamins are not added until the solution is ready to use.

ADMINISTRATION OF PARENTERAL NUTRITION

Administration of hypertonic PN solutions requires an easily placed, well-tolerated central venous access device (CVAD) that can be used for extended periods. Infusion into a large vein with high blood flow to dilute the solution rapidly is desirable to reduce phlebitis, venous thrombosis, pain, and hemolysis.

Vascular Access and Catheter Insertion

A variety of CVADs are options for short-term or long-term access to administer PN. Short-term access is usually obtained using percutaneously placed central catheters, although these are not routinely replaced and may remain in place for several weeks (CDC, 2011). Long-term access from months to years is available for PN administration using a peripherally inserted central catheter (PICC), a tunneled CVAD, or an implanted port (Penney-Timmons & Sevedge, 2004; Pittiruti et al., 2009). Standards of practice must be followed for site selection, catheter selection, and insertion (CDC, 2011; INS, 2011). The nurse is the patient advocate to ensure that all infection prevention procedures are followed, such as chlorhexidine solution skin cleansing, maximal sterile barrier precaution, and, always, hand hygiene (CDC, 2011). Institutional protocols for the insertion and maintenance of CVADs should be established and followed according to all applicable standards. Insertion complications are infrequent when the physician/LIP is knowledgeable about anatomy and skilled in the technique. Complications are infrequent, but the patient should be closely monitored after catheter insertion, particularly for signs of respiratory distress, pain, slowly increasing hematoma, or any unexplainable symptom. Insertion complications and complications of indwelling CVADs are addressed in Chapter 14.

EVIDENCE FOR PRACTICE

- Use the fewest number of lumens to achieve the desired infusion therapy.
- No recommendation can be made for using a designated lumen for PN; it is an unresolved issue.
- Do not administer dextrose-containing solutions or PN through the pressure monitoring circuit of hemodynamic pressure monitoring catheters in adults or children.
  From Centers for Disease Control and Prevention (CDC). (2011). Guidelines for the prevention of intravascular catheter-related infections. http://www.cdc.gov/hicpac/pdf/guidelines/bsi-guidelines-2011.pdf

---

Short-length peripheral catheters and midline catheters are the options of last resort to administer PN due to the necessary restrictions to avoid complications. PN solutions that have a final concentration of 10% dextrose or lower and an osmolarity of <600 mOsm may be administered via these peripheral catheters for a limited time. Careful and frequent assessments are necessary to identify phlebitis early, although actions are needed to reduce this occurrence. These include adding heparin and steroids to the PN, coadministration with fat emulsion, cyclical administration, and changing the catheter site every 24 to 48 hours (INS, 2011).

Catheter Tip Placement Verification

Because of the nature of PN infusions, having this infusate flowing into areas other than the central vasculature is a serious complication. PN should never be initiated until catheter tip placement has been confirmed. The catheter tip should be in the distal superior vena cava; it is unacceptable for the tip to be located in the heart, inferior vena cava, or any extrathoracic vessel. Atrial rupture, valvular damage, myocardial irritability with arrhythmias, and cardiac tamponade are some of the reported complications when the catheter tip is located in the heart. An increased incidence of catheter-induced thrombosis and occlusion is associated with tip placement in the subclavian, jugular, inferior vena cava, or narrower extrathoracic vessels.

Considerations include verification of catheter tip placement before use and any time there is a question of tip position. Displacement may occur during insertion from coiling or misdirection, overinsertion or underinsertion, aberrant route on catheter advancement, venous thrombosis or stenosis, and venous or atrial perforation. The catheter tip may become displaced spontaneously at any time, from days to months later because of a change in intrathoracic pressure as with coughing or vomiting, a rapid infusion, or random body movement.

Preparation to Administer PN

All institutions should have specific protocols for the administration, monitoring, and discontinuation of PN, which should be reviewed annually. A.S.P.E.N. has published comprehensive standards for nutritional support of all patients, regardless of the clinical setting in which care is delivered. Safe administration of PN depends on strict adherence to these protocols and the safe practices guidelines.

Normally, PN solutions are refrigerated immediately after preparation or refrigerated at 4°C until used. The acceptable length of time for refrigeration is based on the stability of the admixture. Lipid emulsions are stored at room temperature no higher than 25°C; they should not be frozen. If frozen, discard. The recommended maximum hang time for PN solutions is 24 hours. PN solutions should be inspected for signs of precipitate or instability before hanging. The label also should be matched with the PN orders to ensure accuracy. The volume and infusion rate are usually noted on the label by the pharmacy.

INFUSION TUBING AND FILTERS

Primary IV tubing set changes should be established in organizational policy and procedures, based on appropriate guidelines (CDC, 2011; INS, 2011). Tubing used to administer lipid emulsions and TNA solutions should be changed every 24 hours (CDC). If these solutions are administered in a cyclic regimen, the administration set should be discarded after each unit. If the solution contains only dextrose and amino acids, the administration set does not need to be replaced more frequently than every 72 hours (CDC). It is most efficient to standardize the time of tubing and filter changes to coincide with the daily start time for the day's solution. This eliminates additional breaks in the line. Luer-lock connections are required to avoid accidental disconnection. The use of needleless systems is recommended.

The need for in-line filtration of PN solutions is apparent given the recommendations of the U.S. Food and Drug Administration. A 0.22-μm filter is recommended for traditional dextrose–amino acid solutions, with the lipids piggybacked below the filter. These filters effectively retain bacteria, fungi, and particulate matter. TNA solutions require use of a 1.2- or 5.0-μm filter that effectively eliminates microprecipitates, *Candida*, and some bacteria. Bacterial contamination of PN solutions is rare. The justification for use of in-line filters centers on the removal of microprecipitates rather than microorganisms. Microprecipitates are commonly not visible on inspection, particularly in TNAs. A filter should not be used with only-lipid emulsion infusions (INS, 2011).

A risk of contamination always exists when IV tubing and filters are changed. Therefore, precautions need to be taken and aseptic technique strictly followed. All connections should be swabbed thoroughly for 15 seconds and allowed to dry with 2% chlorhexidine solution, povidone–iodine, or alcohol before the tubing is changed. It is also a good idea to swab the end of the catheter hub to remove any dried blood or sticky residue. The nurse must clamp the catheter before changing the tubing to avoid the risk of air embolism. If a clamp is not available, the patient should be positioned flat in bed and advised to perform the Valsalva maneuver during the tubing change.

ADMINISTERING PN

PN should be administered at a constant rate. Any changes in rate should be gradual. Current rate recommendations advise a gradual rate introduction of approximately 60 to 80 mL/h for the first 24 hours with a 20 mL/h incremental increase every 24 to 48 hours. Changes in the rate of administration should be gradual because fluctuations in glucose levels can occur if the infusion is interrupted or irregular in rate. An electronic infusion device should be used to maintain consistency and accuracy of the infusion, as well as prevent inadvertent sudden infusion (INS, 2011).

Many institutions have established standard start times for PN (e.g., 2 PM) to simplify management of infusions and promote clear communication among departments. This also allows the pharmacy to establish standard times for admixing the solutions and delivery to the nursing unit. Orders for PN are usually required in the pharmacy several hours before the established start time. A clinician should demonstrate core competencies in administering PN (Box 16-4).

Glucose Tolerance

Glucose tolerance may be compromised by sepsis, stress, shock, hepatic and renal failure, starvation, diabetes, pancreatic disease, and administration of some medications, particularly steroids and some diuretics. Age is another variable; the elderly and the very young are particularly susceptible to glucose intolerance and hyperglycemia. For these patients, administration of exogenous insulin is often necessary. In addition, a sliding-scale subcutaneous insulin coverage schedule should be implemented. Box 16-5 provides considerations in managing and preventing hyperglycemia in patients receiving PN. The blood glucose (BG) level should continue to be monitored closely because insulin needs may decrease as the stress or sepsis subsides or as steroids are decreased and discontinued. BG should be maintained at <200 mg/dL during PN administration. One study also found that dextrose infusion rates >4 to 5 mg/kg/min increase the risk of hyperglycemia. Avoidance of the extremes of hyperglycemia and hypoglycemia is important.

Impact of Stress

The average nonstressed individual requires 23 kcal/kg/d to maintain body weight. Changes in physical activity increase this requirement to 28 kcal/kg/d. The need is increased in skeletal trauma, sepsis, burns, and those who are septic. Hypermetabolic patients are also subjected to an increased drain on the body's protein stores. Daily nitrogen losses in fasting patients are

- Elective postsurgical patients: 7 to 9 g N
- Skeletal trauma or septic patient: 11 to 14 g N
- Severe burns: 12 to 18 g N

Extra caution should be used when infusing PN in patients undergoing peritoneal dialysis or propofol infusions. Peritoneal dialysis can provide significant amounts of dextrose calories. The dextrose calories in dialysate solution should be calculated and a comparable amount subtracted from the dextrose ordered in the PN solution to avoid overfeeding and hyperglycemia from excess dextrose. Propofol is a lipid-based sedative that provides 1.1 kcal/mL. It is widely used in critical care units. Infusion of propofol or any other lipid-based drug must be

BOX 16-4　CORE COMPETENCIES FOR NURSES ADMINISTERING AND MONITORING PN

- Demonstrates appropriate use of standard precautions and aseptic technique
- Verbalizes knowledge of nursing policies and procedures related to administering PN
- States awareness of the impact of other dextrose sources (IV infusions, IV medications), lipid-based medications (e.g., propofol), and dialysate on the development and exacerbation of hyperglycemia
- Demonstrates correct procedure of PN administration
- Indicates knowledge of complications associated with PN administration and their management
- Verbalizes knowledge of pharmacy, nursing, and hospital policies related to PN ordering (who can order, when orders need to be received in pharmacy, what to do if changes are needed, start time)
- Verbalizes understanding that no medications or additives can be added to PN on the nursing unit (only in the pharmacy)
- Verbalizes knowledge of instances when the physician/LIP should be notified
- Demonstrates appropriate documentation of PN administration and patient response

Cycling PN

- Demonstrates appropriate use of standard precautions and aseptic technique
- Verbalizes understanding of nursing policies and procedure related to cycling PN
- Demonstrates appropriate use of glucose monitoring device
- States knowledge of acceptable glucose monitoring parameters and management of hypoglycemia and hyperglycemia
- Verbalizes knowledge of parameters to be monitored and the frequency (i.e., intake and output, vital signs, weight, blood analyses, central venous access device site, infusion pump)
- Verbalizes knowledge of potential complications related to cycling and their management
- Expresses knowledge of instances when the physician/LIP should be notified
- Demonstrates appropriate documentation of cycling and patient response

Discontinuing PN

- Demonstrates appropriate use of standard precaution and aseptic technique
- Verbalizes knowledge of nursing policies and procedures related to discontinuing PN
- States understanding of monitoring the patient for signs of rebound hypoglycemia during and after discontinuation of PN
- Displays knowledge of need to hang dextrose 5% in water solution at same rate as PN solution if PN must stop abruptly (i.e., because of no orders, signs of complications, central venous access device malfunction)
- Verbalizes knowledge of instances when physician/LIP should be notified
- Demonstrates appropriate documentation of discontinuing PN and patient response

BOX 16-5   MANAGING HYPERGLYCEMIA IN PATIENTS RECEIVING PN

Goals

- Maintain serum glucose levels between 100 and 200 mg/dL, with an optimal range of 100 to 150 mg/dL
- Avoid overfeeding

Initiating Parenteral Nutrition

- Limit to no more than 200 g dextrose in the first few days until glycemic control is achieved.
- If baseline fasting BG level is >180 to 200 mg/dL, or if the patient is a diabetic patient previously treated with insulin or oral agent, add 0.1 U regular insulin per gram of dextrose (i.e., 15 U/L 15% dextrose [150 g/L]; 20 U/L 20% dextrose [200 g/L]).
- In general, do not increase dextrose concentration in PN until serum glucose level is consistently <200 mg/dL for 24 hours.

Ongoing

- Adjust insulin accordingly whenever the concentration of dextrose increases or decreases.
- Check serum glucose level by reflectance meter every 4 to 6 hours initially, then every 8 hours once the patient's levels are stable.
- Increase regular insulin in PN by 0.05 U/g dextrose daily if serum glucose was consistently >200 mg/dL in previous 24 hours.
- Use subcutaneous (SQ) regular insulin to supplement PN insulin according to the following algorithm:

Glucose (mg/dL)	SQ Regular Insulin Dose (Units)
200–250	2–3
251–300	4–6
301–350	6–9
>350	8–12

- If serum glucose is consistently >200 mg/dL with PN insulin and adherence to the SQ insulin algorithm, a separate IV infusion may be helpful in achieving glycemic control.
- Once the patient's glucose level is stable, frequency of glucose monitoring can be decreased.
- Monitor and assess daily to anticipate effects of PN on glucose level (i.e., patient's clinical status, fluid status, medication/IV profile, peritoneal dialysis, and dextrose volume).

monitored closely when given with PN to avoid the pitfalls of overfeeding and hypertriglyceridemia. PN solutions need to be manipulated when excessive calories are provided in these drugs. Daily calculation of dextrose or lipid calories provided by dialysate or lipid-based drugs with appropriate adjustments in the dextrose or lipids provided in PN should be mandatory.

Consideration should also be given to dextrose administered in crystalloid IV solutions. Many patients on PN need supplemental infusions of crystalloids to correct hypernatremia or because of medication compatibility. When possible, non–dextrose-containing crystalloids should be used. If significant amounts of dextrose-containing crystalloids are needed, insulin may be added to decrease the risk of hyperglycemia.

If PN solutions are interrupted or unavailable, standing orders should be available to infuse 5% dextrose solutions at the same rate, either through the central line or peripherally if the central line is removed or lost. This prevents the sudden hypoglycemia caused by the high endogenous insulin secretion that is associated with hypertonic PN solutions. Although some institutions and physicians/LIPs still prefer to use a 10% dextrose solution in these situations, it has been deemed unnecessary.

Cycling Parenteral Nutrition

Long-term continuous PN can be associated with fatty liver, hepatic indices, and hepatomegaly caused by hyperinsulinism. Therefore, cyclic PN is widely used for those patients who require long-term PN support. This also allows for increased mobility during the day, giving the patient some time to participate in normal daytime activities and offering an improved sense of well-being and quality of life. Cycling may also benefit certain patients by allowing maximum freedom for ambulation and physical therapy. Cyclic administration is often indicated for patients who have been in stable condition on continuous PN, patients who are on HPN, and patients who require PN for only a portion of their nutritional needs.

Once tolerance to 24-hour continuous PN has been established, a transition to cyclic infusions can be initiated. Cycling from 24 hours of nutritional therapy to 12 to 16 hours is usually done over several days with a gradual reduction in the hours of infusion. The infusion time is decreased approximately 4 hours at a time as the infusion rate is increased to maintain nutrition goals for calories and protein. Cyclic PN is usually not infused at a rate >200 mL/h. The patient's ability to tolerate the glucose and fluid volume determines the hourly rate. Close monitoring for fluid status and BG alterations is essential. Most patients tolerate this well without development of rebound hypoglycemia. BG levels during the accelerated infusion rates for cyclic PN may be up to 250 mg/dL. Normoglycemia is usually present during the hours when the patient is receiving PN.

Discontinuing Parenteral Nutrition

PN should not be stopped without alternate plans for therapy so that nutritional status can be maintained or continue to improve. Nor should reductions in PN begin until an alternate source of nutritional intake, such as enteral nutrition, is initiated. Tapering of PN can begin when EN is able to meet 33% to 50% of nutrient requirements. PN can be discontinued once EN is tolerated and able to meet >75% of nutrient requirements (Table 16-10). Accurate calorie counts are essential to the successful transition from PN to enteral or oral intake.

TABLE 16-10	DISCONTINUING PARENTERAL NUTRITION

Equipment

Syringe with appropriate amount of normal saline solution
Povidone–iodine wipes
Syringe with appropriate amount of heparin flush solution
Lock device (Luer lock, male adapter)

Action	*Rationale*
Explain procedure to the patient.	Explanation allays anxiety.
Maintain standard precautions and aseptic technique.	Deters spread of microorganisms
Follow these principles when discontinuing PN:	Avoids abrupt cessation of nutrients in the absence of any other source of glucose (oral, IV, or enteral) and avoids rebound hypoglycemia
• Reduce PN infusion rate in conjunction with an increase in caloric intake by oral or enteral route.	Ensures adequacy of nutrient intake
• Be sure that the patient can take half of the estimated nutrient requirements either enterally or orally before PN discontinues.	Same as above
• Fluid intake may also decrease as the PN is decreased, so provide adequate fluids by other routes.	Prevents dehydration
• Decrease PN by 50% for 2 h prior to discontinuation for unstable patients and patients with glucose intolerance or a high dextrose concentration.	Prevents rebound hypoglycemia
Discontinue PN before surgery: Decrease rate to 40 mL/h the night before surgery, and discontinue infusion at least 4 h before surgery. Any 5% dextrose solution can be infused. Keep in mind that potassium shifts may occur with hyperglycemia. Also ensure adequate preoperative hydration.	Stress of surgery may increase BG levels, and signs and symptoms of hyperglycemia are not easily monitored or detected in the anesthetized patient.
Verify physician/LIP's order to stop infusion.	Ensures that PN is to be discontinued
Hang dextrose 5% in water at the same rate as PN if PN must stop abruptly (e.g., no orders, suspected infection, central venous access device [CVAD] malfunction).	Prevents rebound hypoglycemia
Cleanse CVAD lumen–PN tubing connection with povidone–iodine wipe for 30 s. Allow to dry.	Antibacterial and antifungal cleansing of hub deters spread of microorganisms
Disconnect PN tubing and discard. Then, flush lumen per established protocol and attach lock device to end of CVAD.	Maintains patency and prevents occlusion
Document procedure in appropriate records.	Accurate and comprehensive documentation reflects nursing care given.

NURSING MANAGEMENT

Clinical assessment and monitoring are imperative for the safe administration of PN, which should be considered in the same manner as medication administration. The nurse should be familiar with the solution composition, the expected metabolic response, and the potential complications of therapy. A good knowledge base should enable the nurse to identify patients who are at risk for metabolic complications in order to monitor the patient's response. Catheter site care, dressing changes, and monitoring PN administration are also in the domain of nursing management. The importance of clear and thorough documentation of care cannot be overemphasized. Nutritional Support Teams and Infection Prevention and Control departments track outcomes of PN, such as number of days on PN, glucose levels remain in range, infections, and other adverse outcomes. This supports quality improvement processes, quality patient outcomes, and adequacy of therapy. Patient outcomes should be reviewed quarterly by the team with improvement strategies identified as needed.

Catheter and Site Management

Catheter site care is one of the most important measures for preventing catheter-related infections, especially for PN, since these infusions are the nutritional source for patients. Strict adherence to hand washing and aseptic technique is critical. Clean skin before dressing changes. Any of the skin solutions may be used for dressing change skin preparation, including 2% chlorhexidine-based solution, povidone–iodine, or 70% alcohol (CDC, 2011). Allow the antiseptic to dry prior to dressing.

ANTIMICROBIAL OINTMENTS AND DRESSINGS

Routine use of prophylactic topical antibiotic ointments or creams on the insertion or exit site is not recommended because of their potential to promote fungal infections and antimicrobial resistance (CDC, 2011). (Hemodialysis catheters have different recommendations from CDC.)

The catheter should be stabilized with a sutureless catheter securement device (INS, 2011). This prevents catheter movement within the vein, which irritates the vein lining and promotes mechanical phlebitis.

Transparent or gauze dressings are the two preferred materials for CVAD dressings. Transparent dressings allow the insertion site to be observed without disturbing the dressing. They are more comfortable for the patient and require dressing changes no more than every 7 days (CDC, 2011). Gauze and tape dressings preclude site inspection, are usually more uncomfortable for the patient, and require changing every 48 hours (CDC). Either type of dressing should be changed when the device is removed or replaced, when the dressing becomes damp, loose, or soiled, or any time the integrity of the dressing is compromised. CDC guidelines recommend gauze dressing when the patient is diaphoretic or when the site is oozing or bleeding. No recommendation has been made for the necessity of a dressing on a well-healed exit site of a tunneled catheter (CDC, 2011).

Site care and dressings are completed using sterile technique. Prepackaged sterile dressing change kits, which include all necessary equipment, are typically used. Some kits may include instructions as well. A careful review of the literature and all standards and guidelines should be done when establishing dressing change protocols.

SITE ASSESSMENT

The insertion site should be palpated daily for tenderness and induration; it should be observed through the transparent dressing for erythema, swelling, or exudate. The catheter site should be directly inspected without the dressing if the patient has a fever without obvious source or symptoms of BSI (CDC, 2011). If symptoms are present, physician/LIP notification and further evaluation are warranted.

If the PN is being administered through a short-length peripheral IV catheter, frequent site assessment is recommended by the INS (Gorski et al., 2012). Frequency is based on patient condition, the type of infusate, and whether the infusion is intermittent or continuous (Chapter 13, Box 13-2).

INJECTION PORT CLEANSING

Injection port management is just as important as catheter site care. The injection port should be cleansed with 2% chlorhexidine solution, 10% povidone–iodine, or 70% alcohol before accessing the system (CDC, 2011). Minimizing manipulation of the hub and tubing connection can also decrease the risk of infection.

MAINTAINING CATHETER PATENCY

Anticoagulant locking solutions (heparinized saline) may be used to maintain catheter patency. Some controversy still exists regarding the concentration of heparin, appropriate volume, and frequency of flush. However, the lowest effective concentration of heparin in a volume two times the internal volume of the catheter should be used (INS, 2011). A concentration of 10 U/mL, 3 mL, has been shown to maintain catheter patency. It is imperative to know specific information about the catheter being used, including catheter material, flushing volume, and pressure and syringe size limitations. Studies have found that normal saline is as effective as heparin in maintaining patency of peripheral catheters.

PATIENT SURVEILLANCE

Nurses play a vital role in monitoring patients on PN. Patient monitoring is as important as proper administration in preventing serious metabolic complications (Table 16-11). Accurate measurements of the patient's daily body weight, measured at the same time of day, using the same scale, and with the patient wearing the same amount of clothing, are important. A baseline weight should be obtained and then the patient should be weighed daily thereafter. Intake and output records should also be scrupulously maintained and recorded. These measures are necessary to assess fluid balance and adequacy of the prescribed nutrients.

Vital signs should be obtained and recorded at least twice a day and more often if the patient is unstable or the temperature is >100°F (37.7°C) orally or 101°F (38.3°C) rectally. Certain drugs and disease states suppress the normal febrile response, and affected patients must be assessed individually.

BG levels should be monitored according to physician/LIP order, the patient's level of glycemic control, or minimally every 6 hours. This practice has become easier with the use of glucose monitors on nursing units. Biochemical monitoring is also important to assess the adequacy of the PN regimen and the presence of any metabolic complications. Nutritional profiles or standing laboratory tests are recommended for routine PN monitoring. Routine laboratory tests and their frequency are outlined in Table 16-12. Ideally, a full chemical profile, including glucose, electrolytes, urea nitrogen, creatinine, albumin, transferrin, calcium, magnesium, phosphorus, liver function, prothrombin time, and complete blood count,

TABLE 16-11	MONITORING PARENTERAL NUTRITION
Action	**Rationale**
Explain procedures to the patient.	Patient understanding will allay anxiety.
Check vital signs every shift. If temperature >100.5°F, take vital signs q4h and monitor BG level q4–6h. BG level should be maintained at <200 mg/dL.	Discloses signs of complications or infection during PN infusion; notify physician/LIP if critical value
After 1 wk, stable patients (BG <200 mg/dL) can be monitored less frequently if ordered by physician/LIP.	Determines need to increase or decrease insulin if added to PN and patient not receiving other types of insulin
Monitor blood work as ordered. Notify physician/LIP of any critically abnormal values.	Assesses need to adjust PN regimen and detects complications early
Strictly measure intake and output:	Monitors fluid balance and avoids complications; notify physician/LIP of significant changes
• Intake includes PN, other IV solutions, IV medication volume, and any oral intake. • Output includes urine and any other output (nasogastric tube, ostomies, fistula, drainage); unplanned diuresis.	
Obtain baseline weight, and then weigh daily. (Stable patients on prolonged PN can be weighed weekly.)	Points to adequacy of therapy (weight maintenance or weight gain)
Observe central venous access device (CVAD) site for and notify physician/LIP if: • Erythema, edema, exudate • Intact dressing or sutures • Pain at insertion site • Securely taped catheter and PN tubing that relieves tension on CVAD	Discloses complications early and establishes patency of sutures, if present
Monitor infusion rate and pump for signs of possible malfunction.	Ensures ordered infusion and prevents complications
Monitor for and notify physician/LIP: • If patient's temperature >101°F • If BG >200 mg/dL or for critical laboratory values • Presence or increase in edema • Weight gain ≥2 lb/wk • Edema over insertion site, neck, face, chest, either arm • Any significant changes in clinical status: vital signs, intake or output, mental status, convulsions, or coma	Identifying and treating complications early avoids more serious effects.
Adhere to all policies related to PN administration and CVAD management.	Maintains established standards of care
Culture catheter tip if signs/symptoms of infection are present.	Identifies catheter as source of infection for suspected catheter sepsis
Accurately document all monitoring activities in appropriate patient medical records. Also document any abnormal laboratory results and adverse reactions.	Documentation should be accurate and comprehensive to: communicate with all team members and promote continuity of care.
Include actions taken and the patient's response to treatment.	

TABLE 16-12	LABORATORY MONITORING OF PARENTERAL NUTRITION			
Frequency	Daily until stable, then Monday, Wednesday, Friday			
Test	Blood sugar	BUN	Creatinine	Electrolytes
Frequency	Baseline, then weekly (e.g., every Monday)			
Test	CBC	PT	Albumin	ALT
	AST	Alkaline phosphatase		Calcium
	Cholesterol	LDH	Magnesium	Phosphorus
	Transferrin	Total bilirubin	Total protein	Triglycerides

ALT, alanine transaminase; AST, aspartate transaminase; BUN, blood urea nitrogen; CBC, complete blood count; LDH, lactic dehydrogenase; PT, prothrombin time.

should be obtained before initiating PN. Critically ill and unstable patients may require more frequent monitoring. Other studies may be warranted depending on the clinical status of the patient.

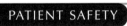

> **PATIENT SAFETY**
>
> Nurses need to demonstrate core competencies when monitoring patients receiving PN; some competencies need initial successful demonstration, whereas others need periodic skill or knowledge demonstration.
> - Demonstrate appropriate use of standard precautions and aseptic technique.
> - Demonstrate appropriate use of BG monitoring device.
> - Verbalize knowledge and understanding of acceptable BG parameters and management of hypoglycemia/hyperglycemia.
> - Verbalize knowledge of parameters to be monitored and frequency (i.e., intake/output, vital signs, weight, blood analyses, central venous access device care, infusion pump).
> - Verbalize knowledge of abnormal assessments and when the physician/LIP should be notified.
> - Demonstrate appropriate documentation.

COMPLICATIONS OF PARENTERAL NUTRITION

Complications associated with PN are divided into two categories: catheter related and metabolic. These complications can be minimized or even avoided with the establishment of and adherence to strict protocols as well as knowledgeable surveillance.

Catheter-Related Complications after Placement

After the catheter is successfully inserted, tip placement is verified, and no insertion-related complications are evident; ongoing concerns with an indwelling intravascular catheter are related to

- Infection and sepsis
- Catheter occlusion
- Thrombosis
- Air embolism

INFECTIOUS AND SEPTIC COMPLICATIONS

Preventing infection will minimize the need for additional hospitalization, antibiotics, and line replacement. In addition, infections that are associated with a blood clot around the catheter can limit the available sites for catheter placement, which can become a major issue in patients who require long-term PN. When a patient experiences a break or a hole in the catheter, one of the complications can be infection as well as catheter or air embolism.

Catheter-related sepsis associated with PN is a serious and potentially lethal complication, particularly in high-acuity patient populations. An estimated 250,000 to 500,000 intravascular device–related BSIs occur in the United States associated with mortality rates of 12% to 25% (Crnich & Maki, 2002; Maki et al., 2000). Central venous catheters (CVCs) pose the greatest risk of BSI. It has been reported that up to 75% of CRBSIs originate from CVCs of various types. CRBSIs increased continuously in the 1980s but declined 30% to 40% in the 1990s through increased adherence to CDC Guidelines for the Prevention of Intravascular Device–Related Infections. The current version of the Guidelines was published in 2011.

Most CRBSIs are associated with short-term, noncuffed, single-lumen, or multilumen catheters inserted into the subclavian or internal jugular vein (CDC, 2011). Migration of skin organisms at the insertion site is the most common route of infection for short-term percutaneously inserted catheters. Hub contamination is the most likely source of infection in long-term catheters. Other causes of catheter-related infections include multiple line violation and manipulation, improper technique during catheter insertion, and hematogenous seeding of the catheter by blood-borne organisms from infection at a distant site.

Meticulous admixing protocols make the incidence of solution contamination rare. PN solutions are poor growth media for bacteria owing to the low pH and hypertonicity of amino acid and dextrose solutions. PN may also contain large quantities of acetate, which is bacteriostatic. When albumin is added to a solution, bacteria and fungi growth increase. *Candida albicans* is a common fungus in standard solutions. Resistance of *Candida* spp. to commonly used antifungal agents is increasing (CDC, 2011). Data from the classic Surveillance and Control of Pathogens of Epidemiologic Importance (SCOPE) Program documented that 10% of *C. albicans* bloodstream isolates from hospitalized patients were resistant to fluconazole (Pfaller, Jones, Messer, Edmond, & Wenzel, 1998). Another 48% of *Candida* BSIs were caused by nonalbicans species that are more likely to demonstrate resistance to fluconazole and itraconazole. Three-in-one solutions have significantly higher microorganism growth than standard solutions. Lipid emulsions support growth of gram-positive, gram-negative, and fungal species at room temperature.

Descriptions and treatment options for catheter-related infections are presented in Table 16-13. CRBSI is indicated by bacteremia/fungemia in a patient with an intravascular catheter with at least one positive blood culture obtained from a peripheral vein, clinical manifestations of infections, and no apparent source for the BSI except the catheter. One of the following should be present: a positive semiquantitative or quantitative culture whereby the same organism is isolated from the catheter segment and peripheral blood; simultaneous

TABLE 16-1   CATHETER-RELATED INFECTIONS

Infection Type	Description	Treatment
Insertion site infection	Erythema, induration, tenderness, and purulence localized to an area within 2 cm of the catheter insertion site	Daily site care Warm, moist compresses Possibly oral antibiotics
Pocket site infection	Erythema, tenderness, and induration over the port reservoir site; possibly necrosis; purulent exudate from the subcutaneous pocket	Warm, moist compresses Oral or IV antibiotics Port removal
Tunnel infection	Erythema, tenderness, induration, or purulence extending more than 2 cm from the site along the course of the subcutaneous tunnel	Catheter removal Infection may respond poorly to other treatment attempts
Catheter-related bloodstream infection	Isolation of the same organism (identical species, antibiogram) from semiquantitative or quantitative cultures of the catheter tip and peripheral blood of a patient with clear signs of BSI and no other identifiable sources of infection (selected symptoms include temperature ≥101.5°F, chills, rigors, malaise, and temperature defervescence with catheter removal)	Catheter removal Systemic antibiotics by catheter Antibiotic lock

quantitative blood cultures with a 3:1 ratio CVC versus peripheral; differential period of CVC culture versus peripheral blood culture positivity of >2 hours (Abad & Safdar, 2011).

Catheter-related sepsis may present in the patient as fever, chills, hypotension, change in mental status, and leukocytosis. Metabolic acidosis and hyperglycemia may be early signs of sepsis in critically ill patients receiving PN. A complete fever workup is necessary. All potential sources of infection need to be cultured.

Options for managing catheter-related sepsis include exchange of the catheter over guidewire, catheter salvage, and catheter removal. The decision is determined by the patient's clinical status, culture results, and the nature of the offending organism. Catheter removal remains the treatment of choice for short-term catheters. Guidewire exchange is indicated only if the catheter is malfunctioning and there is no sign of catheter site infection (CDC, 2011). If infection is suspected and if there is no evidence of catheter site infection and the patient is not floridly septic, the catheter may also be exchanged over a guidewire and the catheter tip sent to the laboratory for culture. If the culture results are positive for colonization or infection, the catheter should be removed and a new catheter inserted in a different location. If the patient is septic, the catheter should be removed immediately (Bodey, 2005). In either situation, empiric antibiotics are often started once all appropriate specimens for culture are obtained.

Tunneled catheters and implanted ports pose additional problems because they cannot be changed over a guidewire or readily replaced, and they often serve as lifelines for patients with limited sites for central venous access. Catheter salvage is a desired option in these instances. Many of these infections can be successfully treated with antibiotics without removing the catheter (Mermel et al., 2009). The use of an antibiotic lock technique has been successful in several instances. Various drugs in a wide range of concentrations for varying durations have been used. Prophylactic vancomycin is not recommended, and in many institutions, *Candida* infection is automatic grounds for catheter removal, regardless of type.

The use of a chlorhexidine-impregnated sponge dressing around the CVC and exit site is recommended by the CDC (2011) only for short-term catheters, in patients older than 2 months, "if the CLABSI rate is not decreasing despite adherence to basic prevention measures, including education and training, appropriate use of chlorhexidine for skin antisepsis, and maximal sterile barrier precautions during insertion" (p. S5).

Vigilant observation of protocols for insertion, use, and maintenance of CVADs is necessary to minimize the incidence of infection and catheter-related sepsis. A recent study supported the use of a dedicated team for PN and care of those catheters used solely for PN; colonization was lower for those short-term CVADs used for PN and cared for by a team (Dimick et al., 2003).

CATHETER OCCLUSION

Partial or complete catheter occlusion may result from fibrin sheath formation or thrombus at the tip of the catheter, blood clots, lipid deposits, precipitates, kinking or malposition, pinch-off syndrome, and rupture or breakage of the device. Increased difficulty in infusing fluids may be the first indication of fibrin sheath formation. The fibrin sheath may cause a partial occlusion of the catheter by acting as a "flap valve" to prevent withdrawal of blood but allow infusions. It may eventually encase the entire catheter, causing complete occlusion of all lumens. The sheath may also become seeded with microorganisms, serving as a focus for infection.

Occlusion of the CVAD may also occur from drug precipitates or lipid deposition. Precipitate occlusion may occur from inadequate flushing between medications, simultaneous administration of incompatible medications or solutions, and medications admixed in concentrations exceeding that required for stability. Calcium and phosphorus precipitates are a common cause of occlusion with PN solutions. Occlusions from drug precipitates or lipid deposition typically result in sudden occlusion of the catheter either during or immediately after an infusion. Occlusion with lipid depositions is also a liability, especially with the use of TNAs. Chapter 14 outlines interventions for catheter occlusions.

VENOUS THROMBOSIS

The development of venous thrombosis may occur with any type of CVAD secondary to injury to the vein wall during insertion or by movement of the catheter against the vein wall after insertion. Catheter thrombogenicity may depend on the type of catheter material and the surface characteristics. Predisposing risk factors for venous thrombosis include hypovolemia, venous stasis, and hypercoagulable states (e.g., pregnancy, cancer, hypovolemia, bone marrow transplantation). Chemically induced thrombosis can result from infusion of hypertonic solutions, including PN, and small-volume antibiotics or chemotherapy admixtures and vesicants administered through CVADs whose tips are in the upper arm, subclavian, or innominate veins. Intermittent or long-term infusion of these solutions should be delivered through catheters whose tips terminate in the superior vena cava. A lower incidence of thrombosis has been noted in catheters whose tips lie in the distal superior vena cava.

Patients with venous thrombosis may be asymptomatic, making careful observation for early signs imperative. Signs may include increased anterior chest venous pattern, arm or neck swelling, external jugular distention, or fluid leaking from the insertion site during infusion (caused by backflow). Diagnosis may be made by arm venography, contrast studies through the catheter, Doppler duplex imaging, magnetic resonance imaging, and radionucleotide studies. Treatment of catheter-induced venous thrombosis remains controversial and depends on the extent of thrombus formation, the severity of the symptoms, the current clinical conditions, and the future access needs of the patient. Conservative treatment without device removal consists of IV anticoagulant therapy followed by warfarin therapy for 3 or more months. Catheter removal followed by anticoagulant therapy may be necessary for more severe symptoms. Some practitioners advocate using prophylactic low-dose warfarin to reduce the risk of thrombosis for patients who are at increased risk.

The major complication of catheter-associated venous thrombosis is pulmonary embolism. This complication should be treated with catheter removal plus standard therapy for that disorder, including anticoagulation or thrombolysis at the discretion of the treating physician/LIP.

AIR EMBOLISM

Air embolism is fortunately rare because its occurrence is the most lethal complication of catheter insertion or maintenance. Air embolism is a potential danger whenever the central venous system is open to the air, such as during insertion, IV tubing or cap changes, accidental disconnection, or through a tract left after catheter removal. This is most likely to occur on deep inspiration when the patient is in an upright position, dehydrated, or hypovolemic. Symptoms occur with an air entry rate of 20 mL/s. Death can occur with an air entry rate of 75 to 150 mL/s; a 70- to 300-mL air volume may be lethal (Drewett, 2000). Signs and symptoms vary depending on the severity; they may include dyspnea, apnea, hypoxia, disorientation, tachycardia, hypotension, pulmonary wheeze, or a precordial murmur. Severe neurologic deficits, including hemiplegia, aphasia, seizures, and coma, are associated with air embolism. This is attributed to direct access of air into the cerebral circulation in most situations.

Immediate treatment aims to prevent obstruction of the right ventricular outflow tract by air. The patient should immediately be placed on the left side in deep Trendelenburg position (right side up). This keeps the air in the right atrium and out of the pulmonary circulation. Needle aspiration of air through the catheter or by direct intracardiac approach may be necessary. Oxygen therapy should be initiated.

Precautions should be taken during catheter insertion, tubing and cap changes, and catheter removal to prevent air embolism. Tubing junctions should be properly secured. Catheter removal should be immediately followed by placement of occlusive gauze dressing with an ointment over the site. The ointment occludes the tract and assists with healing. This dressing is usually needed for 24 to 48 hours or until the tract is totally closed.

Metabolic Complications

Metabolic complications arise when PN causes imbalances in any of the electrolytes and/or trace elements. Metabolic complications are the most frequently observed adverse effects with PN and can be avoided when PN orders are written by knowledgeable physicians/LIPs and laboratory studies are meticulously monitored. Frequent metabolic monitoring can ensure that potential metabolic complications are prevented or documented and treated. The nurse is in a key position to monitor for these changes and report them to the appropriate physician/LIP. Table 16-14 cites the most frequently observed metabolic complications. Only the most life threatening is discussed more fully in the following sections.

TABLE 16-14	POTENTIAL METABOLIC COMPLICATIONS OF PARENTERAL NUTRITION	
Cause(s)	**Prevention**	**Treatment**
Hyperglycemia		
Carbohydrate intolerance Too rapid infusion of PN Too much carbohydrate load Insulin resistance—stress, sepsis, diabetes, steroids	AccuChek q6h Be aware of medications that may cause glucose intolerance (i.e., steroids) Start PN infusion slowly	Decrease PN rate or dextrose concentration/amount Increase proportion of calories as lipids Add insulin to the solution or use sliding-scale insulin coverage Maintain BG 100–150 mg/dL
Hypoglycemia		
Abrupt decrease or cessation of PN Excessive insulin administration Weaning steroids	Wean or slow down PN infusion when stopping Hang $D_{10}W$ at the same rate of PN if unable to hang PN Maintain infusion rate; use an infusion pump Monitor serum glucose levels	Hang $D_{10}W$ at the same rate of PN if unable to hang PN Give IV glucose STAT; 50% dextrose may be needed; maintain proper flow rate
Hyperglycemic hyperosmolar nonketotic coma		
Untreated glucose intolerance causes hyperosmolar diuresis, electrolyte imbalances, coma, death (40%–50% mortality rate) Increased risk in elderly, diabetes malnourishment, steroid therapy, and with stress or sepsis	Appropriate glucose monitoring Frequent chemistry profiles to assess electrolytes, osmolarity	Monitor closely Discontinue PN Rehydrate with normal saline or other isotonic solution Correct electrolyte imbalances, especially potassium and bicarbonate Monitor ABGs Insulin as needed
Hyperkalemia		
Excessive potassium replacement Renal disease—potassium cannot be excreted Leakage of potassium from cells after severe trauma	Monitor serum potassium and renal function Accurate I/O to evaluate fluid balance	Stop or decrease potassium in solution Assess for other sources of potassium Monitor for arrhythmias Administer infusion of $D_{50}W$
Hypokalemia		
Excessive potassium losses (increased GI losses with diarrhea, fistulas) Diuretic therapy Large doses of insulin Increased requirement with anabolism Refeeding severely malnourished patients	Monitor serum potassium Anticipate potential potassium depletion with large GI losses Monitor I/O Be aware of drugs that cause excessive potassium loss Be aware that patients severely malnourished are susceptible (refeeding syndrome)	Add potassium to PN solution May need additional IVPB potassium run over 4–6 h to correct severe deficiency Monitor pulse for tachycardia/arrhythmia Monitor for metabolic alkalosis (potassium loss may cause sodium retention)

POTENTIAL METABOLIC COMPLICATIONS OF PARENTERAL NUTRITION   (*Continued*)

Cause(s)	Prevention	Treatment
Hypernatremia		
Dehydration Diarrhea Diabetes insipidus Excessive replacement	Maintain I/O Monitor serum sodium Be aware of drugs that cause sodium retention (i.e., steroids)	Decrease sodium or provide salt-free solution until corrected Provide enough free water to meet needs Treat or correct cause
Hyponatremia		
Diuretics GI losses (vomiting, fistula) Congestive heart failure, renal failure, cirrhosis Water intoxication	Accurate I/O Urine specific gravity Accurate weights (assess fluid shifts)	Fluid restriction Add sodium to PN Minimize GI loss if possible Close metabolic monitoring
Hyperphosphatemia		
Renal failure Excessive replacement	Accurate I/O Monitor serum levels and renal status	Low or no phosphate added May need dialysis
Hypophosphatemia		

Inadequate in PN
Insulin therapy
Disease states:
  Alcoholism
  Respiratory alkalosis
  Renal problems
  Severe diarrhea
  Malabsorption associated with low calcium
  and magnesium levels
  Increased requirements
  Refeeding severely malnourished patients
	Be aware of potential
	disease states that cause low
	phosphate levels
	Frequent laboratory
	monitoring, especially if low
	levels/depleted
	Be aware of medications
	that may lower phosphates
	(Carafate, magnesium and
	aluminum hydroxide, steroids)
		Replace phosphate in PN
		May need additional IVPB of
		phosphate over 4–6 h
		Replace calcium as needed
		(repletion of phosphate may
		cause calcium to drop)
		Discontinue PN if patient
		symptomatic

Hypocalcemia		
Vitamin D deficiency Insufficient replacement Pancreatitis Hypomagnesemia Hyperphosphatemia Hypoalbuminemia	Monitor serum levels Be aware of disease states, medications, malnutrition that can cause hypocalcemia	Replace by adding calcium to PN May require IVPB of calcium to correct severe deficiency Correct hypomagnesemia Monitor ionized calcium
Hypomagnesemia		
Insufficient magnesium in PN Excess GI or renal losses (diarrhea, fistula, diuretics) Certain drugs (aminoglycosides, diuretics, cisplatin) Disease states (chronic alcoholism, pancreatitis, diabetic acidosis, sepsis/infection, burns)	Monitor serum levels closely Be aware of disease states or drugs that can cause hypomagnesemia	Increase magnesium in PN If very low, IVPB replacement Discontinue PN if patient symptomatic Monitor for cardiac arrhythmia

(Continued)

TABLE 16-14	POTENTIAL METABOLIC COMPLICATIONS OF PARENTERAL NUTRITION *(Continued)*	
Cause(s)	**Prevention**	**Treatment**
Hypermagnesemia		
Excess magnesium in PN	Monitor serum levels	Decrease or delete from PN
Renal failure	Monitor renal function	Calcium salts
Metabolic acidosis		
Renal insufficiency; acute/chronic renal failure	Monitor ABGs, electrolytes	Give bicarbonate or replace
Diabetic ketoacidosis	Monitor renal function	some or all of chloride with
Diarrhea	Be aware of disease states that	acetate in PN
Lactic acidosis (shock)	may cause metabolic acidosis	Monitor vital signs
Potassium-sparing diuretics		
Massive rhabdomyolysis		
Metabolic alkalosis		
Gastric losses	Replace GI losses	Increase chloride content
Thiazide and loop diuretics	Monitor ABGs	Decrease acetate content
Mineralocorticoids	Be aware of acetate content of	
Amino acid solutions	amino acids	

ABGs, arterial blood gases; D$_5$W, dextrose 5% in water; GI, gastrointestinal; I/O, intake and output; IVPB, intravenous piggyback.

COMPLICATIONS RELATED TO GLUCOSE LEVEL

Glucose intolerance has already been discussed. The sudden development of hyperglycemia in a patient who was previously glucose tolerant may indicate impending infection or sepsis. Hyperglycemia and glycosuria may precede clinical signs of sepsis by 12 to 24 hours. Patients with preexisting diabetes or significant physiologic stress may develop hyperglycemia on initiation of PN. Because hyperglycemia has been shown to be associated with decreased immune function and increased risk of infectious complications, efforts to monitor and control BG during specialized nutritional support are prudent.

Blood sugars should be maintained between 100 and 150 mg/dL. Studies have demonstrated that tighter control (80 to 120 mg/dL) may decrease mortality in the ICU patients (Van De Berghe, Wouters, Weekers, et al., 2001).

Progressive hyperglycemia, if not detected or if inadequately treated, can lead to the life-threatening complication of hyperglycemic hyperosmolar nonketotic coma. If untreated, marked hyperglycemia and glycosuria may lead to an osmotic diuresis accompanied by dehydration, electrolyte imbalance, and a decreasing level of consciousness that can result in seizures and coma and death. Reversal of this state requires immediate discontinuation of the PN solution, aggressive fluid and electrolyte replacement, correction of hyperglycemia by insulin administration, and correction of acidosis with bicarbonates. During treatment, frequent monitoring of BG, electrolyte, and arterial blood gas levels and vital signs is essential (Turina, Fry, & Polk, 2005).

Hypoglycemia is chemically defined as a serum glucose level of <50 mg/dL. Many patients may be asymptomatic at this level. Symptoms include weakness, headache, chills, tingling in the extremities or mouth, cold and clammy skin, thirst, hunger, apprehension, diaphoresis, decreased levels of consciousness, and changes in vital signs. Hypoglycemia during PN may occur with excess insulin administration. Insulin needs decrease when steroids are tapered and discontinued, and as sepsis resolves, and should be adjusted in the PN solution accordingly. Abrupt cessation of PN may also result in rebound hypoglycemia, more particularly in children less than 3 years of age (Stout & Cober, 2011). Unstable patients and those with glucose intolerance may benefit from a 1- to 2-hour taper to avoid rebound hypoglycemia (Raymond & Ireton-Jones, 2012). If a PN solution must be discontinued abruptly, D_{10} should be infused for 1 to 2 hours to avoid possible rebound hypoglycemia (Bloch & Mueller, 2004).

COMPLICATIONS RELATED TO ELECTROLYTES

The infusion of hypertonic dextrose results in the intracellular shift of potassium, magnesium, phosphorus, and calcium. Requirements for these electrolytes, particularly potassium and phosphorus, may be increased. Increased losses or requirements related to the patient's clinical status or treatment may also increase electrolyte requirements. Conversely, renal failure may require restriction of potassium, magnesium, and phosphate. Careful monitoring of electrolyte levels and adjustments to the PN solution are essential to maintain electrolyte balance.

The refeeding syndrome describes metabolic complications seen when severely malnourished patients receive aggressive administration of nutritional support. Rapid infusion of carbohydrate calories can result in hypophosphatemia, hypokalemia, and hypomagnesemia. A rapid expansion of extracellular volume can result in heart failure. Alternatively, significant hyperglycemia may cause osmotic diuresis and dehydration. Hypophosphatemia is considered a hallmark of the refeeding syndrome. Careful initiation and close monitoring of serum phosphate, magnesium, potassium, and glucose are imperative when providing specialized nutritional support to chronically malnourished patients.

COMPLICATIONS RELATED TO LIPIDS

EFAD and potentiation of inflammatory response by rapid infusion were discussed previously. Elevated liver enzyme levels may be commonly observed in patients receiving PN. Causes are multifactorial and include drugs, sepsis, shock, surgery, and anesthetics. Mild elevations may appear on days 9 to 14 of PN infusion, usually returning to normal once PN is discontinued. Overfeeding of calories is often responsible and should be avoided. Slow, continuous infusion of lipids over 16 to 24 hours has also been associated with better tolerance and clearance of lipids.

Hypertriglyceridemia usually is owing to an alteration in lipid clearance and occurs most frequently in critically ill patients and those with sepsis. It has been identified as a possible etiologic factor in the development of pancreatitis, immunosuppression, and altered pulmonary hemodynamics in patients receiving PN. Acceptable serum triglyceride levels are <400 mg/dL for continuous lipid infusion. For levels >400 mg/dL, lipid and dextrose amounts should be reduced and/or eliminated from the PN solution. If serum triglyceride levels remains >400 mg/dL for >2 weeks, provide approximately 1 g/kg of lipid emulsion twice each week to prevent EFAD (Seidner & Fuhrman, 2001).

COMPLICATIONS RELATED TO PROTEIN

Adjustments in protein concentrations should be made according to the patient's tolerance, clinical response, and laboratory results. Prerenal azotemia can occur if excess protein is administered, causing a rise in blood urea nitrogen because of excess urea production. The amount of amino acid in PN should be reduced for patients who develop amino acid intolerance such as prerenal azotemia, hepatic encephalopathy, or hyperammonemia. Special solutions are available for patients with liver disease and renal disease.

PATIENT SAFETY

Nurses are legally accountable for providing safe and appropriate care to patients. This includes knowledge of and adherence to established guidelines, standards of care, and institutional policies and procedures. Literature should be evaluated and policies and procedures reviewed annually with staff nurse participation.

HOME PARENTERAL NUTRITION

Advanced technology, care management, and consumer demand have contributed to making HPN a successful alternative for many patients who require prolonged or lifelong PN.

Two of the primary indications for HPN include short bowel syndrome and inflammatory bowel disease; PN is required when these patients do not have enough gut to maintain fluids, electrolytes, and/or nutrition. PN can also be indicated on a short-term basis for patients who have complicated surgical problems and enterocutaneous fistulae; surgeons may prescribe PN for a few months to calm the gut and improve the patient's nutritional status, and then, these patients can undergo a takedown of their fistula.

Regardless of the health care setting, all patients should be evaluated to determine their eligibility for and the appropriateness of HPN. Standards for home nutrition support should be followed.

HPN may be provided as a continuous or a cyclic infusion. Cyclic infusion over 12 to 14 hours, as previously discussed, is preferred, especially for ambulatory patients. Most home infusion companies prefer to provide TNAs for HPN. The teaching program should be individualized for a patient's learning needs, capabilities, and home care environment. Patients should be encouraged to assume as much responsibility for self-care as possible. Doing so enhances their sense of control.

Nurses have a primary role in preparing the patient for HPN. The prospect of HPN may seem overwhelming to the patient and family or caregiver, and thorough preparation and teaching is essential because of the complexity of the procedures to be learned. Careful assessment of the patient and caregiver's willingness and ability to perform the procedures and assume responsibility for managing this therapy should be a priority. One nurse should be selected as the primary teacher because a lack of consistency can confuse the learner and extend the learning period. Survival skills should be taught in the hospital and full education for PN initiated in the home.

Education should include verbal instructions and demonstration of all procedures. Return demonstration by the patient or primary caregiver is essential so that the instructor can assess competency. A manual of written instructions should be provided to all patients. The verbal and written instructions should include the following (A.S.P.E.N., 2007a, 2007b):

- All appropriate procedures related to the administration of PN and care and maintenance of the CVAD
- Use, maintenance, and troubleshooting of the infusion pump
- Storage, management, and disposal of solutions and supplies
- Self-monitoring form for HPN (Figure 16-3)
- Problem-solving techniques

HOME PARENTERAL NUTRITION LOG

Instructions   Name:_____

Keep a daily log to record your results. Fill in the boxes. Put an "X" in the box when you do not
need the information. Your home care nurse will review this log with you on each visit.

	Sun	Mon	Tues	Wed	Thurs	Fri	Sat
Date							
Weight							
Temperature AM							
PM							
Blood sugar							
Urine sugar / acetone AM							
PM							
Rate / amount of PN infused							
Lipids (if separate)							
Oral / IV fluids taken							
Urine output							
Other output							
Stool							
Antibiotics							
Site (or dressing appearance): C = clean /dry D = drainage S = swelling R = red P = pain							
Comments							

FIGURE 16-3 Self-monitoring form for HPN.

- Emergency interventions
- Expectations of home care and follow-up plans

A social worker, discharge planner, or case manager may be helpful to patients and families who have questions and concerns about financial considerations and community

---

BOX 16-6   PRINCIPLES FOR SELF-ADMINISTRATION OF PN

1. The patient/caregiver understands the disorder and rationale for therapy:
   - Agrees to home therapy and the associated benefits and risks
   - Understands alternatives, consequences if therapy not accepted, advantages and disadvantages
   - Understands short- and long-term goals and the expected duration of treatment
2. The patient/caregiver has the visual acuity, manual dexterity, cognitive ability, and mobility to perform procedures related to PN therapy:
   - A backup caregiver is identified and trained in case the patient needs assistance.
   - Adaptive/assistive devices are available if needed.
3. The patient's physical environment is safe and appropriate for home therapy:
   - Adequate work area with water supply, refrigeration, storage area for supplies
   - Grounded outlets or adapters available
4. The patient/caregiver verbalizes and demonstrates knowledge and understanding of PN administration:
   - Aseptic technique
   - Solution storage and handling
   - Solution inspection, preparation, and addition of vitamins or other medications as ordered; attachment of administration set
   - Infusion pump operation, maintenance, and troubleshooting
   - Connection and disconnection from CVAD, including appropriate flushing and locking
   - Administration schedule and importance of compliance with established schedule and protocols (including written instructions provided)
   - Self-monitoring guidelines and record keeping
   - Recognition and treatment of potential complications
   - Emergency interventions
   - When/whom to call for questions or assistance
   - Identify emergency 24-hour on-call number
   - CVAD care and monitoring
5. The patient/caregiver understands and agrees to follow-up care as scheduled by the physician/LIP/nutrition support team:
   - Home nursing visits
   - Follow-up in physician/LIP's office or clinic

resources. Psychosocial support is also essential. Principles for self-administration of TNAs are given in Box 16-6.

Arrangements for a home infusion provider should be determined as early as possible. Ideally, the home infusion nurse visits the patient and family in the hospital to establish rapport and discuss learning needs, feelings and concerns, health status, and the regimen prescribed by the physician/LIP. In many cases, the home infusion nurse provides all the teaching in the home.

Documentation should include patient eligibility data and the indication for therapy. It should also incorporate the patient's nutritional therapy objectives into the care plan. Short- and long-term goals should be included and updated as applicable. Patient progress and monitoring parameters, as well as any problems, should be carefully recorded. Evaluation of the nutritional prescription, readiness for transitional feeding, and periodic nutritional assessments also should be included in the documentation (Ireton-Jones, DeLegge, Epperson, & Alexander, 2003).

Quality nutrition support may be delivered in all clinical settings by highly skilled and credentialed infusion nurses. Specialized certification through the National Board of Nutrition Support Certification further ensures competencies. Nurses and nursing play a key role in maintaining nutritional support and ensuring positive, safe patient outcomes.

Review Questions   *Note: Questions below may have more than one right answer.*

1. Which of the following visceral proteins is most useful in monitoring the effectiveness of nutritional support because of its shorter half-life and sensitivity to acute changes in protein status?
   A. Albumin
   B. Transferrin
   C. Prealbumin
   D. Total protein

2. What is the minimum amount of glucose needed to meet the obligate needs for glucose by the brain, central nervous system, red blood cells, WBCs, active fibroblasts, and certain phagocytes?
   A. 50 to 75 g
   B. 150 to 200 g
   C. 250 to 300 g
   D. 350 to 400 g

3. All of the following are adverse reactions to IV lipids *except*
   A. Dyspnea
   B. Chest pain
   C. Headache
   D. Leg cramps

4. BMI relates a patient's weight to height and to weight-related health problems.
   A. True
   B. False

5. Which of the following complications is not associated with placement of the CVC tip into the heart?
   A. Thrombosis
   B. Cardiac tamponade
   C. Valvular damage
   D. Cardiac dysrhythmias

6. During PN administration, the serum BG level should be maintained at less than
   A. 50 mg/dL
   B. 80 mg/dL
   C. 100 mg/dL
   D. 200 mg/dL

7. If symptoms of an air embolism occur, the patient should be placed in which of the following positions?

A. On the back, in semi-Fowler's

B. On the left side, in deep Trendelenburg

C. On the right side, in deep Trendelenburg

D. On the left, in semi-Fowler's

8. Symptoms of hyperglycemic hyperosmolar nonketotic coma include all of the following *except*

A. Glycosuria

B. Seizures

C. Coma

D. Anuria

9. During PN administration, the refeeding syndrome is associated with which of the following electrolyte abnormalities?

A. Hypophosphatemia

B. Hypermagnesemia

C. Hypercalcemia

D. Hyponatremia

10. Infectious complications are more frequently associated with which type of central venous access device?

A. Cuffed tunneled central catheter

B. Cuffed tunneled port

C. Noncuffed PICC

D. Noncuffed, short-term, multilumen catheter

References and Selected Readings *Asterisks indicate references cited in text.*

*Abad, C.L., & Safdar, N. (2011). Catheter-related bloodstream infections. *Infectious Disease*, 84–98. Retrieved from http://www.idse.net/download/BSI_IDSE11_WM.pdf

Alexander, M., Corrigan N., Gorski, L., Hankins, J., & Perucca, R. (2010). *Infusion Nursing: An evidence-based practice approach* (3rd ed.). St. Louis, MO: Saunders Elsevier.

Allison, S.P. (2003). History of nutritional support in Europe pre-ESPEN. *Clinical Nutrition*, 22(Suppl. 2), 53–65.

*American Society for Parenteral and Enteral Nutrition (A.S.P.E.N.). (2007a). The A.S.P.E.N. Nutrition Support Patient Education Manual. https://www.nutritioncare.org/Information_for_Patients/Information_for_Patients/

*American Society for Parenteral and Enteral Nutrition (A.S.P.E.N.). (2007b). Special report. *Journal of Parenteral and Enteral Nutrition*, 31(5), 441–443.

*American Society for Parenteral and Enteral Nutrition (A.S.P.E.N.). (2009a). Board of Directors and Clinical Practice Committee. *Definition of terms, style, and conventions used in A.S.P.E.N. Board of Directors–approved documents.* http://www.nutritioncare.org/Library.aspx

*American Society for Parenteral and Enteral Nutrition (A.S.P.E.N.). (2009b). A.S.P.E.N. enteral nutrition practice recommendations. *Journal of Parenteral and Enteral Nutrition*, 33(2), 122–167.

American Society for Parenteral and Enteral Nutrition (A.S.P.E.N.). (2011). Clinical guidelines: Nutrition screening, assessment, and intervention in adults. *Journal of Parenteral and Enteral Nutrition*, 35, 16–24.

A.S.P.E.N. Board of Directors and Task Force on Parenteral Nutrition Standardization. (2007). A.S.P.E.N. statement on parenteral nutrition standardization. *Journal of Parenteral and Enteral Nutrition*, 31(5), 441–448.

*Barker, L.A., Gout, B.S., & Crowe, T.C. (2011). Hospital malnutrition: Prevalence, identification and impact on patients and the healthcare system. *International Journal of Environmental Research and Public Health*, 8(2), 514–527.

*Bloch, A.S., & Mueller, C. (2004). Enteral and parenteral nutrition support. In K. L. Mahan & S. Escott-Stump (Eds.), *Krause's food, nutrition, & diet therapy* (11th ed., pp. 533–553). Philadelphia, PA: W.B. Saunders.

*Bodey, G.P. (2005). Managing infections in the immunocompromised patient. *Clinical Infectious Diseases*, 40(Suppl. 4), S239.

Braga, M., Ljungqvist, I., Soeters, P., Fearon, K., Weimann, A., Bozzetti, F., et al. (2009). ESPEN guidelines on parenteral nutrition: Surgery. *Clinical Nutrition*, 28, 378–386.

*Brogden, B.J. (2004). Clinical skills: Importance of nutrition for acutely ill hospital patients. *British Journal of Nursing, 13*(15), 914–920.

Btaiche, I.F., Carver, P.L., & Welch, K.B. (2011). Dosing and monitoring of trace elements in long-term home parenteral nutrition patients. *Journal of Parenteral and Enteral Nutrition, 35*(6), 736–747.

*Carney, D.E., & Meguid, M.M. (2002). Current concepts in nutritional assessment. *Archives of Surgery, 137,* 42–45.

*Casaer, M.P., Mesotten, D., Hermans, G., Wouters, P.J., Schetz, M., Meyfroidt, G., et al. (2011). Early versus late parenteral nutrition in critically ill adults. *The New England Journal of Medicine, 365,* 506–517.

*Centers for Disease Control and Prevention (CDC). (2011). Guidelines for the prevention of intravascular catheter-related infections. http://www.cdc.gov/hicpac/pdf/guidelines/bsi-guidelines-2011.pdf

*Cresci, G.A. (2002). Nutrition assessment and monitoring. In S. A. Shikora, R. G. Martindale, & S. D. Schwaitzberg (Eds.), *Nutritional considerations in the intensive care unit* (pp. 21–29). Dubuque, IA: Kendall/Hunt.

*Cresci, G.A. (2005). *Nutrition support for the critically ill patient: A guide to practice* (p. 612). Boca Raton, FL: CRC Press, Taylor & Francis Group.

*Crnich, C.J., & Maki, D.G. (2002). The promise of novel technology for the prevention of intravascular device-related bloodstream infection, I: Pathogenesis and short-term devices. *Healthcare Epidemiology, 34,* 1232–1242.

*Dimick, J.B., Swoboda, S., Talamini, M.A., Pelz, R., Hendrix, C., & Lipsett, P. (2003). Risk of colonization of central venous catheters: Catheters for total parenteral nutrition vs other catheters. *American Journal of Critical Care, 12,* 328–335.

*Drewett, S. (2000). Complications of central venous catheters: Nursing care. *British Journal of Nursing, 9*(3), 465–477.

Driscoll, D.F. (2005). Stability and compatibility assessment techniques for total parenteral nutrition admixtures: setting the bar according to pharmacopeial standards. *Current Opinion in Clinical Nutrition and Metabolic Care, 8*(3), 297–303.

Driscoll, D.F. (2008). Hospital pharmacists and total parenteral nutrition: Current status and trends. *The European Journal of Hospital Pharmacists, 14*(1), 64.

Dudrick, S.J. (2009). History of parenteral nutrition. *Journal of the American College of Nutrition, 28*(3), 243–251.

*Galica, L.A. (1997). Parenteral nutrition. *Nursing Clinics of North America, 32,* 705–718.

*Gerlach, A.T., Thomas, S., Murphy, C.V., Stawicki, P.S., Whitmill, M.L., Pourzanjani, L., et al. (2011). Does delaying early intravenous fat emulsion during parenteral nutrition reduce infections during critical illness? *Surgical Infection, 12,* 43–47.

*Gorski, L.A., Hallock, D., Kuehn, S.C., Morris, P., Russell, J.M., & Skala, L.C. (2012). INS Position Paper: Recommendations for frequency of assessment of the short peripheral catheter site. *Journal of Infusion Nursing, 35,* 290–292.

*Grant, A., & DeHoog, S. (2008). *Nutrition assessment support and management* (2nd ed.). Burlington, VT: Elsevier Academic Press.

*Hammond, K.A. (2004). Dietary and clinical assessment. In K.L. Mahan & S. Escott-Stump (Eds.), *Krause's food, nutrition, & diet therapy* (11th ed., pp. 407–431). Philadelphia, PA: W.B. Saunders.

*Infusion Nurses Society. (2011). Infusion nursing standards of practice. *Journal of Infusion Nursing, 34*(Suppl. 1), S1–S110.

*Ireton-Jones, C.S. (2002). Estimating energy requirements. In S. A. Shikora, R. G. Martindale, & S. D. Schwaitzberg (Eds.), *Nutritional considerations in the intensive care unit* (pp. 31–36). Dubuque, IA: Kendall/Hunt Publishing.

*Ireton-Jones, C.S., DeLegge, M., Epperson, L., & Alexander, J. (2003). Management of the home parenteral nutrition patient. *Nutrition in Clinical Practice, 18,* 310–317.

*Jeejeebhoy, K.N. (2012). Parenteral nutrition in the intensive care unit. *Nutrition Reviews, 70*(11), 623–630.

*Jensen, G.L., Mirtallo, J., Compher, C., Dhaliwal, R., Forbes, A., Grijalba, R.F., et al. (2010). Adult starvation and disease-related malnutrition: A proposal for etiology-based diagnosis in the clinical practice setting from the International Consensus Guideline Committee. *Journal of Parenteral and Enteral Nutrition, 34*(2), 156–159.

Kirby, D.F. (2012). Improving outcomes with parenteral nutrition. *Gastroenterology & Hepatology, 8*(1), 39–41.

*Kochevar, M., Guenter, P., Holcombe, B., Malone, A., Mirtallo, J., & A.S.P.E.N. Board of Directors and Task Force on Parenteral Nutrition Standardization. (2007). A.S.P.E.N. statement on parenteral nutrition standardization. *Journal of Parenteral and Enteral Nutrition, 31*, 441–448.

*Kris-Etherton, P.M., Taylor, D.S., Yu-Poth, S., et al. (2000). Polyunsaturated fatty acids in the food chain in the United States. *American Journal of Clinical Nutrition, 71*(1 Suppl.), 179S–188S.

Kruizenga, H.M., Van Tulder, M.W., Seidell, J.C., Thijs, A., Ader, H.J., & M.A. Van Bokhorst-de van der Schueren (2005). Effectiveness and cost-effectiveness of early screening and treatment of malnourished patients. *American Journal of Clinical Nutrition, 82*, 1082–1089.

Litchford, M.D. (2012). Clinical: Biochemical assessment. In L.K. Mahan, S. Escott-Stump, & J.L. Raymond (Eds.), *Krause's food and the nutrition care process* (13th ed., pp. 191–208). St. Louis, MO: Elsevier Saunders.

Maki, D.G., Kluger, D.M., & Crnich, C.J. (2006). The risk of bloodstream infection in adults with intravascular devices: A systematic review of 200 published prospective studies. *Mayo Clinic Proceedings, 81*(9), 1159–1171.

*Maki, D.G., Mermel, L.A., Kluger, D., Narins, L., Knasinski, V., Parenteau, S., et al. (2000). The efficacy of a chlorhexidine-impregnated sponge (Biopatch) for the prevention of intravascular catheter-related infection—A prospective, randomized, controlled, multicenter study. Paper presented at the 40th Interscience Conference on Antimicrobial Agents and Chemotherapy. Toronto, Ontario, Canada.

Manzanares, W., Dhaliqal, R., Jurewitsch, B., Stapleton, R., Jeejeebhoy, K., & Heyland, D. (2013). Parenteral fish oil lipid emulsions in the critically ill: A systematic review and meta-analysis. *Journal of Parental and Enteral Nutrition.* http://pen.sagepub.com/content/early/2013/04/19/0148607113486006.abstract

*McClave, S.A., Martindale, R.G., Vanek, V.W., McCarthy, M., Roberts, P., Taylor, B., et al. (2009). Guidelines for the provision and assessment of nutrition support therapy in the adult critically ill patient: Society of Critical Care Medicine (SCCM) and American Society for Parenteral and Enteral Nutrition (A.S.P.E.N.). *Journal of Parenteral and Enteral Nutrition, 33*, 277–316.

Meisel, J.A., Le, H.D., DeMeijer, V.E., Nose, V., Gura, K.M., Mulkern, R.V., et al. (2012). Comparison of 5 intravenous lipid emulsions and their effects on hepatic steatosis in a murine model. *Journal of Pediatric Surgery, 46*(4), 666–673.

*Mermel, L.A., Allon, M., Bouza, E., Craven, D.E., Flynn, P., O'Grady, N.P., et al. (2009). Clinical practice guidelines for the diagnosis and management of intravascular catheter-related infection: 2009 update by the Infectious Diseases Society of America. *Clinics in Infectious Disease, 49*(1), 1–45.

Moriyama, B., Henning, S.A., Jin, H., Kolf, M., Rehak, N.N., Danner, R.L., et al. (2010). Physical compatibility of magnesium sulfate and sodium bicarbonate in a pharmacy-compounded bicarbonate-buffered hemofiltration solution. *American Journal of Health-System Pharmacy, 67*(7), 562.

*Mueller, C., Compher, C., Ellen, D.M., & American Society for Parenteral and Enteral Nutrition (A.S.P.E.N.) Board of Directors. (2011). A.S.P.E.N. clinical guidelines: Nutrition screening, assessment, and intervention in adults. *Journal of Parenteral and Enteral Nutrition, 35*(1), 16–24.

*Penney-Timmons, E., & Sevedge, S. (2004). Outcome data for peripherally inserted central catheters used in an acute care setting. *Journal of Infusion Nursing, 27*(6), 431–436.

*Pfaller, M.A., Jones, R.N., Messer, S.A., Edmond, M.B., & Wenzel, R.P. (1998). National surveillance of nosocomial blood stream infection due to species of *Candida* other than *Candida albicans*: Frequency of occurrence and antifungal susceptibility in the SCOPE program. *Diagnostic Microbiology and Infectious Disease, 30*, 121–129.

*Pittiruti, M., Hamilton, H., Biffi, R., MacFie, J., Pertkiewicz, M., & ESPEN. (2009). ESPEN guidelines on parenteral nutrition: Central venous catheters (access, care, diagnosis and therapy of complications). *Clinical Nutrition, 28*, 365–377.

*Probst, Y., & Tapsell, L. (2005). Overview of computerized dietary assessment programs for research and practice in nutrition education. *Journal of Nutrition Education and Behavior, 37*(1), 20–26.

Raymond, J.L., & Ireton-Jones, C.S. (2012). Food and nutrient delivery: Nutrition support methods. In L.K. Mahan, S. Escott-Stump, & J.L. Raymond (Eds.), *Krause's food and the nutrition care process* (13th ed., pp. 306–324). St. Louis, MO: Elsevier Saunders.

*Rodriguez, L. (2004). Nutritional status: Assessing and understanding its value in the critical care setting. *Critical Care Nursing Clinics of North America, 16*(4), 509–514.

*Rychlec, G., Edel, J., Murray, M., Schurer, W., & Tomko, M.M. (2000). Nutrition assessment of adults. In B. Hornick (Ed.), *Manual of clinical dietetics* (6th ed., pp. 3–33). Chicago, IL: American Dietetic Association.

*Seidner, D.L., & Fuhrman, P.M. (2001). Nutrition support in pancreatitis. In M. M. Gottschlich (Ed.), *The science and practice of nutrition support: A case-based core curriculum* (pp. 553–565). Dubuque, IA: Kendall/Hunt Publishing.

Seres, D. (2013). *Nutrition support in critically ill patients: Parenteral nutrition. UptoDate.* Wolters Kluwer Health. www.uptodate.com.

Smyth, N.D., Neary, E., Power, S., Feehan, S., & Duggan, S. (2013). Assessing appropriateness of parenteral nutrition usage in an acute hospital. *Nutrition in Clinical Practice, 28*(2), 232–236.

*Somanchi, M., Tao, X., & Mullin, G.E. (2011). The facilitated early enteral and dietary management effectiveness trial in hospitalized patients with malnutrition. *Journal of Parenteral and Enteral Nutrition, 35,* 209–216.

Souba, W.W. (1997). Nutritional support. *The New England Journal of Medicine, 336,* 41–48.

Stanberry, L., Mias, G.I., Haynes, W., Higdon, R., Snyder, M., & Kolker, E. (2013). Integrative analysis of longitudinal metabolomics data from a personal multi-omics profile. *Metabolites, 3,* 741–760.

Stout, S.M., & Cober, M.P. (2011). Cyclic parenteral nutrition infusion: Considerations for the clinician. *Practical Gastroenterology, 35*(7), 11–24.

Tajchman, S.K., & Bruno, J.J. (2010). Prolonged propofol use in a critically ill pregnant patient. *Annals of Pharmacotherapy, 44*(12), 2018–2022.

*Trissel, L.A. (2013). *Handbook on injectable drugs* (17th ed.). Bethesda, MD: American Society of Health-System Pharmacists.

*Turina, M., Fry, D.E., & Polk, H.C. Jr. (2005). Acute hyperglycemia and the innate immune system: Clinical, cellular, and molecular aspects. *Critical Care Medicine, 33,* 1624–1633.

Van den Berghe, G., Wilmer, A., Hermans, G., Meersseman, W., Wouters, P. J., Milants, I., et al. (2006). Intensive insulin therapy in the medical ICU. *The New England Journal of Medicine, 354,* 449–461.

*Vanek, V.W., Borum, P., Buchman, A., Fessler, T.A., Howard, L., Jeejeebhoy, K., et al. (2012). A.S.P.E.N. position paper: Recommendations for changes in commercially available parenteral multivitamin and multi-trace element products. *Nutrition in Clinical Practice, 27,* 440–491.

*Vanek, V.W., Seidner, D.L., Allen, P., Bistrian, B., Collier, S., Gura, K., et al. (2012). A.S.P.E.N. position paper: Clinical role for alternative intravenous fat emulsions. *Nutrition in Clinical Practice, 27,* 150–192.

Walshe, C., Bourke, J., Lynch, M., McGovern, M., Delaney, L., & Phelan, D. (2012). Culture positivity of CVCs used for TPN: Investigation of an association with catheter-related infection and comparison of causative organisms between ICU and non-ICU CVSs. *Journal of Nutrition and Metabolism, 2012,* 257959.

*Wilmore, D.W., & Dudrick, S.J. (1968). Growth and development of an infant receiving all nutrients exclusively by vein. *Journal of the American Medical Association, 203,* 860–864.

Young, A.M., Kidston, S., Banks, M.D., Mudge, A.M., & Isenring, E.A. (2013). Malnutrition screening tools: Comparison against two validated nutrition assessment methods in older medical inpatients. *Nutrition, 29*(1), 101–106.

Blood and Blood Component Therapy

Molly Hendricks
Valerie Kolmer

BLOOD AND BLOOD COMPONENT THERAPY—21ST CENTURY CONSIDERATIONS

Opportunities are endless to transform and improve the administration of blood and blood components. With more than 5 million patients requiring these products per year, transfusion therapy needs to be safe and address innovative therapeutics while being cost-effective and efficient. Depending on the geographical location, blood donation continues to be in a high demand as the supply continues to fluctuate due to unexpected events such as mass casualties, hurricanes, and earthquakes (U.S. Department of Health and Human Services [HHS], 2011). Maintaining a 3-day supply of blood remains imperative to meet the transfusion demands of blood and blood components. With over 15 million transfusions provided in 2008, it is essential to instill trust in the blood collection and transfusion process for the recipient (HHS, 2011).

Regulatory bodies such as The Joint Commission (TJC) have focused efforts on safe transfusion practices through their National Patient Safety Goals (TJC, 2013). Blood transfused to the wrong patient is a major cause of patient complications; therefore, specific attention should focus on improving the process of blood verification and administration (American Association of Blood Banks [AABB], 2011). Safe transfusions are possible through strictly adhering to regulations and continually improving blood component testing.

One of the most important steps is identification of the patient for each procedure in the transfusion process. As a critical component to reduce adverse effects, correct identification has been at the forefront of discussions with the AABB, U.S. Food and Drug Administration (FDA), as well as donation and transfusion services. A current mandate is that patients must be identified using two identifiers, such as the patient name and date of birth (TJC, 2013). Accurate identification of the patient and verification of the correct blood component allow the correct patient to receive the correct blood. Realizing it was imperative to correctly identify the right patient; multiple requirements have been set forth since 2004. The FDA instituted a "bar code rule" in 2004 stating that some drug and all blood-related packaging must provide a bar code label. In the same statement, the FDA required machine-readable information. The intention was to prepare for technology-related identification of patients and blood components such as machine-readable bar codes. Recognizing the difficulty of implementing such a system with limited funds, the FDA began revisiting ideas to facilitate its role in patient safety. The FDA acknowledged both the positive and negative aspects of implementing such a system. Although in a 20-year span, bar coding would prevent nearly 500,000 adverse events and transfusion errors, the cost would total $93 billion (HHS, 2013).

PATIENT SAFETY

Bar coding for positive patient identification enhances patient safety by limiting some human errors.

Another technological advancement for safer blood transfusion practices is **radiofrequency identification devices (RFID)**. A small chip can be implanted into wristbands, laboratory tubes, and blood component bags. The transmitter functions over radio waves and alerts the transfusionist of incompatibility instead of relying on the precise optical reading requirements of the bar coding technology (Brooks, 2008; Davis, Geiger, Gutierrez,

Heaser, & Veeramani, 2009). Current research is focused on feasibility and cost-effectiveness of RFID for the entire transfusion process (Hohberger, Davis, Briggs, Gutierrez, & Veeramani, 2012).

Although enhanced technology assists in positive patient identification, there was a need to make blood and blood component labeling universal and reduce errors related to misread labels. In 2008, all accredited facilities implemented a standardized system called the International Society of Blood Transfusion (ISBT 128) bar code labels. Continued exploration of technology and processes are needed to make transfusion therapy safer and efficient at the bedside.

Nurses will also need to maintain their knowledge and competence with each new blood and blood component product. Recent advances in transfusion therapy such as hematopoietic growth factors, blood substitutes, cord blood, gene therapy, and cellular engineering are improving patient outcomes. Nurses are the last checkpoint to ensure safe administration of transfusion therapy. Along with the patient, nurses are the first to identify possible transfusion reactions and can intervene appropriately. Nursing care is the surveillance, assessment, problem identification, and intervention that keep patients safe.

The future of health care leans on interprofessional collaboration to provide a safe patient environment. Through interprofessional interactions, nurses must encourage patient-centered care (Institute of Medicine, 2011). As current and future research continues to advance transfusion therapy, nurses must understand the importance of their role in including patients in their care. As advocates for patient safety and improving quality of care, nurses must work closely with patients requiring one or more transfusions. Nurses need to be aware of these innovations to explain how blood is made safe and to be alert to the potential for the patient's reactions to a blood-processing methodology. By understanding the patient's concerns related to blood transfusions, nurses can assist by evaluating patient education materials and by involving patients in the decision-making process.

 PATIENT SAFETY

Care for each patient must be customized to ensure his or her safety and enhance engagement.

Nurses are integral health care partners in transfusion therapy. Along with providers in their own facilities, nurses work with many regulatory agencies to improve care. Some of these agencies in the United States include the Centers for Disease Control and Prevention (CDC), the FDA, the Occupational Safety and Health Administration, the AABB, the Clinical Laboratory Improvement Act, and TJC. The AABB sets standards that represent accepted performance guidelines for the provision of safe blood banking, transfusion, transplantation, and work environments for personnel. Professional organizations also assist in the maintenance of standards, both for professionals and health care agencies, such as the American Nurses Association (ANA), the American Association of Critical-Care Nurses (AACN), the Infusion Nurses Society (INS), and the Oncology Nursing Society (ONS). Adhering to the standards of these agencies instills confidence in providers and patients that care is current and policies and procedures are followed. The future for transfusion therapy is filled with opportunities. Nurses can provide the safest therapy for patients and minimize risks when working collaboratively with all health care colleagues toward this common goal.

BASIC IMMUNOHEMATOLOGY

Immunohematology is the science that deals with antigens of the blood and their antibodies. **Antigens** (also called agglutinogens because they can cause blood cell agglutination, or clumping) are substances capable of stimulating the production of antibodies in response to their presence on the blood cell. An **antibody** is a protein in the plasma that reacts with this specific antigen. People who have been exposed to the red blood cells (RBCs) or leukocytes of other people through transfusion, transplantation, or pregnancy (maternal–fetal hemorrhage) may produce antibodies to the antigens carried on those foreign cells.

Antibodies are named for the antigen that stimulated their formation and with which they react. For example, an antibody against the Rh, or "D" antigen, formed after the transfusion of an Rh (D)-positive unit to an Rh (D)-negative recipient, is called *anti-D*. Antibodies formed in response to exposure to foreign antigens are called *immune antibodies*.

Numerous antigens have been discovered on human blood cells, some more commonly encountered, such as Kell, Duffy, and Kidd. There are, however, hundreds of antigens that are rarer. Most of these are weak and of minimal importance in transfusion. Leukocytes also carry antigens on their surfaces, the most important being **human leukocyte antigens (HLA)**. The groups most likely to cause transfusion reactions are the ABO and Rh systems of antigens.

The **ABO system**, discovered by Karl Landsteiner in 1901, is the most important group of antigens for transfusion as well as for transplantation. The synthesis of these antigens, which are located on the surface of RBCs, is under the control of the A, B, and O *genes*. There are four ABO blood types: In the presence of the A gene, a person makes A antigen and is classified as group A; group B people have B antigens on their RBCs; group AB people have both; and group O people have neither. These antigens, inherited genetically, determine the person's blood group.

Some blood group antibodies are formed without exposure to **allogeneic** (from another person) RBCs. The most important of these so-called naturally occurring antibodies, or isoagglutinins, are anti-A and anti-B. During the first few months of life, infants make antibodies to whichever of the ABO antigens they lack. For example, a group A infant makes anti-B (Table 17-1). These isoagglutinins can produce rapid hemolysis of RBCs with the corresponding antigen, forming the basis of ABO incompatibility.

The **Rh system**, discovered in 1940 by Stetson and Levine, is the second most clinically important system for transfusion. The Rh system is so-called because of the discovery of this substance in the RBCs of the Rhesus monkey. The antigens of the human Rh system are of great

TABLE 17-1	ABO CLASSIFICATION OF HUMAN BLOOD				
	Cell Antigens		Plasma Antibodies		
Group	A	B	A	B	% US Population
O	−	−	+	+	44
A	+	−	−	+	42
B	−	+	+	−	10
AB	+	+	−	−	4

clinical significance because they often are responsible for transfusion incompatibility and hemolytic disease of the newborn (HDN). Approximately 85% of the white population has the D antigen on their RBCs and are classified as Rh positive, and 92% of African Americans are Rh positive (AABB, 2010). In the remainder of the population, the D antigen is missing; these people are classified as Rh negative and can readily form anti-D after exposure to the antigen. Severe hemolytic reactions and HDN result from this antigen–antibody reaction.

Mechanism of Immune Response

When a patient is transfused with allogeneic blood bearing foreign (i.e., nonself) antigens, the immune system may respond by producing antibodies. Phagocytic cells called *macrophages* play an important role in this response by capturing and processing foreign antigens. The macrophages then present the processed antigens to other members of the immune system, called *T* and *B lymphocytes*, which begin to produce antibodies specific for the antigens presented. Stimulated by the foreign antigen, the B cell swells, changes its internal structure, and differentiates into plasma cells or memory B cells that produce the antibodies to bind and aggregate foreign cells and ensure their removal (Sommer, 2009). Each plasma cell then produces large quantities of antibodies specific to the particular antigen as genetically programmed into the cell. The cells secrete the antibodies into a variety of body fluids, including the blood plasma. The T lymphocytes act as helpers or suppressors of B-lymphocyte function. The intertwined relationship between B and T lymphocytes regulates the type and sensitivity of the immune response.

Mechanism of Red Blood Cell Destruction

Two mechanisms of RBC destruction are known: intravascular **hemolysis** and extravascular hemolysis. Intravascular hemolysis occurs within the vascular compartment. This mode of RBC destruction results from the sequential binding of an antibody to a foreign antigen on the surface of a RBC. This reaction then activates the complement system. When the complement system cascade is triggered, a resulting lytic complex forms on the RBC membrane, which leads to rupture of the RBC and the rapid release of free hemoglobin into the intravascular compartment overwhelming the system. The most frequent cause of this type of RBC destruction is transfusion of ABO-incompatible blood. Mostly immunoglobulin (IgM) antibodies, anti-A and anti-B, are capable of engaging the complement, coagulation, and kinin systems when they bind with their corresponding antigens. The consequences of this type of hemolysis are usually immediate, severe, and often fatal.

The other mechanism of RBC destruction, extravascular hemolysis, is more commonly seen as a result of incompatibilities in blood group systems other than the ABO. In contrast to anti-A and anti-B, antibodies to these other blood group antigens are usually immunoglobulin G (IgG) and bind to RBCs with the corresponding antigen. Phagocytic cells of the reticuloendothelial system, particularly in the spleen, bind the IgG-coated RBCs, ingest them, and destroy them extracellularly—hence the term *extravascular hemolysis*. These IgG antibodies also may fix some amount of complement, but not enough to lyse the RBCs. Instead, the phagocytic cells of the liver, the Kupffer cells, clear the complement-coated RBCs from the circulation and destroy them intracellularly. Although the rapid clearance of red cells can induce systemic inflammation and cytokine storm, the consequences of extravascular hemolysis are less severe than those of intravascular hemolysis. Extravascular hemolysis is recognizable by a drop in the hematocrit, an increase in the bilirubin level, and perhaps the clinical signs of fever or malaise.

Blood Group Systems

As discussed, the ABO system is the only system in which antibodies (anti-A and anti-B) are consistently and predictably present in the sera of people whose RBCs lack the corresponding antigen(s). The ABO system is the foundation of pretransfusion testing and compatibility.

Antibodies to the Rh (D) antigen are not present unless a person has been exposed to D-positive RBCs, through either transfusion or pregnancy. Because of the ease with which antibody D is made, grouping is done on all donors and recipients to ensure that D-negative recipients receive D-negative blood, except for reasonable qualifying circumstances. D-positive recipients may receive either D-positive or D-negative blood. People who develop Rh antibodies have detectable levels for many years. If undetected, subsequent exposure may lead to a secondary immune response. Occasionally, weak variants of the Rh (D) antigen are found, which are identified by special serologic tests. These people are termed weak D or Du positive, but they are considered Rh positive both as donors and recipients.

Other blood group systems have been defined on the basis of the cell's reactions to antigens. Antibodies to antigens in the Kell, Duffy, and Kidd systems are encountered frequently enough to be clinically important. Antibodies to the blood group antigens in most other systems are found so infrequently that they do not cause everyday problems. When present, these antibodies may produce hemolytic reactions. Once demonstrated, precautions must be taken to ensure that the patient receives compatible blood lacking the corresponding antigen. When difficulty arises in cross-matching or when a transfusion reaction occurs, these systems acquire special significance. Today, systems to identify, validate, and ensure ABO and Rh groupings are set up on computer databases. Confirmatory testing must be in place according to AABB guidelines.

PRETRANSFUSION TESTING, BLOOD DONATION, AND BLOOD PRESERVATION

The Donor

Consistent with American Red Cross (ARC) guidelines, a donor may donate whole blood or red cells no more than every 8 weeks. A double red cell donation may be made no sooner than 16 weeks (ARC, 2013). Platelets may be donated every 7 days but donation frequency cannot exceed a maximum of 24 times per year (ARC, 2013). A donation shall be no more than 10.5 mL/kg body weight. In addition to ABO and Rh group determination and a screen for unexpected antibodies, several other tests are performed on donors, including a physiologic health assessment, questionnaire, and blood sample. These tests must be negative for the antibodies identified (Box 17-1) before any blood or component is released for patient use.

The Recipient

Tests performed on the intended transfusion recipient include ABO and Rh group determination and screening for unexpected antibodies. Before the administration of whole blood or RBC components, a major cross-match (combining donor RBCs and recipient serum or plasma) is

---

BOX 17-1 DONOR AND RECIPIENT BLOOD TESTING REQUIREMENTS FOR TRANSFUSION THERAPY

Allogeneic Donor

ABO group
Rh type
Antibodies to HbsAg (hepatitis B surface antigen)
Antibodies to HBc (hepatitis B core antigen)
Antibodies to HCV (hepatitis C virus)
Antibodies to HIV-1 and -2
STS (serologic test for syphilis)
Antibodies to HTLV I/II (human T-cell lymphotropic virus)
Antibodies to CMV (cytomegalovirus) (performed on the cellular blood component donated for an immunocompromised patient)

Recipient

ABO group
Rh type
Unexpected antibodies to red cell antigens
Cross-match against donor red cells

Adapted from American Association of Blood Banks. (2010). *Primer of blood administration.* Bethesda, MD: Author.

---

performed to detect serologic incompatibility. The AABB requires that if a patient has been transfused in the preceding 3 months with blood or a blood component containing RBCs, has been pregnant within the preceding 3 months, or the history is uncertain or unavailable, the sample must be obtained from the patient within 3 days of the scheduled transfusion (AABB, 2010). This requirement is made to rule out the possibility of missing a newly formed antibody.

In situations in which delaying the provision of blood may jeopardize life, blood may be issued before completion of routine tests according to AABB standards (AABB, 2011). Recipients whose ABO group is not known must receive group O RBCs. Physicians/licensed independent practitioners (LIPs) must indicate in the record that the clinical condition is sufficiently urgent to release blood before the completion of compatibility testing. The tag or label must conspicuously indicate that compatibility testing is not completed, and standard compatibility tests should be completed as promptly as possible. Recipients whose ABO group has been determined by the transfusing facility without reliance on previous records may receive ABO group–specific whole blood or ABO group–compatible RBC components before other compatibility tests have been completed (Box 17-1).

Directed Donations

The risk of transfusion-transmitted diseases has generated programs whereby prospective patients may designate their own blood donors. Blood centers and hospitals have increased the availability of this program, known as **directed donation**, for the public. Each donor enters the same process as any other, but the blood is labeled for a specific recipient provided screening tests are appropriate and the unit is compatible. Units are specifically labeled for the intended recipient; however, the component may be used for allogeneic donation if not needed by the individual for whom the donation was intended.

The primary benefit of this program may be to reduce the fear of disease transmission in recipients who feel reassured knowing who their donors are. If the donor is a blood relative of the recipient, the cellular components must be irradiated to prevent graft versus host disease (GVHD) (AABB, 2010). These programs must address cost-effectiveness, staffing, quality assessment measures, and legal considerations.

Autologous Donation

Autologous transfusion is the collection, filtration, and reinfusion of a person's own blood; thus, the donor and recipient are the same individual. There are several types of autologous donation, all of which eliminate the risk of disease transmission as well as alloimmunization, although other mechanical and nonhemolytic reactions can occur. Autologous transfusion takes on several different meanings and methods and is accepted practice for appropriate candidates in a specific setting based on the patient's clinical condition.

Autologous transfusion is a conservative approach. In the 1980s and early 1990s, the acquired immunodeficiency syndrome (AIDS) epidemic and increased awareness of bloodborne disease transmission created interest and demand for autologous blood collection. This interest, however, decreased to only 1.5% of the total donations in 2008 (AABB, 2011) because of improved donor screening and public perception of a safe blood supply. As the possibility of new transfusion-transmitted diseases is identified or significant reductions in the blood supply occur, the demand for autologous donations may rise (AABB, 2011).

Although receiving one's own blood is the safest transfusion, careful administration of autologous blood is still required. To avoid any errors, those administering the blood must verify all aspects of the component, including proper identification. Verification procedures should be identical to those for giving homologous transfusions. All products of autologous donation must be labeled "For Autologous Use Only."

The AABB endorses all modalities of blood conservation, including the goals of autologous transfusions. Autologous transfusion can be accomplished by preoperative donation, acute normovolemic hemodilution, intraoperative salvage, and postoperative blood salvage.

PREOPERATIVE AUTOLOGOUS DONATION

This technique is best used when a patient is planning an elective surgical procedure that normally would cause the loss of a significant number of units of blood. The patient may plan periodic visits to a donor center for phlebotomies to store his or her own blood for later use. Consideration should be made for patients donating preoperatively to include receiving recombinant erythropoietin to rebuild red cell mass prior to surgery and decrease the likelihood of receiving perioperative transfusion.

ACUTE NORMOVOLEMIC HEMODILUTION

In this procedure, the patient's blood is collected, stored at room temperature for up to 8 hours in the operating room, and returned to the patient at the time of blood loss. Deterioration of platelets and coagulation factors is minimal in this time frame. To maintain plasma volume, the patient receives infusions of a crystalloid or colloid solution. The benefit of this technique is that it reduces the patient's hematocrit by dilution before surgical blood loss so that the patient loses a smaller number of red cells. Frequently used in cardiac surgery, hemodilution may be limited by the patient's blood volume or other hemodynamic considerations. Because the hematocrit is reduced, patients with lung disease or hypooxygenation require close monitoring.

INTRAOPERATIVE BLOOD COLLECTION

This frequently used method of autologous transfusion involves recovering blood during surgical procedures associated with significant blood loss from clean wounds. Blood is aspirated from the operative site, washed using cell-washing machines, and reinfused to the patient. The process may be performed completely in the operating room. It is most frequently used in cardiovascular, thoracic, orthopedic, neurologic, and hepatic surgery, including transplantations. The technique makes large volumes of blood immediately available when bleeding occurs in a clean operative procedure. The procedure is contraindicated in patients with malignancy or infection because reinfusion of contaminated cells may disseminate the tumor cells or infectious organism.

Sterile technique is mandated to prevent infectious agents from entering the system. Initial equipment and personnel costs can be high, but improved medical care outweighs the disadvantages. Institutions that provide intraoperative blood collection require policies, processes, and procedures that address day-to-day operations.

POSTOPERATIVE BLOOD COLLECTION

This technique involves salvaging blood shed from surgical drains after cardiac, trauma, orthopedic, and plastic surgery. Other clinical conditions also may be appropriate. The advantage of this technique is that it can be done for planned surgery or emergency operations and trauma. Postoperative shed blood is collected through special equipment for reinfusion. If the blood in the sterile canister is not reinfused within 6 hours, it must be discarded. This technique is safe, simple, and cost-effective. Combined with other methods of autologous transfusions described, the goal of avoiding homologous blood transfusions is nearer.

Blood Preservation

Blood is routinely collected in sterile plastic bags that contain different anticoagulant–preservative solutions. Whole blood may be collected in anticoagulant citrate–phosphate–dextrose solution (CPD), citrate–phosphate–dextrose–dextrose solution (CP2D), or anticoagulant citrate–phosphate–dextrose–adenine solution (CPDA-1). Since patients may suffer an adverse reaction to an anticoagulant–preservative, it is important to be knowledgeable of chemicals used in the solutions. Citrate is an anticoagulant that binds with free calcium in the donor's plasma. Since blood requires calcium to clot, the presence of citrate inhibits the coagulation cascade. Phosphate buffers the pH, preventing a decrease in 2,3-diphosphoglycerate (2,3-DPG), thus facilitating the oxygen-carrying capacity of the blood. Dextrose (glucose) prolongs the life of the RBCs by providing a nutrient source. Blood cells may be stored in CPD for 21 days at 1°C to 6°C. CPDA-1 contains adenine, which helps the RBCs synthesize adenosine triphosphate (ATP) during storage and lengthens the shelf life of the blood to 35 days. The RBC depends on ATP to maintain cell surface ion pumps.

The duration of time for storage is based on the standard that a minimum of 75% of the transfused RBCs (stored for 35 days) must be present in the bloodstream of the recipient 24 hours after the transfusion. Providing a nutrient biochemical balance to RBCs during storage is important to maintain viability and function of the components in the blood and to prevent physical changes. To minimize bacterial proliferation, specific temperatures are maintained.

A second group of anticoagulant–preservative systems labeled as additive solutions is similar to CPDA-1. They differ, however, in that once the platelet-rich plasma is removed from the unit within 8 hours, an additive solution of 100 mL containing saline, dextrose, and adenine is added to the packed RBCs. These additive systems permit storage for up to 42 days. FDA-approved solutions include AS-1 (Adsol), AS-3 (Nutricel), and AS-5 (Optisol).

WHOLE BLOOD

Whole blood contains RBCs, white blood cells, platelets, plasma (blood proteins, antibodies, water, and waste), and electrolytes. The usual volume is 450 to 550 mL/unit. Transfusions of whole blood are rare and indicated only in acute, massive blood loss for the purpose of expanding blood volume and increasing the oxygen-carrying capacity. If possible, blood loss should be managed with other blood components, crystalloids, or colloidal solutions.

Administration of whole blood subjects the patient to the possibility of complications such as fluid volume excess, especially in patients with a compromised cardiac status. In addition, after 24 hours of storage, cell breakdown can result in elevated potassium levels; the formation of microaggregates, nonviable platelets, and granulocytes; and decreased levels of the clotting factors, factor V and factor VIII. In patients with a severely damaged liver, massive whole-blood transfusions can result in a calcium deficit owing to the presence of citrate anticoagulant. Monitoring the patient's potassium level before and after the transfusion is important. Hemoglobin and hematocrit levels may be inaccurate owing to fluid shifts during active bleeding. Whole blood transfusion must be ABO *identical* with that of the recipient because of the presence of antibodies. One unit of whole blood increases hemoglobin by about 1 g/dL and hematocrit by about 3 to 4 percentage points (American Association of Blood Banks, American Red Cross, America's Blood Centers, & the Armed Services Blood Program [AABB, ARC, ABC & ASBP], 2009).

Whole blood is stored at a temperature of 1°C (34°F) to 6°C (43°F) within 8 hours after collection. Expiration depends on the anticoagulant–preservative. The rate of administration for whole blood should be as rapid as necessary to correct and maintain the hemodynamic status. In massive hemorrhage, one or more large-gauge catheters, such as 14 or 16 gauge, allow a free-flow infusion of blood, although whole blood can be administered through either an 18- or a 20-gauge catheter. Electronic infusion devices do not deliver high enough rates to meet the needs of a clinical crisis. In this instance, pressure cuffs applied to the bag of blood may be required for rapid infusion. Further information is in the section on Blood Administration.

Irradiated Whole Blood and Blood Components

Irradiated whole blood and blood components have been exposed to a measured amount of radiation in order to prevent lymphocytes from replication. Irradiated blood components are used to prevent GVHD in patients with Hodgkin's or non-Hodgkin's lymphoma also known as Hodgkin's or non-Hodgkin's lymphoma, acute leukemia, and congenital immunodeficiency disorders, patients with malignant tumors who are being treated with immunosuppressive therapy such as chemotherapy or radiation, low birth weight neonates, and patients treated with intrauterine infusions (AABB, 2010). Irradiated units pose no risk to a transfusionist or the recipient. Because irradiation may damage and reduce the viability of RBCs, the original expiration date of the component prevails.

RED BLOOD CELLS

Packed Red Blood Cells

Packed RBCs are prepared by removing platelet-rich plasma from a unit of whole blood, by either centrifugation or apheresis. These processes pack the RBCs and separate most of the platelet-rich plasma (Figure 17-1). The RBC concentrate contains the same RBC mass as whole blood, 20 to 100 mL of the original plasma, and some leukocytes and platelets. Depending on the anticoagulant–preservative used, RBCs usually have a hematocrit of between 55% and 65%; thus, the viscosity of the unit is decreased compared to RBCs without anticoagulant–preservative solutions or additives. Each unit of RBCs contains about 50 to 80 g of hemoglobin or 160 to 275 mL of pure red cells. A unit designated as a low-volume collection will contain at least 50 g of hemoglobin. One unit of packed RBCs provides the same amount of oxygen-carrying RBCs as a unit of whole blood but at a reduced volume.

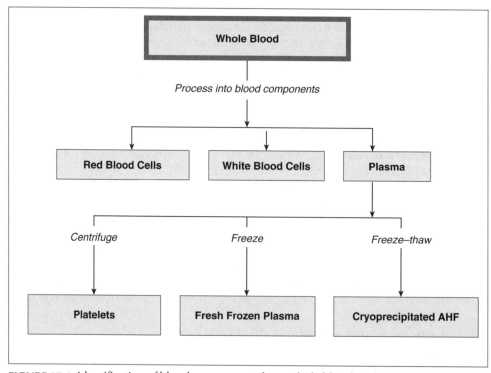

FIGURE 17-1 Identification of blood components from whole blood. (Adapted from American Association of Blood Banks. (2010). *Primer of blood administration*. Bethesda, MD: Author.)

Each unit of packed RBCs is expected to raise the hematocrit by 3 percentage points and the hemoglobin level 1 g/dL in the average 70-kg person.

The major indication for packed RBCs is to restore or maintain the oxygen-carrying capacity, as in cases of acute or chronic blood loss, symptomatic anemia, trauma, and chemotherapy when nutrition, drug therapy, and treatment of the underlying disease cannot achieve an improved RBC count (ARC, 2012). Criteria for transfusion are based on the patient's symptoms, time frame, amount of blood loss, and levels of hemoglobin and hematocrit. Patients with chronic anemia usually adjust to a lower hemoglobin level and are transfused only when symptomatic and/or alternative treatments, such as medication or supplements, are ineffective. RBCs should not be given to treat anemia that responds to iron or recombinant erythropoietin.

Because of the reduced volume of a unit of RBCs, the danger of circulatory overload is decreased with advantages for the patient with renal failure or heart failure and for the elderly or debilitated patients (AABB, 2011). Because RBCs have reduced amounts of plasma, less citrate is infused and there are fewer by-products of cell breakdown such as potassium and ammonia.

The expiration time of packed RBCs is 21 to 42 days, depending on the anticoagulant–preservative or additive solution used. RBCs may be frozen for extended storage (AABB et al., 2009). Typing and cross-matching is still required. Group O may be given to other blood groups. In emergencies, when time does not permit ABO determination, group O RBCs may be given (Table 17-2).

Red Blood Cells, Leukocytes Reduced

RBCs, leukocytes reduced, are used in patients with symptomatic anemia who have previously experienced febrile reactions from leukocyte antibodies and cytokines released during storage (AABB, 2010). This component prevents recurrent febrile, nonhemolytic transfusion reactions and reduces the incidence of HLA alloimmunization and the risk of transfusion-transmissible cytomegalovirus (CMV) (AABB et al., 2009). Leukocyte-reduced RBCs are not to be used to prevent GVHD.

A unit of leukocyte-reduced RBCs contains $< 5 \times 10^6$ white blood cells as compared with a unit of whole blood, which contains ≥ 1 to 10×10^9 cells. Leukocyte reduction may be accomplished either at the bedside or during processing. At the bedside, leukocyte reduction is done by filtering blood with a special filter that can remove as much as 99.9% of the white blood cells. An acute hypotensive reaction may occur in patients during this procedure and taking angiotensin-converting enzyme (ACE) inhibitors (AABB, 2010). Currently, leukocyte reduction is more commonly completed prior to storage in efforts to decrease transfusion-related infections or adverse reactions. At least 85% of the original red cells remain present in leukocyte-reduced RBCs. Washing the RBCs will also remove the leukocytes but may reduce the number of RBCs by 20% and is an expensive and time-consuming process. Washed RBCs must be refrigerated and used within 24 hours. The ABO compatibility is the same as for packed RBCs.

Red Blood Cells, Rejuvenated, and the Use of Anticoagulants

RBCs prepared from whole blood and collected with appropriate anticoagulants can be rejuvenated at any time during storage for up to 3 days after expiration. The FDA-approved rejuvenating solution consists of inosine, phosphate, and adenine, which restores 2,3-DPG and ATP to normal levels. However, they must be washed before infusion to remove the inosine, which may be toxic. If not administered within 24 hours, these RBCs must be glycerolized and frozen (AABB et al., 2009). The ABO compatibility is the same as for packed RBCs.

Red Blood Cells, Deglycerolized

Deglycerolized RBCs are prepared for freezing by removing plasma and adding glycerol, which enters the cell and protects it from cell dehydration and ice formation in its frozen state. The purpose of this process is to preserve rare units of blood or autologous donor units. They may be frozen for up to 10 years. At the time the unit is needed, it is thawed and the glycerol is removed by washing the cells with successively lower concentrations of sodium chloride until the final suspension is 0.9% sodium chloride injection (USP). Deglycerolized RBCs carry the risk of hemolysis if the deglycerolization process is inadequate (AABB, 2011). After thawing, the component should be administered within 24 hours of the washing process in an open system and 14 days in a closed system. The finished product has virtually all the leukocytes, plasma, and platelets removed. It contains minimal original donor platelets and leukocytes and has a hematocrit of approximately 80%.

TABLE 17-2 ABO COMPATIBILITIES FOR RED BLOOD CELL COMPONENTS, FRESH FROZEN PLASMA, AND WHOLE BLOOD

Donor: Red Blood Cell Components

Universal donor is O− and Universal recipient is AB+

Recipient	First Choice	Second Choice	Third Choice
O+	O+	O−	—
A+	A+	O+, A−	O−
B+	B+	O+, B−	O−
AB+	AB+	AB−, A+, B+	O+, A−, B−, O−
O−	O−	—	—
A−	A−	O−	—
B−	B−	O−	—
AB−	AB−	A−, B−, O−	—
Recipient	**Donor: Fresh Frozen Plasma**		
O	O, A, B, or AB	—	—
A	A or AB	—	—
B	B or AB	—	—
AB	AB	—	—
Recipient	**Donor: Whole Blood** (must be ABO identical)		
O	O	—	—
A	A	—	—
B	B	—	—
AB	AB	—	—

Adapted from American Association of Blood Banks. (2010). *Primer of blood administration.* Bethesda, MD: Author.

This component is not used as a routine red cell replacement but is useful to preserve blood from donors with rare blood groups. It is also useful to patients who are sensitized to IgA or other plasma proteins because the cellular components have been removed. The major disadvantage is the substantial additional cost related to the process of preparing and storing the component. The ABO compatibility is the same as for packed RBCs.

PLATELETS

Platelets are indicated for the control or prevention of bleeding in the presence of thrombocytopenia or abnormal platelet function. There are two preparations for platelets: random donor concentrates made from pooled units of platelets from several donors and concentrates obtained by platelet apheresis of a single donor. Units may be combined into a single bag before release from the blood bank. Platelets should not be infused through the same tubing as RBCs since some platelets are not ABO specific and may cause coagulation in the tubing. Platelets contain **factor III** (tissue thromboplastin), a phospholipid that enhances the conversion of prothrombin to thrombin, which forms one of the most important steps in the coagulation process. Table 17-3 describes coagulation factors.

Platelets, Pooled

Clinical conditions that adversely affect platelet function include sepsis, diseases of the liver and kidney, some bone marrow disorders, and congenital and acquired platelet disorders (AABB et al., 2009). Platelet transfusions are indicated for thrombocytopenia caused by

TABLE 17-3 COAGULATION FACTORS	
Name	Function
Fibrinogen (factor I)	Adhesive protein forming the fibrin clot
Prothrombin (factor II)	Main enzyme of coagulation is the activated form
Tissue factor (factor III)	Lipoprotein initiator—extrinsic pathway
Calcium ions (factor IV)	Cations needed for coagulation reactions
Factor V (Labile)	Activates prothrombin > thrombin
Factor VII (proconvertin)	Initiates extrinsic pathway with factor III
Factor VIII (antihemophilic)	Cofactor for intrinsic activation of factor X
Factor IX (Christmas)	Enzyme for intrinsic activation of factor X
Factor X (Stuart-Prower)	Enzyme for final common pathway activation of prothrombin
Factor XI (plasma thromboplastin)	Intrinsic activator of factor IX
Factor XII (Hageman)	Normally starts the aPTT-based intrinsic pathway
Factor XIII (fibrin stabilizing)	Transamidase to cross-link fibrin clot
High molecular weight kininogen (Fitzgerald, Flaujeac, or William)	Cofactor
Prekallikrein (Fletcher)	Participates at inception of the aPTT-based intrinsic pathway

Adapted from Lefkowitz, J. B. (2008). Coagulation pathway and physiology. In *Hemostasis physiology*. Northfield, IL: College of American Pathologists. www.cap.org/apps/docs/cap_press/hemostasis_testing/coagulation_pathway.pdf

hemorrhage with platelet counts of <50,000/μL, surgery with a platelet count of <50,000/μL, antineoplastic therapy with platelet counts of ≤10,000/μL, and in patients without bleeding whose counts are <15,000 to 20,000/μL and are rapidly decreasing. Major invasive procedures require platelet counts of at least 50,000/μL.

The decision to transfuse platelets must be based on the clinical condition of the patient, the cause of the thrombocytopenia, and the ability of the patient to produce platelets. Patients who are stable and are thrombocytopenic may tolerate platelet counts of <5,000/μL with minor (but not serious) bleeding. Platelets are not routinely indicated for patients with conditions in which rapid platelet destruction occurs such as in idiopathic thrombocytopenic purpura (ITP) or untreated disseminated intravascular coagulation (DIC), except in the presence of life-threatening bleeding (AABB et al., 2009). For patients with thrombotic thrombocytopenic purpura (TTP) and heparin-induced thrombocytopenia with thrombosis, transfusion with platelets should be avoided due to the risk of fatal thrombosis, except in the setting of life-threatening hemorrhage.

Platelet concentrate prepared from whole blood contains a minimum of 5.5×10^{10} platelets in 40 to 70 mL of plasma (AABB et al., 2009). Each unit is expected to increase the platelet count of a 70-kg adult by 5,000 to 10,000/μL. The usual dose in an adult is 4 to 6 units and may be repeated in 1 to 3 days owing to the short life span of 3 to 4 days. Routinely, random donor platelets are pooled and transfused, and patients are the recipients of multiple allogeneic donors (AABB, 2010).

Since ABO antigen is present on the platelet membrane, it is ideal to give ABO identical platelets. However, if a matching unit is not available and prompt transfusion is required, patients may receive any ABO group (AABB, 2011). Platelet concentrates do not require cross-matching before infusion; however, documentation of the patient's ABO and Rh status is necessary to make appropriate selection decisions. D-negative patients should receive compatible platelets, however, if available. Platelets may be infused as fast as the patient tolerates but must be infused within 4 hours after release from the blood bank (AABB, 2010). Platelets may be stored at 20°C to 24°C for 5 days with gentle agitation. Platelets are never put into a refrigerator or cooler.

Platelets, Single Donor

Because of immune or nonimmune mechanisms, as many as 70% of patients who receive repeated platelet transfusions will become refractory to platelet transfusions and will not have an adequate sustained rise in their platelet counts after transfusion. This is due to the destruction of platelets by HLA antibodies soon after the transfusion is completed (AABB, 2010). Causes of refractoriness to platelets also include DIC, drug therapies, ITP, and sepsis (AABB, 2010). These patients are more likely to benefit by receiving HLA-compatible blood transfusions or receiving platelets that lack the antigens to which the recipient's antibodies will not react.

EVIDENCE FOR PRACTICE

Studies related to pulmonary complications have been published in the literature. How may algorithms facilitate detection of transfusion-related complications and what is the role of the infusion clinician?

Single-donor platelets are collected by platelet pheresis from a single donor who is HLA compatible with the recipient. Family is often a more suitable match; however, a nonrelated donor may be found. Pheresis platelets contain approximately $\geq 3 \times 10^{11}$ per bag in about 250 mL of plasma. The platelet infusion volume may be between 100 and 500 mL supplied in a large plastic pack or in two connected packs to improve platelet viability by providing more surface area for gas exchange. The exact number of platelets in the unit can be obtained from the blood bank. Reactions to platelets may include disease transmission, GVHD, alloimmunization, febrile or allergic effects, and circulatory overload.

Platelets, Leukocytes Reduced

Leukocyte-reduced platelets are used to prevent recurrent febrile, nonhemolytic transfusion reactions that are caused when the donor white cell antigens and/or cytokines released during storage react to the recipient white cell antibodies (AABB, 2010). Leukocyte removal may be accomplished by filtration resulting in the removal of 99.9% of the leukocytes at the bedside. The manufacturer's guidelines for priming the filter must be adhered to for effective administration. Leukocyte reduction RBC filters and leukocyte reduction platelet filters are not interchangeable (AABB, 2010). Again, acute hypotension may occur when leukocyte reduction is completed at the bedside, particularly in patients taking ACE inhibitor medication. Leukocyte-reduced platelets are also used to decrease the incidence of HLA alloimmunization in patients who may require long-term platelet replacement or transplantation in the future.

GRANULOCYTES

Granulocytes, administered infrequently, are most often collected from donors stimulated by corticosteroids (AABB, 2011). Single-donor units are generally reserved for neonates due to the small number of granulocytes per unit. Previously prescribed for gram-negative sepsis, the emergence of new antibiotic regimens, new recombinant growth factors, and improved management of infections have greatly decreased the use of this component. Granulocytes are used in neutropenic patients with absolute neutrophil counts $<500/\mu L$. Granulocytes migrate toward, phagocytize, and kill fungi and bacteria. Patients receive granulocytes when they have infections not responsive to antibiotics and have a reasonable chance of recovery of bone marrow function or for neonatal sepsis. Cultures to identify the offending organism should be done. Granulocyte transfusion is not effective in localized infections or infections caused by agents other than bacteria. These transfusions only temporarily improve the patient's condition. There is a renewed interest in granulocyte transfusions owing to improved cell doses that can be obtained from donors using sedimenting agents and granulocyte colony–stimulating factors (AABB, 2011).

A unit of granulocytes contains variable amounts of lymphocytes, platelets, and RBCs suspended in 200 to 300 mL of anticoagulant and plasma. The number of granulocytes in each concentrate is usually $>1 \times 10^{10}$. The granulocyte donor must be ABO and Rh compatible because a unit of granulocytes contains a significant amount of donor RBCs (AABB et al., 2009).

Hydroxyethyl starch (HES) may be used as a red cell–sedimenting agent and will be present in the final component (AABB et al., 2009). Granulocytes are administered through a standard blood filter over 2 to 4 hours for both adult and pediatric patients. Depth-type microaggregate filters and leukocyte reduction filters should not be used.

Patients undergoing granulocyte transfusions are acutely ill, and adverse effects are common. Fever, chills, allergic reactions, alloimmunization, and pulmonary reactions may occur and can be managed with diphenhydramine, nonaspirin antipyretics, steroids, and slow administration of the unit. The transfusion should not be stopped unless severe life-threatening symptoms occur. If the recipient is seronegative and severely immunosuppressed, donor CMV-seropositive granulocytes should not be given. Granulocytes are generally irradiated to prevent GVHD (AABB et al., 2009).

Granulocytes are stored at 20°C to 24°C (68°F to 75°F) for no more than 24 hours without agitation (AABB et al., 2009). Granulocytes should be administered as soon after collection as possible because of the deterioration of granulocyte function during short-term storage. Granulocytes are never put into a refrigerator or cooler.

PLASMA

Plasma is the liquid content remaining after the RBCs have been removed from a unit of whole blood. It contains water, electrolytes, proteins (principally albumin), globulin, and coagulation factors. Plasma plays an important role in the treatment of trauma, the reversal of anticoagulation therapy in patients with moderate to severe bleeding without coagulopathy or in coagulated patients needing to undergo an invasive procedure.

Liquid Plasma

Although rarely used in the United States, liquid plasma is indicated for acute bleeding. Primarily, patients require plasma therapy to reverse the anticoagulation effects of warfarin (Benjamin & McLaughlin, 2012). However, this component has reduced amounts of factor VIII, which limits its use in some patients (AABB et al., 2009). Single-donor liquid plasma is stored at 1°C to 6°C for no more than 5 days after the expiration of whole blood (AABB, 2011). Thawed plasma expires 5 days from date of thaw if collected and stored in a closed system. Some of the clotting factor activity may be lost during storage. Under ordinary circumstances, single-donor plasma should be compatible with the recipient's RBCs. Because it lacks anti-A and anti-B agglutinins, AB plasma may be used for all ABO groups and in emergencies when the patient's blood group is unknown.

Fresh Frozen Plasma

Fresh frozen plasma (FFP) is used to replace coagulation factors in patients with coagulation disorders or deficiencies secondary to DIC, liver disease, or dilutional coagulopathy resulting from volume replacement or volume overload. It is also used to reverse warfarin sodium overdose, in patients who are to undergo an invasive procedure when there is not adequate time to administer vitamin K, or to stop the drug. Patients with antithrombin III deficiency, TTP, C1 esterase deficiency, protein S deficiency, and those with deficiencies for which there are no concentrates available may also receive FFP. It is beneficial to patients with demonstrated multiple coagulation deficiencies, inherited or acquired bleeding disorders, and, on occasion, to treat active bleeding owing to vitamin K deficiency.

FFP contains albumin, globulins, antibodies, and clotting factors in addition to around 200 to 250 mg fibrinogen. It has a shelf life of 1 year when stored at a temperature of −18°C or 7 years at −65°C when frozen within 8 hours of collection and stored in CPD, CP2D, or

CPDA-1. Plasma stored in acid-citrate-dextrose solution (ACD), must be frozen within 6 hours at − 18°C or colder (AABB, 2011). The volume is dependent on the method of collection used but can contain usually 500 to 800 mL when single-donor automated plasmapheresis. Kept frozen until the time of transfusion, FFP is then thawed in a water bath at 30°C to 37°C (98.6°F) and gently agitated. FFP should be administered within 4 to 6 hours, but no more than 24 hours after thawing to minimize the loss of the most labile clotting factors, factor V and factor VIII. To provide factors V and VIII, the component should be used within the 1st year of storage for treatment of coagulation disorders.

FFP is an isotonic volume expander, and patients receiving multiple units should be monitored closely to prevent fluid overload. FFP should never be used for volume expansion or as a nutrient supplement; these situations are more safely treated with crystalloid or colloid solutions that lack the risk of transmitting disease and are less expensive than FFP. Other safe volume expanders are albumin and plasma substitutes, which do not carry the risk of viral disease transmission.

FFP may be administered slowly in the first 5 minutes and then, if no reaction noted, as rapidly as tolerated through a standard blood filter (AABB, 2011). The unit must be ABO compatible, but Rh matching is not required. If the recipient's blood type is unknown, group AB can be safely given (Table 17-2). Although a cross-match is not required, the component should be compatible with the recipient's RBCs. Generally, 5 to 20 mL/kg are needed to bring coagulation factor levels up to sufficient concentrations to achieve hemostasis and to bring fibrinogen levels and activated partial thromboplastin time levels within the normal hemostatic range (generally ≤1.5 times the midrange of the normal value).

Solvent–Detergent-Treated Plasma

Somewhat controversial, solvent–detergent-treated plasma has been approved again in 2013 by the FDA for congenital or acquired TTP. Referred to as PLAS + SD (pooled plasma, solvent–detergent treated) or SDP, this plasma component is prepared from ABO blood group–specific donor-pooled plasma. The solvent–detergent process inactivates the viruses by stripping away their lipid coating (AABB, 2011). It is the only human blood plasma product treated to inactivate human immunodeficiency virus (HIV), hepatitis C virus (HCV), and hepatitis B virus (HBV). It is thought that the process used to treat the plasma adds another layer of protection for the public from disease transmission.

Two main disadvantages of SDP are cost and a potential greater risk of nonenveloped virus transmission such as hepatitis A virus (HAV) and parvovirus because of pooling of plasmas. All coagulation factors are also reduced by at least 10%.

An alternative to SDP is nonpooled FFP, donor retested. This method requires the donor to be retested after a minimum of 90 days after collection. Used extensively in Europe, advantages and disadvantages are still being evaluated in the United States because, to date, the risk/benefit and cost/benefit ratios are not favorable compared with a single unit of FFP. Table 17-4 contains a summary of the blood and blood components described.

Plasma Derivatives and Plasma Substitutes

Normal Serum Albumin and Plasma Protein Fraction

Albumin and plasma proteins are referred to as *protein colloids* and are the most abundant solutes in plasma; albumin is the most abundant, making up 54% of the plasma proteins (Gaspard, 2009a). These protein colloids are collected from blood, serum, and human

TABLE 17-4	BLOOD COMPONENTS AND WHOLE BLOOD: ACTION AND USE, VOLUME AND INFUSION GUIDE, AND SPECIAL CONSIDERATIONS AND RISKS		
Blood Component	**Action and Use**	**Volume and Infusion Guide**	**Special Considerations and Risks**
RBCs	• Increases the oxygen-carrying capacity • For symptomatic anemia, aplastic anemia, or bone marrow failure caused by malignancy or antineoplastic therapy • Expected to increase the hematocrit 3% and the hemoglobin level 1 g/dL in the average 70-kg person	225–350 mL As tolerated but no longer than 4 h from the time of release from blood bank	Hemolytic, allergic, and febrile reactions GVHD Infectious disease transmission TACO TRALI
RBCs, leukocyte reduced	• To prevent recurrent febrile, nonhemolytic transfusion reactions • Reduces the incidence of HLA alloimmunization and the risk of transfusion-transmissible CMV	250–300 mL	Infectious disease transmission
RBCs, deglycerolized	• To preserve rare units of blood or autologous donor units • Used in patients sensitized to IgA/plasma proteins causing anaphylaxis • Expected to increase the hematocrit 3% and the hemoglobin level 1 g/dL in the average 70-kg person	200–250 mL	Hemolytic, allergic, and febrile reactions GVHD Infectious disease transmission TACO TRALI Substantial cost related to preparation
Platelets, pooled	• Thrombocytopenia or platelet function abnormality • Improves hemostasis • Increases platelet count by 5,000/mL per each unit (30,000–60,000/mL for a 6-unit pool)	50–70 mL/unit Usual dose 4–6 units; units must be infused within 4 h after release from laboratory/blood bank	Infectious disease transmission GVHD Allergic/febrile reactions TRALI TACO May need to be repeated every 1–3 d
Platelets, single donor	• To prevent platelet destruction • Platelets are from a single donor who is HLA compatible • Increase platelet count as above	100–500 mL Unit must be infused within 4 h after release from laboratory/blood bank	GVHD Febrile/allergic reactions

TABLE 17- **BLOOD COMPONENTS AND WHOLE BLOOD: ACTION AND USE, VOLUME AND INFUSION GUIDE, AND SPECIAL CONSIDERATIONS AND RISKS** *(Continued)*

Blood Component	Action and Use	Volume and Infusion Guide	Special Considerations and Risks
Platelets, leukocyte reduced	• To prevent recurrent febrile, nonhemolytic transfusion reactions • Reduces the incidence of HLA alloimmunization and the risk of transfusion-transmissible CMV • Increase platelet count as above	30–50 mL/unit Usual dose 6–8 units; units must be infused within 4 h after release from laboratory/blood bank	Infectious disease transmission GVHD Allergic/febrile reactions TACO TRALI May need to be repeated every 1–3 d
Granulocytes or irradiated granulocytes	• Rarely used • Neutropenia with infection; unresponsive to antibiotic	200–300 mL Administer slowly over 2–4 h	Hemolytic, allergic, and febrile reactions common; requires premedication to control reactions GVHD TACO TRALI
Fresh frozen plasma	• Replace coagulation factors in patients with DIC, liver disease, factor V or XI deficiencies, reversal of warfarin	200–250 mL Unit must be infused within 4 h after release from laboratory/blood bank	Infectious disease transmission Allergic reactions Does not provide platelets
Cryoprecipitated AHF	• von Willebrand disease • Hemophilia A • Factor XIII deficiency • Fibrinogen deficiency	Pooled units contain several units of about 15 mL Must be infused within 4 h after release from laboratory/blood bank	Infectious disease transmission Allergic reactions
Whole blood	• Rarely used • Indicated for volume expansion in massive acute blood loss • Increases oxygen-carrying capacity • Increases Hgb 1 g/dL and Hct 3%–4%	450–500 mL As fast as tolerated through large-gauge catheter but <4 h	Fluid volume overload Hyperkalemia Decreased clotting factors Hemolytic, allergic, and febrile reactions GVHD TACO TRALI
Whole blood, irradiated	• As above and also used to prevent GVHD in patients with Hodgkin, non-Hodgkin lymphoma, and acute leukemia and in patients receiving immunosuppressive therapy		Infectious disease transmission All risks as above except no risk for GVHD

Adapted from American Association of Blood Banks. (2010). *Primer of blood administration.* Bethesda, MD: Author.

placentas and are heated at 60°C (140°F) for 10 hours to inactivate viruses including HIV, HBV, and HCV. Albumin is available in two concentrations, 5% in 250 or 500 mL saline and 25% in 50 mL saline. It may replace plasma in some clinical conditions (McLeod, 2012).

Albumin 5% is isotonic; it is osmotically equivalent to an approximately equal volume of citrated plasma and may be used to provide volume and colloid in the treatment of shock and burns. Initially, after a burn, large volumes of crystalloid solution are needed to correct extracellular fluid losses because of fluid leakage into the intracellular compartment. Smaller amounts of colloid are required at this time. After 24 hours, increased amounts of albumin may be used to maintain intravascular volume and avoid hypoproteinemia while smaller amounts of crystalloid are then infused.

Albumin 25% is hypertonic and depends on additional fluids, either drawn from the tissues or administered separately, for its maximal osmotic effect; 50 mL of 25% albumin is osmotically equivalent to 250 mL of citrated plasma. Albumin 25% must be administered with caution because a rapid infusion may cause an increase in intravascular oncotic pressure. This may result in circulatory overload and pulmonary edema or in the development of interstitial dehydration unless adequate amounts of supplemental fluids are administered. Other uses for specific patient conditions include therapeutic apheresis, large-volume paracentesis, diuresis, and subarachnoid hemorrhage. Albumin 25% is not appropriate for hypovolemia unless there is an associated condition such as hypoalbuminemia, malnutrition, chronic nephrosis or hepatic failure, or peripheral edema. The rate of administration for albumin varies depending on the indication of administration, the patient's blood volume, and the patient response (McLeod, 2012).

Administration of 5% and 25% albumin requires strict aseptic handling (Table 17-5). Once the container is punctured or opened, it must be used within 4 hours or discarded because albumin has no preservatives. Drugs should not be added to albumin, nor should albumin be added to IV solutions. Albumin is a good culture medium, and bacterial contamination is rare. If a reaction is suspected, the product should be held, the lot number recorded, and the manufacturer and the FDA notified. More frequently, adverse reactions are caused by improper administration. Both products have been heat treated to eliminate transfusion-transmitted diseases (McLeod, 2012).

Plasma protein fraction (human) 5% is an isotonic solution of protein consisting of 88% albumin and 12% alpha and beta globulins. Similar to albumin, it is used for emergency treatment of shock or other conditions in which there is a circulatory volume deficit. Plasma protein fraction is given IV without dilution and is available as a 5% solution; each 100 mL contains 5 g of selected plasma proteins. Again, the dose and rate of administration are dependent on the patient's condition but should not exceed 10 mL/min because too rapid administration may cause hypotension. For treatment of shock, the minimum effective dose is usually 250 to 500 mL, depending on the patient's condition and response.

Neither albumin nor plasma protein fraction has any clotting factors, nor should they be considered plasma substitutes. There is no ABO or Rh matching for albumin or plasma protein fraction.

PLASMA SUBSTITUTES

Several types of infusions are available to expand vascular volume, including crystalloids such as isotonic saline or plasma expanders such as dextran and colloidal solutions. Dextran 40, dextran 70, and hetastarch (HES) are nonprotein colloids that do not require blood typing and remain in circulation longer than the crystalloids.

TABLE 17-   ADMINISTRATION OF ALBUMIN

1. Maintain hand hygiene. Assemble equipment: albumin 5% or 25%; vented administration set; blunt cannula, if connecting to primary IV; alcohol prep pad; equipment for performing IV access if the patient does not have an IV line.
2. Verify written order for correct product (concentration) and prescribed rate of administration.
3. Verify signed transfusion consent form. Check your institution's policies; some health care facilities do not require consent for albumin.
4. Make positive patient identification per institution policy.
5. Close clamp on the albumin set.
6. Remove closure disk from the albumin bottle and prepare entry port with an alcohol pad.
7. Squeeze the drip chamber of the albumin set and insert spike of the set into the center of the stopper of the albumin bottle.
8. Suspend the albumin bottle from the IV pole, release the drip chamber, and flush all air from line. Close clamp.
9. Attach an appropriate blunt cannula to the albumin set.
10. Do not administer through any IV line containing any medications.
11. Scrub the injection site of the primary IV with alcohol prep pad and insert the blunt cannula into the injection site. Secure catheter tightly.
12. Regulate albumin to the prescribed administration rate using an electronic infusion device.
13. Document vital signs before the start, during, and after the transfusion. Record date, time, and signature of transfusion on blood requisition that accompanies the blood component. Place in appropriate part of the patient's record. Document the patient's response and record the volume of infusion.

NOTE: Procedure can be converted for institutions using multilead blood administration sets. This procedure also may be modified for the administration of plasma and single-donor platelets.

CRYOPRECIPITATED AHF

Cryoprecipitated AHF (antihemophilic factor) is a plasma precipitate containing fibrinogen, factor VIII:C, factor VIII:vWF (von Willebrand factor), factor XIII, and fibronectin (AABB, 2011). Cryoprecipitated antihemophilic factor (AHF) is indicated for treatment of fibrinogen and factor XIII deficiency. It is used for the treatment of von Willebrand disease and hemophilia A (factor VIII:C deficiency) only if virus-inactivated factor VIII concentrates are not available.

Cryoprecipitated AHF is prepared by thawing FFP between 1°C and 6°C, gathering the precipitate, and refreezing within 1 hour (AABB et al., 2009). Pooled units contain several units of cryoprecipitated AHF. This component should be kept at room temperature and transfused as soon as possible within 6 hours or 4 hours if units have been pooled. Each unit of cryoprecipitate should contain at least 80 international units of factor VIII:C and 150 mg of fibrinogen in about 5 to 20 mL of plasma (AABB et al., 2009). ABO compatibility is preferred. For treatment of hemophilia A, a rapid loading dose may be required to produce the desired level of factor VIII:C followed by a maintenance dose every 8 to 12 hours. For fibrinogen deficiency, close monitoring of fibrinogen assays helps identify the need for continued therapy (AABB et al., 2009).

The patient must be closely monitored during and after the transfusion to assess and identify signs and symptoms of potential reactions. Most immediate adverse effects are preventable and caused by improper administration, failure to comply with standards, or lack of knowledge of the procedure or impact of the therapy. Thoroughly following written procedures and complying with policy are crucial for safe transfusion therapy.

Antihemophilic Factor (Human)

AHF is a sterile, purified, dried concentrate prepared from the cold-insoluble fraction of pooled FFP by a variety of methods, including fractionation by physiochemical techniques to provide factor VIII concentrates, and extraction and purification from plasma using monoclonal antibodies to factor VIII. These newer techniques offer a higher activity of AHF and are less likely to transmit disease. The levels of AHF vary depending on the technique used to make the component. Various processes used to inactivate viruses have yielded a safer product and greatly decreased the incidence of viral infection after transfusion. The discovery of the molecular structure of factor VIII has led to the creation of genetically engineered products that are produced using recombinant DNA technology. There are several concentrates of recombinant factor VIII available in the United States.

The clinical use of AHF concentrate is the treatment of hemophilia A, a hereditary bleeding disorder characterized by deficient coagulant activity. Infusions offer a temporary replacement of the deficient clotting factor to prevent bleeding episodes or provide coagulant activity when emergency or elective surgery is performed on hemophiliac patients.

Plasma-based AHF is obtained from a fresh human plasma cryoprecipitate and has been tested to be free from hepatitis virus and HIV. Recombinant AHF is genetically engineered and is purified, removing the risk of viral transmission as it is not derived from human blood. These are supplied as a powder, and preparations are labeled in international units per bottle. The concentrate is provided with a sterile diluent and a filter. Users should adhere to sterile technique and guidelines supplied by the manufacturer. Plastic syringes should be used to prevent binding to glass surfaces. No ABO or Rh matching is required. The dosage to be administered is calculated based on knowing that one international unit of factor VIII per kilogram of patient weight will raise the level of factor VIII in the blood by about 2%. The site and severity of hemorrhage are also considered in dosing (Gahart & Nazareno, 2012).

Factor IX Concentrate

The clinical indication for factor IX concentrate is the prevention and control of bleeding in patients with hemophilia B, also known as Christmas disease. This disorder resembles hemophilia A. The cause of the deficiency of factor IX is an abnormal gene that leads to defective synthesis of factor IX or an acquired factor IX deficiency. To achieve therapeutic levels of factor IX, large volumes of FFP would be required. Factor IX concentrates are the only treatment available for patients with this deficiency. The product, in conjunction with activated factor VIII, results in the conversion of prothrombin to thrombin. Thrombin then converts fibrinogen to fibrin, with clot formation as the end result.

Several preparations of factor IX concentrate are available. One product is available in the United States; it is produced by recombinant DNA technology and is free from the risk of transmission of human blood-borne pathogens such as HIV, hepatitis viruses, and parvovirus. The product is not derived from human blood and contains no preservatives or human components. Other preparations are made from fresh human plasma and are irradiated and dried by specific processes to reduce risks of transmission of viral infection (Gahart & Nazareno, 2012).

Preparation cautions vary from one product to another. It is important for users to adhere to sterile preparation and administration guidelines supplied by the manufacturer.

Plastic syringes should be used to prevent binding to glass surfaces. The number of units of factor IX is printed on each vial. The rate of administration is determined by the patient's condition, and the concentrate may be infused by either an IV push method or an infusion that should not exceed 10 mL/min.

Intravenous Immune Globulin

Intravenous immune globulin (IVIG) is a highly purified solution of human IgG for IV use. It is prepared by a manufacturing process that eliminates contaminants such as bacteria and viruses. Many different preparations are available from different manufacturers and are ordered for specific patient populations. One brand should not be substituted for another. The properties and side effects of IVIG can vary from patient to patient as well as between manufacturers (Gahart & Nazareno, 2012).

The primary use of IVIG is to supply IgG antibodies passively to patients who are unable to produce sufficient amounts of their own antibodies. The FDA has control over IVIG as a drug and has approved its use for the following conditions: ITP, primary immunodeficiencies, secondary immunodeficiency owing to chronic lymphocytic leukemia, pediatric HIV, prevention of infection, and in Kawasaki syndrome. Additionally, there are off-label uses for IVIG that have emerged through research, many of which are controversial. The off-label indications amount to 70% of IVIG usage (AABB, 2011).

Some IVIG products are liquid, and some are powders that need to be reconstituted before administration. Manufacturers of IVIG indicate the individual product's storage requirements as some products need to be refrigerated. Follow the manufacturer's guidelines, and if provided, use the infusion kit supplied with the product. IVIG should be administered promptly after the vial is reconstituted. IVIG should not be mixed with other medications or IV solutions. If required, filtration is provided by most manufacturers. Filtration may be required as the solution is drawn into a syringe or as the product is administered through IV tubing (Gahart & Nazareno, 2012) (Table 17-6).

TABLE 17-6   ADMINISTRATION OF INTRAVENOUS IMMUNE GLOBULIN

1. Maintain hand hygiene. Assemble equipment: IV immune globulin; vented IV administration set; infusion pump, if needed; alcohol prep pad; blunt cannula.
2. Allow the product to warm to room temperature.
3. Verify written order for transfusion and rate of administration. (Note: Adverse reactions are frequently rate related.)
4. Make positive patient identification.
5. Calculate the dosage and rate based on weight of the patient.
6. Infusion with an IV pump:
   a. Insert spike of the IV administration set into the bottle. Prime as directed.
   b. Secure the IV administration set to the injection site closest to the IV site.
7. Initiate infusion at a specified rate and monitor the patient. Increase the rate as indicated.
8. The patient must be monitored before infusion, at every rate change, midpoint of the infusion, at the end of the infusion, and several times after the infusion completed.
9. Record date, time, and signature on requisition, which accompanies the blood component. Place in appropriate part of the patient's record. Document the patient's response. Record the volume of infusion.

Dosage varies depending on the patient's response and may be repeated every 3 to 4 weeks. IVIG should be administered by an electronic infusion device using a large peripheral vein or central venous access to reduce infusion site discomfort. A slow rate of infusion of IVIG, antihistamines, and/or steroids can reduce the risk for reactions (AABB, 2011). Most reactions are rate related, so caution is necessary. IVIG containing sucrose may lead to renal insufficiency (Gahart & Nazareno, 2012). Other reactions are mild and self-limiting.

INTRAVENOUS CYTOMEGALOVIRUS IMMUNE GLOBULIN (HUMAN)

Intravenous CMV immune globulin (CMV-IVIG) is a purified pooled plasma product containing a standardized amount of antibody to CMV. It is derived from plasma selected for high titers of the antibody and is primarily indicated as an adjunct to antiviral therapy in organ transplantation (Gahart & Nazareno, 2012). Solid organ transplant recipients who are seronegative for CMV and receiving an organ from a CMV-seropositive donor are at risk of CMV disease. The risk of actual virus transmission may be reduced when CMV-IVIG is combined with prophylaxis use of ganciclovir.

Because the product does not contain preservatives, infusion should begin within 6 hours after preparing the dose and be completed within 12 hours after entering the vial. The recommended initial rate of infusion is 15 mg/kg/h, increasing to a maximum of 60 mg/kg/h at specified intervals if the patient experiences no adverse reactions. No infusion should exceed 75 mL/h (Gahart & Nazareno, 2012). An electronic infusion pump is necessary to maintain a constant infusion.

Most reactions are rare and are usually rate related. When flushing, chills, muscle cramps, nausea, back pain, fever, or hypotension are observed, the infusion should be slowed or temporarily stopped. Close observation and vital signs should be completed on a scheduled basis.

RH IMMUNE GLOBULIN

Rh immune globulin (RIG) is a concentrate of anti-D immune globulin that is derived from plasma. It is used to prevent an Rh-negative individual from becoming sensitized (isoimmunized) to the Rh (D) antigen when exposed to the antigen by transfusion or, more commonly, pregnancy.

Rh antibody is produced by the Rh-negative mother in response to the D antigen in an Rh-positive infant and is the cause of Rh HDN. Prophylaxis against this sensitization was developed in the 60s and 70s. Since antepartum administration of RIG was introduced in 1968, the incidence of pregnancy-associated isoimmunization and HDN has decreased. RIG is given at 28 weeks' gestation and again at 72 hours postpartum. This reduces the risk of isoimmunization to 0.1% (AABB, 2011). Mothers are not candidates for RIG if the fetus is Rh negative or there is evidence that the mother is already sensitized. A standard 300-µg dose of RIG will prevent maternal sensitization in most cases; however, in situations such as fetomaternal hemorrhage, higher dosages may be needed (AABB, 2011). In addition to antepartum and postpartum use, RIG is used for other outcomes of pregnancy (abortion, miscarriage) or amniocentesis when a fetomaternal hemorrhage could occur.

Use of RIG may be appropriate when an Rh-negative recipient receives Rh-positive RBCs or components, such as platelets or granulocytes, which may contain sufficient cells to cause immunization. Individual situations dictate prophylaxis for RBC transfusions because the dose required is extremely large and causes discomfort.

Several commercial preparations of RIG are available. RIG is primarily administered by intramuscular injection; however, there are now several RIG products available that can be given IV (Gahart & Nazareno, 2012). RIG is usually given intramuscularly in the deltoid, but the manufacturer's recommendations for administration and patient observation should be followed closely. Although use of RIG is not associated with viral transmission, no drug is risk free, and informed consent is recommended as this is a product that is derived from human plasma (AABB et al., 2009).

Transfusion Reactions

Significant improvements in the collection, testing, and storage of blood and blood components, together with growing knowledge in the field of immunohematology, have increased the safety of transfusion therapy. An inherent risk still exists, however, with every unit of transfused blood. The transfusionist, the primary nurse (if different from the transfusionist), and the patient should be aware of the risks and remain alert for symptoms of untoward events. Since the patient is often the first person to recognize a change in how he or she feels, it is important to involve the patient in all aspects of the transfusion, if possible. ABO and Rh compatibility testing cannot eliminate all reactions to administered blood.

A transfusion reaction is defined as "any unfavorable event that occurs in a patient during or following transfusion of blood or blood components and that can be related to that transfusion" (AABB, 2010). Any unfavorable sign or symptom experienced by the patient during or following a transfusion should be considered serious, the transfusion should be stopped, and the patient should be evaluated. Box 17-2 outlines the objective signs and subjective symptoms that may be observed, need assessment, and require intervention. Table 17-7 describes the key interventions that should be performed for a suspected transfusion reaction. Urticarial reactions need treatment but may not require blood testing; they should be reported to the blood bank or transfusion service per institutional procedure. Institutional policy will outline the specific course of action that must be followed when a transfusion reaction is suspected (AABB, 2010).

Transfusion reactions may be divided into two main classes: acute and delayed. These may each be further divided into immunologic and nonimmunologic (Box 17-3). Some reactions are common, and actions can be taken to reduce the patient's discomfort—for example,

---

BOX 17-2 HEMOLYTIC TRANSFUSION REACTION SIGNS AND SYMPTOMS

Objective Signs	Subjective Symptoms
Fever	Pain in abdomen, chest, flank, or back
Chills, with or without rigor	Headache
Dyspnea	Nausea, vomiting
Hypotension, shock	Pain at the IV site or along the vein
Hemoglobinuria, oliguria, anuria	
Bleeding, generalized oozing	

TABLE 17-7	INTERVENTION FOR SUSPECTED TRANSFUSION REACTION

1. At an initial sign or symptom of a suspected transfusion reaction, *stop* the transfusion.
2. Immediately set up an infusion of 0.9% sodium chloride. Prime the new administration set with the 0.9% sodium chloride.
3. Disconnect the blood or component and blood administration set from the hub of the catheter and replace with the set primed with sodium chloride. Put a sterile cap on the blood component tubing and save for possible restart of infusion. If using a Y-tubing blood set, *do not open* the lumen infusing sodium chloride because this causes more blood to be infused.
4. Begin infusion of sodium chloride solution.
5. Notify the physician/LIP and the blood bank or transfusion service of the patient's symptoms and vital signs.
6. If the physician/LIP determines the need for a transfusion reaction evaluation, initiate the following steps: Gather remaining equipment to draw blood and package the blood administration bag and set.
7. Draw blood samples as directed by institutional protocol and send to the blood bank. Blood samples are tested to determine the cause of the reaction.
8. Confirm that the blood component set is tightly clamped and distal end is covered to prevent leakage of blood. Place the blood component bag with any residual fluid, attached administration set with an IV solution, filter, and all related tags and labels in a plastic bag. Secure the bag and send to blood bank or transfusion service with suspected transfusion reaction report and other related forms. Report must be on the outside of the plastic bag.
9. Send a urine sample for hemoglobinuria if ordered by the patient's physician/LIP or institutional protocol.
10. Continue to monitor the patient closely for any further signs and symptoms of reaction.
11. Document any signs and symptoms observed and the time of recognition. Note the type of the component, amount infused, amount remaining, and nursing interventions performed. Record that the remaining component and suspected transfusion reaction report were sent to blood bank or transfusion service.

a mild allergic reaction—whereas other adverse effects need to be prevented, such as circulatory overload.

Acute Transfusion Reactions

Acute adverse effects of transfusion therapy usually occur during the transfusion or within hours (<24 hours) after the completion of a transfusion. Therefore, the patient must be closely monitored during and after the transfusion to assess and identify signs and symptoms of impending reactions. Most immediate adverse effects are preventable and caused by improper administration, failure to comply with standards, or lack of knowledge of the procedure or impact of the therapy. Thoroughly following written procedures and complying with policy are crucial for safe transfusion therapy and to protect patients from harm.

ACUTE IMMUNOLOGIC REACTION

Antigen–antibody reactions from RBCs, leukocytes, or plasma proteins are responsible for adverse effects in the recipient. They are usually produced by the body's response to foreign proteins.

| BOX 17-3 | ACUTE AND DELAYED IMMUNOLOGIC AND NONIMMUNOLOGIC TRANSFUSION REACTIONS |

Acute Reactions

Immunologic

Acute hemolytic reaction

Febrile nonhemolytic reaction

Transfusion-related acute lung injury (TRALI)

Urticaria (mild allergic reaction)

Anaphylaxis

Nonimmunologic

Transfusion-associated circulatory overload (TACO)

Air embolism

Citrate toxicity

Hypothermia

Electrolyte disturbances

Bacterial contamination

Delayed Reactions

Immunologic

Delayed hemolytic reaction

Posttransfusion Purpura (PTP)

Transfusion-associated graft versus host disease (TA-GVHD)

Nonimmunologic

Infectious organism transmission

Iron overload

ACUTE HEMOLYTIC REACTION

Acute hemolytic transfusion reactions occur when an antigen–antibody reaction occurs in the recipient as the result of an incompatibility between the recipient's antibodies and the donor's RBCs (intravascular). Incompatibilities in the ABO blood group system are responsible for most deaths from acute hemolytic transfusion reactions and may occur with administration of as little as 10 to 15 mL of incompatible blood.

The interaction of the isoagglutinins and ABO-incompatible RBCs activates the complement, kinin, and coagulation systems. The entire complement system is activated in the ABO mismatch, causing intravascular hemolysis. If the amount of free hemoglobin released from the destruction of RBCs exceeds the quantity that can combine with haptoglobin in the plasma, the excess hemoglobin filters through the glomerular membrane into the kidney tubules and hemoglobinuria occurs. The kinin system is activated by the antigen–antibody complex and produces bradykinin, which increases capillary permeability, dilates arterioles, and decreases systemic blood pressure. The coagulation system activates the intrinsic clotting cascade, causing small clots in the circulation, and may trigger DIC, which results in formation of thrombi in the microvasculature.

Intravascular hemolytic reactions are often fatal. Investigation of fatal hemolytic transfusion reactions shows that the most common causes are clerical or other errors in the identification of (a) the recipient sample sent to the blood bank, (b) the blood unit, or (c) the recipient. Hemolytic transfusion reactions may be accompanied by chills, fever, dyspnea, facial flushing, a burning sensation along the vein in which the blood is being infused, lumbar or flank pain, chest pain, frequent oozing of blood at the injection site and surgical areas, or shock. The severity of symptoms is related to the amount of incompatible blood transfused (AABB, 2011). When reactions occur, the transfusion must be stopped at once and the vein kept open with 0.9% sodium chloride. When Y tubing is used, a new setup (container of fluid and a new administration set) should be connected directly to the patient's intravascular device (i.e., peripheral IV or central venous catheter). The flow to the normal saline hanging with the Y tubing should not be opened; to do so could result in the patient receiving additional incompatible blood cells contained in the Y tubing.

Vigorous treatment of hypotension and promotion of adequate renal blood flow are imperative. Therapy may consist of administration of volume, diuretics, and volume expanders to promote diuresis and to minimize renal damage. Urinary flow rates in adults should be maintained above 1 mL/kg/h (AABB, 2011). Vasopressors, such as dopamine in low doses (<5 µg/kg/min), dilate the renal vasculature while increasing cardiac output (AABB, 2011). Their use requires careful monitoring of the patient's urinary flow, cardiac output, and blood pressure. A diuretic agent such as furosemide is recommended to be administered concurrently with adequate IV fluid replacement. The drug improves renal blood flow, thus minimizing the possibility of renal tubular ischemia and renal failure. The use of heparin therapy for the resulting DIC remains controversial and is addressed after evaluation of all consequences of the acute hemolytic reaction. Prevention is the hallmark of therapy for this severe reaction.

Extravascular hemolysis occurs when an antigen–antibody reaction occurs as an incompatibility between the recipient's RBCs and the donor's plasma. Signs and symptoms of extravascular hemolysis are chills, fever (typically several hours after the transfusion is completed), and a positive direct antiglobulin test. Relief of symptoms is the goal of treatment.

PATIENT SAFETY

If a transfusion reaction is suspected, essential interventions are universal:

- Stop the transfusion.
- Keep the IV access open with normal saline.
- Notify the physician/LIP.
- Notify the blood bank or transfusion service.

FEBRILE NONHEMOLYTIC REACTION

Febrile nonhemolytic reactions (FNHR) are usually the result of transfusion of cellular components in the absence of hemolysis, whereby antileukocyte antibodies in the recipient are directed against the donor's white blood cells. Even though some leukocytes break down rapidly during storage, the membrane fragments are still capable of sensitizing patients in the same manner as intact leukocytes. Patients who have been sensitized by numerous transfusions or multiple pregnancies are more likely to have a FNHR.

A FNHR is characterized by a rise in temperature of 1°C or 2°F or more without any other clinical reason and may occur immediately or within several hours of completion of the transfusion. Febrile reactions, which occur in 1% of transfusions (AABB et al., 2009), may be accompanied by chills, rigors, change in blood pressure, and anxiety. These reactions are most often benign, and symptom management will aid in recovery and reduce discomfort. As the name implies, no RBC hemolysis occurs. Antipyretics are used for treatment. When this reaction is anticipated, acetaminophen may be given 30 minutes before the blood or component is started or as ordered by the physician/LIP. Documentation of the reaction is important for prevention of future adverse effects. This reaction can be prevented through the use of leukocyte-reduced components, which usually are produced by filtration techniques. Deglycerolized RBCs and washed RBCs are also relatively depleted of leukocytes. All febrile responses should be clinically monitored because other reactions may occur.

ANAPHYLACTIC REACTIONS

Fortunately, anaphylactic reactions are rare, estimated to occur in 1 per 20,000 to 50,000 units (AABB, 2011). There are potentially several causes, but most appear to be due to sensitization to a foreign protein. They may occur in patients who are IgA deficient and who have developed anti-IgA antibodies. Early signs of an impending anaphylactic reaction may include apprehension, abdominal cramping, and warm, burning feeling of skin. Symptoms may occur rapidly and with only a few milliliters of blood or plasma infused. No fever is associated with transfusion-related anaphylactic reactions. Bronchospasm, respiratory distress, abdominal cramps, vascular instability, shock, and perhaps loss of consciousness characterize the reaction. This medical emergency requires immediate resuscitation of the patient along with administration of epinephrine and steroids. Close observation during the first 15 minutes of the transfusion and continuing surveillance throughout the transfusion are important to monitor for signs of this reaction. Patient education will alert the patient to signs and symptoms that may occur once the patient is home and must be reported to the physician/LIP.

Since an anaphylactic reaction is more likely to present in an IgA-deficient patient, prevention includes the use of autologous transfusions, washed cellular components, or obtaining units from donors who lack IgA. Reducing the plasma content of RBC and platelet transfusions may also be effective in reducing the severity of this reaction.

ALLERGIC REACTIONS

These reactions are relatively common and are based on a hypersensitivity response to foreign plasma proteins in the donor plasma. Allergic reactions can range from mild to severe. Reactions are characterized by local erythema, hives, and itching, wheezing, and laryngeal edema in varying degrees of intensity. Treatments for these reactions are based on the severity of the patient's symptoms. In mild allergic reactions, such as urticaria, the transfusion may be stopped temporarily and then continued after the patient has responded to antihistamine therapy. In severe allergic reactions, the transfusion is stopped until a diagnosis is made. The goal of treatment is to alleviate the patient's symptoms.

TRANSFUSION-RELATED ACUTE LUNG INJURY

Transfusion-related acute lung injury (TRALI) is a clinical syndrome associated with the transfusion of whole blood, packed RBCs, FFP platelet concentrate, cryoprecipitate, and, rarely, IGIV. It is often undiagnosed and underreported; yet among transfusion-related deaths in the United States, TRALI is the most common cause (AABB et al., 2009). It is important to recognize the signs and symptoms of TRALI and treat it promptly and aggressively.

Although the specific cause of TRALI remains unknown, the cause is suspected to be linked to a reaction between the donor high-titer antileukocyte antibodies and recipient leukocytes. The reaction can result in leukoagglutination. The leukoagglutinins may become trapped in the pulmonary microvasculature and cause massive leakage of fluids and proteins into the alveolar spaces and interstitium (AABB, 2011). This reaction causes severe respiratory distress unassociated with circulatory overload and without evidence of cardiac failure. Acute onset of hypoxemia is a strong clinical indicator of TRALI. The severity of the respiratory distress is usually disproportional to the volume of blood infused and is related to the degree of hypoxemia. Chest radiography reveals bilateral pulmonary infiltrates consistent with pulmonary edema but without other evidence of left heart failure. Clinical signs and symptoms other than respiratory distress include chills, fever, cyanosis, hypotension, and normal pulmonary capillary wedge pressure. These symptoms can occur during or within 1 to 2 hours after the transfusion but must present within 6 hours posttransfusion to meet TRALI criteria. Treatment begins by discontinuing the transfusion and providing aggressive respiratory and blood pressure support measures (Kleinman, Gajic, & Nunes, 2007).

After thorough investigations of TRALI incidents, antileukocyte antibodies were identified as being related to the reactions. Female blood donors with previous pregnancies frequently have HLA antibodies; these increase with the number of previous pregnancies; and a relationship was identified to donated plasma components. Thus, in a goal toward prevention, blood centers have focused on male donors for plasma components. Further research is still encouraged to identify patient risk factors related to TRALI (Triulzi, 2009).

Acute Nonimmunologic

Acute nonimmunologic adverse effects are caused by external factors in the administration of blood: bacterial infection of the patient, contamination of the donor blood, improper handling of blood, administration through a small-gauge IV catheter, and administration of a hypertonic fluid or medications with the transfusion. An antigen–antibody reaction is absent.

Circulatory Overload

Transfusion-associated circulatory overload (TACO) may occur when blood or its components are infused at a rate exceeding the recipient's cardiac output. The consequence is volume overload resulting in pulmonary edema. Patients receiving whole blood may be more at risk than those receiving RBCs due to higher volume infused without increased oxygen-carrying capacity. Patients susceptible to this adverse effect are the young and elderly and those with cardiac disease or renal disease, and chronic anemia. Symptoms include a pounding headache, dyspnea, constriction of the chest, coughing, hypertension, engorged neck veins, pulmonary edema, and heart failure. The transfusion must be stopped and the patient placed in a sitting position. Rapid-acting diuretics and oxygen usually relieve the symptoms.

Prevention consists of lung auscultation at the initiation of the transfusion and frequent monitoring during the transfusion for those patients susceptible to heart failure, the administration of diuretics before and/or between units, and the slow administration of concentrated components. Additionally, the blood bank can be requested to divide the unit into two aliquots for slower administration; each aliquot can be administered over 2 to 4 hours, thus decreasing the risk of fluid overload. This adverse effect is preventable.

Air Embolism

The use of plastic bags has dramatically reduced this complication of transfusion therapy, which may result from faulty technique in changing equipment or plastic bags, careless use of Y-type administration sets, air infused from one of the containers when fluid and blood are pumped together, or when infusing blood under pressure before the container is empty (AABB, 2010). If air does enter the patient, acute cardiopulmonary insufficiency occurs. Symptoms are the same as those for circulatory collapse: cyanosis, cough, dyspnea, shock, and occasionally cardiac arrest. The infusion should be stopped immediately and the patient turned on the left side, with the head down. This position traps air in the right atrium, preventing it from entering the pulmonary artery; the pulmonic valve is kept clear until the air can escape gradually. It may be necessary for the physician/LIP to aspirate the air with a transthoracic needle. This adverse effect is emergent and preventable.

CITRATE TOXICITY

Patients at risk for development of citrate toxicity or a calcium deficit are those who receive infusions of plasma, whole blood, or platelets at rates >100 mL/min; patients with kidney or liver disease; or neonates. The liver, unable to keep up with the rapid administration, cannot metabolize the citrate, which chelates calcium, reducing the ionized calcium concentration. Hypocalcemia may induce cardiac arrhythmia. This adverse effect may be encountered in emergency departments and operating rooms when large amounts of blood and blood components have been administered rapidly. Symptoms of hypocalcemia include tingling of the fingers, muscular cramps, convulsions, tetanus, hyperactive reflexes, carpopedal spasm, laryngeal spasm, and cardiopulmonary arrest (AABB, 2010). Treatment consists of slowing the rate of infusion and the administration of calcium chloride or calcium gluconate solution. However, the calcium must never be added to any IV administration set infusing blood.

HYPOTHERMIA

Hypothermia occurs when large volumes of cold blood or blood components are infused rapidly. Rapid infusions may cause chills, hypothermia, peripheral vasoconstriction, ventricular arrhythmias, and cardiac arrest. Clinically, it is important to be certain that central catheters, if placed, are not positioned in the right atrium, a situation that can stimulate arrhythmias if rapid infusions are given. In many situations, warming blood to 37°C with automatic blood warmers during rapid, massive replacement prevents hypothermia. However, time does not always permit the equipment to be set up.

ELECTROLYTE DISTURBANCES

Electrolyte disturbances may occur in patients as a result of chronic infusions or the infusion of multiple units over a short time, exemplified by the hypocalcemia of citrate toxicity mentioned earlier in this section.

Hyperkalemia is a rare complication of blood transfusion. It can occur in premature infants and newborns, patients with renal disease, and patients requiring massive transfusions. The total extracellular potassium is 0.5 mEq in a fresh unit of packed RBCs and 5 to 7 mEq in a unit of packed RBCs at its expiration date (AABB, 2011). Signs and symptoms include cardiac rhythm changes, a slow heartbeat, nausea, muscle weakness, diarrhea, flaccid paralysis and paresthesia of extremities, apprehension, and cardiac arrest.

BACTERIAL CONTAMINATION

Bacterial contamination of blood may occur at the time of donation or in preparing the component for infusion. In addition to skin contaminants, cold-resistant gram-negative bacteria and some gram-positive bacteria may contribute to this untoward event. *Staphylococcus*,

Klebsiella, *Acinetobacter*, and *Escherichia coli* species are some of the organisms identified in contaminated blood and blood products (CDC, 2011). These organisms, capable of proliferating at refrigerator temperatures, and those using citrate as a nutrient (AABB et al., 2009), release an endotoxin that initiates this rare, potentially fatal reaction.

Inspecting the unit before administration can prevent this complication. Observation of any discoloration or abnormal color of the blood or plasma, clumping, gas bubbles, extraneous material, or obvious clots should be reported to the blood bank. Clinical manifestations of a septic reaction include high fever ($\geq 2°C$ or $\geq 3.5°F$ increase in temperature), chills, hypotension, flushing of the skin, "warm" shock, hematuria, renal failure, and DIC (AABB, 2010). These signs and symptoms are similar to those of an acute hemolytic reaction, so diagnosis must be made quickly. The transfusion should be discontinued; immediate therapy, including aggressive management of shock and antibiotics, is required. Cultures obtained of the patient's blood, the suspected component, and all IV solutions determine whether the blood or an IV-related infection caused the bacteremia.

Many of the reactions discussed thus far are preventable. Treating of comorbid conditions may mask signs and symptoms of bacteremia related to a transfusion. Quality improvement and monitoring measures can assist in avoiding other errors, along with computerized methods of verifying necessary data.

Delayed Effects from a Transfusion

These complications occur days, weeks, months, or years after the transfusion and usually are the result of alloimmunization or transmitted disease.

DELAYED IMMUNOLOGIC

DELAYED HEMOLYTIC REACTION

Delayed hemolytic reactions, caused by an immune antibody created in response to a foreign antigen (e.g., Rh, Kell, Duffy, Kidd), are classified as primary and secondary. The primary or initial reaction usually is mild and may occur between 2 and 14 days after the transfusion.

ALLOIMMUNIZATION

Blood or blood components contain additional substances such as red cells, white cells, or plasma proteins not identified on the label and antigens occur. *Primary alloimmunization* rarely produces symptoms, may be clinically insignificant but could present itself days to weeks following the transfusion. The degree of hemolysis depends on the quantity of antibody produced. The secondary reaction occurs in a patient previously immunized by transfusion or pregnancy. These patients have formed a RBC alloantibody, but the level of this alloantibody has become so low that it is serologically undetectable. On a later occasion, when the donor RBCs possessing the corresponding antigen are infused, they provoke a rapid increase in the specific antibody. The incompatible RBCs survive until sufficient antibody is present to initiate a rejection response. The reaction is called a *secondary* or *anamnestic* (memory) response and is caused by reexposure to the same antigen. These reactions are rarely caused by ABO incompatibility. Manifestations of a delayed hemolytic reaction include fever, mild jaundice, hemoglobinuria, and an unexplained drop in hemoglobin. Treatment is usually not necessary, although monitoring the patient's renal function may be needed. These coated cells are removed from the body by the reticuloendothelial system (extravascular hemolysis). A direct antiglobulin test may detect the antibody, and future donor units are selected that lack the corresponding antigen to the antibody formed.

POSTTRANSFUSION PURPURA

Posttransfusion Purpura (PTP) is a rare syndrome identified 7 to 10 days after the transfusion in a patient with sensitivity to blood or blood components. Thrombocytopenia, platelet counts <10,000/μL, occurs in a rapid and self-limited manner. Symptoms include bleeding from mucous membranes and the gastrointestinal tract. In more severe cases, intracranial hemorrhage occurs.

Whole-blood exchange, plasma exchange, and steroids have all been used to treat PTP; however, current treatment for PTP may include high-dose immune globulin intravenously (AABB, 2010). To prevent the recurrence of PTP, autologous donations and directed donations are preferred.

TRANSFUSION-ASSOCIATED GRAFT VERSUS HOST DISEASE

Transfusion-associated graft versus host disease (TA-GVHD) is a complex, rare, and often fatal immunologic reaction. It most commonly occurs in a severely immunocompromised patient with the transfer of immunocompetent T lymphocytes in blood components. It may also occur due to a transfusion from a blood relative (AABB et al., 2009). The donor lymphocytes engraft and multiply in a severely immunodeficient recipient. These engrafted cells react against the foreign tissue of the host recipient (AABB, 2011). Leukocyte-reduced components continue to pose a risk for TA-GVHD as T lymphocytes are still present.

The onset of TA-GVHD is usually 8 to 10 days after transfusion (AABB, 2011). Signs and symptoms may include rash, fever, diarrhea, elevated liver function tests, and pancytopenia. TA-GVHD is associated with a mortality rate > 90% of affected patients, and bone marrow suppression and infection are the causes of death.

The only approved method to prevent or reduce the incidence of TA-GVHD is gamma irradiation of all blood components containing lymphocytes. Pretransfusion inactivation of lymphocytes by irradiating cellular components reduces the risk of TA-GVHD in the following situations:

a. Fetuses receiving intrauterine transfusions
b. Selected immunoincompetent or immunocompromised recipients
c. Recipients of donor units known to be from a blood relative
d. Recipients who have undergone bone marrow or peripheral blood progenitor cell transplantation
e. Neonates undergoing exchange transfusion or use of extracorporeal membrane oxygenation
f. Patients with Hodgkin disease (AABB, 2011; Brooks, 2008)

DELAYED NONIMMUNOLOGIC REACTION

CYTOMEGALOVIRUS INFECTION

Recognized to be present in blood and transmitted by transfusion, CMV poses little problem to most immunologically intact transfusion recipients. CMV is in the herpes virus family, and white cells are the major reservoir of CMV transmitted by blood (AABB et al., 2009). With up to 70% of donors being CMV seropositive, blood donations are not limited to

CMV-seronegative donors. Patients most at risk for serious consequences of the infection are those who have not been previously exposed and are immunocompromised. These patients should receive CMV-seronegative products. These include low birth weight neonates, patients with malignancies who are immunosuppressed as a result of therapy for their disease, patients with AIDS, and recipients of bone marrow and solid organ transplants. Many of these patients have depressed cell-mediated immunity and are at risk for development of systemic CMV infections, including pneumonia, hepatitis, retinitis, and mononucleosis-like symptoms. Careful screening of donors and use of blood from CMV-seronegative donors or those with depleted leukocytes are effective steps to reduce CMV infection in specific patient populations.

Hepatitis

Hepatitis often presents clinically with self-limiting fever, fatigue, and jaundice but may lead to progressive inflammation of the liver, resulting in cirrhosis or hepatic cancer. The clinical outcome of hepatitis, manifested by elevated liver enzymes and abnormal liver function tests, results in anorexia, fatigue, malaise, dark urine, fever, nausea, and jaundice; it usually resolves within 4 to 6 weeks. Treatment of symptoms is the aim of hepatitis management. Some patients demonstrate few symptoms, whereas others may become extremely ill and die of fulminating hepatic failure.

Posttransfusion hepatitis (PTH) has been recognized since the 1960s as a complication of receiving blood and potentially can be caused by HAV, HBV, HCV, hepatitis B–associated D virus (HDV), and hepatitis E virus (HEV). HAV and HEV are exceedingly rare causes of PTH, largely because the virus is present only during the acute phase of the disease and there is no carrier state. HDV needs HBV to replicate and must be transmitted at the same time as HBV into a person already infected with HBV. HDV usually is transmitted through IV drug use or sexual contact with an infected person and, as a superinfection, may worsen the course of chronic hepatitis B infection. The viruses predominantly responsible for PTH are HBV and HCV, although the risk of these infections from transfusions has been substantially reduced. The incidence of PTH has decreased dramatically since 1995 because of the thorough screening of donors and the use of more sensitive laboratory tests to identify at-risk donors.

Hepatitis B Virus. HBV accounts for only a small proportion of cases of PTH. The primary reasons for this low incidence are screening of donors for behaviors that expose them to viral hepatitis and the testing of all donations for HBsAg and anti-HBc. The ARC estimates the risk of PTH attributed to HBV as 1 in 280,000 to 1 in 357,000 per unit transfused (AABB, 2011).

The average incubation period for HBV infection is >50 days. Although most patients clear the virus, a proportion of patients remain chronically infected without symptoms. Becoming an HBsAg carrier is age dependent. It has been estimated that more than 90% of infants infected become carriers prior to immunization and routine prophylactic immunoglobulin infusion (AABB, 2011). Hepatitis B can be transmitted directly by percutaneous needle inoculation or by transfusion of infected blood. It can be transmitted indirectly by infectious serum, saliva, or semen through minute cuts or abrasions on the skin or mucosal surfaces. Health care workers are strongly advised to be immunized with hepatitis B vaccine to reduce the risk of acquiring HBV infection.

Hepatitis C Virus. HCV is the major etiologic agent of PTH. The estimated risk of PTH attributed to HCV as 1 in 1.1 million per unit transfused (AABB, 2011). At least 50% of HCV carriers have evidence of chronic liver disease, but most remain asymptomatic. Screening blood donors for antibody to HCV has been in place since 1998. An enzyme immunoassay (EIA) for antibodies to HCV is used to identify blood donors who have been exposed. Donors found to be repeatedly active by EIA are deferred. A supplemental test, the recombinant immunoblot assay, may be used to determine which reactive EIA results are true positives because the EIA screening test is extremely sensitive but not completely specific for HCV.

The modes of transmission of HCV appear to be similar to those of HBV; however, the route of HCV infection in many infected people is unknown. The incubation period for HCV ranges from 2 to 26 weeks. The initial and acute illness is usually milder than in HBV and is often subclinical. Approximately 75% of patients are anicteric. Liver abnormalities persisting after 1 year indicate chronic hepatitis and predispose the patient to cirrhosis and liver failure. Chronic HCV infection also predisposes patients to hepatocellular carcinoma. Clinical management of chronic HCV infections may include a combination of antiretroviral agents and interferons (Porth, 2009).

HUMAN IMMUNODEFICIENCY VIRUS (HIV)

HIV is a retrovirus that infects and kills CD4-positive lymphocytes (helper T cells), thereby disabling the cellular immune system. It produces severe immunosuppression and renders the infected person vulnerable to opportunistic infections and other symptoms such as fever, night sweats, weight loss, and skin lesions. HIV-2 (type 2) is similar to HIV-1 (type 1), but the incubation period appears to be longer and transmission is less efficient than for HIV-1 (Faulhaber & Aberg, 2009).

HIV-1 and HIV-2 can both be transmitted by transfusions. Their existence has necessitated aggressive work to safeguard the blood supply. The first test for HIV antibody was developed and testing initiated in 1985. Since then, very few cases of HIV transmission by transfusion have occurred. The current estimated risk of posttransfusion HIV in the United States is 1 in 1.5 million per unit transfused (AABB, 2011). Donated blood is tested for antibodies to the virus (anti–HIV-1 and anti–HIV-2) using an EIA (AABB, 2011). The confirmatory test for repeatedly reactive anti-HIV EIA tests is the Western blot.

Of concern are donors who may have been recently infected with HIV and are able to transmit the disease but have not yet seroconverted. Since 1996, donated blood has also been tested for HIV-associated antigen p24, which appears sooner than HIV antibodies and reduces the *infectious window* by 6 days (AABB, 2011). More sensitive tests based on nucleic acid technologies (NATs) are being used to test for HIV-infected donors. These tests have reduced the infectious window to as soon as 9 days (AABB, 2011). Current testing has virtually eliminated transmission of enveloped viruses such as HBV, HCV, and HIV via blood components, but rare cases continue to be reported as a result of window periods (Brooks, 2008). Techniques also have been developed to inactivate viruses in plasma derivatives, such as AHF, IVIG, and others.

HUMAN T-CELL LYMPHOTROPIC VIRUSES

Type I and II human T-cell lymphotropic viruses (HTLVs) are spread through viable lymphocytes in blood. HTLV type I is associated with adult T-cell lymphoma/leukemia and a neurologic disorder called HTLV-associated myelopathy or tropical spastic paraparesis (AABB, 2011). Transmission is by breast milk, sexual contact, and exposure to blood. The prevalence of this disease varies widely geographically and is most common in Japan and other Pacific regions, Central and South America, and parts of Africa. The only disease known to be associated with the retrovirus HTLV-II is HTLV-associated myelopathy, but its occurrence is less frequent than with HTLV-I (AABB, 2011). The virus is prevalent in some high-risk populations such as those previously infected with HIV and IV drug users in the United States.

Testing for HTLV-I has been ongoing since 1988, and seropositive donors have been removed from donor pools. Testing for antibodies to HTLV-II began in 1997. Combination HTLV-I/II testing began in 1998 and offers more sensitive detection of both anti–HTLV-I and anti–HTLV-II, further reducing the risk of transfusion-transmitted HTLV-I/II. The frequency of transfusion-transmitted HTLV is quite low in the United States, with an estimate at 1 in 1, 364,000 units transfused (ARC, 2012). The only FDA-approved donor test for HTLV infection is screening for the IgG assay to HTLV-I/II.

MALARIA

Nearly eradicated in the United States and Canada, malaria is still prevalent in other parts of the world. The number of cases of transfusion-transmitted malaria reported in the United States is 0.6 cases per million transfusions (AABB, 2011). Monitoring for this complication of transfusion is ongoing because of increased travel, immigration, and the continued presence of malaria in many areas of the world. No laboratory test is used widely to screen blood donors for malaria, and donors are excluded through donor questioning. The patient may have a high fever, chills, and headache, which reflect the lysis of infected RBCs as they release the parasites into the bloodstream. Prevention is accomplished through donor questioning and by excluding donors from regions of the world where malaria is prevalent.

Prospective donors who have actually had malaria are deferred for 3 years after becoming asymptomatic (AABB, 2011). Travelers who have visited an endemic area are deferred for 1 year. Immigrants, refugees, and citizens from endemic countries may be accepted as blood donors 3 years after departure from the area if they are asymptomatic. Donors with a history of babesiosis or Chagas disease are deferred permanently.

SYPHILIS

Although refrigerated storage of RBC components has nearly eradicated the transmission of syphilis due to the effect of low temperatures on the survival of the spirochete, STS is required on all donations. Positive STS results also may denote immunologic abnormalities unrelated to syphilis or inadequately treated syphilis, a fact that may be more helpful to the donor than to the recipient (AABB, 2011). There have been no reports of transfusion-transmitted syphilis in several decades.

WEST NILE VIRUS

West Nile virus (WNV), which first appeared in the United States in 1999, is a seasonal infection transmitted by the bite of an infected mosquito. It was not until 2002 when WNV was identified as a transfusion-associated infection (Brooks, 2008). The virus is not spread by human-to-human contact but by mosquitoes and carriers such as birds, cats, horses, squirrels, and rabbits. In response to the increase in WNV infections, investigational NATs were deployed to test for the West Nile viral genome in 2003. These NATs are performed regionally, and positive results have been reported in volunteer blood donors. WNV has a relatively small transmission window occurring early in the infection. Elderly and immunocompromised individuals have the greatest risk of contracting the virus.

IRON OVERLOAD

Iron overload or hemosiderosis may occur in patients with hemoglobinopathies who are receiving chronic transfusions. Each unit of packed RBCs contains 250 mg of iron. Signs and symptoms include hepatic failure and cardiac toxicity. Treatment involves the administration of iron chelator agents, such as deferoxamine mesylate (Desferal), to bind ferric ions to remove iron without reducing the patient's circulating hemoglobin.

Blood Administration

The administration of blood and blood components can be a lifesaving therapy; in contrast, fatal consequences can result from error or improper technique (Table 17-8). Nurses must be well versed in every phase of therapy as well as knowledgeable about the administration of components and monitoring of patients during and after the transfusion. The patient's safety depends on adherence to specific rules regarding safe administration. Some institutions

---

TABLE 17- ADMINISTRATION OF WHOLE BLOOD OR RBC COMPONENTS

---

1. Maintain hand hygiene. Obtain vital signs before blood arrives on the unit; this ensures prompt and timely administration. If the patient's temperature is 38.8°C or 100°F or greater, notify the physician/LIP before requesting the blood or component from the blood bank. An elevated temperature is not a contraindication to the transfusion, but it may make assessment and decisions regarding blood reactions difficult (AABB, 2011). Assemble equipment: whole blood or RBC component; blood recipient set; blunt cannula if connecting to primary IV; alcohol prep pad; electronic infusion device, if needed; equipment for performing IV access if the patient does not have IV access established.
2. Verify the written order for transfusion.
3. Verify the signed transfusion consent form.
4. Verify the blood component for donor/recipient ABO and Rh compatibility.
5. Confirm that blood numbers on the component match with those on transfusion requisition.
6. Check the expiration date of the component.
7. Two qualified health professionals use two identifiers for positive patient identification. Confirm that blood numbers on the component match numbers on the patient's identification band.
8. At bedside set up equipment for transfusion. Clamp-on the blood recipient set should be closed.
9. Open one tab port of the component bag and insert the spike of the blood recipient set into this port.
10. Invert and hang the component bag on IV pole.
11. Prime entire surface of filter for best flow rates. Fill drip chamber of the blood recipient set half full. Open clamp and flush all air from the line. Close clamp.
12. Attach appropriate blunt cannula to the blood set if blood will be infusing by primary IV. Sodium chloride 0.9% should be used to flush any set that may contain a drug incompatible with RBCs.
13. Scrub the injection site with alcohol prep pad and attach the blunt cannula into the injection site. Secure catheter tightly.
14. Regulate the component to the prescribed rate or set pump to the desired rate. All blood must be infused within 4 h from the time it was released from the blood bank.
15. Take vital signs prior to the start of the infusion, after the first 15 min of the infusion, and at the conclusion of the transfusion. Record date, time, and signature on blood requisition that accompanies the blood component. Place in appropriate part of the patient's record. Document the patient's immediate response to initial administration of RBCs, whole blood, or other blood component.

NOTE: This procedure can be converted for institutions using multilead blood administration sets. This procedure also may be modified for the administration of plasma and single-donor platelets.

have delegated the administration of blood and blood components to a restricted group of specially trained personnel. If so, competency must be evident in knowledge and skill demonstration for all aspects of transfusion (Box 17-4). Ultimately, it is the nurse who has the accountability to advocate for the patient, conduct appropriate assessments, prevent complications, and intervene when there are reactions. Outcomes for the patient would include safe therapy, effective treatment, and patient satisfaction.

Blood Samples

Mislabeled specimens can contribute to transfusion-related deaths. The intended recipient must be identified positively at the time of blood sample collection at the patient's bedside. Labeling requirements are aimed at preventing a potentially tragic outcome in patient care and significantly decrease errors in blood grouping. Labels must be affixed to the blood tubes and contain the institution's required information related to the recipient, including the date of sample collection, two independent identifiers (i.e., name, medical record number), and identification of the person drawing the specimen. Although an institution may define the length of time samples may be used, the general ruling is that samples intended for use in cross-match should be collected no more than 3 days before the intended transfusion. This helps ensure that the sample reflects the recipient's current immunologic status (AABB, 2011).

Issue and Transfer of Blood and Blood Components

Patient and blood identification is of paramount importance in preventing reactions from incompatible blood. The risk of identification error is reduced by the use of a triplicate requisition or an online ordering system. Such requisitions, identifying the patient, indicating the amount and kind of blood required, and time needed, are usually sent to the blood bank with the blood sample.

BOX 17-4   RESPONSIBILITIES OF A CLINICIAN

- Verifying the presence of a written physician/LIP order for the transfusion
- Verifying that documented informed consent has been obtained from the patient
- Verifying ABO and Rh compatibility between the donor and recipient
- Performing procedures relevant to the patient and blood identification
- Inspecting the unit before administration
- Explaining the procedure to the patient
- Taking pretransfusion vital signs
- Selecting and using proper technique and equipment
- Observing the patient for 15 minutes at the beginning of the transfusion and monitoring vital signs for changes
- Monitoring the patient throughout the transfusion or notifying the primary nurse of this accountability
- Documenting the transfusion according to established policy
- Taking posttransfusion vital signs

The mode of transfer of blood components to the nursing unit depends on institutional policy. It may involve a pneumatic tube system, a messenger service, hospital personnel, or the person who will administer the blood. One of the most common causes of a hemolytic reaction is the accidental administration of incompatible blood to the patient. To prevent administration of incompatible blood, only 1 unit should be transported by a person at a time.

Patient and Blood Identification

Improper identification leads to 1 in every 19,000 units transfused to the wrong patient (AABB, 2011). In fact, patients have a higher risk of receiving an ABO-incompatible transfusion than a blood component with any undetected virus (Brooks, 2008). Omission of any of the validation steps can allow for misidentification. Absolute and positive identification of the donor blood and the patient must be made. All personnel handling the blood should be responsible for checking patient and blood identification. The nurse makes the final check and must decide whether to administer the blood or question it. ABO and Rh compatibility identification is made by comparing the patient's previous ABO and Rh determination with the patient's and donor's ABO and Rh on the compatibility tag; and also the blood identification number on the blood container with the identification number on the blood tag and the blood unit itself. Many health care facilities have incorporated computer information and validating systems to link the patient to the blood bank for more reliable checking. Bar coding continues to be implemented throughout hospitals in the United States as a method for validating the administration of compatible units.

Patient identification is made by checking two identifiers, and neither of the identifiers can be a room number. Each institution will have a policy naming the two identifiers. If able, the patient must identify himself or herself by complete name. Identity should never be made by addressing the patient by name and awaiting a response. Errors can occur from faulty response of medicated patients. Patients unable to respond may be identified by the primary or attending nurse. Hospital numbers on the identification bracelet must match hospital numbers on the tag to prevent errors in cases of similar names. Any discrepancy must be investigated and corrected before the blood is administered. Blood must never be administered to a patient who has no identification bracelet.

In summary, the person performing the transfusion is responsible for the verification of information regarding the component, proper patient identification, administration, and documentation (see Box 17-4). Transfusion information is part of the patient's permanent record.

Reducing Blood Exposure and High-Risk Injuries

Needleless Devices

Health care workers are at risk for acquiring blood-borne infections through needlestick exposure to blood-filled hollow-bore needles commonly used for vascular access and blood sampling. Of greatest concern are HIV, HBV, and HCV. Shielded or self-blunting needles for vacuum tube phlebotomy, shielded butterfly needles, automatically retracting fingerstick/heelstick lancets, and plastic capillary tubes should be used for blood sampling. When the nurse needs to obtain IV access for the administration of the transfusion, IV catheters designed to prevent stylet injuries should be used. When connecting the transfusion to a primary line, blunted or integrated safety devices designed to reduce injury should be used.

BARRIER PROTECTION

Barrier protection must be used when exposure to blood may occur. Minimal protection consists of gloves for handling any blood component; liquid-resistant gowns and protective eyewear may be advisable in emergency and trauma settings. In addition, electronic infusion devices used to administer blood and blood components should have tight, Luer-locking connections to prevent high-pressure rupture, thus avoiding the risk of blood exposure. Latex-free gloves and equipment are strongly recommended and required for any patient with a history of latex sensitivities.

Handling Blood

To prevent excessive warming, blood transfusion must be initiated within 30 minutes of the time it leaves the blood bank. If blood is not maintained at 1°C to 10°C (34°F to 50°F) while outside the control of the blood bank, it cannot be reissued. Banked blood stored at 1°C to 6°C (34°F to 43°F) will exceed 10°C (50°F) in approximately 30 minutes at room temperature; blood that cannot be administered immediately should be returned to the blood bank within this time. Blood should never be placed in the patient care unit refrigerators because they are not controlled and contain no alarms to warn of temperature fluctuation.

If warmed blood is ordered, an FDA-approved blood-warming device that maintains a controlled temperature should be used to warm the blood. Equipment should have a visible thermometer and an audible warning alarm. Temperatures must not rise above 37°C. These warming devices should be available in emergency departments, where it is common to administer blood rapidly. Patients receiving multiple units of cold blood rapidly (i.e., 100 mL/min) reportedly have increased incidences of cardiac arrest. Hot water and standard microwave ovens must never be used to warm blood.

Before the blood component is administered, the expiration date should be noted to avoid infusion of an outdated component. Sodium chloride injection, USP 0.9% (normal saline), may be used to initiate the infusion and flush administration sets at the completion of the transfusion of RBCs, whole blood, platelets, or leukocytes. Hypotonic or hypertonic solutions should not be used to dilute blood. Extreme hypotonicity causes water to invade the RBCs until they burst (i.e., hemolysis). Hypertonic solutions dilute blood, resulting in reversal of this process with shrinkage of the RBCs. Solutions containing calcium such as Lactated Ringer's should never be used in conjunction with blood or blood components containing citrate. Additionally, IV solutions containing dextrose can destroy red cells due to loss of water by the red cell.

Unless approved for use by the FDA, no medication or IV fluid (with the exception of 0.9% sodium chloride) should be added to blood or administered simultaneously through the same set.

Venipuncture

Peripheral veins with an adequate diameter should be used to ensure the flow of viscous components. The lower extremities are avoided in adults because thrombosis and blood pooling may occur. Areas of joint flexion should also be avoided. The peripheral IV site should be checked frequently during the infusion for early detection of infiltration. RBCs and whole blood can usually be administered through an 18- or 20-gauge catheter, although smaller gauges may be used for other components. A 22- or 24-gauge catheter may be used for pediatric patients. When a smaller catheter is used, infuse the blood or components at a slow constant rate to reduce hemolysis of cells.

Blood and blood components may be administered through central venous catheters, including short-term catheters such as a subclavian catheter and long-term access devices such as tunneled catheters or implanted ports. Increasing numbers of peripherally inserted central catheters and midline catheters are being placed in patients receiving long-term IV therapy. In most situations, components infuse in a timely manner through 20- to 22-gauge or larger peripherally inserted central catheters. If a dual-lumen catheter has been placed, the larger lumen should be reserved for transfusions. It is necessary to flush the catheter adequately with normal saline at the conclusion of the transfusion. A minimum of 10 mL normal saline should be used to flush the catheter vigorously after transfusion.

Rate of Infusion

The rate of infusion is governed by the clinical condition of the patient, the type and viscosity of the component being infused, and the catheter's internal diameter (gauge). Nurses have an important role in assessing the patient's clinical condition and ensuring a proper rate of administration. Macrobore IV administration sets should be used and changed after every unit or every 4 hours. Infusions should be set at a slow rate for the first 15 minutes to avoid infusion of a large quantity of blood in case of an immediate reaction. Adverse reactions may occur with a small volume of the blood or blood component administered. If the patient experiences discomfort related to the cold blood infusion, consider alternative warming methods to warm the patient not the blood.

Most patients can tolerate infusions of 1 unit of RBCs over 1 to 2 hours (AABB, 2011). Patients in heart failure or at risk of fluid overload require infusions given over a longer time, but not to exceed 4 hours from the time the blood or component was released from the blood bank. If necessary, the blood bank can divide a unit of RBCs into two aliquots that are given as two separate infusions. Each aliquot may be given over 3 to 4 hours to reduce fluid overload. Large-gauge catheters should be used when it is necessary to infuse blood rapidly; approved external pressure devices may be used if necessary. Physicians/LIPs need to be readily available because certain risks are inherent in rapid volume replacement. Electronic infusion devices for the administration of blood and its components are frequently required and especially important for slow rates of infusion to elderly, pediatric, and neonatal patients.

Blood Filters

A standard (usually 170 to 260 μm), sterile, pyrogen-free blood filter designed to remove debris, including clots, is acceptable for administration of most blood components. For best flow rates, the entire surface area of the filter should be filled with the component. A single filter may be used to infuse 2 to 4 units of blood. If the initial transfusion lasts >4 hours, it is recommended to not reuse the same filter in subsequent transfusions. Filters need to be added to dedicated infusion pump sets. Once the blood filter contains debris, it should be discarded. Continued use of such filters may result in bacterial contamination, a slower rate of infusion, or hemolysis of the blood at room temperature.

Microaggregate Filters

The demonstration of microaggregates, composed of leukocytes, platelets, and fibrin, led to the manufacture of microaggregate filters in the early 1960s. Overtime, the filters evolved into depth filters with high efficiency. Pore size is 20 to 40 µm, and they are used for the administration of RBCs. These filters retain fibrin strands and clumps of dead cells. The volume required for priming is significant; thus, flushing the set with isotonic saline at completion of the transfusion is recommended. Pediatric microaggregate filters are useful because of the small priming volume rather than the removal of debris.

Leukocyte Removal Filters

RBC and platelet leukocyte removal filters are available to reduce a number of transfusion-associated complications: HLA alloimmunization and platelet refractoriness, transmission of cell-associated viruses, and febrile nonhemolytic reactions. Clinical conditions where benefit is realized include patients with cancer and those with renal disease, who may become immunocompromised and are at risk of alloimmunization. These filters, which remove approximately 99.9% of leukocytes and are quick and convenient to prime, may be used for filtration at the bedside. Most institutions filter RBCs or platelets prior to storage for better monitoring of the filtration process. The filters are efficient and effective and provide a convenient method of removing leukocytes. Filters are designed for either RBCs or platelets and should not be interchanged. These filters have no effect on the shelf life of the unit.

Patient Monitoring and Education

After initiation of the transfusion, the nurse transfusionist should observe the patient for the initial 15 minutes of the infusion or longer based on professional judgment (AABB et al., 2009). Staying with the patient or being in close observation is critical to detect a reaction and be immediately responsive. Many of the fatal incompatible transfusion reactions produce symptoms early in the course of the infusion. Primary nurses also share a responsibility for safe transfusion administration. They must be familiar with the various transfusion reactions, be able to recognize adverse reactions, and know what procedures to follow. Changes in vital signs or objective signs are other indicators. Critical points in this process are outlined in Box 17-5. The patient's report of his or her subjective symptoms is often the first indication of a reaction. The patient and/or caregiver should be educated on the possible signs and symptoms associated with a transfusion reaction.

Documenting the Transfusion

All data relevant to the transfusion should be recorded in the patient's clinical and transfusion records. The time the transfusion was complete, the volume of fluid infused, and the condition of the patient should be noted. Observation of the patient periodically for 4 to 6 hours after the transfusion is recommended, but minimum documentation of observation should be 1 hour posttransfusion. Posttransfusion monitoring of vital signs and laboratory values ensures that the clinical goal was achieved. Latex sensitivity or any other comments about the transfusion should be noted. Legal and safety issues are summarized in Box 17-6.

BOX 17-5 KEY COMPONENTS OF PATIENT EDUCATION

Patient Transfusion History

- Previous reactions may trigger the need to premedicate the patient. Review the patient record and interview the patient to identify previous reactions and interventions.
- Goal: Lessen potential reactions, relieve anxiety.

Latex Sensitivity

- Use only latex-free equipment.
- Goal: Eliminate any progression of a reaction.

Signed Transfusion Consent Form From the Patient

- All patients must be informed of administration of blood or blood components. The patient or parent must sign forms, which a physician/LIP must witness. Some institutions grant privileges to nurse practitioners to witness transfusion consents.
- Goal: Patient awareness and participation in the course of therapy.

Patient Education

- Inform the patient of the steps involved in having a transfusion; include length of time for the transfusion and expected outcomes.
- Instruct the patient regarding signs and symptoms that could indicate a reaction.
- Share with the patient how important his or her personal report is to detect reactions early.
- Goals: early identification of potential reactions; lessen anxiety.

Disposal of Equipment

Sharps must be disposed of in specially designed, puncture-resistant, leak-proof containers located near the area of use. All transfusion-related equipment should be placed in biohazard containers. Administration sets used to infuse blood components should be discarded within 4 hours after use. Bacterial growth may occur on the trapped proteins and debris contained in the set. Institutional guidelines for observing standard precautions should be followed.

Increased Prothrombotic Factors

FACTOR V LEIDEN DEFICIENCY

Factor V Leiden is a variant of the protein factor V, which is needed for blood clotting. People who have a factor V deficiency are more likely to bleed severely, whereas people with factor V Leiden have blood that has an increased tendency to clot. Those who carry the factor V Leiden gene have a greater risk of developing thrombosis than do the rest of the population. However, only 10% of individuals with the factor V Leiden gene will develop blood clots.

Factor V Leiden is the most common hereditary blood coagulation disorder in the United States. It is present in 3% to 7% of the White population and far less prevalent in Black and Asian populations (Gahart & Nazareno, 2012).

BOX 17-6 LEGAL AND SAFETY ISSUES FOR TRANSFUSION THERAPY

- All health care institutional policies and procedures address the standards and guidelines of the AABB, the FDA, and those of professional health care–related agencies (such as the INS, the Institute of Medicine, the National Patient Safety Foundation, and the ONS) as appropriate.
  - Policies and procedures incorporate standards and guidelines for all facets of patient care across all settings as needed.
  - Policies and procedures are jointly reviewed and approved by the nurse executive and staff nurse committee, the blood bank or transfusion service, and the medical director or medical executive committee.
- Patients are identified using two methods of identification and two health care providers, one of whom is the transfusionist.
- Informed consent is obtained for blood and blood components; the patient refusal would include all blood components.
- Standard precautions should specify how to draw blood samples and administer the transfusion to prevent exposure to blood-borne pathogens.
  - Latex-free equipment is available for latex-sensitive patients and personnel.
  - Policy is established and equipment is provided to prevent accidental blood exposure and needlestick injury.
- The entire transfusion and the patient's reactions are documented according to institutional practice.
- Monitoring for quality and safety is ongoing.

Factor V Leiden increases the risk of venous thrombosis by a factor of 5 to 10 for **heterozygous** (one inherited gene) individuals and substantially more of a risk factor, 50 to 100, for **homozygous** (two inherited genes) individuals. Areas for clots and other complications of factor V Leiden are outlined in Box 17-7.

BOX 17-7 COMPLICATIONS ASSOCIATED WITH FACTOR V LEIDEN

- Venous thrombosis blood clots in veins, such as
  - Deep vein thrombosis, veins in the arms and legs
  - Superficial thrombophlebitis
  - Sinus vein thrombosis, veins around the brain
  - Mesenteric vein thrombosis, intestinal veins
  - Budd-Chiari syndrome, liver veins
- Pulmonary embolism, blood clots in the lungs
- Arterial clots (stroke, heart attack) in selected patients (some smokers)
- Possibly with stillbirth or recurrent unexplained miscarriage
- Preeclampsia and/or eclampsia (toxemia while pregnant)

PROTHROMBIN GENE G20210A

The prothrombin 20210A mutation is the second most common inherited clotting abnormality. It is present in 1% to 2% of the white population. In fact, in 3% to 8% of patients with a venous thromboembolism, the prothrombin 20210A mutation is found. It is only a mild risk factor for clots, but together with other risk factors such as oral contraceptives or combined with other clotting disorders (like factor V Leiden), the risk of clotting increases dramatically (Figure 17-2).

TREATMENT FOR HYPERCOAGULABILITY STATES

Treatment of a patient with increased prothrombotic factors depends on the individual patient's risk of recurrent thromboembolic disease. When one has a venous clot, regardless of what thrombophilic state(s) one may have, that person will receive anticoagulation. This is accomplished by several different medications: heparin, warfarin, and low molecular weight heparins. These medications are generally used for 3 to 6 months. Further continuation is generally not indicated in hypercoagulable states after a single thromboembolic episode, given the risk of bleeding associated with anticoagulation. Patients who have had multiple thromboembolic episodes or are at high risk of further episodes (e.g., those with

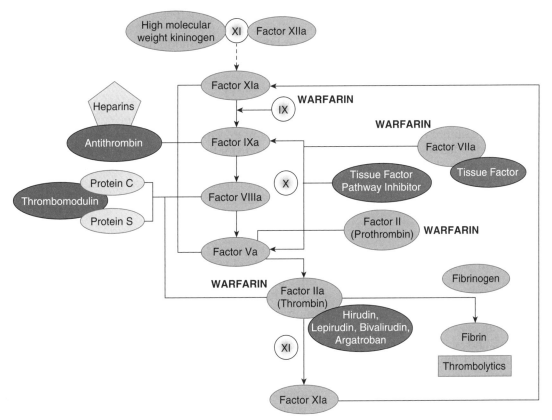

FIGURE 17-2 The clotting cascade.

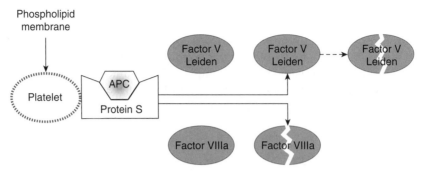

FIGURE 17-3 The effect of factor V Leiden on activated protein C (APC). The formation of APC is not altered by the presence of factor V Leiden. However, the complex of APC and protein S on the platelet phospholipid's surface cannot inactivate factor V Leiden as efficiently as it normally can (occurs about 80 times slower than normal). It is able to inactivate factor VIIIa normally. This is known as APC resistance.

multiple deficiencies or factor V Leiden homozygotes) are likely started on long-term anticoagulation (Weinstein, 2009). The use of Lovenox may be indicated prior to long plane flights and other activities that increase the risk of clotting.

Long-term anticoagulation has risks associated with it. Beginning long-term anticoagulation is influenced by the patient's overall risk of recurrent thrombosis balanced against the risks associated with long-term anticoagulation on an individual basis.

Terminology

The terms heterozygous (*hetero*, different) and homozygous (*homo*, same) are used in genetics. The human genome contains two copies of the information. If the copies are the same, they are homozygous; if the copies are different, they are heterozygous. For example, take a protein called A. The normal genome would code for the protein as AA. This is homozygous for the normal protein. If there is a variation of the protein called "a," there are two possible ways to get "a." The genome could be Aa, which is called heterozygous, or the genome could be aa, which is called homozygous (Figure 17-3).

SUMMARY

Transfusion of blood saves life. An error in blood transfusion, at the same time, takes life. Nurses being responsible for the final bedside check before transfusion, have the final opportunity to prevent a mistransfusion (Mole, Hogg, & Benvie, 2007). Blood and blood component therapies are commonly ordered within diverse health care settings. Today's health care consumer is more aware than ever before of the inherent dangers of transfusion and will advocate on behalf of himself or a family member. Published literature has validated the consequences of blood transfusion errors and the element of human error involved in such wrong transfusions including administration to the wrong recipient, phlebotomy errors, testing of wrong specimen, and failure to detect at the bedside before transfusion of the wrong unit. A nurse, by profession, has opportunities to ensure safe blood and blood component therapy.

Review Questions   *Note: Questions below may have more than one right answer.*

1. The antigen in the ABO system that denotes a person's blood group is located
   A. On the RBC
   B. In the plasma
   C. In the serum
   D. On body tissue

2. Which of the following may stimulate a reaction?
   A. Antigen A combining with anti-A antibody
   B. Antigen AB combining with anti-AB antibody
   C. Antigen B combining with anti-A antibody
   D. Antigen D combining with anti-D antibody

3. A febrile nonhemolytic reaction is characterized by
   A. Anxiety
   B. Change in blood pressure
   C. Chills and rigors
   D. All of the above

4. The most important intervention for patients with IVIG-associated nonallergic reactions is to
   A. Slow the infusion rate
   B. Discontinue the infusion
   C. Continue the rate because the reaction will resolve
   D. Stop the infusion for 4 to 8 hours and then resume therapy

5. A patient, group O, may receive RBCs from a donor who is
   A. Group A only
   B. Group O only
   C. Group A or O
   D. Any group

6. A patient, group AB, may receive plasma from a donor who is
   A. Group A, AB, or O
   B. Group AB or O
   C. Group AB only
   D. Any group

7. Intravascular hemolytic reactions are potentially caused by
   A. ABO incompatibility
   B. Rh incompatibility
   C. ABO and Rh incompatibility
   D. None of the above

8. The primary cause of PTH is
   A. HAV and HBV
   B. HBV and HCV
   C. HAV and HDV
   D. HBV only

9. Leukocyte-reduced blood and blood components are ordered to prevent which transfusion reaction?
   A. Anaphylaxis
   B. Citrate toxicity
   C. Febrile, allergic reaction
   D. Febrile, nonhemolytic reaction

10. An elderly patient with a history of heart failure is most at risk for which potential transfusion reaction from a unit of packed RBCs?
    A. Acute hemolytic reaction
    B. Circulatory overload
    C. Hypersensitivity reaction
    D. Iron overload

References and Selected Readings   *Asterisks indicate references cited in text.*

*American Association of Blood Banks. (2010). *Primer of blood administration*. Bethesda, MD: Author.

*American Association of Blood Banks. (2011). *Technical manual* (17th ed.). Bethesda, MD: Author.

American Association of Blood Banks. (2012). *Standards for blood banks and transfusion services* (28th ed.). Bethesda, MD: Author.

*American Association of Blood Banks, American Red Cross, America's Blood Centers, & the Armed Services Blood Program.. (2009). *Circular of information for the use of human blood and blood components*. Bethesda, MD: Author.

*American Red Cross. (2012). *Compendium of transfusion practice guidelines* (1st ed.). Washington, DC: Author.

*American Red Cross. (2013). Donating blood. http://www.redcrossblood.org/donating-blood

*Benjamin, R.J., & McLaughlin, L.S. (2012). Plasma components: Properties, differences, and uses. *Transfusion*, *52*, 9S–19S.

*Brooks, J.P. (2008). Quality improvement opportunities in blood banking and transfusion medicine. *Clinical Laboratory Medicine*, *28*, 321–337.

*Centers for Disease Control and Prevention. (2011). Blood safety. http://www.cdc.gov/bloodsafety/

*Davis, R., Geiger, B., Gutierrez, A., Heaser, J., & Veeramani, D. (2009). Tracking blood products in blood centres using radio frequency identification: A comprehensive assessment. *Vox Sanguinis*, *97*, 50–60.

*Faulhaber, J., & Aberg, J.A. (2009). Acquired immunodeficiency syndrome. In C. M. Porth (Ed.), *Pathophysiology: Concepts of altered health states* (8th ed., pp. 427–447). Philadelphia, PA: Wolters Kluwer Health/Lippincott Williams & Wilkins.

*Gahart, B.L., & Nazareno, A.R. (2012). *2013 Intravenous medications: A handbook for nurses and health professionals* (29th ed.). St. Louis, MO: Elsevier Mosby.

*Gaspard, K.J. (2009a). Blood cells and the hematopoietic system. In C. M. Porth (Ed.), *Pathophysiology: Concepts of altered health states* (8th ed., pp. 254–261). Philadelphia, PA: Wolters Kluwer Health/Lippincott Williams & Wilkins.

Gaspard, K.J. (2009b). Disorders of hemostasis. In C. M. Porth (Ed.), *Pathophysiology: Concepts of altered health states* (8th ed., pp. 262–277). Philadelphia, PA: Wolters Kluwer Health/Lippincott Williams & Wilkins.

Gaspard, K.J. (2009c). Disorders of red blood cells. In C.M. Porth (Ed.), *Pathophysiology: Concepts of altered health states* (8th ed., pp. 278–300). Philadelphia, PA: Wolters Kluwer Health/Lippincott Williams & Wilkins.

Grody, W.W., Griffin, J.H., Taylor, A.K., Korf, B.R., Heit, J.A., et al. (2007). *Consensus statement on factor V Leiden mutation testing*. http://www.acmg.net/resources/policies/pol-009.asp

*Hohberger, C., Davis, R., Briggs, L., Gutierrez, A., & Veeramani, D. (2012). Applying radio-frequency identification (RFID) technology in transfusion medicine. *Biologicals*, *40*, 209–213.

Infusion Nurses Society. (2011). Infusion nursing standards of practice. *Journal of Infusion Nursing*, *34*, S1–S110.

*Institute of Medicine. (2011). *The future of nursing: Leading change, advancing health*. Washington, DC: National Academies Press.

*Kleinman, S., Gajic, O., & Nunes, E. (2007). Promoting recognition and prevention of transfusion-related acute lung injury. *Critical Care Nurse*, *27*, 49–53.

Lefkowitz, J.B. (2008). Coagulation pathway and physiology. In *Hemostasis physiology*. Northfield, IL: College of American Pathologists. www.cap.org/apps/docs/cap_press/hemostasis_testing/coagulation_pathway.pdf

*McLeod, B.C. (2012). Plasma and plasma derivatives in therapeutic plasmapheresis. *Transfusion*, *52*, S38–S44.

*Mole, L.J., Hogg, G., & Benvie, S. (2007). Evaluation of a teaching pack designed for nursing students to acquire the essential knowledge for competent practice in blood transfusion administration. *Nurse Education in Practice*, *7*(4), 228–237.

Morrison, A.P., Tanasijevic, M.J., Goonan, E.M., Lobo, M.M., Bates, M.M., Lipsitz, S.R., et al. (2010). Reduction in specimen labeling errors after implementation of a positive patient identification system in phlebotomy. *American Journal of Clinical Pathology*, *133*, 870–877.

Murphy, M.F., Fraser, E., Miles, D., Noel, S., Staves, J., Cripps, B., et al. (2012). How do we monitor hospital transfusion practice using an end-to-end electronic transfusion management system? *Transfusion*, *52*, 2502–2512.

Pandey, S., & Vyas, G.N. (2012). Adverse effects of plasma transfusion. *Transfusion, 52,* 65S–79S.

*Porth, C.M. (2009). Disorders of white blood cells and lymphoid tissue. In C.M. Porth (Ed.), *Pathophysiology: Concepts of altered health states* (8th ed., pp. 301–321). Philadelphia, PA: Wolters Kluwer Health/Lippincott Williams & Wilkins.

*Sommer, C. (2009). Innate and adaptive immunity. In C.M. Porth (Ed.), *Pathophysiology: Concepts of altered health states* (8th ed., pp. 347–376). Philadelphia, PA: Wolters Kluwer Health/Lippincott Williams & Wilkins.

*The Joint Commission. (2013). *National patient safety goals.* http://www.jointcommission.org/hap_2013_npsg/

*Triulzi, D.J. (2009). Transfusion-related acute lung injury: Current concepts for the clinician. *Anesthesia and Analgesia, 108,* 770–776.

*U.S. Department of Health and Human Services. (2011). The 2009 national blood collection and utilization survey report. http://www.aabb.org/programs/biovigilance/nbcus/Pages/default.aspx

*U.S. Department of Health and Human Services. (2013). Updating regulations in recognition of changing technology. http://www.hhs.gov/open/execorders/13563/highlights/6a1-updatingregs.html

University of Illinois–Urbana/Champaign. (2001). Clotting cascade. http://www.med.illinois.edu/hematology/PtClotInfo.htm

University of Illinois–Urbana/Champaign. (2001). Factor V Leiden. http://www.med.illinois.edu/hematology/PtFacV2.htm

*Weinstein, S. (2009). Factor V Leiden: Impact on infusion nursing. *Journal of Infusion Nursing, 32*(4), 219–223.

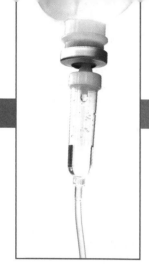

CHAPTER 18

Pharmacology Applied to Infusion Therapy

Lindsey M. Ladell
Sherry A. Tennies

KEY TERMS

Double
 Decomposition
Drug Concentration
Half-life
Hydrolysis
Incompatibility
Laminar Flow
Leaching

Oxidation
pH
Pharmacokinetics
Plasma Concentration
Precipitation
Receptor Site
Reduction
Therapeutic Index

ADMINISTERING DRUG THERAPY BY THE INTRAVENOUS ROUTE

The administration of medications via the intravenous (IV) route is common across health care settings. The nurse whose patients receive IV drug therapy needs to be well versed in the advantages and disadvantages of drug therapy delivered by the IV route. The nurse also needs to be a skilled practitioner who can administer IV drugs safely, monitor the patient's response to therapy, instruct the patient regarding the prescribed medication therapy, and prevent potential adverse events. Nurses must have a comprehensive understanding of IV drug therapy to ensure patient safety and quality patient outcomes.

PATIENT SAFETY

Nurses are in a unique position to improve IV drug administration due to their proximity to the patient, insight to identify potential problems and to be a part of safety solutions.

This chapter is intended to expand the nurse's knowledge about pharmacology as it relates to the safe preparation and delivery of IV drug therapy. The Institute of Medicine (IOM), in its hallmark report, demonstrated that the most common type of medical error is related to medication administration (IOM, 1999); thus, each section will address related patient safety matters. The first section offers a review of infusion therapy, including advantages and disadvantages of the IV route. The second section addresses patient considerations during IV medication delivery. The third section discusses pharmacokinetics and selected parameters for IV drugs. The fourth section details drug dosage and flow rate calculations.

ADVANTAGES OF THE INTRAVENOUS ROUTE

The IV route of drug administration offers pronounced advantages:

- Offers an alternate route for medication administration in patients who are unable to take medications orally or for those who need medications that cannot be absorbed by any other route
- Allows drugs to be administered to a patient who cannot tolerate fluids and drugs by the gastrointestinal route
- Allows for the capacity to control the rate of administration of medications and the ability to slow or stop drug delivery at once if sensitivity reactions occur
- Provides the route of administration for drugs that would not otherwise be able to be absorbed by the gastrointestinal route due to large molecular size or due to instability of the medication in the presence of gastric juices destroying the drug
- Provides the route of administration for medications that have irritating properties and cause pain and trauma when given intramuscularly or subcutaneously
- Provides rapid drug action via the vascular system since the drug bypasses processing in the gastrointestinal system and circulates directly in the bloodstream
- Offers better control over the rate of administration of drugs; prolonged action can be provided by administering a dilute infusion intermittently or over a prolonged period

Understanding the basics of pharmacokinetics, pharmacodynamics, and pharmacotherapeutics provides an insight into how the IV route offers rapid drug action and better control over the duration of action.

PATIENT SAFETY

Even with the advantages of the IV route, there remains the potential for infection from the insertion site, catheter, or infusate. On a daily basis, review the need for IV access (CDC, 2011).

Pharmacokinetics and Selected Parameters for Intravenous Drugs

Pharmacokinetics refers to the way in which a medication reacts in the body and includes how a drug is absorbed, distributed, metabolized, and eliminated by the body. The pharmacokinetic basis of therapeutics relies on various factors, such as the drug's route and frequency of administration, to achieve and maintain a proper **drug concentration** at the **receptor site**, where the drug exerts its action. If an insufficient amount of drug reaches this site of action, the drug may appear to be ineffective, and the therapy may therefore be discontinued. Conversely, the typically appropriate dosage of a drug may produce toxicity, and therefore therapy may be discontinued simply because excessive amounts are in the body. An awareness of how drug pharmacokinetics affects the body is an essential part of preventing or lessening potential toxicity. Factors influencing the pharmacokinetics of drugs are presented in Box 18-1. Some aspects of pharmacokinetics that are particularly relevant to IV drug administration are therapeutic index, plasma concentration, and drug distribution.

THERAPEUTIC INDEX

The **therapeutic index** is the margin between a drug's therapeutic and toxic concentrations at the receptor site. Some medications, such as warfarin, are considered to have a narrow therapeutic index, meaning that the margin between therapeutic and toxic concentrations is small. Pharmacokinetic models describe and predict drug amounts and concentrations in various body fluids and the changes in these quantities over time.

PLASMA CONCENTRATIONS

Plasma concentration is a measurement representing a drug that is bound to plasma protein plus a drug that is unbound or free. Two factors determine the degree of plasma protein binding. The first is the binding affinity of the drug for the plasma proteins; the second is

---

BOX 18-1   FACTORS INFLUENCING THE PHARMACOKINETICS OF DRUGS AND PATIENT RESPONSE

Patient Characteristics

Age, sex, body weight, dietary habits, smoking habits, alcohol consumption, coingestion of other drugs, other treatment protocols

Disease States

Hepatic disease, renal disease, congestive heart failure, infection, fever, shock, severe burns

the number of binding sites available or the concentration of plasma protein. An acidic drug, such as salicylate or phenytoin, may be bound to the protein, albumin. A basic drug, such as lidocaine or quinidine, may be bound to serum globulins. Calculated plasma concentrations may assist the provider in evaluating the effectiveness or potential for toxicity of the therapy. Figure 18-1 shows concentration–time curves after IV drug injection at three different rates.

THERAPEUTIC CONCENTRATION AND LOADING DOSE

The drug concentration level may be calculated after the dosage regimen is initiated to ensure that the selected dosage produces the drug concentration desired. It may also be measured periodically to ensure that the dosage continues to produce the desired target concentration or to determine if the therapeutic regimen is failing. Table 18-1 highlights therapeutic drug concentrations and toxic values.

The loading dose is the initial dose of drug ordered and is used to decrease the time it takes for a drug to reach a target or the therapeutic, concentration. Loading doses are not always practical or safe but necessary at times. For example, when administering vanco-mycin, the first dose may be given as a loading dose to assure that the drug concentration reaches the appropriate therapeutic level to kill bacteria.

DRUG HALF-LIFE

The term **half-life** denotes the time required for the plasma concentration of a drug or the total amount of drug in the body to decline by one half. The half-life of a drug depends on its volume of distribution (the distribution between the plasma and the various other fluids and tissues, and the actual nature of distribution and clearance). Upon discontinuation of

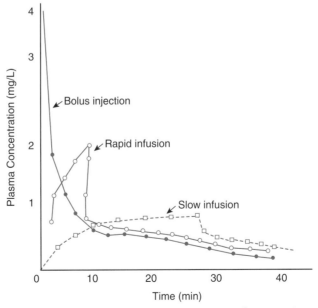

FIGURE 18-1 Concentration–time curves after IV injec-tion at three different rates.

TABLE 18-1	SELECTED THERAPEUTIC DRUG CONCENTRATIONS AND TOXIC VALUES	
Drug	**Therapeutic Concentration**	**Toxic Value**
Amikacin (Amikin)	25–35 µg/mL (peak level) or 43–60 µmol/L	> 35–40 µg/mL or > 60–68 µmol/L
Nitroprusside (Nipride)	0.5–1.5 µg/mL or 2.7–4.1 µmol/L	> 10 µg/mL or > 27.0 µmol/L
Procainamide (Pronestyl)	4–10 µg/mL or 17–42 µmol/L	10–12 µg/mL or > 42–51 µmol/L
Theophylline (Slo-Phyllin)	9–20 µg/mL or 44–111 µmol/L	> 20 µg/mL or > 111 µmol/L
Tobramycin (Nebcin)	8–10 µg/mL (peak level) or 17–21 µmol/L	> 10 µg/mL or 21–26 µmol/L
Vancomycin (Vancoled)	20–40 µg/mL (peak level) or 14–28 µmol/L	> 80–100 µg/mL or 55–69 µmol/L

a medication, the drug concentration is reduced by 50% after one half-life; it is reduced by 75% after two half-lives; it is reduced by 87.5% after three half-lives; and the drug concentration is reduced by 93.75% after four half-lives.

DISADVANTAGES OF THE INTRAVENOUS ROUTE

Despite the advantages of the IV route, there are certain actual or potential hazards. They include the following:

- Therapeutic incompatibilities: may occur when one or more drugs are added to the IV solution, including antagonism, synergism, and potentiation (Turner & Hankins, 2010).
- Anaphylaxis: a hypersensitive reaction induced by preliminary drug injection.
- Speed shock: an adverse systemic reaction to a substance rapidly injected into the bloodstream.
- Vascular irritations and subsequent problems: including phlebitis, infiltration, extravasation, infection, and air embolism.
- Rapid onset of action: inability to recall a drug once it enters the bloodstream.
- Precipitate formation: may occur when one or more drugs are added to a parenteral solution. The precipitate does not always form when the solution is prepared, which increases the challenge of IV administration. Some drugs that are stable for a limited time degrade and may or may not precipitate as they become less therapeutically active. If administered IV, fluids containing insoluble matter carry the potential danger of embolism, myocardial damage, and harmful effects on other organs such as the liver and the kidneys.

Incompatibilities

The number of possible drug combinations is overwhelming, as is the potential for incompatibility. Incompatibility is the undesired reaction occurring between the drug and the solution, the container, or another drug (Turner & Hankins, 2010). Manufacturers provide an ever-increasing number of new drug products for the treatment of disease processes.

Compounding drugs for IV administration is usually performed as a component of a hospital-based or home infusion pharmacy. Today, admixture programs have expanded their service base to provide compounding services for extended care, ambulatory care, and any clinical setting in which infusion therapies are delivered.

All people responsible for mixing and compounding IV drugs must be alert to the hazards involved. Compatibility charts are provided through admixture services to alert the nurse to potential problems, particularly when additions to infusions in progress are made on a nursing unit or added in a patient's residence.

A factor related to compatibility is the composition of the solution container. Box 18-2 lists drugs affected by increased *adsorption* (adhesion to the surfaces of substances with which they are in contact) when infused in polyvinyl chloride (PVC) containers (Trissel, 2013). Factors affecting the compatibility of drugs include order of mixing, quantity of the drug and solution, room temperature, and light. Incompatibilities are not always obvious to the naked eye. They may be classified as physical, chemical, or therapeutic and are described in Box 18-3.

Leaching is the release of di(2-ethylhexyl)phthalate (DEHP) from PVC containers into the medication in solution. DEHP has a wide range of toxic effects, especially in male neonates where the infant's reproductive system can be compromised. Products like lipid emulsions and cyclosporine exacerbate leaching.

CHEMICAL

The most common incompatibilities are the result of certain chemical reactions (FDA, 2012)—for example, hydrolysis is the process in which water absorption causes decomposition of a compound. In preparing solutions of salt, the nurse should understand that certain salts, when placed in water, hydrolyze, forming a strong acid and a weak base or a weak acid and a strong base. Because pH is a significant factor in the solubility of drugs, the increased acidity or alkalinity from hydrolysis of a salt may result in an incompatibility if another drug is added. For example, the acid salt sodium bicarbonate when placed in water

---

BOX 18-2   DRUGS WITH INCREASED ADSORPTION WHEN INFUSED USING PVC CONTAINERS

Diazepam

Hydralazine (Apresoline)

Insulin

Lorazepam

Nitroglycerin

Phenothiazine tranquilizers (Thorazine, Compazine)

Thiopental sodium

Urokinase

Vitamin A acetate (nonpalmitate form)

Warfarin sodium

BOX 18-3   TYPES OF INCOMPATIBILITIES

Physical—Those in which an undesirable change is physically observed, such as sodium bicarbonate and calcium chloride forming an insoluble precipitate (see http://www.fda.gov/downloads/Drugs/GuidanceComplianceRegulatoryInformation/Guidances/ucm292362.pdf)

Chemical—Those occurring in the molecular structure or pharmacologic properties of a substance (note: They may or may not be physically observed), such as penicillin and ascorbic acid lowering the pH

Therapeutic—Those in which an undesirable reaction results from the overlapping effects of two drugs given together or closely together, such as penicillin and tetracycline inhibiting the bactericidal effect of penicillin

---

hydrolyzes to form a strong alkali (sodium hydroxide) and a weak and unstable acid (carbonic acid). Many organic acids are known as weak acids because they ionize only slightly.

Reduction is the process whereby one or more atoms gain electrons at the expense of some other part of the system (ASHP, 2013).

Oxidation is the corresponding loss of electrons occurring when reduction takes place. Antioxidants are often used as preservatives to prevent oxidation of a compound.

Double decomposition is the chemical reaction in which ions of two compounds change places and two new compounds are thus formed (ASHP, 2013). A great many salts act by double decomposition to form other salts, and this process accounts for a large number of incompatibilities. For example, calcium chloride is incompatible with sodium bicarbonate; the double decomposition results in the formation of the insoluble salt, calcium carbonate.

PHYSICAL

Precipitation may occur in some parenteral solutions; some commonly prescribed drugs precipitate when added to IV solutions. Differences in the physical and chemical properties of each of these solutions may affect the stability of any drug introduced.

Moreover, a compound that is soluble in one solution may precipitate in another. Sodium ampicillin deteriorates in acid solutions. This drug, when added to isotonic sodium chloride at a concentration of 30 mg/mL, loses < 10% activity in 8 hours. However, when it is added to 5% dextrose in water, usually a more acid solution, its stability is reduced to a 4-hour period.

pH AND STABILITY

Because pH plays an important role in drug solubility, stability, and compatibility, a definition is in order. The term **pH** stands for the degree of concentration of hydrogen ions or the acidity of the solution. The weight of hydrogen ions in 1 L pure water is 0.0000001 g, which is numerically equal to 10^{-7}. For convenience, the negative logarithm is used. Because it is at this concentration that the hydrogen ions balance the hydroxyl ions, a pH of 7 is neutral. Each unit decrease in pH represents a 10-fold increase in hydrogen ions.

The greatest number of drug incompatibilities may be produced by changes in pH (ASHP, 2013). For example, precipitation occurs when a compound is insoluble in solution.

The degree of solubility often varies with the pH. A drastic change in the pH of a drug when added to an IV solution suggests an incompatibility or a decrease in stability.

Solutions with a high pH appear to be incompatible with solutions with a low pH and may form insoluble free acids or free bases. A chart denoting the pH of certain drugs and certain solutions to be used as a vehicle is helpful in warning of potential incompatibilities. A broad pH range (3.5 to 6.5) of dextrose solutions is allowed by the *United States Pharmacopeia (USP)*. A drug may be stable in one bottle of dextrose 5% in water and not in another (FDA, 2012).

Again, whereas one drug may be compatible in a solution, a second additive may alter the established pH to such an extent as to make the drugs unstable (Box 18-4). Buffers or antioxidants in a drug may cause two drugs, however, compatible, to precipitate. For

---

BOX 18-4   FACTORS AFFECTING THE STABILITY OF INTRAVENOUS DRUGS AND SOLUTIONS

Precipitation of Parenteral Solution

- Some commonly prescribed drugs precipitate when added to IV solutions.
- Differences in the physical and chemical properties of each of these solutions may affect the stability of any drug introduced.
- A compound soluble in one solution may precipitate in another. Sodium ampicillin deteriorates in acid solutions. This drug, when added to isotonic sodium chloride at a concentration of 30 mg/mL, loses <10% activity in 8 hours. However, when it is added to dextrose 5% in water, usually a more acid solution, and its stability is reduced to a 4-hour period.

pH

- A broad pH range (3.5 to 6.5) of dextrose solutions is allowed by the USP. A drug may be stable in one bottle of dextrose 5% in water and not in another.

Additional Drugs

- One drug may be compatible in a solution, but a second additive may alter the established pH to such an extent as to make the drugs unstable.

Buffering Agents in Drugs

- Presence of buffers or antioxidants, which may cause two drugs, however, compatible, to precipitate. For example, ascorbic acid, the buffering component of tetracycline, lowers the pH of the product and therefore may accelerate the decomposition of a drug susceptible to an acid environment.

Preservatives in the Diluent

- Sterile diluents for reconstitution of drugs are available with or without a bacteriostatic agent.
- The bacteriostatic agents usually consist of parabens or phenol preservatives.
- Certain drugs, including nitrofurantoin, amphotericin B, and erythromycin, are incompatible with these preservatives and should be reconstituted with sterile water for injection.

BOX 18-4 FACTORS AFFECTING THE STABILITY OF INTRAVENOUS DRUGS AND SOLUTIONS (*Continued*)

Degree of Dilution

- Solubility often varies with the volume of solution in which a drug is introduced. For example, tetracycline hydrochloride, mixed in a small volume of fluid, maintains its pH range over 24 hours. However, when added to a large volume (1 L), it degrades after 12 hours, becoming less therapeutically active.

Length of Time Solution Stands

- Decomposition of substances in solution is proportional to the length of time they stand. For example, sodium ampicillin with the high pH of 8 to 10 becomes unstable when maintained in an acid environment over time.

Order of Mixing

- The order in which drugs are added to infusions often determines their compatibility.

Light

- Light may provide energy for chemical reactions to occur.
- Certain drugs, such as amphotericin B and nitrofurantoin, once diluted must be protected from light.

Room Temperature

- Heat provides energy for reactions.
- After reconstitution or initial dilution, refrigeration prolongs the stability of many drugs.

---

example, ascorbic acid, the buffering component of tetracycline, lowers the pH of the product and therefore may accelerate the decomposition of a drug susceptible to an acid environment.

Preservatives in the diluent may lead to problems as well. Sterile diluents for reconstitution of drugs are available with or without a bacteriostatic agent. The bacteriostatic agents usually consist of parabens or phenol preservatives.

DILUTION AND SOLUBILITY

Solubility often varies with the volume of solution in which a drug is introduced. For example, tetracycline hydrochloride, mixed in a small volume of fluid, maintains its pH range over 24 hours. However, when added to a large volume (1 L), it degrades after 12 hours, becoming less therapeutically active.

OTHER FACTORS

- The order in which drugs are added to infusions often determines their compatibility.

- Light may provide energy for chemical reactions to occur. Certain drugs, such as amphotericin B and nitrofurantoin, once diluted, must be protected from light.
- Room temperature may affect incompatibility. Heat provides energy for reactions, which is why reconstituted or diluted drugs are refrigerated to prolong stability.

Vascular Irritation

Vascular irritation is a significant hazard of drugs administered IV. Any irritation that inflames and roughens the endothelial cells of the venous wall allows platelets to adhere to the wall and promotes the formation of a thrombus. Thrombophlebitis is the result of the sterile inflammation. When a thrombus occurs, the inherent danger of embolism is always present.

If aseptic technique is not strictly followed, septic thrombophlebitis may result from bacteria that is introduced through the infusion catheter and then trapped within the thrombus. This is much more serious because of the potential dangers of septicemia and acute bacterial endocarditis. Strategies for avoiding vascular irritation are presented in Box 18-5.

SAFEGUARDS TO MINIMIZE HAZARDS OF ADMINISTERING INTRAVENOUS DRUGS

Medication systems in hospitals are complex and multilayered, involving many steps and many people. According to the Institute for Safe Medication Practices (ISMP), this complexity increases the probability of errors (American Hospital Association, 2013; Cohen, 2007).

BOX 18-5   STRATEGIES FOR PREVENTING VASCULAR IRRITATION

Select Most Appropriate Site

- Use veins with ample blood volume.
- Avoid veins in lower extremities.
- Start at the most distal location.

Select Most Appropriate Catheter

- Select a catheter that is appreciably smaller than the lumen of the vein so that smooth blood flow can provide adequate hemodilution.

Infuse Drug Carefully

- Administer isotonic solutions after administering hypertonic solutions to flush irritating substances.
- Infuse slowly; slow administration provides greater dilution of the drug in a large vein.
- Adhere to recommendations for the following: use of filters, inspection of solution for clarity, proper reconstitution, and dilution of additives.

Monitor Regularly

- Change the insertion site at designated intervals and as needed because prolonged catheter insertion increases the risk of phlebitis.

Errors may occur at any stage—prescribing, ordering, dispensing, administering, or monitoring the effects of medication. Common sources of medication errors in health systems are presented in Box 18-6. In Table 18-2, the collaborative responsibilities of health care personnel involved in IV drug therapy are outlined. Ten key elements of medication use, as defined by ISMP are:

BOX 18-6 MEDICATION SAFETY ALERT! COMMON SOURCES OF MEDICATION ERRORS

Unavailable Patient Information

The patient's clinical record lacks critical patient information (laboratory values, allergies).

Unavailable Drug Information

Clinical pharmacy expertise is not provided on-site.

Miscommunication

Failed communication owing to illegible handwriting, confusion of drugs with similar names, confusion of metric and apothecary systems, ambiguous or incomplete orders is a common cause of error.

Problems With Labeling, Packaging, and Nomenclature

Unit dose medications may not be available throughout the health care institution, and drug administration procedures do not ensure that medications remain labeled until they reach the patient.

Poor Storage Procedures

Stocking multiple concentrations or storing drugs in look-alike containers may contribute to error.

Inconsistent Standards

Drug device acquisition, use, and monitoring may be inadequately standardized, leading to use of unsafe equipment or errors.

Work Environment

Excessive interruptions and excessive workload may lead to error.

Limited Staff Education

In-service training should alert staff to potential for errors and serve as a reminder.

Insufficient Patient Education

Patient education is essential to good patient outcomes. Patient engagement and participation in care promote good care and help prevent errors.

Flawed Quality Improvement Processes and Risk Management

Quality systems should include methods for identifying, reporting, analyzing, and correcting errors, as well as measurement systems for tracking the effect of system changes.

TABLE 18-	RESPONSIBILITIES FOR INTRAVENOUS DRUG ADMINISTRATION
Institution	• Provide written policies • Issue approved drug list • Offer continuing education • Provide institutional review board approval of investigational drugs
Licensed Independent Practitioner	• Provide written drug order • Act as overall gatekeeper • Administer drugs not on approved list • Participate in continuing medical education
Pharmacist	• Maintain a drug incompatibility profile • Implement admixture process • Perform safe compounding • Act in clinical pharmacy role • Participate in continuing education
Nurse	• Adhere to seven "rights" of drug administration • Assess and monitor the patient during drug administration • Participate in continuing education • Keep current knowledge base of drug delivery systems • Educate the patients • Update knowledge of antidotes

- Patient information
- Drug information
- Adequate communication
- Drug packaging, labeling, and nomenclature
- Medication storage, stock, standardization, and distribution
- Drug device acquisition, use, and monitoring
- Environmental factors
- Staff education and competency
- Patient education
- Quality processes and risk management

Various safeguards are in place to diminish the potential hazards of IV drug administration. Safeguards affect the activities of all disciplines and departments. These include lists of drugs approved for IV use by an institution's pharmacy, laws regulating the use and availability of potentially dangerous drugs (controlled substances), standards and protocols for admixture preparation, standards for monitoring and documenting patient responses to drugs, resources for accurate dosage calculation, drug expiration dates, regulation of investigational drugs, patient education programs, and safety improvements in drug delivery systems.

Safety improvements in drug delivery systems have been created to improve the IV drug administration process. Process improvements leading to standardization of nursing workspace, patient care processes, and medication products help reduce error and improve safety. "Forcing functions" are process improvements that push or promote the person to do the right thing. For example, when a person is programming a "smart pump" and inadvertently enters a medication dose or rate that is out of the normal range, an alarm will sound and a message provides a visual cue that will not allow programming to continue until the message has been acknowledged. This forces the user to do the right thing and program the pump correctly (Turner & Hankins, 2010).

Approved Drug Lists

Lists of drugs approved for administration by nurses in all clinical care settings must be readily available. In the inpatient setting, the institution's pharmacy and therapeutics committee is the group that usually approves such lists. Infusion nursing professionals are often members of this committee, and protocols are brought to this group for approval before a drug is added to the list. Ideally, the committee provides a list of approved drugs for administration by nurses, a list of drugs approved for addition to infusions in progress, and a list of investigational agents approved for administration (ASHP, 2013; Spath, 2011). In the alternative care environment, home health agencies, infusion centers, and clinics may also develop lists that are subsequently approved by their medical directors before acceptance by the nursing community.

Controlled Substances Act

This act established five categories of controlled substances, known as *schedules*, based on their potential for abuse, the medical indications, and the potential for dependence on the drug. Many of the drugs administered for pain control are Schedule II drugs. Their safe use is regulated by specific prescription and record-keeping requirements.

Safe Admixture Preparation

IV additives and solutions are best prepared in an IV additive station of the institution's pharmacy to ensure sterility and accuracy. Nurses may also prepare drugs in emergencies or when medications must be mixed immediately prior to administration. Aseptic technique is observed and enhanced by a clean-room approach. A laminar flow hood, proper illumination, and handwashing facilities must be readily available in such a setting. Appropriate manufacturing guidelines including cleaning, environmental testing, and expiration guidelines must be strictly adhered to in order to ensure safety (INS, 2011).

USE OF LAMINAR FLOW HOOD

Laminar flow confines airflow to a specific area. The entire body of air within that area moves with uniform velocity along parallel flow lines (INS, 2011). Laminar flow hoods play a vital role in eliminating the hazard of airborne contamination of IV solutions and admixtures. Nurses should be familiar with the general operating guidelines of the hood. Vertical and horizontal hoods are available. Laminar flow hoods should be used according to state and federal guidelines as well as the recommendations of the American Society for Health-System Pharmacists (ASHP).

ADMIXTURE PREPARATION POLICIES AND PROCEDURES

The infusion policies and procedures addressing admixing should define potential hazards, compatibility, stability requirements, and the types of admixtures in the scope of practice. The following are some safeguards that may be implemented to protect both patients and health care personnel from potential health hazards associated with the admixing of medications:

- Aseptic technique is imperative. Bacterial and fungal contamination of drug products and parenteral solutions must be avoided.
- Proper dilution of lyophilized drugs is essential. Two special cautions to ensure complete solubility in the reconstitution of drugs must be observed: the specific diluent recommended by the manufacturer should be used, and the drug should be initially diluted in the volume recommended.
- Introduction of extraneous particles into parenteral solutions must be avoided. Fragments of rubber stoppers are frequently cut out by the needles used and accidentally injected into solutions. Large-bore (15-gauge) needles are practical for use in the nurses' station and appear to have fewer disadvantages than smaller needles, for several reasons. Smaller needles may deposit particles that may be difficult to see on inspection of the solution. The particles may be so small that they can advance through the indwelling catheter. Using filtered aspiration needles when preparing admixtures can remove extraneous particles.
- Any solution that contains visible fragments of rubber must be discarded.

See Table 18-3 for more information on compounding and administering medications in parenteral solutions.

EVIDENCE FOR PRACTICE

Beaney, A. (2010). Preparation of parenteral medicines in clinical areas: How can the risks be managed—A UK perspective? *Journal of Clinical Nursing*, 19, 1569–1577.

A tool was developed to "allow the preparation of parenteral medicines to be scored for risk." This action moves the highest-risk medication preparation from the clinical unit to the pharmacy (Beaney, 2010). Although this study has not been replicated as of this writing, it provides support for nurses adhering to the INS (2011) standard of compounding.

Improved Drug Delivery Systems

Manufacturers have kept pace with demands for improved drug delivery systems for use in all clinical settings in which infusion therapy is administered. Standard methods of drug delivery and terminology still apply.

Intermittent infusion allows drugs to be administered on an intermittent basis through a slow, keep-vein-open infusion, using a secondary container, single-dose additive, or multidose admixture connected to a controlled volume set. The intermittent infusion may also be given through a self-contained administration system such as an elastomeric pump.

TABLE 18-	COMPOUNDING AND ADMINISTERING PARENTERAL MEDICATION

Preparations

1. Check and recheck the order with the drug label.
2. Inscribe order for drug additive directly from original order to medication label or submit electronically to pharmacy.
3. Verify drug orders with the drug product and the parenteral solution.
4. Inspect the solution for extraneous particles.
5. Check the drug product:
   - Expiration date—do not use outdated drugs, which may have lost potency or stability. Check the expiration dates of the drug and of the diluent.
   - Method of administration—intramuscular (IM) preparations are seldom used for IV administration because they may contain components, such as anesthetics or preservatives, not meant for administration by the vascular route. In addition, some are packaged in multidose vials, which may contribute to contamination, and the dosage recommended for IM administration may be inappropriate for IV administration.
   - Clarify any questions or doubts with the patient's physician/LIP
6. Clean the injection site of both the drug product and the diluent with an accepted antiseptic.
7. Use a sterile syringe and needle.
8. Reconstitute medication according to the manufacturer's recommendation.
9. Make sure that the diluted drug is completely dissolved before adding to the parenteral solution.
10. After adding to the solution, invert the solution container to mix the additive completely.
11. Clearly and properly label the solution container with the following (ISMP, 2013):
    - Name of the patient
    - Generic drug name; patient-specific dosage
    - Route of administration; dosing frequency
    - Date and time of compounding; expiration date
    - The preparer's and checker's initials
12. As an added precaution to prevent errors, recheck the label with used drug ampules before discarding ampules.

Administering

1. Inspect the solution for precipitates. If any precipitates are present, discard the solution.
2. Make sure that the drug is compatible with the IV solution if it is administered through a primary line. If incompatible, clamp the set and flush the injection port with compatible fluid. Do not use sterile water. (Note: Electronic infusion devices may be set to flush the line automatically following medication administration.)
3. Also make sure that the drug is compatible with heparin when a heparinized lock is used. If incompatible, flush the lock with a compatible fluid before and after the IV injection.
4. Verify identity of the patient with the solution prepared.
5. Wear gloves when preparing medications and administering infusion therapy. (If latex allergy is a concern, keep in mind that glove manufacturers have developed alternative materials to lessen this concern.)
6. Perform venipuncture consistent with institutional policy and standards of the Infusion Nurses Society (2011).
7. Ensure placement within the lumen of the vessel.
8. Ensure first-dose delivery of the drug in a clinically monitored environment and administer the medication at an evenly divided rate over the length of time recommended by the manufacturer, using a watch with a second hand.
9. Observe the patient for a few minutes after the initial IV administration of any drug that may cause anaphylaxis.
10. Use added caution in administering any drug whose fast action could produce untoward reactions.
11. Document medication administration and patient response in the patient medical record.

Intermittent infusions are typically given through an intermittent infusion device (heparin or saline lock) to conserve veins, allow freedom of motion between infusions, and provide a minimal amount of infusate for the patient whose intake may be restricted.

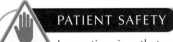

PATIENT SAFETY

Innovations in catheter, tubing, and solution containers/bags have increased patient safety; for example, epidural solution containers/bags cannot be spiked with regular IV tubing. This prevents a possibly highly concentrated drug from being delivered systemically.

Peripheral and central vascular access devices (CVAD) are adaptable as intermittent infusion devices by the addition of a catheter plug or resealable adapter. Patency of these lines is maintained by administering an amount of flush solution sufficient to fill the internal diameter of the line in use. Short peripheral catheters should be flushed with preservative-free 0.9% sodium chloride following each use for adults and children. Heparin lock solution, 10 units/mL heparin, is the preferred lock solution following intermittent use of a CVAD due to the cost and risks associated with these devices (Gorski, Perucca, & Hunter, 2010). Antibiotic lock solutions are not recommended as routine prophylactic practice due to the possibility of developing resistant strains of microorganisms (INS, 2011).

Intravenous push is the direct injection of a medication into the vein. It may be administered through the distal Y site of an administration set, through the intermittent infusion device, or by catheter. The terms *IV push* and *bolus* may be confusing. Substances such as radiopaque dye (contrast media) used to visualize the cardiac chamber must be injected as a bolus (defined as a discrete mass). Most medications ordered for an IV-push or bolus administration must be administered slowly (up to 30 minutes), depending on the drug itself. Rapid injection increases the drug concentration in the plasma, which may reach toxic proportions, flooding the organs rich in blood—the heart and the brain—and resulting in shock and cardiac arrest. The rate of administration, included with the order for the medication, can reduce any misconceptions and prevent the potential risk of a life-threatening reaction from too rapid administration of the drug.

Because delivery of drugs by IV push instantly increases the drug levels in the blood, IV push offers immediate relief to the patient. Nurses in many special care units are trained and authorized to administer specific IV pushes. In the past, the IV push was restricted to the intensive care unit, where the patient was monitored and where a potential crisis might arise requiring its immediate use in the absence of a physician/licensed independent practitioner (LIP). Today, nurses frequently administer IV-push injections.

Many drugs given as IV injections can be potentially dangerous to the patient. The nurse must understand the action of the drug and assess the patient's condition before administering the medication (see Box 18-7 and the next section, Monitoring Response to Treatment).

Continuous administration is the term applied to medications mixed in a large volume of infusate and infused continuously over several hours to several days. Continuous infusion is useful when a medication must be highly diluted or when large volumes of fluids or

> ## BOX 18-7   IMPORTANT SAFETY CHECKPOINTS IN INTRAVENOUS DRUG ADMINISTRATION
>
> ### The Drug
>
> - Understand the expected therapeutic effect of the medication.
> - Know the recommended dosage range and the length of time required for administration.
> - Understand the side effects and toxic symptoms that can occur.
> - Be skilled in using proper antidotes and have appropriate antidotes readily available.
>
> ### The Patient
>
> - Ensure positive identification of the patient: Use two patient identifiers. Do not rely solely on the patient's verbal identification of himself or herself.
> - Ascertain allergy history (food and drug).
> - Assess the patient's condition and be aware of any factors that can affect the drug action.
> - Know what other medications the patient is receiving; be aware of therapeutic incompatibilities that may occur between any other medication the patient is receiving and the IV medication.
> - Watch for the patient's response during and after injection of the medication.

electrolytes require replacement (Turner & Hankins, 2010). The infusion of IV medications can be impacted by patient-specific factors such as:

- Decreased cardiac output
- Reduced renal flow or poor glomerular filtration
- Diminished urinary output
- Pulmonary congestion
- Systemic edema

Greater dilution of the drug and a longer infusion time can prevent drug accumulation, reduce venous irritation caused by a low pH, and allow time to assess the patient's response and detect early reactions. Conversely, possible fluid overload and potential incompatibilities between the infusion and other IV drugs infused through the same access devise are disadvantages to continuous infusion (Turner & Hankins, 2010). Use of the manufacturer's recommended diluent is most important because different drugs require different diluents.

Monitoring Response to Treatment

Knowing the expected therapeutic effects of the medication, the recommended dosage range, untoward drug responses, and symptoms of toxic reactions is essential. Untoward drug responses are undesired and unexpected responses to a medication and can include

---

BOX 18-8   UNTOWARD DRUG RESPONSES

Accumulation—increased concentrations of drug in circulation when the rate of administration is greater than the rate of drug metabolism

Dependence—the need for continued drug administration to prevent withdrawal symptoms

Allergic reaction—hypersensitivity resulting from previous exposure to a drug and manifested by symptoms as mild as itching or hives or as serious as life-threatening anaphylaxis

Idiosyncratic reaction—unpredictable response not attributed to hypersensitivity

Tachyphylaxis—rapidly developing tolerance after few doses

Tolerance—increasing amounts of a drug needed to produce same therapeutic effect

---

tolerance, accumulation, dependence, or drug allergy (Simpson, 2010). Major reactions may consist of respiratory distress, anaphylaxis, cardiac dysrhythmias, and convulsions. Reactions must be detected and reported at once so that proper treatment can be administered. Untoward responses are described in Box 18-8.

Nurses who administer IV medications should be knowledgeable about various antidotes and their use. Emergency supplies of antidotes should be readily available. Many are prepared in prefilled syringes for emergency use. Sterile cartridge needle units, with accurately machine-measured doses, provide a closed-injection system ready for instant use.

Accurate Calculations

An integral component of IV nursing practice is the ability to perform the mathematical calculations required to administer correct doses of the medication and solution to the patients. Accuracy is a priority when medications are administered IV. Guidelines to ensure safety in calculating doses are presented in Box 18-9.

BOX 18-9   DOSAGE CALCULATION

When to calculate the base dose:
- At the start of your shift
- When titrated medications are started and when a transferred patient is receiving titrated medications

Consider the patient's fluid replacement and duration of infusion

Stronger concentrations may be needed to avoid fluid overload

Titrate the drug to the patient's condition and note the response

Use an electronic infusion device to ensure delivery of the prescribed dose

FLOW RATE CALCULATIONS

Flow rate calculations require the following basic information:

- Amount of the solution to be infused
- Duration of the administration
- Drop factor of the set to be used

First, the amount of solution to be administered is determined, and then that number is divided by the delivery time:

$$\frac{1,000\,\text{mL}}{8\,\text{h}} = 125\,\text{mL}/\text{h}$$

Next, the drop factor of the set being used is noted. A macrodrip set takes 10, 15, or 20 drops to deliver 1 mL of solution:

$$\frac{\text{No. of drops}/\text{mL of set}}{60(\text{minutes in an hour})} \times \text{total hourly volume} = \text{no. of drops}/\text{min}$$

$$\frac{\text{mL}/\text{h} \times \text{drop factor of set}}{60} = \text{drops}/\text{min}$$

For microdrip or pediatric systems, the equation is:

$$\frac{\text{mL}/\text{h} \times \text{drop factor}}{60} = \text{drops}/\text{min}$$

DRUG DOSAGE CALCULATIONS

Ratio and proportion or "desired over have" (D/H) may be easily applied to calculation of drug dosages for infusion therapy. The rate of administration of IV drugs may be calculated in units per hour. For example, there are 12,500 units of heparin sodium in 250 mL IV solution. The dose ordered is 800 units/h:

$$X = \frac{250}{12,500}$$
$$X = 0.02$$

Then, calculate the rate of the prescribed dosage:
0.02 mL × 800 units = 16 mL/h

In this example, the nurse has 200 mg drug in 500 mL of dextrose 5% in water and wants to know the number of milligrams of drug the patient is receiving per hour. The amount of drug per milliliter of solution is determined by D/H or:

$$\frac{500}{20} = 25$$
$$\frac{200}{25} = 8\,\text{mg}/\text{h}$$

BOX 18-10   ELEMENTS OF INFORMED CONSENT REGARDING INVESTIGATIONAL THERAPY

- Written by the investigator
- Approved by the institution's review board or ethics committee
- Signed by the subject (patient or volunteer) or authorized representative
- Witnessed

PERCENT SOLUTIONS

The relationship between the amount of solute and the total quantity of solution is expressed as a percentage or ratio. Percentage strength of solution may be calculated in one of three ways:

- Percent weight in weight (w/w)—the weight of the solute (drug) compared with the weight of the solution (g drug/100 g solution)
- Percent weight in volume (w/v)—the weight of the solute compared with the volume of the total solution (g drug/100 mL solution)
- Percent volume in volume (v/v)—the volume of the solute compared with the volume of the total solution (mL drug/100 mL solution)

Expiration Dates

To ensure safe and effective drug therapy, drug containers are labeled with expiration dates that identify when a medication or product is no longer acceptable for use. Institutional policy and procedure should state that medications must not be administered beyond their

---

BOX 18-11   PHASES OF CLINICAL DRUG TRIALS

Phase I: Clinical Pharmacology and Therapeutics

- Evaluate drug safety.
- Determine an acceptable single dosage or levels of patient tolerance for acute multiple dosing of the drug.

Phase II: Initial Clinical Investigation for Therapeutic Effect

- Evaluate drug efficacy.
- Conduct a pilot study.

Phase III: Full-Scale Evaluation of Treatment

- Evaluate the patient population for which the drug is intended.

Phase IV: Postmarketing Surveillance

- Provide additional information about the efficacy or safety profile.

expiration dates. Expiration dates should be verified by the nurse before drugs and infusates are given to patients.

Regulation of Investigational Drugs

Administration of investigational agents is governed by state and federal regulations. Signed informed consent is required before the patients can participate in the investigation (Box 18-10). An informed consent must be written by the investigator, approved by the institutional review board, signed by the subject, and witnessed. Before approval by the U.S. Food and Drug Administration (FDA), drug studies are conducted in four phases (Box 18-11). Policies and procedures should be developed pertaining to the administration of investigational agents, regardless of the clinical setting in which care is provided.

Review Questions *Note: Questions below may have more than one right answer.*

1. Responsibilities for drug administration are shared by which of the following?
   A. Nurse and pharmacist
   B. Institution and physician/LIP
   C. A only
   D. A and B

2. Common sources of error in drug administration include all of the following *except*
   A. Packaging
   B. Work environment
   C. Readily available drug information
   D. Miscommunication

3. Which of the following disease states influences pharmacokinetics of drugs?
   A. Hepatic and renal failure
   B. Congestive heart failure
   C. Presence of infection
   D. Burns

4. Potential hazards of vascular irritation can be minimized by all of the following *except*
   A. Using veins with ample blood volume
   B. Selecting a large catheter
   C. Slowing the rate of administration
   D. Changing the insertion site

5. Before preparing the medication, the nurse should implement which of the following measures?
   A. Question the patient regarding allergy
   B. Check and recheck order with the drug label
   C. Use the manufacturer's diluents as directed
   D. Clarify order with the pharmacist

6. Untoward drug responses include which of the following?
   A. Dependence
   B. Allergic reaction
   C. Accumulation
   D. All of the above

7. Drugs with increased adsorption when infused via PVC containers include
   A. Insulin
   B. Thiopental sodium
   C. A only
   D. A and B

8. The term *half-life* refers to which of the following?
   A. Time of the initial dose of the drug administered
   B. Target concentration of the drug divided by two
   C. Time for plasma concentration of the drug to decline by one half
   D. Time for distribution to occur

9. Quality improvement processes in drug administration include which of the following?

A. Identifying

B. Reporting

C. Analyzing and correcting errors

D. All of the above

10. Which of the following is true of the Controlled Substances Act?

A. It classifies drugs based on potential for abuse

B. It classifies drugs according to medical indications and potential for dependence

C. A only

D. A and B

References and Selected Readings *Asterisks indicate references cited in text.*

*American Hospital Association. (2013). *Quality and patient safety*. Chicago, IL: Author. http://www.aha.org/advocacy-issues/quality/index.shtml

*American Society of Health-System Pharmacists. (2013). *American hospital formulary service*. Bethesda, MD: Author. http://www.ahfsdruginformation.com/

*Centers for Disease Control and Prevention (CDC). (2011). Guidelines for the prevention of intravascular catheter-related infections. http://www.cdc.gov/hicpac/pdf/guidelines/bsi-guidelines-2011.pdf

*Cohen, M.R. (2007). *Medication errors* (2nd ed.). Washington, DC: American Pharmacists Association.

Dougherty, L., Sque, M., & Crouch, R. (2011). Decision-making processes used by nursing during intravenous drug preparation and administration. *Journal of Advanced Nursing, 68*(6), 1302–1311.

*Gorski, L., Perucca, R., & Hunter, M.R. (2010). Central venous access devices: Care, maintenance, and potential complications. In M. Alexander, A. Corrigan, L. Gorski, J. Hankins, & R. Perucca (Eds.), *Infusion nursing: An evidence-based approach* (pp. 495–515). St. Louis, MO: Saunders.

Hicks, R.W., & Becker, S.C. (2006). An overview of intravenous-related medication administration errors as reported to MEDMARX, a national medication error-reporting program. *Journal of Infusion Nursing, 29*(1), 20–27.

Hughes, R.G., & Ortiz, E. (2005). Medication errors: Why they happen and how they can be prevented. *American Journal of Nursing, 105*(3 Suppl.), 14–24.

*Infusion Nurses Society. (2011). Infusion Nursing Standards of Practice. *Journal of Infusion Nursing, 34*(Suppl. 1), S1–S110.

Institute for Safe Medication Practices. (2010). ISMP Medication Safety Alert! Nurse Advise-ERR [Newsletter]. http://www.ismp.org/Newsletters/nursing/default.asp

*Institute for Safe Medicine Practices. (2013). Principles of designing a medication label for intravenous piggyback medication for patient specific, inpatient use. http://www.ismp.org/Tools/guidelines/labelFormats/Piggyback.asp

*Institute of Medicine (IOM). (1999). *To err is human: Building a safer health system*. Washington, DC: National Academies Press.

Leape, L.L., Kabcenell, A.I., Gandhi, T.K., Carver, P., Nolan, T.W., & Berwick, D.M. (2000). Reducing adverse drug events: Lessons from a breakthrough series collaborative. *Joint Commission Journal on Quality and Patient Safety, 26*(6), 321–331.

Nicholas, P., & Agius, C. (2005). Toward Safety IV Medication Administration: The narrow safety margins of many IV medications make this route particularly dangerous. *American Journal of Nursing, 105*(3), 25–30.

Nuckols, T.K., Paddock, S.M., Bower, A.G., Rothschild, J.M., Fairbanks, R.J., Carlson, B., et al. (2008). Costs of intravenous adverse drug events in academic and nonacademic intensive care units. *Medical Care, 46*(1), 17–24.

Richards, J. F., & Creamer, L. (1999). Med errors: Solving the microgram/kilogram puzzle. *American Journal of Nursing, 99*(10), 11–12.

*Simpson, M.H. (2010). Pain management. In M. Alexander, A. Corrigan, L. Gorski, J. Hankins, & R. Perucca (Eds.), *Infusion nursing: An evidence-based approach* (pp. 372–390). St. Louis, MO: Saunders.

*Spath, P.L. (2011). *Error reduction in health care: A systems approach to improving patient safety* (2nd ed.). San Francisco, CA: Jossey-Bass.

*Trissel, L.A. (2013). *Handbook on injectable drugs* (17th ed.). Bethesda, MD: American Society of Health-System Pharmacists.

*Turner, M.S., & Hankins, J. (2010). Pharmacology. In M. Alexander, A. Corrigan, L. Gorski, J. Hankins, & R. Perucca (Eds.), *Infusion nursing: An evidence-based approach* (pp. 263–298). St. Louis, MO: Saunders.

*U.S. Department of Health and Human Services/Food and Drug Administration. (2012). Clinical pharmacology. http://www.fda.gov/downloads/Drugs/GuidanceComplianceRegulatoryInformation/Guidances/ucm292362.pdf

Westbrook, J.I., Rob, M.I., Woods, A., & Parry, D. (2011). Errors in the administration of intravenous medications in hospital and the role of correct procedures and nurse experience. *British Medical Journal Quality and Safety*, 20(12), 1027–1034.

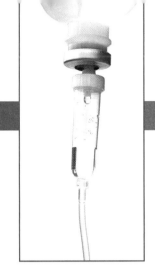

CHAPTER 19

Antineoplastic Therapy

Kerry A. Twite
Jayme L. Cotter
Sol A. Yoder

KEY TERMS

Adjuvant
Alkylating Agents
Alopecia
Anticancer
Antimetabolite
Antineoplastic
Biotherapy
Bolus
Cell Cycle
Cytotoxic
Extravasation
Interferons

Interleukins
Investigational
   Protocol
Monoclonal
   Antibodies
Nadir
Neoadjuvant
Plant Alkaloids
Targeted Therapy
Toxicity
Vesicant

ROLE OF THE INTRAVENOUS NURSE IN CHEMOTHERAPY/ BIOTHERAPY EDUCATION

Antineoplastics, which include both chemotherapeutic and biologic agents used in cancer treatment, present a challenge to nurses responsible for their administration. Many nurses point to the reputation of antineoplastics as intimidating and express anxiety about administering them. Success with these drugs usually is ensured, however, for nurses with refined intravenous (IV) skills, sensitive patient preparation practices, and keen awareness of how and why chemotherapy and biotherapy work. The Infusion Nursing Standards of Practice echo that the nurse who administers antineoplastic agents is competent and has the knowledge of protocols for prescribed therapies (INS, 2011).

Approximately 85% of all patients with cancer will receive antineoplastic therapy that may include either chemotherapy or biotherapy or a combination of both in the course of treatment. Successful administration of an IV cancer treatment regimen depends on adequate patient preparation and education, the competence and skill of the nurse, mutual understanding of the patient and nurse on the current goal of therapy (cure, control, or palliation), and finally, the nurse's broad knowledge of indications, administration, and side effects of the cancer treatment. The nurse is critical to the experience and outcomes of the patient when receiving chemotherapy/biotherapy. Nurses who are committed to the care of patients undergoing cancer treatment can make a difference in the lives of these patients.

Education for Nurses Administering Antineoplastic Drugs

The privilege of administering antineoplastic agents is preceded by extensive exposure to standardized educational preparation and practical experience. To provide consistently safe, appropriate, and high-quality patient care, many centers mandate comprehensive training programs leading to credentialing in chemotherapy administration.

To ensure consistency in practice, the Oncology Nursing Society (ONS) has developed a chemotherapy/biotherapy course that is presented nationwide. ONS members who become trainers for the course are selected based on criteria that include experience in administering chemotherapy and presenting educational content. The book, *Chemotherapy and Biotherapy: Guidelines and Recommendations for Practice* (Polovich, Whitford, & Olsen, 2009), provides a standardized framework for the didactic education to handle cytotoxic (cell-killing) agents and for the care of the patient undergoing cancer treatment. The instructional component is comprehensive and includes content covering the disease, drug treatment and administration, and side effects. An outline of the ONS chemotherapy/biotherapy major subject areas needed to prepare for chemotherapy administration is included in Box 19-1 (ONS, 2011).

The participant in the course must also achieve a passing score on a test in order to demonstrate requisite knowledge and receive a Chemotherapy/Biotherapy Provider card. Individual employers determine clinical competence. Course information is applied during a practicum phase at an institutional level where clinical skills are exercised and evaluated. Within the *ONS Guidelines*, the clinical practicum is described and an evaluation tool is included. The clinical practicum emphasizes clinical skills and allows the nurse to demonstrate competence in the safe administration of chemotherapy and biotherapy (Polovich et al., 2009).

Safe delivery of IV antineoplastic agents is only one part of caring for patients receiving chemotherapy/biotherapy. A nurse who specializes in oncology needs a solid foundation of specialized knowledge. See Box 19-2 for a list of areas of emphasis in a basic oncology online education program for nurses (ONS, 2013a, 2013b). With specialty knowledge plus clinical experience, the oncology nurse can prepare for professional certification through the Oncology Nursing Certification Corporation (ONCC). Certification is a formal recognition of the nurse who possesses specialized knowledge, skills, and experience required to provide quality patient care (INS/INCC, 2009; ONS, 2013a, 2013b).

BOX 19-1 PREPARATION OF THE PROFESSIONAL NURSE TO CARE FOR PATIENTS RECEIVING CHEMOTHERAPY/BIOTHERAPY

Major subject areas to be mastered by nurses who administer chemotherapy/biotherapy are based on *Oncology Nursing Society Position on the Education of the Nurse Who Administers Chemotherapy and Biotherapy* (1/2011)

I. Didactic Component

A. Cancer review covering tumor cell kinetics and angiogenesis

B. The drug development process, legal, and ethical issues related to cancer therapy

C. Indications, pharmacology, molecular biomarkers, and protectants related to chemotherapy and biotherapy

D. Principles of cancer chemotherapy and biotherapy

E. Types, classifications, and routes of administration of chemotherapy and biotherapy agents

F. Specific drug administration, as well as administration schedules, dose determinations, drug response, and drug delivery systems

G. Administration procedures, including administration schedule, dose, and route; patient consent; and appropriate medical record documentation

H. Safe handling practices: use and disposal of personal protective equipment (PPE) drugs

I. Safe mixing, storage, and labeling, transportation, and disposal of chemotherapeutic and biologic agents

J. Side effects (acute, late, and long term), as well as principles of management into survivorship, and patient/family education

II. Clinical Practicum (Completed under the auspices of the nurses' institution)

A. Drug calculation and dose verification

B. Drug preparation, handling, and spill management

C. Drug storage, transport, and disposal of drugs and equipment

D. Prechemotherapy patient physical and laboratory assessment

E. Drug administration techniques, including peripheral IV access, central vascular access device (CVAD).

F. Extravasation and hypersensitivity management

G. Acute drug side effect management

H. Appropriate medical record documentation

I. Patient and family teaching and follow-up

Adapted from Oncology Nursing Society (ONS). (2011). *Education of the RN who administers and cares for the individual receiving chemotherapy and biotherapy*. Pittsburgh, PA: Author.

BOX 19-2 BASIC EDUCATION FOR ONCOLOGY NURSES BASED ON THE *CANCER BASIC ONLINE COURSE* (ONS, 2013A, 2013B)

Comprehensive Understanding of Cancer

- Disease statistics
- Carcinogenesis, including cell structure and cell cycle
- Primary and secondary prevention of cancer
- Seven warning signs of cancer

Current Treatment of Cancer

- Diagnostic evaluation and staging of cancer
- Treatment goals: cure, control, and palliation
- Treatment modalities: indications and side effects
  - Radiation therapy
  - Chemotherapy
  - Biotherapy
  - Molecular-targeted therapy
  - Antiangiogenesis therapy

Patient Care Management and Treatment-Related Symptoms

- Patient assessment and evaluation
- Performance status
- Nutritional status
- Pain assessment and control
- Hematologic assessment
- Psychosocial assessment (coping skills and support systems)
- Systems review (cardiac, renal, hepatic, pulmonary, GI), comorbidities

Complications and Toxicities

- Short-term side effects: alopecia, GI reactions, bone marrow suppression, dermatologic and cutaneous disturbances, allergic reactions, phlebitis and extravasation, psychosocial changes
- Long-term side effects: genetic, oncogenetic, immunosuppression, reproductive alterations, psychosocial changes
- Specific organ toxicities: cardiac, renal, pulmonary, hepatic, GI, neurologic, dermatologic, reproductive

Nursing Care

- Early detection and prevention of complications
- Delivery of expert care
- Patient and family education
- Psychosocial support throughout the continuum of care (new diagnoses remission, recurrence, end of life, survivorship)
- Follow-up support needs: complete remission, disease control, survivorship, hospice

Adapted from Oncology Nursing Society (ONS). (2013). *Cancer basics online course*. Pittsburgh, PA: Author. http://www.ons.org/CourseDetail.aspx?course_id=20

CLINICAL CHALLENGES

The remarkable progress of antineoplastic agents as a major treatment modality poses a growing series of challenges to infusion nurses. Ongoing and vigorous clinical investigations from cooperative groups are dedicated to drug development and discovering new therapeutic methods of delivering cytotoxic drugs. The use of the oral route has expanded. Nurses who specialize in oncology have a responsibility to maintain up-to-date expertise through study of current professional literature along with continuing education programs.

Certification is an excellent demonstration of one's knowledge in antineoplastic therapy. The Infusion Nurses Society (INS) supports certification in infusion nursing through the Infusion Nurses Certification Corporation (INCC). One of the nine major content areas on the infusion nurse's examination is antineoplastic therapy. Nurses successful in the test receive the designation of CRNI (Certified Registered Nurse Infusion). The CRNI who possesses an RN license and has 1,000 hours of clinical practice in infusion nursing may renew every 3 years through testing or recertification units. The ONS Chemotherapy/Biotherapy Provider card is renewed every 2 years through completion of online self-study and testing. The ONCC offers one general oncology nursing certification. The CPOHN designation is awarded to the Certified Pediatric Hematology Oncology Nurse. Additionally, two national certifications for advanced practice oncology nurses are offered: one for Advanced Oncology Clinical Nurse Specialists and the other for Advanced Oncology Nurse Practitioners. Oncology Certification is renewed every 4 years by practice hours and exam, practice hours, or exam along with professional development points [known as ONC-PRO] (ONCC, 2013).

Patient Education

The nurse caring for an oncology patient can make all the difference in the patient's experience with treatment. The nurse acts as the coordinator of care, collaborating with all providers to ensure the highest quality of care. It is critical that patients are actively involved and informed of all aspects of their care to ensure patient satisfaction and a sense of control during treatment. The nurse's role is to advocate for and empower patients and family members to seek information and to ensure informed consent and understanding of their treatment plans. The nurse needs to evaluate whether the patient and significant other have a clear understanding of the treatment goals. Is the goal of treatment to cure, control, or offer palliative relief of symptoms? The patient and significant other should be educated in all aspects of the disease process and treatment methods. When administering antineoplastic agents, the nurse should establish open communication with the patient in all phases of care, even to the extent of actively soliciting patient assistance in clinical functions such as assessing vein status. The astute nurse listens to, and is guided by, patient statements like, "The nurse tried that vein two times last week, and it didn't work." In addition to providing a sense of patient involvement and control, the nurse can capitalize on a patient's intimate knowledge of his or her own body.

It is important to inform a patient that, as IV solutions are infused, it is normal to detect a sense of coolness along the venous pathway. Likewise, it is prudent to alert a patient to early signs of **extravasation** (pain, burning, stinging, a feeling of tightness, tingling, numbness, and any other unusual sensations) when vesicant (tissue-damaging) agents are infused because patients can usually detect them before they are apparent to the nurse.

Some antineoplastic and biotherapy drugs are associated with localized and generalized anaphylactic reactions. When signs and symptoms are reported early and treated properly, their course can be reversed or minimized. Particularly with these agents, patients should be encouraged to report unusual symptoms of generalized tingling, chest pains or sensations, shortness of breath, or light-headedness. Education must be tailored to the individual patient based on the patient's learning needs. It is important that the patient understands some side effects can occur once treatment is completed or anytime during the course of their specific treatment, such as alopecia, bone marrow suppression, diarrhea, fatigue, mucositis, nausea and vomiting, depression, reproductive and sexual side effects, and changes in taste sensations. It is critical that patients are educated on side effects before treatment begins. This not only allows the patient to make an informed decision on the treatment plan but also reduces fear and anxiety when delayed reactions occur. Education needs to be ongoing with each interaction with your patient and to be multifaceted in delivery.

Patients with a cancer diagnosis experience dramatic life changes and loss of control. It is important for the nurse to partner with the patient to give the patient a sense of control. Once a relationship is established, the nurse usually finds that patients implicitly trust in the skill and judgment of the nurse with whom he or she is most familiar. During the active treatment phase, the staff and nurses offer security, hope, and stability to the patient and his or her extended family. It is important to connect with your patients and guide the patient and family through these uncertain times in their lives. Nurses administering chemotherapy and biotherapy have a tremendous opportunity to minimize treatment-related morbidity (and thus to enhance their patients' quality of life) through competent patient education. Patient, family, and caregiver education is integral to the cancer treatment; teaching identification of signs and symptoms, appropriate self-care activities, and when to report sign and symptoms to the provider are critical.

Safe and competent delivery of antineoplastics is only half the job of contemporary IV therapy nursing professionals. The more sensitive (and sometimes more influential) part of the art revolves around the relationship with the patient, and then their education, individualized to address a patient's situation. Nurses need to adhere to the scope of practice and standards of care established by the ONS. Key components to be included in patient/family education include the following:

- The patient is able to describe his or her understanding of extent of disease and current treatment at a level consistent with cultural and educational background and emotional state.
- The nurse and patient (and family) agree on learning outcomes based on the patient's needs.
- The patient participates in decision making regarding plan of care and life activities if desired or possible.
- The nurse selects educational methods and materials consistent with the patient's and family's learning needs and abilities.
- The nurse considers how, when, and by whom teaching will be done.
- The nurse continuously evaluates the patient's and family's comprehension, with reference to original learning outcomes.

- The nurse conscientiously documents all components of the education process. An organized and systematic form in the medical record is an efficient and effective way to ensure that this phase of therapy is up to date and critical components are not missed.

Multiple psychosocial, emotional, cultural, and physiologic barriers come into play because of the nature of the disease and public perceptions of cancer and cancer therapy. A nurse's primary concern is that the patient not only has adequate information but has absorbed sufficient information to provide legitimate informed consent. When assessing your patients, it is important to address their psychosocial status. How are they and their family members coping? Do they feel they have an adequate support system in place? Patients should be encouraged to communicate their feelings on coping with a cancer diagnosis and referred to appropriate community resources.

Some barriers to the patient learning (Table 19-1) can be overcome by methods as simple as teaching in a physical environment that reduces anxiety, including the family in the educational process, and providing patient-appropriate materials. Often it is wise to allow a span of time between a scheduled teaching session and treatment itself so that the patient has time to assimilate important information and form questions concerning areas that are unclear. Certainly, the patient education is an ongoing process, from the outset and for the duration of therapy. The process may sort itself into a natural division of three phases, with the common outcome of all phases an increased patient understanding of antineoplastic therapy. Table 19-2 summarizes the essential components of the education process. The following guidelines are for nurses involved in the patient education. They can be used to

TABLE 19- POTENTIAL BARRIERS TO SUCCESSFUL PATIENT LEARNING

Type of Barrier	Examples
Emotional	Anxiety related to cancer diagnosis, anticipation of cancer therapy, concern over insurance coverage, family concerns Depression related to disease process and treatment Denial, used as a coping mechanism External locus of control—learned helplessness and powerlessness
Physical	Pain, nausea and vomiting, fatigue, restlessness, irritability, impaired hearing or vision
Psychosocial	Altered consciousness caused by disease process or medications Cultural attitudes, beliefs, roles, or values contributing to unwillingness to learn ("My wife/husband takes care of this kind of thing.") Refusal to claim ownership of self-care Lack of inquisitiveness in effort to be perceived as a "good patient"
Functional	Compromised literacy level or language differences Being overwhelmed by new information, names of drugs, disease jargon, personnel names, schedules, sequence, and so forth Age, undeveloped or decreased data retention or memory
Environmental	Busy, rushed, and distracting Unusual or foreign, high-tech, frightening, or threatening surroundings Restrictive and depersonalized surroundings in close proximity to personnel and other patients

TABLE 19-2	EDUCATIONAL ESSENTIALS FOR PATIENTS RECEIVING CHEMOTHERAPY
Outcomes	**Nursing Interventions**

Pretreatment Phase

• Presentation of sufficient information for the patient to give valid informed consent • Provision of a nonthreatening environment conducive to learning and to accepting chemotherapy confidently	• Provide written, patient-appropriate educational materials explaining specific chemotherapeutic agents and their effects before the treatment begins. Allow for extended learning period, if necessary • Thoroughly discuss expectations of the therapy • Discuss anticipated procedures and administration technique, including the need for central venous access, potential side effects, and planned interventions for symptom management • Encourage the patient's involvement in decision making regarding care and treatment plan. Have the patient bring pretreatment question list to clinic or office • Conduct patient teaching in a quiet, comfortable, and private environment • Offer opportunity for the patient and family to tour the treatment area • If possible, introduce the patient to the IV nurse assigned to the patient • Provide nutritional counseling • Encourage the patient to express fears, concerns, and comprehension of situation • Emphasize variability and reversibility of side effects such as alopecia and offer patient assistance and alternatives • Be absolutely honest with the patient • Review drug and food allergy history (document this before first treatment)

Treatment Phase

• Provision of sufficient and enabling information, allowing the patient to cope effectively with immediate effects of chemotherapy • Enhancement of the patient's sense of participation in and control over care	• Explain how chemotherapy works (e.g., cytotoxic effect of drugs) • Instruct the patient to report immediately any discomfort, pain, or burning during the administration of chemotherapy • Review the antiemetic schedule, foods to avoid, and hydration requirements • Identify known side effects of each drug in use • Discuss precautions to take against potential adverse effects • Assess potential for multiple drug therapy complications/incompatibilities, and caution the patient to take only medications ordered by a physician/LIP • Instruct the patient to maintain oral hygiene and to use non–alcohol-based mouth rinses • Provide a calendar with schedule of treatments, appointments with physicians/LIPs, laboratory tests, and expected time line for neutropenia or thrombocytopenia • Assist the patient in energy conservation program and in setting realistic goals for work and social activities • As appropriate, discuss contraceptive measures, potential for infertility, and sperm banking

TABLE 19- EDUCATIONAL ESSENTIALS FOR PATIENTS RECEIVING CHEMOTHERAPY *(Continued)*	
Outcomes	Nursing Interventions
Posttreatment or Ongoing Treatment Phase • Provision of sufficient information to allow the patient to demonstrate self-management strategies to control side effects and to promote functioning at maximum realistic potential	• Explain self-care measures to use in managing side effects of each drug treatment • Explain reasons for follow-up studies to evaluate disease response • Remind the patient not to travel alone immediately after treatment in most cases • Instruct the patient to report temperature >100.4°F (38°C) and other signs and symptoms of complications, such as increased bruising, blood in urine or stool, bleeding gums, rashes, fatigue, shortness of breath, sore throat, oral lesions, change in bowel habits, numbness or tingling in the fingers or toes • Stress the importance of good personal hygiene and hand washing, and avoidance of rectal thermometers, enemas, anal sex, and people with known communicable diseases • Encourage the patient to call for assistance with any new or unusual signs or symptoms • Provide information on how to reach appropriate health care personnel 24 h a day • Confirm return appointments and assist with patient transport services, if needed or possible • Phone the patient after the first and subsequent treatments when there is a potential for problems • Solicit questions from the patient and caregivers • Review and reinforce previous information related to diagnosis, disease, and treatment

evaluate teaching content and technique by assessing the degree to which expected patient outcomes are achieved:

1. The patient demonstrates knowledge related to diagnosis and disease process:
   - States diagnosis and explains disease process
   - Describes previous experience with cancer and treatments
   - Acknowledges the need for treatment
   - States alternatives to prescribed treatment
2. The patient demonstrates knowledge related to rationale for chemotherapy and/or biotherapy:
   - Verbalizes the need for chemotherapy/biotherapy
   - Expresses attitude toward and expectations about cancer treatment
   - States understanding of use of chemotherapy or biotherapy alone or with other treatment modalities, if applicable
   - Identifies treatment protocol
3. The patient demonstrates knowledge related to potential therapeutic side effects of chemotherapy/biotherapy:
   - States diagnosis and expected response to treatment
   - Identifies specific effect of treatment with antineoplastic agents

4. The patient demonstrates knowledge of treatment plan and schedule:
   - Identifies drugs to be given
   - States frequency and duration of treatment
   - Identifies studies, tests, and procedures required before treatment
   - Identifies follow-up tests, studies, and procedures needed to evaluate treatment results
5. The patient demonstrates knowledge of potential drug side effects:
   - States mechanism of drug action
   - Defines reason for side effects
   - Identifies specific side effects that may occur with each drug
   - States self-management interventions to control side effects
   - Verbalizes signs and symptoms reportable to health care professionals
   - Identifies procedures for reporting signs and symptoms
6. The patient demonstrates knowledge of techniques to manage antineoplastic treatment:
   - Maintains nutritional status to best of ability
   - Follows oral, body, and environmental hygiene measures
   - Maintains optimal rest and activity pattern
   - Uses safety precautions to prevent injury
   - Seeks and uses resources as necessary
   - Verbalizes reduced anxiety related to treatment
   - States intention to comply with treatment plan
7. The patient demonstrates knowledge relative to various access devices, if applicable.

Oncology nurses are encouraged to refer to and follow the ONS *Statement on the Scope and Standards of Oncology Nursing Practice* (Brant & Wickham, 2004). Additionally, adhering to the ONS *Standards of Oncology Education: Patient/Significant Other and Public* (Blecher, 2004) will ensure thorough patient and family education in the disease process, treatment, toxicities, and symptom management.

Legal Considerations Related to Education

A thorough understanding of legal responsibilities and implications is an essential element of professional education for the nurse administering antineoplastic agents. Nurses need to know the specific regulations related to chemotherapy administration in their own state's Nurse Practice Act.

It is in a nurse's best interest to request a written definition of the institution's scope of practice and to explore details of medical liability insurance covering the practice. Many employers provide adequate coverage for care administered when the nurse is on duty. All nurses—especially LIPs, instructors, or those working in a physician/LIP's offices—may opt for personal malpractice coverage. Nurses who assume greater responsibility in administering cancer chemotherapy are at greater risk for litigation.

Meticulous adherence to the details of defined statutes and standards of care may minimize that risk. The ANA, individual departments of professional regulation for the state's Nurse Practice Act, INS, and ONS can provide more details on legal statutes that govern nursing practice pertaining to administration of chemotherapeutic agents.

LEGAL ISSUES

Legal Considerations Pertinent to Cancer Chemotherapy

- *Clinical education:* Before treating any patient, the nurse's successful education and competency assessment in IV therapy and drug administration, specifically chemotherapy and biotherapy should be documented and available in personnel files.
- *Lines of supervision:* The nurse should have a clear, written statement of the lines of supervision.
- *Standards of care:* The nurse should have a clear, written statement of the employing facility's standards of care, including a definition of reasonable care in each pertinent area of practice. Facility-specific policies and procedures and job descriptions should be based on nationally established standards from professional organizations, including but not limited to the Infusion Nurses Society (INS, 2011), ONS, and American Nurses Association (ANA).
- *Patient and family education:* The nurse should initiate and complete patient and family education regarding treatment goals, all medications in the treatment regimen, side effects, length of therapy, and follow-up restaging. Evaluation of the patient's understanding and response to teaching should be documented.
- *Informed consent:* Patients who are participating in clinical drug trials must sign an informed consent form before administration of the **investigational** (experimental) **protocol**. Specific regulations regarding written informed consent for noninvestigational protocols vary from state to state. Although obtaining informed consent is a physician/licensed independent practitioner's (LIP) responsibility in most states, a nurse should make sure that consent has been granted before administering chemotherapy. The hospital or institution may be held liable if treatment is administered without the informed consent of the patient or responsible parties. Failure to obtain a patient's consent may constitute battery, defined as any physical contact of a patient without his or her permission.

Because a patient's clinical record is a legal document that can be used as evidence in a lawsuit, it is a fundamental legal nursing responsibility to ensure that documentation is accurate, comprehensive, and current and reflects the care given to the patient. The essentials of adequate documentation include time of a significant incident, a thorough and objective description of the care provided, the patient's status, and the exact nature of physician/LIP involvement.

The expert oncology nurse frequently practices more autonomously than nursing colleagues in other specialties, which implies increased legal vulnerability. For example, because extensive telephone contact is common with patients with cancer, the nurse should therefore be mindful of the accepted scope of practice when responding to patient needs. Telephone protocols related to symptom management may serve as guidelines for the nurse in responding to calls from patients. Telephone conversation, especially if the nurse provides advice or instructions, should be documented in the medical record (Polovich, 2009).

The nurse commonly is a key clinician involved in clinical trials that call for take-home investigational drugs. By law, only a pharmacist or physician/LIP may dispense medication. Therefore, packaging and delivering investigational drugs are not usually legal functions for nurses. Finally, knowledge of common dosing and scheduling of each common chemotherapeutic agent is the best protection (for the patient and nurse) from delivering an incorrect and possibly lethal drug dose.

SAFE PREPARATION, HANDLING, AND DISPOSAL OF CHEMOTHERAPEUTIC AND BIOLOGIC AGENTS

In 2004, the U.S. National Institute for Occupational Safety and Health (NIOSH) issued an alert entitled "Preventing Occupational Exposures to Antineoplastic and Other Hazardous Drugs in Health Care Settings." Drugs are classified as *hazardous* if animal or human studies indicate that exposure to them has the potential for causing cancer, developmental or reproductive toxicity, or harm to organs (NIOSH, 2004). Antineoplastic drugs are among the agents considered hazardous. Personnel, who prepare, handle, administer, and dispose of chemotherapy and biotherapy drugs risk exposure to hazardous agents. Although the therapeutic benefits outweigh the risks of side effects for ill patients, health care workers who are exposed to hazardous drugs risk these same side effects without the therapeutic benefit. Guidelines have been established since 1986 for handling antineoplastics safely (Occupational Safety and Health Administration [OSHA], 1986). The 2004 NIOSH alert summarized the health effects associated with hazardous drugs and provided recommendations for safe handling. Subsequent NIOSH alerts expanded the list of hazardous drugs so health care workers had an up-to-date reference (NIOSH, 2012).

Adherence to recommendations for safe handling of these agents minimizes potential routes of exposure through skin or mucous membrane contact via absorption, inhalation, ingestion, or accidental needlestick (Polovich et al., 2009), as well as contact with body fluids of the patient who has received antineoplastic agents within the past 48 hours. Occupational exposures to hazardous drugs can result in skin rashes, skin and mucous membrane irritation, nasal sore, blurred vision, light-headedness, dizziness allergic reactions, headache, abdominal pain, nausea and vomiting, and alopecia (hair loss). Long-term exposure can result in liver dysfunction, chromosomal abnormalities, reproductive risks, and increased risk of cancer (Itano & Taoka, 2005). These manifestations appear in direct relationship to the time, amount, and method of exposure to specific classes of antineoplastics. Health care professionals can minimize their potential health risks by strict adherence to safe handling guidelines embedded in antineoplastic policies and procedures, along with cautions during drug preparation and administration. Employees who are pregnant, planning pregnancy, or breast-feeding should be allowed to refrain from preparation and administration of hazardous agents or from caring for the patient during treatment with them (NIOSH, 2004; Polovich et al., 2009).

OSHA recommends that workers handling hazardous drugs be monitored through a medical surveillance program that includes medical and exposure history, physical examination, and some laboratory tests (NIOSH, 2004). A list of all employees who are exposed to hazardous drugs should be maintained with careful documentation of spills, spill cleanup, and accidental exposures. Initial training and periodic review of drug preparation and administration practices that include risks of exposure and strategies to minimize exposure can ensure that all staff members have the necessary education to handle hazardous agents in the workplace (Polovich et al., 2009). Successful administration of chemotherapy and biotherapy calls for expert judgment based on scientific evidence. Expert technical skills aside, the safe administration of these agents requires knowledge of preparation, administration, and disposal of hazardous drugs (Box 19-3). A basic understanding of the indications for use and mechanisms of action of antineoplastic drugs is pivotal to the quality of patient care an IV nurse provides. In 2008, the ONS and the American Society of Clinical Oncology partnered together to develop recommendations to improve the quality and safety of

---

BOX 19-3   ADMINISTRATION OF ANTINEOPLASTIC AGENTS: SAFE HANDLING, PREPARATION, ADMINISTRATION, AND DISPOSAL

Drug Preparation

All antineoplastic drugs should be prepared by specially trained personnel in a centralized area to minimize interruptions and risks of contamination.

- Prepare drugs in a Class II type B or Class III vertical airflow biologic safety cabinet. Air is exhausted to the outside through HEPA (high-efficiency particulate absorption) filters. The fan remains on at all times. The hood is serviced and certified by a qualified technician at least every 6 months (Polovich, 2009) according to the manufacturer's recommendations.
- Cover the work surface with a plastic-backed absorbent pad to minimize contamination as long as it does not interfere with the airflow. Change the pad immediately in the event of contamination and at the completion of drug preparation each day or shift.
- Use aseptic preparation technique and mix according to the order, other pharmaceutical resources, or both.
- Use unpowdered, disposable, good-quality gloves made of latex, nitrile, polyurethane, neoprene, or other materials that have been tested with hazardous drugs. Inspect gloves for visible defects. Use double gloves when preparing hazardous drugs. Tuck the inner glove under the gown sleeve; the cuff of the outer glove extends over the gown sleeve. Change gloves after each use, immediately if torn, punctured, or contaminated with drug or after 30 minutes of wear (ASHP, 2006; NIOSH, 2004; Polovich, 2009).
- Wear a disposable long-sleeved gown made of lint-free fabric with knitted cuffs and a solid front during drug preparation. Laboratory coats and other cloth fabrics absorb fluids, so they are an inadequate barrier to hazardous drugs and are not recommended (Polovich, 2009). Discard gown after drug preparation, after handling cytotoxic drugs, and if visibly contaminated. Gowns should not be reused (NIOSH, 2004).

(Continued)

> **BOX 19-3** **ADMINISTRATION OF ANTINEOPLASTIC AGENTS: SAFE HANDLING, PREPARATION, ADMINISTRATION, AND DISPOSAL** *(Continued)*
>
> - Wear a plastic face shield (protect eye, mouth, and nasal opening) or goggles (only protect eyes) when the possibility of splashing is evident. Use a powered air-purifying respirator or NIOSH-approved face mask when cleaning up cytotoxic spills. Surgical masks do not provide respiratory protection from aerosolized powders or liquids (Polovich, 2009).
> - Use needles, syringes, tubing, and connectors with Luer-lock connections (Polovich, 2009).
> - Guard against potential chemical contamination by priming all IV tubing under the protection of the laminar airflow hood with a compatible, nondrug solution before adding hazardous drugs (Polovich, 2009). This prevents potential exposure when connecting IV tubing.
> - Guard against drug leakage during drug preparation; use special care when reconstituting agents packaged in the following:
>   - **Ampules:** Clear drug from neck of ampule; break top of the ampule away from the body using a gauze or alcohol pad as protection; withdraw the drug through a filter needle with ampule upright on a flat surface; change the needle before administration (ASHP, 2006).
>   - **Vials:** Avoid the buildup of pressure within the vial. Use of a closed system (such as PhaSeal [Baxa Corp., Englewood, CO]) limits aerosolization of the drug and worker exposure to sharps when withdrawing hazardous drugs from vials (NIOSH, 2004).
> - Avoid overfilling syringes (Polovich, 2009).
> - After reconstituting the drug, label it according to institutional policies and procedures. Include the drug's vesicant properties and hazardous drug warning on the label.
> - Transport antineoplastic drugs in an impervious packing material, such as a zippered bag, and mark the bag with a distinctive warning label stating "Cytotoxic Drug" or similar warning (Polovich, 2009).
> - Dispose of gowns, gloves, and preparation equipment in appropriately labeled puncture-proof containers.
> - Be informed on procedures to follow in the event of drug spillage.
>
> ## Drug Administration
>
> Chemotherapeutic agents are administered by registered professional nurses who have been specially trained and designated as qualified according to specific institutional policies and procedures.
>
> - Ensure that informed consent has been completed before administering any chemotherapeutic agent; also clarify any misconceptions the patient may have regarding the drugs and their side effects, and assure that education has been completed.
>   - Review laboratory test results (e.g., complete blood count, renal and liver function values) for acceptable levels. Drug dosages may need to be adjusted by the physician/LIP according to laboratory values. Cardiac (ECG or multiple-gated acquisition [MUGA] scan) and pulmonary function tests (PFTs) may need to be evaluated based on the drug's side effect profile.

BOX 19-3 ADMINISTRATION OF ANTINEOPLASTIC AGENTS: SAFE HANDLING, PREPARATION, ADMINISTRATION, AND DISPOSAL (Continued)

- Determine the vesicant/irritant potential of drugs and implement measures to minimize acute side effects of the drugs before drug administration.
- Assess orders for completeness, for example, hydration and premedications such as antiemetics, antianxiety, antihypersensitivity agents (Polovich, 2009).
- Have available a chemotherapy spill kit, extravasation management information and antidotes and equipment, and emergency drugs and equipment in case of adverse reactions, such as anaphylaxis.
- Review the order. Compare with the formal drug protocol or reference source; check for completeness (schedule, route, admixture solution, etc.; Itano & Taoka, 2005).
- Determine drug dose. Verify actual height and weight. Calculate body surface area (BSA) or appropriate dose calculations (e.g., milligrams per kilogram or area under the curve [AUC]).
- Perform *independent* double check on dosage calculations (pharmacist and chemotherapy-credentialed nurse and/or two chemotherapy-credentialed nurses) and verify dose against the physician/LIP's order. Verify that the dose is appropriate for the patient, diagnosis, and treatment plan (Polovich, 2009).
- Check the syringe, IV bag, or bottle against the original medication order to verify medication, dose, route, time, and patient identification, using two different patient identifiers. Perform double check with two chemotherapy-credentialed nurses.
- Wear PPE, including nonpowdered surgical latex, nitrile, polyurethane, or neoprene disposable gloves and a disposable gown made of a lint-free, low-permeability fabric with a solid front, long sleeves, and elastic or knit closed cuffs. Double gloving is recommended (NIOSH, 2004). Change gloves after each use, tear, puncture, or contamination or after 30 minutes of wear. Use gloves when handling oral antineoplastic agents. Use face shield if there is a risk of splashing, for example, intravesical instillation (Polovich, 2009).
- Gather all supplies needed for drug administration. Protect the work surface with a disposable absorbent pad. Perform all work below eye level. Don PPE and inspect drug container within delivery bag for leaks prior to removing the hazardous drug from the delivery bag. Do not prime or expel air of intravenous (IV), intramuscular (IM), or subcutaneous (SQ) injection syringes (Polovich, 2009).
- Confirm patency of line.
- Administer the drug or drugs according to established institutional policies and procedures and the physician/LIP's order, using safe handling precautions.
- When infusion has completed, flush IV with a compatible flush solution.
- Document drug administration, including any adverse reaction, in the medical record.
- Establish a mechanism for identifying the patient receiving antineoplastic agents for the 48-hour period after drug administration.
- Implement chemotherapy precautions (gowns, double gloves) when handling body secretions such as urine, stool, blood, or emesis of patients who received hazardous drugs within the prior 48 hours. Dispose of PPE after each use or when it becomes contaminated (NIOSH, 2004).

(Continued)

> **BOX 19-3 ADMINISTRATION OF ANTINEOPLASTIC AGENTS: SAFE HANDLING, PREPARATION, ADMINISTRATION, AND DISPOSAL** *(Continued)*
>
> - In the event of accidental exposure, remove contaminated gloves or gown immediately and discard according to institutional procedures.
> - Wash the contaminated skin with soap and water. Refer to MSDS for agent-specific interventions (Polovich, 2009).
> - For accidental eye exposure, flood the eye immediately with water or isotonic eyewash for at least 15 minutes. Areas where hazardous drugs are routinely handled should be equipped with an eye wash station (Polovich, 2009).
> - Obtain a medical evaluation as soon as possible after exposure and document the incident according to institutional policies and procedures.
>
> ### Drug Disposal
>
> Regardless of the setting (hospital, ambulatory care, the physician's/LIP's office, or home), all equipment and unused drugs are treated as hazardous and disposed of according to the institution's policies and procedures.
>
> - Hazardous drug waste containers should be available in all areas where hazardous drugs are prepared and administered. Any item that comes in contact with a hazardous drug during preparation or administration is considered potentially contaminated and must be disposed of as hazardous waste (Polovich, 2009).
> - Discard all contaminated equipment, including needles, intact to prevent aerosolization, leaks, and spills. Dispose of contaminated sharps in a puncture-proof hazardous waste container.
> - Place contaminated materials including PPE in a sealable 4-mm polyethylene or 2-mm polypropylene bag and dispose of in a leak-proof, puncture-proof container with a distinctive warning label identifying "Hazardous Waste" (NIOSH, 2004; Polovich, 2009).
> - Put linen contaminated with bodily secretions of patients who have received chemotherapy/biotherapy within the previous 48 hours in a specially marked laundry bag with a distinctive biohazard warning label.
> - Follow established institutional policies and procedures for management of spills. The size of the spill might dictate who is to conduct the cleanup and decontamination and how the cleanup is managed. A small spill is one that is <l5 mL. A large spill is >5 mL.
>
> (Adapted from Polovich, M., Whiteford, J. M., Olsen, M. (Eds.). (2009). *Chemotherapy and biotherapy: Guidelines and recommendations for practice* (3rd ed.). Pittsburgh, PA: Oncology Nursing Society.)

chemotherapy administration. The published 2009 Chemotherapy Administration Safety Standards included 31 voluntary standards focused on the outpatient setting (Jacobson et al., 2009). The ONS/ASCO 2011 revisions expanded the scope of recommendations to include inpatient settings (Jacobson et al., 2012). The next area this collaborative group will look at is the safety of oral chemotherapy (Box 19-4).

BOX 19-4   ASCO/ONS CHEMOTHERAPY ADMINISTRATION SAFETY STANDARDS

Staffing Standards

- Policies/procedures are in place for verification of training and continuing education.
  - Qualified physicians/LIPs write and sign orders for parenteral and oral chemotherapy.
  - Qualified pharmacists, pharmacy technicians, and nurses prepare chemotherapy drugs (oral and parenteral).
  - Chemotherapy is administered only by qualified physicians/LIPs or registered nurses.
  - A comprehensive educational program is in place for new staff administering chemotherapy; includes competency assessment. The education includes all routes of administration. The ONS Chemotherapy/Biotherapy course meets this criteria.
  - Annual competency reassessment is done for all staff who administer chemotherapy.
  - All clinical staff maintain current basic life support (BLS) certification.

Chart Documentation

- Available chart documentation prior to the first administration of a new chemotherapy regimen includes the following:
  - Pathology report confirming or verifying the initial diagnosis of cancer
  - Initial cancer stage and current status of the patient's disease since diagnosis
  - Medical history and physical, which includes height, weight, and assessment of organ function specific to the planned antineoplastic regimen
  - Allergies and history of hypersensitivity reactions
  - The patient's understanding of the disease and planned medication regimens and associated medications are documented in chart
  - Psychosocial assessment, identifying concerns, need for support, and interventions taken
  - Chemotherapy treatment plan (chemotherapy drugs, doses, anticipated durations, and goals of care)
  - Treatment plan for oral chemotherapy includes schedule of office visits and monitoring based on the antineoplastic drugs and the individual patient

General Chemotherapy Practice

- Standard chemotherapy regimens are defined by diagnosis with available references. All chemotherapy regimens have identified sources, including research protocols.
- Deviations from standard regimens are supported by a reference. Dose modification or exception orders include the reasons for alterations.
- Regimen-specific laboratory tests are determined, and their intervals are determined by evidence-based national guidelines, site practitioners, or as part of the standard chemotherapy orders.
- Informed consent for chemotherapy is obtained and documented.
- Quality control is maintained for chemotherapy that is mixed off-site.

(Continued)

BOX 19-4   ASCO/ONS CHEMOTHERAPY ADMINISTRATION SAFETY STANDARDS   *(Continued)*

Chemotherapy Orders

- New orders and changes in chemotherapy orders are made in writing. There are no verbal orders except to hold or stop chemotherapy administration.
- Parenteral chemotherapy orders are a standardized, regimen based in either a preprinted format or as electronic forms in e-prescribing software.
- Orders list all medications by generic names and avoid all Joint Commissions' prohibited abbreviations. All chemotherapy drugs in the regimen with their dosing are listed in the orders.
  - Complete orders include the patient's name/second identifier, date, diagnosis, regimen name and cycle number, treatments conditions (lab results and toxicities) to be met to treat, allergies, established standards for dose calculation, height, weight, dosage, route and rate of administration, length of infusion, premedications, hydration, growth factors, and hypersensitivity medications, sequence of drug administration, time limit to ensure evaluation at designated intervals.

Drug Preparation

- A second chemotherapy-credentialed practitioner verifies each order prior to preparation, confirming two patient identifiers, drug names, doses, volumes, rate and route of administration, dose calculations, and cycle and day of cycle.
- Chemotherapy drugs are labeled upon preparation with the patient's full name and second identifier, generic drug name, route, total volume required to give dose, date of administration, and date/time of preparation and expiration.
- A policy for administration of intrathecal medications includes separate preparation from other drugs, stored after preparation in an isolated area with a unique intrathecal medication label, and delivery of the medication to the patient only with other medications for the central nervous system (CNS).

The Patient Consent and Education

- The patient consent information includes diagnoses, goals of treatment, drugs, schedule, and length of treatment, short- and long-term side effects, drug-specific symptoms that trigger contact with the provider, and how to contact the provider and plan for follow-up and monitoring.
- Informed consent is documented prior to initiation of the chemotherapy administration.
- Patients prescribed oral chemotherapy are taught preparation, administration, and disposal of oral chemotherapy. Written information is provided to the patient and family and caregivers who will be assisting the patient in managing the therapy.

Administration of Chemotherapy

- Prior to chemotherapy administration, confirm with the patient planned therapy before each cycle.

BOX 19-4   ASCO/ONS CHEMOTHERAPY ADMINISTRATION SAFETY STANDARDS   *(Continued)*

- Two chemotherapy-credentialed practitioners verify the accuracy of drug names, dose, volume, rate, route, expiration dates/times, appearance, and physical integrity of drugs. This verification is documented in the medical record.
- In front of the patient, two individuals verify the identity of the patient using two identifiers.
- Extravasation procedures are current and referenced. Orders and access to antidotes are ensured.
- A physician/LIP is on-site and immediately available during all chemotherapy administration.

Assessment and Monitoring

- Response protocols are established and reviewed annually to manage life-threatening emergencies that include BLS and transfer to location for higher acuity patient support.
  - At each clinical visit or day of treatment: Assess and document clinical status, performance status, vital signs, weight, allergies, previous reactions, toxicities (NCI or WHO toxicity criteria), current medication list including OTV meds, complimentary/alternative therapies. Review and document medication changes.
- Assess psychosocial concerns, identify needs, and refer to appropriate psychosocial and other support services.
- Follow-up with patients who miss appointments and/or scheduled chemotherapy treatments.
- Policy/procedure is in place for 24/7 access to a provider/department for care of side effects. A process for hand-off communication allows for written/verbal communication of toxicities across settings to provide continuity of care.
- Cumulative doses of specific drugs, for example, doxorubicin, are tracked to determine the risk of cumulative toxicity.
- The patient response to treatment is monitored using evidence-based standard disease-specific criteria.

(Adapted from Jacobson, J. O. Pelvic, M., Gilmore, T. R., Schulmeister, L., Esper, P., LeFebvre, K. B., et al. (2012). Revisions to the 2009 American Society of Clinical Oncology/Oncology Nursing Society Chemotherapy Administration Safety Standards: Expanding the Scope to Include Inpatient Settings. *Oncology Nursing Forum*, *39*(1), 31–38.)

OVERVIEW OF ANTINEOPLASTIC THERAPY

Before the discovery of chemical and biologic agents to treat cancer, surgery and radiation therapy were the primary cancer treatment techniques. Surgery and radiation therapy provide an important approach to the treatment of local or regional cancers. These modalities treat localized tumors that can be surgically removed or destroyed by radiating the genetic material in the cancer cells in a particular part of the body.

In many cases, cancer is a systemic disease that requires *systemic therapy* (drugs distributed through the body by the blood stream). By nature, cancer cells deviate from normal cells in structure, function, and production; therefore, a characteristic of cancer is the cell's ability to invade surrounding tissue, blood, and lymphatic vessels and spread beyond the localized region of the primary disease site (DeVita, Lawrence, & Rosenberg, 2011). The ability of these aberrant cells to metastasize forms the basis for systemic antineoplastic therapy. Antineoplastic therapy includes chemotherapy, hormonal therapies, biotherapy, and targeted therapies. These systemic modalities are indicated for hematologic malignancies or for solid tumors that either have the potential to spread or have already metastasized.

Chemotherapy

Chemotherapy agents work by disrupting cellular events occurring within the cell cycle of both cancer cells and normal cells. Chemotherapy controls cancer with cytotoxic (cell killing) effects. Chemical agents are designed to kill rapidly dividing cancer cells with minimal impact on cells with normal, healthy mitotic characteristics. Because of the effect on normal cells as well as cancer cells, the side effects that are experienced are related to the rapidly proliferating normal cells. Chemotherapy is limited by the toxic effects on normal cells.

Chemotherapy drugs are grouped according to their specific effect on cancer cell chemistry and the cell cycle phase in which they interfere. The cell cycle refers to a series of phases in normal cell and cancer cell growth. Cell cycle time is the length of time needed for a cell to replicate.

Chemotherapy agents fall into two categories: cell cycle phase–specific agents are active only during a particular phase in the cell proliferation cycle; cell cycle phase–nonspecific agents are active at any point of the cell proliferation cycle. Regardless of whether the chemotherapy is cell cycle specific or cell cycle nonspecific, the basic mechanism of antineoplastic action is the same: to disrupt DNA synthesis. This disables cell reproduction, so the cancer cells die. Chemotherapy generally is most effective when the cell is actively dividing.

Chemotherapeutic agents are further categorized into major groups: alkylating agents; nitrosoureas; antimetabolites; antitumor antibiotics; plant alkaloids such as, camptothecins; epipodophyllotoxins; taxanes; Vinca alkaloids; and miscellaneous (Polovich et al., 2009). Within each of these categories is a spectrum of agents with various toxicities, all of which relate to their antineoplastic properties.

Chemotherapy drug toxicities can be appreciated by understanding that these agents are designed to destroy rapidly dividing cells; therefore, the toxicities that are seen occur in cells that divide rapidly, such as bone marrow, hair follicles, gastrointestinal mucosa, and reproductive tissues. Thus, the most frequent side effects of these drugs include cytopenias, alopecia, mucositis, nausea, vomiting, and infertility.

Table 19-3 provides a quick reference chemotherapy guide for drug handling, dosing, administration, side effects, and major toxicities. Comprehensive tables are available and should be used for more detailed information on indications for use, drug preparation, pharmacokinetics, and protocols.

Biotherapy

Biotherapy refers to systemic treatment with agents from biologic sources or those agents that affect biologic responses. As a class, these agents are known as biologic response modifiers because of their ability to influence and change the relationship of the tumor and the host, resulting in therapeutic effects. Biologic agents are classified by their action: agents

TABLE 19- QUICK REFERENCE TO COMMONLY ADMINISTERED PARENTERAL CHEMOTHERAPEUTIC AGENTS

Drug	Usual Dose	Usual Administration Technique	Comments and Major Toxicities
Amifostine (Ethyol) Chemoprotectant	910–740 mg/m² (nephroprotectant) 200–340 mg/m² (reduction of xerostomia)	IVPB over 15 min, 30 min prior to chemotherapy agents IVP over 3 min, 15–30 min prior to radiation Subcutaneous	Nausea and vomiting (dose dependent)—antiemetic medication, including dexamethasone and a serotonin 5-HT$_3$ receptor antagonist, is recommended prior to amifostine Transient hypotension (dose dependent)—monitor blood pressure Sneezing, flushing, hypocalcemia, hiccups, cutaneous reactions
Arsenic trioxide (Trisenox) Novel arsenical differentiation agent	Induction: 0.15 mg/kg until bone marrow remission (up to 60 doses) Consolidation: 0.15 mg/kg × 25 doses over a period up to 5 wk	IVP (D$_5$W, NS) in 100–250 mL over 2 h	"Differentiation syndrome" characterized as leukocytosis, fever, dyspnea, chest pain, tachycardia, hypoxia, and sometimes death. Corticosteroids seem to benefit this syndrome (dose limiting) QT prolongation (common) Avoid other drugs that prolong the QT interval Rash, pruritus, headache, arthralgias, anxiety, bleeding, nausea, vomiting (common) Liver and renal toxicity (uncommon)
Asparaginase (Elspar, Erwinaze) Antineoplastic enzyme	6,000–25,000 units/m² as a single dose 200 units/kg/d for 28 d	IVPB (D$_5$W, NS) over no <30 min IM (if more than 2 mL, give in multiple injections)	Hypersensitivity (life threatening, requiring anaphylaxis precautions, and a 2-unit test dose) IM reduces incidence of anaphylaxis Coagulopathy is common and requires monitoring Nausea, vomiting, abdominal cramps, anorexia, elevated liver function tests, transient renal insufficiency (common) Depression, lethargy, drowsiness, fatigue, confusion Fever, pancreatitis
Azacitidine (Vidaza) DNA demethylation agent	Initial cycle: 75 mg/m² daily for 7 d Subsequent cycles: 75–100 mg/m² daily for 7 d Recommended minimum 4–6 cycles	IVPB (NS, lactated Ringer's) over 10–40 min. Infusion must be completed within 1 h of vial reconstitution Subcutaneous. Gently roll the syringe between the palms to mix the medication immediately prior to administration. Divide the dose >4 mL into two syringes and inject into two sites. Rotate sites	Myelosuppression (dose limiting) Prolonged leukopenia Nausea, vomiting, diarrhea (common) Mucositis (rare) Liver enzymes elevated and liver function compromised (common) Transient azotemia Lethargy, confusion, coma have been reported

(Continued)

TABLE 19-			
QUICK REFERENCE TO COMMONLY ADMINISTERED PARENTERAL CHEMOTHERAPEUTIC AGENTS *(Continued)*			
Drug	**Usual Dose**	**Usual Administration Technique**	**Comments and Major Toxicities**
Bendamustine (Treanda) Alkylating agent	100 mg/m² on days 1 and 2 every 28 d × 6 cycles (chronic lymphocytic leukemia) 120 mg/m² on days 1 and 2 every 21 d × 8 cycles (non-Hodgkin lymphoma)	IVPB (D$_5$W, NS) over 30–60 min	Myelosuppression (dose limiting) Nausea, vomiting, diarrhea Rash, pruritus Pyrexia, fatigue, asthenia Hyperuricemia, infections Infusion reactions (if reaction with the first dose, consider administering subsequent doses with acetaminophen, diphenhydramine, and corticosteroid)
Bleomycin (Blenoxane) Antitumor antibiotic	10–20 units/m² every week or twice weekly Cumulative lifetime dose should not exceed 400 units	IVP IM Subcutaneous IVPB (rare)	Reversible or irreversible pulmonary fibrosis (dose limiting) Hypersensitivity (administer a test dose) Fever and chills (premedicate with acetaminophen) Pruritic erythema, hyperpigmentation, photosensitivity (common) Alopecia, nausea, and vomiting Renal or hepatic toxicity Mucositis, myelosuppression (rare)
Bortezomib (Velcade) Proteasome inhibitor	1.3 mg/m² twice weekly for 2 wk followed by a 10-day rest period	IVP over 3–5 s Subcutaneous	Myelosuppression Nausea, vomiting, diarrhea, constipation, anorexia Peripheral neuropathy (dose limiting) Hepatic and renal toxicity Rash, flu-like symptoms, fever, fatigue Orthostatic hypotension
Busulfan (Busulfex) Alkylating agent	Induction: 4–8 mg/d Maintenance: Usually 1–3 mg/d but can range from 2 mg/wk to 4 mg/d	IVPB (D$_5$W, NS) over 2 h Diluent volume should be 10 times busulfan, volume to final concentration of approximately ≥ 0.5 mg/mL Also available in oral tablets	Nadir: 11–30 d; recovery 24–57 d Prolonged myelosuppression with slow recovery (dose limiting) Severe thrombocytopenia, anemia, electrolyte imbalances Nausea, vomiting, anorexia, mucositis, hyperpigmentation, elevated liver function tests (common) Hypertension, tachycardia, thrombosis, vasodilatation Interstitial lung disease

TABLE 19-   QUICK REFERENCE TO COMMONLY ADMINISTERED PARENTERAL CHEMOTHERAPEUTIC AGENTS   (Continued)

Drug	Usual Dose	Usual Administration Technique	Comments and Major Toxicities
Cabazitaxel (Jevtana) Antimicrotubule agent	20–25 mg/m² every 3 wk Premedication with antihistamine, corticosteroid, and H₂ antagonist	IVPB (D₅W, NS) over 1 h	Myelosuppression, especially neutropenia (dose limiting) Peripheral neuropathy, dizziness, dysgeusia, headache Diarrhea, nausea, vomiting, constipation, abdominal pain, dyspepsia Hematuria, dysuria Fatigue, asthenia, pyrexia, anorexia, back pain, dyspnea, cough, alopecia Hypersensitivity reactions. Do not give if the patient has a history of a severe hypersensitivity reaction to cabazitaxel or to other drugs formulated with polysorbate 80
Carboplatin (Paraplatin) Alkylating agent	360–400 mg/m² every 4 wk The dose is commonly based on a desired area under the curve (AUC) using a specific formula (Calvert formula: Total dose (mg) = target AUC × (GFR + 25))	IVPB (D₅W, NS) over at least 15 min to 24 h May dilute to as low as 0.5 mg/mL Intraperitoneal (IP) Intra-arterial	FDA recommendation to cap the GFR at a maximum of 125 mL/min; it is not necessary to cap the GFR value when it is actually measured Nadir at day 21; recovery by days 28–30 Myelosuppression, especially thrombocytopenia (dose limiting) Nausea, vomiting, anorexia Ototoxicity, hypersensitivity reaction (later cycles) Increase in creatinine and blood urea nitrogen *Do not use aluminum needles*
Carfilzomib (Kyprolis) Proteasome inhibitor	20 mg/m²/d on 2 consecutive days each week for 3 wk (days 1, 2, 8, 9, 15, and 16) followed by 12 d of rest (days 17–28) for cycle 1; if tolerated, escalate the dose to 27 mg/m²/d in cycle 2 and continue The dose is calculated using the patient's ACTUAL BSA at baseline. Maximum BSA > 2.2 m²	IVPB (D5W) in 50 mL over 10 min IVP undiluted over 2 to 10 min Premedicate with dexamethasone 4 mg prior to all doses during cycle 1 and prior to all doses during the first cycle of dose escalation to reduce the severity of infusion reactions The manufacturer confirms that while medication cannot be admixed in 0.9% NS, flushing with either 0.9% NS or D5W prior to or following administration is safe	Death due to cardiac arrest within 1 day of administration; new-onset congestive heart failure (NYHA III/IV, myocardial infarction within 6 mo excluded from trial); pulmonary arterial hypertension Thrombocytopenia, leukopenia, anemia (dose limiting) Tumor lysis syndrome, hypokalemia, hypomagnesemia, hypercalcemia, hyperglycemia, hypophosphatemia, hyponatremia Headache, back pain, insomnia, dizziness, peripheral neuropathy Nausea, diarrhea, constipation Dyspnea, infusion reactions (up to 24 h post-administration); hepatic toxicity, pneumonia; acute renal failure, pyrexia, upper respiratory infection; cough; arthralgia/spasms If history of herpes zoster infection, consider antiviral prophylaxis

(Continued)

TABLE 19-3	QUICK REFERENCE TO COMMONLY ADMINISTERED PARENTERAL CHEMOTHERAPEUTIC AGENTS *(Continued)*		
Drug	**Usual Dose**	**Usual Administration Technique**	**Comments and Major Toxicities**
Carmustine (BCNU) Alkylating agent Nitrosourea Irritant	150–200 mg/m² every 6 wk as a single dose or divided over a period of 2 d	IVPB (D₅W, NS) Dilute to a concentration of 0.2 mg/mL Stable for 8 h at room temperature Carmustine wafers implanted during surgery	Delayed nadir 4–5 wk after administration and may last 60 d Myelosuppression (slow at onset, cumulative, dose limiting) Severe nausea and vomiting Alopecia, painful/burning venous irritation during administration Hypotension Infiltrates and/or pulmonary fibrosis Azotemia, decreased kidney size, renal failure Impotence, testicular damage causing infertility, facial flushing
Cisplatin (Platinol) Alkylating agent Vesicant if concentrated	20–40 mg/m²/d × 3–5 d every 3–4 wk 20–120 mg/m² given as a single dose every 3–4 wk Closely monitor creatinine clearance (may require dose adjustments) 100–200 mg/m² for IP ovarian cancer	IV infusion (D₅W, NS) in 250–1,000 mL Infuse over 30 min–8 h Prehydrate 1–2 L NS with potassium chloride 20 mEq/L + magnesium sulfate 8 mEq/L (commonly given) Posthydration 1–2 L is also common IP Intra-arterial	Hydration should be adequate to maintain an I/O of 100–150 mL/h before administration of the drug Severe nausea and vomiting—lasting 24–96 h Aggressive antiemetic treatment is required Peripheral neuropathy (dose limiting for cumulative doses) Nephrotoxicity (dose limiting for individual doses) Ototoxicity Nadir on days 18–23 and recovery by day 39 (mild) Alopecia Electrolyte imbalances, especially potassium or magnesium wasting *Do not use aluminum needles* *Protect from light*
Cladribine (Leustatin) 2-CdA antimetabolite	0.09 mg/kg/d × 7 d (hairy cell leukemia) Other malignancies 5–9 mg/m²/d × 5 d	Unstable in D₅W IV 24-hour continuous infusion for 7 d A second cycle of treatment has been given to some nonresponding patients. Can be given as 2-h infusion Subcutaneous	Thrombocytopenia, neutropenia with nadir at 7–14 d Universal lymphopenia Cellulitis at the catheter site, rash, asthenia, fever, chills, fatigue Renal toxicity (dose limiting)

TABLE 19   QUICK REFERENCE TO COMMONLY ADMINISTERED PARENTERAL CHEMOTHERAPEUTIC AGENTS   *(Continued)*

Drug	Usual Dose	Usual Administration Technique	Comments and Major Toxicities
Clofarabine (Clolar) Antimetabolite (purine analog)	52 mg/m^2/d × 5 consecutive days every 2–6 wk, following recovery or return to baseline organ function	IVPB (D$_5$W, NS) over 2 h	Tumor lysis syndrome, cytokine release (systemic inflammatory response), capillary leak syndrome. Recommend continuous IV fluids, allopurinol, and prophylactic steroids (hydrocortisone 100 mg/m^2/d) on days 1–3 Hypotension, tachycardia Neutropenia, anemia, thrombocytopenia Dizziness, headache, anxiety, light-headedness Nausea, vomiting, diarrhea, anorexia, abdominal pain, constipation Dermatitis, erythema, petechiae, pruritus Hematuria, elevated creatinine Arthralgia, myalgia, limb pain, cough, epistaxis, fatigue, pyrexia, elevated LFTs
Cyclophosphamide (Cytoxan) Alkylating agent	May be given as a single dose or in several divided doses, common doses of 500–1,500 mg/m^2 every 3 wk 50 to 200 mg/m^2/d orally for 14 d of a 28-d cycle 400 mg/m^2/d for 4 d every 4–6 wk	IVP over 5–10 min (doses <750 mg) IVPB (D$_5$W, NS) infuse in 100–150 mL over 15–30 min Higher doses require hydration of 500 mL or more of NS	Leukocyte nadir 8–14 d and recovery in 18–25 d Myelosuppression (dose limiting) Nausea and vomiting 6–10 h after treatment Alopecia, nail and skin hyperpigmentation Nasal congestion and burning, metallic taste during infusion Hypersensitivity reactions Testicular atrophy and amenorrhea Acute hemorrhagic cystitis (give the dose in morning) Frequent voiding; hydrate to prevent cystitis Mesna (uroprotectant) for high doses Cardiac necrosis and/or acute myopericarditis with high doses (rare) Secondary malignancies

(Continued)

TABLE 19-3 QUICK REFERENCE TO COMMONLY ADMINISTERED PARENTERAL
CHEMOTHERAPEUTIC AGENTS *(Continued)*

Drug	Usual Dose	Usual Administration Technique	Comments and Major Toxicities
Cytarabine (Ara-C) Antimetabolite	60 to 200 mg/m² IV for 5–10 d 100 mg/m² IV or subcutaneously BID for 5 d every 28 d High dose: 1–3 g/m² every 12 h for 3–6 d 10 mg/m² subcutaneously every 12 h for 15–21 d 10–30 mg/m² intrathecally up to 3 times per week	IVP (low dose) over 1–2 min, or IV in 50 mL or more approximately over 30 min For high dose, IV (D₅W, NS) in 250–500 mL over 1–3 h	Nadir in 5–7 d, leukopenia, thrombocytopenia, anemia (dose limiting) Nausea, vomiting, anorexia, diarrhea (common) Metallic taste, mucositis (common) Rare syndrome of sudden respiratory distress, rapid progression to pulmonary edema Keratoconjunctivitis with high doses (use dexamethasone eyedrops for prevention) Cerebellar toxicity with high doses (lethargy, confusion, slurred speech) Most cases resolve, but in some cases, irreversible and/or even fatal Flu-like symptoms, bone/muscle pain, skin rash, alopecia (common) Concurrent treatment with dexamethasone is recommended for an IT or intraventricular route
Cytarabine liposome (Depocyt) Antimetabolite	Induction: 50 mg intrathecally every 14 d × 2 doses Consolidation: 50 mg intrathecally every 14 d × 3 doses Maintenance: 50 mg intrathecally every 28 d × 4 doses Liposomal cytarabine is different dosing than conventional Cytarabine	Intrathecal over 1–5 min by lumbar puncture or into an intraventricular reservoir Do not filter	Mild neutropenia and thrombocytopenia Headache, confusion, somnolence Nausea, vomiting, constipation Arachnoiditis syndrome (neck pain, N/V, headache, fever, back pain). Give dexamethasone 4 mg BID PO or IV for 5 d beginning on the day of injection Asthenia, peripheral edema
Dacarbazine (DTIC) Alkylating agent Irritant	375 mg/m² on days 1 and 15 (as part of the ABVD regimen for Hodgkin lymphoma) 150–250 mg/m²/d × 5 d every 3–4 wk 650–1,450 mg/m² every 3–4 wk 250 mg/m²/d continuous infusion × 4 d every 3 wk	IVPB (D₅W, NS) in 100 mL or more Infuse over 30–60 min IVP or rapid infusion over 15 min but may increase venous irritation	Nadir at 2–4 wk after treatment, leukopenia, thrombocytopenia, anemia (dose limiting) Severe nausea and vomiting; prevent with aggressive antiemetic support Fever, anorexia, metallic taste (common) Flu-like symptoms with high doses Facial flushing Irritant: Avoid extravasation. Local pain at the injection site. Slow the rate of infusion to decrease the pain from venous spasm Protect from sunlight. Pink solution indicates decomposition

TABLE 19-   QUICK REFERENCE TO COMMONLY ADMINISTERED PARENTERAL
CHEMOTHERAPEUTIC AGENTS   *(Continued)*

Drug	Usual Dose	Usual Administration Technique	Comments and Major Toxicities
Dactinomycin (Cosmegen) Antitumor antibiotic Vesicant	500 mcg/d × 5 d (ovarian) 1,000 mcg/m^2 × 1 day (testicular) 12–15 mcg/kg/d × 5 d (gestational trophoblastic neoplasia)	IVP slowly over 2–3 min IVPB (D$_5$W, NS) in 50 mL over 10–15 min Do not administer IM or SC Regional perfusion: 50 mcg/kg (lower extremity) and 35 mcg/kg (upper extremity)	Leukopenia, thrombocytopenia 1–2 wk after treatment. Nadir at 3 wk (dose limiting) Severe nausea and vomiting (occur 1 h after dose and may last several hours) Erythema, multiforme, hyperpigmentation, alopecia (common) Mucositis, anorexia, diarrhea (uncommon) Skin irritation, erythema, or necrosis in previously irradiated areas ("radiation recall")
Daunorubicin (Cerubidine) Antitumor antibiotic Vesicant	30–90 mg/m^2/d for 2–3 d every 3–4 wk Pediatric doses will vary	Single IV injection or split into a 3- to 5-day schedule running IV over 2–5 min	Nadir between 1 and 2 wk, recovery in 2–3 wk Grade 3–4 neutropenia with higher dosing (dose limiting) Nausea and vomiting 1 h after dose and lasting for several hours (prevented by antiemetics) Alopecia, mucositis (common) Rash, diarrhea, elevated liver enzymes (uncommon) Cumulative cardiotoxicity at maximum lifetime dose of 500–600 mg/m^2 (aggravated by concurrent radiation) Arrhythmias, usually asymptomatic/transient, congestive cardiomyopathy Red urine—advise the patient
Daunorubicin liposomal (DaunoXome) Antitumor antibiotic	40 mg every 2 wk	IVPB (D$_5$W) over 60 min Do not filter	Infusion reaction (triad of symptoms: back pain, flushing, chest tightness), within first 5 min of infusion; subsides with interruption of infusion; generally does not recur if infusion is resumed at a slower rate Myelosuppression Nausea, vomiting, diarrhea, fatigue, abdominal pain, anorexia, headache Fever, chills, hyperuricemia, cough, dyspnea Cumulative cardiotoxicity at a maximum lifetime dose of 320 mg/m^2
Decitabine (Dacogen) Pyrimidine analogue	15 mg/m^2 every 8 h × 3 d every 6 wk 20 mg/m^2/d daily × 5 d every 4 wk	IVPB (D$_5$W, NS) over 1–3 h	Myelosuppression Headache, dizziness, insomnia, confusion, fatigue Nausea, vomiting, diarrhea, constipation, stomatitis, dyspepsia, hyperglycemia, pyrexia Rash, erythema, pruritus, petechiae Fever, edema, rigors, arthralgia, electrolyte imbalance, limb pain, cough

(Continued)

TABLE 19-3	QUICK REFERENCE TO COMMONLY ADMINISTERED PARENTERAL CHEMOTHERAPEUTIC AGENTS *(Continued)*		
Drug	**Usual Dose**	**Usual Administration Technique**	**Comments and Major Toxicities**
Dexrazoxane (Zinecard) Cardioprotectant (Totect) Extravasation Antidote	(For cardioprotectant) Dosage ratio of 10 mg/m² of dexrazoxane for every 1 mg/m² of doxorubicin (10:1 ratio) (For antidote) 1,000 mg/m² (max 2,000 mg) on days 1 and 2, and then 500 mg/m² (max 1,000 mg) on day 3	(For cardioprotectant) Slow IVP or rapid IV infusion (NS, D₅W) over 15–30 min In final concentration of 1.3–5 mg/mL (For antidote) IVPB (NS 1,000 mL) over 1–2 h	*As a cardioprotectant, administer within 30 min before the administration of doxorubicin* *As an extravasation antidote, should be started within 6 h of event* Dexrazoxane may add to myelosuppression Mild nausea, vomiting, anorexia (common) Fever, mucositis, fatigue, anorexia (uncommon) Hypotension, deep vein thrombosis, liver toxicity
Docetaxel (Taxotere) Antimicrotubule agent Irritant Potential vesicant	60–100 mg/m² every 3 wk 40 mg/m² every week × 6 wk followed by 2-wk rest 75 mg/m² every 3 wk *Other doses have been evaluated	IV (D₅W or NS) over 1–3 h Final concentration of 0.3–0.74 mg/mL *Avoid PVC tubing or bags*	Severe neutropenia (dose limiting) Total alopecia (universal) Edema, fluid retention, ascites, pleural effusions are common (dose limiting) *Recommended premedication:* dexamethasone 8 mg BID 1 d prior to docetaxel for a total of 3 d to reduce fluid accumulation and prevent hypersensitivity reactions Capillary leak syndrome in patients after cumulative dose of 400 mg/m² Hypersensitivity or anaphylaxis (uncommon when premedicated with steroids and antihistamines) Peripheral neuropathy, mucositis, diarrhea (mild, common) Rash, hand-foot syndrome, elevated liver functions (uncommon)
Doxorubicin (Adriamycin) Antitumor antibiotic Vesicant	Usual dose of 40–75 mg/m²	Bolus (extravasation precautions) over 2–5 min IVPB (D₅W, NS) in 50–100 mL over 20–30 min via central line Intra-arterial to liver, Intravesicular IP	Nadir at 10–14 d and recovery in 21 d Myelosuppression (universal, dose limiting with individual dose) Alopecia, hyperpigmentation of nail beds and dermal creases, facial swelling (common) Nausea and vomiting, anorexia, mucositis—especially with daily schedule Radiation recall (irritation of previously irradiated areas) Cardiotoxicity: CHF, EKG changes, monitoring of LVEF (dose limiting) Lifetime cumulative dose 550 mg/m² May enhance cyclophosphamide cystitis Red urine up to 24 h after administration Erythematous streak up the vein ("Adria flare") Incompatible with heparin and fluorouracil

TABLE 19- QUICK REFERENCE TO COMMONLY ADMINISTERED PARENTERAL
CHEMOTHERAPEUTIC AGENTS   *(Continued)*

Drug	Usual Dose	Usual Administration Technique	Comments and Major Toxicities
Doxorubicin (Doxil) Liposomal doxorubicin Anthracycline	20 mg/m² every 3 wk (Kaposi sarcoma) 50 mg/m² every 4 wk (ovarian cancer)	IVPB (D₅W) in 250 mL. Doses of 20 mg/m² are given over 30 min, larger doses are given over 1 h	Same toxicities as doxorubicin Mild nausea, mucositis (common) Severe hand-foot syndrome (can be dose limiting) Acute infusion reaction: rate related: flushing, shortness of breath, facial swelling, chest tightness, hypotension—decrease the rate or stop infusion Alopecia (uncommon) Lifetime cumulative dose 550 mg/m²
Epirubicin (Ellence) Anthracycline Antitumor antibiotic Vesicant	100 mg/m²/d on day 1 every 21 d or 60 mg/m²/d on days 1 and 8 every 28 d	Bolus (extravasation precautions) free-flowing line over 2–5 min Continuous infusion through a central line	Epirubicin of ≥90 mg/m² produces a degree of myelosuppression equivalent to doxorubicin 60 mg/m² Leukopenia, expected nadir 10–14 d (dose limiting) Thrombocytopenia, anemia Hyperpigmentation of nail beds and dermal creases, dermatitis, radiation recall Alopecia (expected) Nausea, vomiting, mucositis, fatigue (common) CHF increased the risk with higher doses Lifetime cumulative dose 900 mg/m² Red urine, fevers, anaphylactic reactions, parenthesis, headache *If extravasated, will cause local tissue damage, flush along the vein, facial flush, urticaria, phlebitis
Eribulin mesylate (Halaven)	1.4 mg/m² on days 1 and 8 of a 21-day cycle	IVP or IVPB (NS 100 mL over 2–5 min Do not administer with dextrose-containing solutions	Neutropenia, anemia (dose limiting) Peripheral neuropathy, headache Nausea, constipation, vomiting, diarrhea QT prolongation (observed on day 8, not on day 1) Alopecia, asthenia/fatigue, fever, arthralgia, anorexia, cough, dyspnea

(Continued)

TABLE 19-3 **QUICK REFERENCE TO COMMONLY ADMINISTERED PARENTERAL CHEMOTHERAPEUTIC AGENTS** *(Continued)*

Drug	Usual Dose	Usual Administration Technique	Comments and Major Toxicities
Etoposide (VP-16) Plant alkaloid	50–150 mg/m²/d × 3–5 d 100 mg/m²/d × 5 d every 3 wk (testicular cancer in combination with cisplatin) Oral doses are generally twice the IV dose	IVPB (D$_5$W or NS) over at least 30 min–1 h Dilute to concentration of 0.2–0.4 mg/mL *Final concentrations above 0.4 mg/mL could result in precipitation*	Leukopenia; nadir within 7–14 d and recovery within 20 d (dose limiting) Thrombocytopenia/anemia uncommon Mild alopecia Nausea and vomiting: mild; anorexia (common) Elevated bilirubin and transaminase levels Peripheral neuropathy Transient hypotension associated with rapid administration: Infuse over 30 min–1 h Discontinue infusion if hypersensitivity/bronchospasm occurs
Etoposide phosphate (Etopophos) Plant alkaloid (water-soluble ester of etoposide)	35 mg/m²/d × 4 d to 50 mg/m²/d × 5 d every 3–4 wk 50–100 mg/m²/d on days 1 to 5 or 100 mg/m²/d on days 1, 3, and 5 every 3–4 wk	IV push over 5 min into freely running IV IVPB (D$_5$W, NS) over up to 120 min For high-dose HSCT regimens (off-label use), infuse over 4 h directly into a central venous line. If undiluted etoposide is used, solutions should be prepared in sterile glass containers and administered through non-ABS tubing (e.g., nitroglycerin tubing) to avoid cracking of plastic	Blood pressure changes Alopecia, rash, urticaria, pruritus Anorexia, nausea, vomiting, mucositis, constipation/diarrhea Myelosuppression Anaphylaxis, chills, fever, dyspnea Asthenia, malaise
Floxuridine (FUDR) Antimetabolite	Continuous infusion Intra-arterial infusion via pump (0.1–0.6 mg/kg/d) Hepatic artery infusion via pump (0.4–0.6 mg/kg/d) IV: 0.075–0.275 mg/kg/d × 14 d 30 mg/kg/d × 5 d	Intra-arterial Hepatic arterial infusion IV	Thrombocytopenia, leukopenia, anemia Vomiting, diarrhea, nausea, stomatitis Erythema, alopecia, dermatitis, rash Fever, lethargy, weakness, malaise, anorexia

		Usual Administration	
Drug	Usual Dose	Technique	Comments and Major Toxicities

Drug	Usual Dose	Usual Administration Technique	Comments and Major Toxicities
Fludarabine (Fludara) Antimetabolite	25–30 mg/m²/d for 5 consecutive days every 4 wk	IVPB (NS, D₅W)	Leukopenia; nadir 13 d, thrombocytopenia nadir 16 d (dose related, may be cumulative, and dose limiting) Lymphopenia (common and clinically important) CNS toxicity—delayed blindness, coma, death—can occur up to 21–60 d after the last dose (rare, occurs in extreme high doses, and is dose limiting) Somnolence, confusion, weakness, fatigue Nausea, vomiting (rare), diarrhea, anorexia Tumor lysis syndrome associated with large tumor burdens Cough, pneumonia, dyspnea chills, fever, malaise
Fluorouracil (5-FU) Antimetabolite	Numerous regimens used, including: 300–450 mg/m²/d IVP × 5 d every 28 d 600–750 mg/m² IVP every week or every other week 1,000 mg/m² infused over 24 h × 4–5 d 300 mg/m²/d infused indefinitely	IVP, IVPB, or continuous infusion (NS, D₅W) Intraocular 1 mg/0.1 mL in preservative-free NS Arterial infusion, intracavitary IP Topical Oral when mixed in liquids	Nadir at 9–14 d, with recovery in 21–25 d; less common with continuous infusion Dermatitis, nail hyperpigmentation, alopecia, and chemical phlebitis with long-term infusion Nausea, vomiting, and anorexia Severe diarrhea associated with prolonged infusions (dose limiting) Mucositis (more common with 5-d infusion and bolus dosing) Cerebellar ataxia and headache (rare, with higher doses) *Toxicities are more common and more severe in patients with dihydropyrimidine dehydrogenase deficiency
Gemcitabine (Gemzar) Antimetabolite	1,000 mg/m² every week × 7 wk, and then 1-week rest Combination with cisplatin: 1,000 mg/m²/d on days 1, 8, and 15 of a 28-d cycle 1,250 mg/m²/d on days 1 and 8 of a 21-d cycle	IV over 30 min or a fixed-dose rate of 10 mg/m²/min; prolonged infusion times increase the active metabolite accumulation, which may increase toxicity Use with NS only	Mild to moderate neutropenia, myelosuppression with anemia, recovery within 1 wk (dose limiting) Mild nausea and vomiting, diarrhea, mucositis, flu-like symptoms Fever during administration Rash with pruritus Elevations of hepatic transaminase level, hyperbilirubinemia Peripheral edema Proteinuria, hematuria, elevated BUN (uncommon)

(Continued)

TABLE 19-3 QUICK REFERENCE TO COMMONLY ADMINISTERED PARENTERAL CHEMOTHERAPEUTIC AGENTS *(Continued)*

Drug	Usual Dose	Usual Administration Technique	Comments and Major Toxicities
Glucarpidase (Voraxaze) Antidote for methotrexate toxicity Recombinant enzyme from *E. coli*	50 units/kg	IVP over 5 min. Flush the IV line before and after administration Do not administer leucovorin within 2 h before and after glucarpidase as leucovorin may be inactivated	Pain at the injection site, rash, flushing
Idarubicin (Idamycin) Antitumor antibiotic Vesicant	12 mg/m²/d for 3 d 8–15 mg/m² as a single dose every 3 wk	IVP over 1–5 min (extravasation precautions)	Myelosuppression (dose limiting for each individual dose) Nausea, vomiting, (common) Diarrhea and mucositis (occasional) Alopecia (partial), extravasation reactions, and rash Transient arrhythmias, decreased left ventricular ejection fraction, and CHF increased the risk with higher doses (cumulative dose–limiting toxicity)
Ifosfamide (Ifex) Alkylating agent	1,000–1,200 mg/m² over 5 consecutive days every 3–4 wk Higher doses (2,500–4,000 mg/m²/day) have been given over 2–3 d	IVPB *only* (D₅W, NS) in 250–1,000 mL over 30 min or longer	Leukopenia, thrombocytopenia (dose limiting); anemia Nausea, vomiting, anorexia, constipation and diarrhea, mucositis Alopecia, rash, urticaria, nail ridging Increased ALT, AST, and bilirubin Hemorrhagic cystitis and hematuria (dose limiting) Hydration of 2 L/d to maintain urinary output, frequent voiding. Mesna recommended
Mesna (Mesnex) Uroprotectant	Mesna must be given with Ifosfamide	IVPB over 15 min or continuous infusion (infuse until 12–24 h after ifosfamide completion) Recommended aggressive hydration to reduce the risk of hemorrhagic cystitis Oral	CNS toxicity: somnolence, lethargy, disorientation, confusion, dizziness, malaise, myoclonus, seizures: reversible (dose limiting) Electrolyte imbalance

TABLE 19	QUICK REFERENCE TO COMMONLY ADMINISTERED PARENTERAL CHEMOTHERAPEUTIC AGENTS *(Continued)*		
Drug	**Usual Dose**	**Usual Administration Technique**	**Comments and Major Toxicities**

Irinotecan (Camptosar, CPT-11)
  Topoisomerase I inhibitor
  Irritant
	125 mg/m² every week × 4, then 2-week rest and repeat cycle
	350 mg/m² every 28 d
	If combined with cisplatin: 80 mg/m² on day 1 every 4 wk
	60 mg/m² every week × 3 wk
		IV (D$_5$W preferred) in 500 mL over 60–90 min or longer	Myelosuppression, especially neutropenia and diarrhea (common and dose limiting)
			Consult the manufacturer's recommendations for guidelines
			Diarrhea, "acute cholinergic" along with cramping, nausea, vomiting during or immediately following drug administration, or for several days after drug administration; treated with anticholinergics and antidiarrheal agents
			Moderate to severe nausea, anorexia
			Alopecia, flushing, rash (common)
			Elevated liver enzymes
			Fatigue, fevers, salivation, lacrimation
			Increased prothrombin times of patients taking warfarin
			Advise the patients not to take St. John's wort

Ixabepilone (Ixempra) Mitotic inhibitor	40 mg/m² every 3 wk Premedicate with H$_1$ antagonist and H$_2$ antagonist. If hypersensitivity reaction, add corticosteroid premedication	IVPB (lactated Ringer's 250 mL or adjust to concentration between 0.2 and 0.6 mg/mL) over 3 h *Use non-PVC infusion containers and administration sets with a 0.2- to 1.2-μm filter*	Use with caution in cardiac disease Myelosuppression Asthenia, peripheral neuropathy, dizziness Abdominal pain, diarrhea, constipation, nausea, stomatitis, vomiting Alopecia, hand–foot syndrome Arthralgia, myalgia, fatigue, hypersensitivity reactions Avoid concomitant administration with CYP3A4 inhibitors (e.g., ketoconazole, itraconazole, clarithromycin, atazanavir). If coadministration is necessary, consider reducing ixabepilone dose to 20 mg/m²
Leucovorin, Calcium Tetrahydrofolic acid derivative Nonchemotherapeutic agent	Methotrexate rescue: 10–25 mg/m² every 6 h × 6–8 doses starting up to 24 h after the start of methotrexate To potentiate the cytotoxic effect of 5-FU: 20–500 mg/m² dose	IVP at any convenient rate IM Oral IVPB (D$_5$W, NS) 50–250 mL over 15 min	Rare hypersensitivity reactions Thrombocytosis, nausea, diarrhea, rash, headache Dose adjustments are made based on methotrexate serum levels and serum creatinine levels

(Continued)

TABLE 19-3 QUICK REFERENCE TO COMMONLY ADMINISTERED PARENTERAL CHEMOTHERAPEUTIC AGENTS *(Continued)*

Drug	Usual Dose	Usual Administration Technique	Comments and Major Toxicities
Mechlorethamine (Nitrogen Mustard) Alkylating agent Vesicant	6 mg/m² on days 1 and 8 (MOPP regimen for Hodgkin lymphoma) Up to 0.4 mg/kg as a single agent monthly	IVP over 1–5 min (extravasation precautions) into the tubing of a rapidly running IV Intracavitary injection; usually painful—patients should be given appropriate analgesia IP should be avoided	Leukopenia and thrombocytopenia within 24 h, with a nadir at 6–8 d to 3 wk (dose limiting) Severe nausea and vomiting beginning 1–3 h after treatment (dose limiting); aggressive antiemetic premedication is mandatory Discoloration of the infused vein and phlebitis Alopecia and mucositis Vesicant antidote is sodium thiosulfate if extravasation occurs Metallic taste Amenorrhea and impaired spermatogenesis, sterility (common) Diarrhea, anorexia, jaundice, tinnitus, skin rash (topical application) Secondary malignancy and hearing loss (rare) Incompatible with other antineoplastic agents Short stability
Melphalan (Alkeran) Alkylating agent Vesicant	16 mg/m² 0.1 mg/kg/d for 2–3 wk or up to 6 mg/m² for 5 d every 6 wk (multiple myeloma)	IVPB over 15–20 min 60 min stability Oral tablets	Myelosuppression, prolonged recovery, effects cumulative (dose limiting) Nausea, vomiting Vein reactions, scarring Diarrhea, mucositis (uncommon) Pulmonary fibrosis, alopecia, vasculitis, infertility, secondary leukemia (uncommon)
Mesna Uroprotective agent (nonchemotherapeutic)	20% of ifosfamide dose given just before and at 4 and 8 h after ifosfamide Can be administered with high-dose cyclophosphamide	IVPB (D₅W, NS) 50–100 mL IVP (<100 mg) Oral tablets	Nausea, vomiting, diarrhea, abdominal pain, altered taste, flushing Rash and urticaria Lethargy, headache, joint or limb pain, fatigue

TABLE 19-	QUICK REFERENCE TO COMMONLY ADMINISTERED PARENTERAL CHEMOTHERAPEUTIC AGENTS *(Continued)*		
Drug	**Usual Dose**	**Usual Administration Technique**	**Comments and Major Toxicities**
Methotrexate Antimetabolite	30 mg/wk (psoriasis) 200–500 mg/m^2 every 2–4 wk (leukemias and lymphomas) Low dose: <100 mg/m^2 Moderate dose: 100–1,000 mg/m^2 High dose: >1,000 mg/m^2 Intrathecal: usu- ally 10–15 mg in preservative-free NS or lactated Ringer solution	IVPB (D$_5$W, NS) in 50 mL (up to 500 mL) over 30 min to 1 h Can also be given as 24-h continuous infusions Intrathecally IM	Myelosuppression expected (dose limiting) Mucositis, sore throat, and pruritus with high dose Hematemesis Nausea and vomiting (uncommon) Diarrhea (common) Renal toxicity, dose related, and more likely to occur in patients with compromised renal function; reversible Hepatotoxicity, pulmonary dysfunction (rare) Encephalopathy with multiple intrathecal doses Confusion, ataxia, tremors, irritability, seizures, and coma Hypersensitivity reactions associated with fever, chills, and rash Skin erythema, depigmentation or hyperpigmentation, alopecia, and photosensitivity Doses >80 mg/wk should be accompa- nied by leucovorin rescue
Mitomycin (Mitomycin-C, Mutamycin) Antitumor antibiotic Vesicant	10–20 mg/m^2 every 6–8 wk It is recommended that total cumula- tive doses not exceed 50 mg/m^2 to avoid excessive toxicity	IVP over 2–5 min Use vesicant precautions IVPB (D$_5$W, NS in up to 250 mL) over 30 min Intravesical IP Intraocular Intra-arterial	Leukopenia and thrombocytopenia: delayed, cumulative, and dose limiting; anemia Nadir at 4–5 wk, recovery 2–3 wk later Alopecia (4%), dermatitis, and pruritus Nausea, vomiting, anorexia, fatigue (common) Diarrhea, mucositis, fever (uncommon) Hepatotoxicity; venoocclusive disease (rare) Parenthesis, lethargy, weakness, and blurred vision Interstitial pneumonitis infrequent toxicity but can be severe Bronchospasm, acute SOB when given with a Vinca alkaloid Hemolytic uremic syndrome (rare) Nephrotoxicity at doses >50 mg/m^2

(Continued)

TABLE 19-3	QUICK REFERENCE TO COMMONLY ADMINISTERED PARENTERAL CHEMOTHERAPEUTIC AGENTS (Continued)		
Drug	**Usual Dose**	**Usual Administration Technique**	**Comments and Major Toxicities**
Mitoxantrone (Novantrone) Antitumor antibiotic Irritant	12 mg/m²/d × 3 d (in combination with cytarabine) for induction therapy for AML 12 mg/m² every 3–4 wk	IVP has been used (over ≥ 3 min, dilute in at least 50 mL), but IVPB the preferred route IVPB (D_5W, NS, in at least 50 mL) over 15–30 min or longer	Pain on injection and phlebitis Leukopenia expected, nadir at 10–12 d, with recovery 21–28 d Alopecia (mild), pruritus, and dry skin Nausea, vomiting, diarrhea, and mucositis (mild) Cumulative cardiomyopathy; maximum lifetime dose is 140–160 mg/m² Hypersensitivity: hypotension, urticaria, and rash Blue-green urine, stool, and sclera for 24–48 h after treatment; the vein may be discolored Fever, conjunctivitis, phlebitis, and amenorrhea
Nelarabine (Arranon) Antimetabolite (pro-drug of Ara-G)	1,500 mg/m² on days 1, 3, and 5 every 21 d	IV undiluted over 2 h (adults) or 1 h (pediatrics)	Anemia, thrombocytopenia, neutropenia Altered mental status, severe somnolence, Convulsions, peripheral neuropathy, demyelination, dizziness, headache, paresthesia, seizures Nausea, diarrhea, vomiting, constipation Petechiae, fatigue, pyrexia, asthenia, peripheral edema, infection Anorexia, myalgia, cough, dyspnea, pleural effusion
Oxaliplatin (Eloxatin) Alkylating agent	85 mg/m² on day 1 every 2 wk in combination with fluorouracil 130 mg/m² every 3 wk in combination with the 5-FU protocol Numerous regimens refer to chemo-therapy text for doses/schedules of protocols	IVPB (D_5W in 250–500 mL) of over 2–6 h Should be administered *prior to* fluorouracil	Myelosuppression mild, occasionally dose limiting; the risk of grade 3 and 4 neutropenia is significantly increased with combination of fluorouracil Nausea, vomiting, diarrhea, dehydration, hypokalemia, metabolic acidosis Hand-foot syndrome Elevations of transaminase enzymes, hyperbilirubinemia Tachycardia supraventricular arrhythmia, hypertension, phlebitis, thromboembolism Acute/chronic neurologic symptoms, aggravated with exposure to cold (dose limiting) Hypersensitivity reactions (later cycles) Fatigue, back pain, arthralgia Pharyngolaryngeal dysesthesias

TABLE 19- QUICK REFERENCE TO COMMONLY ADMINISTERED PARENTERAL CHEMOTHERAPEUTIC AGENTS   (Continued)

Drug	Usual Dose	Usual Administration Technique	Comments and Major Toxicities
Paclitaxel (Taxol) Plant alkaloid Taxane Irritant Potential vesicant	Variety of doses/ schedules including: Ovarian: 135–175 mg/m^2 over 3 h every 3 wk or 135 mg/m^2 over 24 h repeated every 3 wk Breast: 175 mg/ m^2 over 3 h every 3 wk (doses up to 200–250 mg/ m^2 have been administered) Non–small cell lung cancer: 135 mg/m^2 as CI over 24 h (higher doses have been given in combination with carboplatin)	IV infusion (NS, D$_5$W) Over 1, 3, or 24 h Concentration of 0.3–1.2 mg/mL in glass, polypropylene, or poly- olefin containers Avoid contact of the undiluted paclitaxel with plasticized PVC equipment Use an in-line filter of 0.22 μm or less, and a non–PVC-containing infusion set	Pancytopenia (dose limiting), shorter infusions produce less neutropenia; mild anemia, infection Premedicate to avoid hypersensitivity reaction, with dexamethasone, diphen- hydramine, and ranitidine (or cimetidine) Hypersensitivity: urticaria, wheezing, chest pain, dyspnea, and hypotension (common) Cardiovascular: hypertension, hypotension, premature contractures, bradycardia—monitor vital signs during the first hour; EKG abnormalities (common) Peripheral neuropathy (increases with cumulative doses) Nausea, vomiting, diarrhea Mucositis (with longer infusions) Alopecia—complete, rash, flushing, nail changes, arthralgia/myalgia Liver toxicity, interstitial pneumonitis (uncommon)
Paclitaxel protein- bound (Abraxane) Taxane Vesicant	260 mg/m^2 every 3 wk 100–250 mg/m^2 on days 1, 8, and 15 of a 28-day cycle	IV over 30 min Extravasation precautions Do not use an in-line filter	Contains human albumin, which may be prohibited in certain religious/cultural beliefs Myelosuppression, primarily neutropenia (dose limiting) Thrombocytopenia (uncommon); anemia (common) Sensory neuropathy (common) Hypersensitivity reactions: dyspnea, flushing, hypotension, chest pain, arrhythmia (uncommon) No premeds needed for hypersensitivity prevention Hypotension and bradycardia during a 30-minute infusion (uncommon) Nausea, vomiting, diarrhea, mucositis (common) EKG abnormalities (common) Dyspnea and cough Ocular/visual disturbances (e.g., keratitis, blurred vision; severe, reversible) Arthralgia/myalgia; transient, resolved within a few days Interstitial pneumonia, lung fibrosis, and pulmonary embolism (rare)

(Continued)

	TABLE 19-	QUICK REFERENCE TO COMMONLY ADMINISTERED PARENTERAL CHEMOTHERAPEUTIC AGENTS *(Continued)*		

Drug	Usual Dose	Usual Administration Technique	Comments and Major Toxicities
Pegaspargase (Oncaspar) Pegylated form of asparaginase	2,500 units/m^2 every 14 d with other agents for induction and maintenance	IM	Acute liver dysfunction, hypercholesterolemia Coagulopathy Hypersensitivity and anaphylaxis can still occur (used when the patient is allergic to asparaginase) Pancreatitis, hyperglycemia, fever, chills, anorexia, lethargy, confusion, headache, seizures, azotemia (same as asparaginase allergy)
Pemetrexed (Alimta) Antimetabolite	500 mg/m^2 every 21 d with cisplatin (75 mg/m^2 over 2 h) to follow 30 min later	IV infusion over 10 min	Myelosuppression, especially neutropenia, thrombocytopenia Fatigue, nausea, vomiting, dyspnea *Side effects reduced with vitamin supplementation:* Administer folic acid 350–1,000 mcg daily starting 1–3 wk prior to the first cycle and daily for 1–3 wk after the final cycle. Vitamin B$_{12}$ injection 1,000 mcg IM given 1–3 wk before the first cycle and repeat every 9 wk until the treatment is completed Dexamethasone 4 mg BID for 3 d starting the day before treatment decreases the incidence of skin rash
Pentostatin (Nipent) Antimetabolite	4 mg/m^2 every 2 wk Dose reduction may be necessary for renal dysfunction exhibited by creatinine clearance <60 mL/min	IV bolus over 5 min IVPB (NS, D$_5$W, in 25–50 mL) over 20 min or longer Recommend hydration of 1–2 L before and after each treatment IVPB (D$_5$W, NS, in 100 mL) or more over 30–60 min	Severe leukopenia; lymphopenia common; can lead to serious infection (dose limiting) Thrombocytopenia, anemia Nausea, vomiting, fever fatigue (common) Anorexia, diarrhea, mucositis, rashes, dry skin, headache (uncommon) Elevated hepatic transaminase levels, nephrotoxicity (uncommon) Keratoconjunctivitis, photophobia, arthralgia, cough Neurotoxicities rare with standard dose, increased with higher dosing Acute tubular necrosis, hepatitis (rare) Cumulative myelosuppression, anemia, leukopenia, and thrombocytopenia

TABLE 19-	QUICK REFERENCE TO COMMONLY ADMINISTERED PARENTERAL CHEMOTHERAPEUTIC AGENTS *(Continued)*		
Drug	**Usual Dose**	**Usual Administration Technique**	**Comments and Major Toxicities**
Pralatrexate (Folotyn) Antimetabolite (folate analog inhibitor)	30 mg/m² once weekly × 6 wk in a 7-week cycle Supplement with vitamin B₁₂ 1 mg IM every 8–10 wk, starting no more than 10 wk prior to first dose, and folic acid 1–1.25 mg PO daily starting 10 d prior to treatment and ending 30 d after the last pralatrexate dose	IVP undiluted over 3–5 min	Thrombocytopenia, anemia, neutropenia Mucositis, nausea, vomiting, constipation, diarrhea Edema, cough, dyspnea, fever, fatigue, epistaxis hypokalemia, rash, severe dermatologic reactions Tumor lysis syndrome, hepatic dysfunction
Romidepsin (Istodax) HDAC (histone deacetylase) inhibitor	14 mg/m² on days 1, 8, and 15 in 28-day cycles	IVPB (NS 500 mL) over 4 h Due to the risk of QT prolongation, potassium and magnesium levels should be within normal range	Thrombocytopenia, neutropenia, anemia EKG T-wave changes Nausea, vomiting, diarrhea, anorexia, constipation Fatigue, fever, infections, hypomagnesemia Coadministration with strong inhibitors of CYP3A4 may increase romidepsin concentrations and coadministration of potent CYP3A4 inducers may decrease concentrations and should be avoided
Streptozocin (Zanosar) Alkylating agent Irritant	500–1,000 × 5 d every 4–6 wk 1,000–1,500 mg/ m²/wk Doses >1,500 mg/ m²/d should not be exceeded owing to an increased risk of nephrotoxicity. Doses should be adjusted for creatinine clearance <50 mL/min	Continuous infusion × 5 d Can be given IVP, recommended slow administration IVPB (NS, D₅W) over 30–60 min or over 6 h	Leukopenia; nadir 10–14 d (dose limiting) Eosinophilia Nausea and vomiting (severe), anorexia, diarrhea, abdominal cramps (potentially dose limiting) Nephrotoxicity (renal tubular damage) with proteinuria (common and potentially dose limiting) Vein irritation during administration; slow infusion to minimize pain Transient increases in ALT, AST, alkaline phosphatase, and LDH Glucose intolerance and glycosuria Fever, delirium, depression (rare)

(Continued)

TABLE 19-3	QUICK REFERENCE TO COMMONLY ADMINISTERED PARENTERAL CHEMOTHERAPEUTIC AGENTS *(Continued)*			
Drug	**Usual Dose**	**Usual Administration Technique**	**Comments and Major Toxicities**	
Temozolomide (Temodar) Alkylating agent	75–200 mg/m² Bioequivalence w/oral form only established when given over 90 min. Infusion over shorter or longer time may result in suboptimal dosing and/ or increase in infusion-related reactions	IV (in an empty 250-mL bag without further dilution) over 90 min	Myelosuppression Nausea, vomiting, constipation, diarrhea Headache, dizziness, convulsions, confusion, somnolence, fatigue, anorexia Dyspnea, coughing, rash, alopecia, fever	
Temsirolimus (Torisel) Kinase inhibitor	25 mg weekly until disease progression or unacceptable toxicity Premedicate with diphenhydramine 25–50 mg IV	IV undiluted over 30–60 min. A non-PVC infusion container should be used due to the polysorbate 80 vehicle. Use an administration set with an in-line polyethersulfone filter not >5 μm	Myelosuppression, especially anemia Insomnia, headache Mucositis, anorexia, nausea, vomiting, diarrhea, constipation Rash, pruritus, hypersensitivity reaction Elevated serum creatinine, acute renal failure Hyperglycemia, hyperlipemia, asthenia, edema, fever, arthralgia, myalgia, cough, dyspnea, elevated LFT's, wound healing complications, interstitial lung disease If patients must be coadministered a strong CYP3A4 inhibitor or CYP3A4 inducer, a dose modification may be warranted	
Teniposide (VM-26) Plant alkaloid	165 mg/m² 2 times/ week for 8–9 doses (with cytarabine protocol) Maintenance dose of 250 mg/m² weekly for 4–8 wk	IVPB (D₅W, NS) over at least 30–60 min Maintain concentration of 0.1–0.4 mg/mL Administer via non-PVC containers or glass IP	Anaphylaxis may occur Mucositis, nausea, vomiting, diarrhea, anorexia (uncommon) Alopecia (mild) Hypotension (rapid IV infusion) Fatigue, seizures, somnolence, fever, renal insufficiency, and secondary malignancies (rare) Leukopenia: nadir at 14 d and recovery after 2–4 wk (dose limiting)	

	TABLE 19-	QUICK REFERENCE TO COMMONLY ADMINISTERED PARENTERAL CHEMOTHERAPEUTIC AGENTS *(Continued)*		

Drug	Usual Dose	Usual Administration Technique	Comments and Major Toxicities
Thiotepa Alkylating agent	Nontransplant: 12–16 mg/m² every 1–4 wk Transplant: 900 mg/m² Intrathecal: 1–10 mg/m² 1–2 times weekly Bladder instillation: 30–60 mg every week × 4 wk Numerous routes of administration	IV over 30 min Intravesically Intrathecally	Anemia, thrombocytopenia Alopecia Hypersensitivity reactions: angioedema, hives, rash, and pruritus Nausea, vomiting, anorexia, mucositis, diarrhea, fever (uncommon) Headache, dizziness, and weakness of lower extremities Paresthesias associated with intrathecal administration Impaired fertility—azoospermia and amenorrhea Dose-limiting neutropenia grade 4 with nadir on days 10–12
Topotecan (Hycamtin) Topoisomerase 1 inhibitor	1.5 mg/m²/d × 5 consecutive days every 21 d for the first four courses of treatment Subsequent treat- ment should be administered at a dose of 1.25 mg/ m²/d × 5 d Numerous other doses have been evaluated	IVPB (D₅W 50 mL) over 60–90 min IVP	Mild thrombocytopenia, anemia (common) Total alopecia Nausea, vomiting, diarrhea (common) Headache, fever, fatigue, anorexia, malaise, elevated liver enzymes (common) Hypertension, tachycardia, urticaria, renal insufficiency, hematuria, dizziness, peripheral neuropathy, mucositis (uncommon) Dyspnea Patients with moderate renal compromise require a dose adjustment
Trimetrexate (Neutrexin) Antimetabolite	45 mg/m² × 21 d with concomitant leucovorin Leucovorin must also be given 3 d after cessation of treatment with trimetrexate Has also been given 110 mg/m² in combination with fluorouracil every week × 6 wk followed by 2 wk of rest	IVP over 1–5 min Extravasation precautions IVPB not recommended	Patients with hypoalbuminemia are more likely to experience severe anemia, muco- sitis, thrombocytopenia Myelosuppression dose related (leucovorin greatly reduces these toxicities) Fever, shaking, chills, malaise Transient elevations of liver enzymes Dose-limiting leukopenia with early nadirs Thrombocytopenia and anemia (uncommon) Extravasation: treat with application of heat

(Continued)

TABLE 19-3   QUICK REFERENCE TO COMMONLY ADMINISTERED PARENTERAL CHEMOTHERAPEUTIC AGENTS   *(Continued)*

Drug	Usual Dose	Usual Administration Technique	Comments and Major Toxicities
Valrubicin (Valstar) Antitumor antibiotic (semisynthetic analog of doxorubicin)	800 mg intravesicularly once weekly × 6 wk Use non-PVC containers and tubing	Intravesical instillation via a urethral catheter. The patient should retain the drug for 2 h before voiding Warming may be required if precipitation occurs	Urinary frequency, urgency, incontinence, dysuria, spasm, pain, hematuria, cystitis Nausea, abdominal pain, dizziness Urinary tract infection, headache, malaise, rash
Vinblastine (Velban) Plant alkaloid Vesicant	6–10 mg/m² every 2–4 wk Also given every week and as a continuous infusion in a dose of 1.7–2 mg/m²/d for 96 h through a central line	IVP over 1 min Occasionally given as a continuous infusion (D_5W, NS)	Rash and photosensitivity Nausea, vomiting, and constipation; abdominal cramping, anorexia Peripheral neuropathy, myalgias, headache, seizures, depression, dizziness, and malaise Acute bronchospasm, dyspnea, chest pain, tumor pain, fever, especially when administered with mitomycin Severe jaw pain, pain in pharynx, bones, back Phlebitis and vein discoloration SIADH and angina pectoris (rare) Leukopenia (mild and rare); thrombocytopenia (rare) Alopecia
Vincristine (Oncovin) Plant alkaloid Vesicant	0.5–1.4 mg/m² every 1–4 wk Usually the maximum dose is 2 mg 0.5 mg/d to 0.5 mg/m²/d over 96 h via a central line	IV syringe (NS, D_5W), IV bag (NS, D_5W, lactated Ringer's)	If extravasated, treat with application of heat Nausea, vomiting (rare); constipation; abdominal pain, anorexia *Intrathecal administration is fatal* Peripheral neuropathy, paresthesias, paralytic ileus, and myalgias (cumulative, dose limiting) Acute bronchospasm, dyspnea when administered with mitomycin Diplopia, ptosis, photophobia, cortical blindness Azoospermia and amenorrhea
Vincristine liposomal (Marqibo) Vinca alkaloid	2.25 mg/m² once every 7 d Use actual BSA	IVPB (D5W, NS to total volume of 100 mL) over 1 h Preparation requires water bath and thermometer	Febrile neutropenia, pyrexia Anemia Peripheral neuropathy, insomnia Constipation, nausea, diarrhea Fatigue, decreased appetite

TABLE 19 QUICK REFERENCE TO COMMONLY ADMINISTERED PARENTERAL CHEMOTHERAPEUTIC AGENTS *(Continued)*

Drug	Usual Dose	Usual Administration Technique	Comments and Major Toxicities
Vindesine (Eldisine) Vinca alkaloid Vesicant	3–4 mg/m²/wk 1–2 mg/m² on days 1–5 (continuous infusion) every 2–4 wk 0.2–2 mg/m² × 5–21 consecutive days Maximum tolerated dose is 4 mg/m²/wk	IVP over 2–3 min IVPB 15–20 min or 24-h continuous infusion	Leukopenia, thrombocytopenia (dose limiting) Pyrexia, malaise, myalgia, alopecia, paresthesia, loss of deep tendon reflexes (dose limiting) Mild nausea and vomiting, constipation
Vinorelbine (Navelbine) Vinca alkaloid Vesicant	30 mg/m²/wk	Infuse over 6–10 min into a side port of a free-flowing IV, flush with 100–200 mL of solution to reduce the risk of phlebitis	Myelosuppression, mostly leukopenia (dose limiting) Acute reversible dyspnea, chest pain, wheezing after IV administration; prevented by premedication with steroids Injection site erythema, pain, phlebitis Fatigue, tumor pain, jaw pain Mild nausea, constipation, diarrhea, stomatitis Hepatic: transient elevated LFTs Chest pain with or without EKG changes
Ziv-aflibercept (Zaltrap) (Aflibercept) Vascular endothelial growth factor (VEGF) inhibitor	4 mg/kg every 2 wk	IVPB (D_5W, NS) over 1 h Final concentration between 0.6 and 8 mg/ mL Use a 0.2-μm filter	Hypertension Dysphonia, epistaxis, dyspnea, oropharyngeal pain, rhinorrhea Neutropenia, leukopenia, thrombocytopenia Headache Palmar–plantar erythrodysesthesia syndrome, skin hyperpigmentation Diarrhea, stomatitis, abdominal pain, hemorrhoids, rectal hemorrhage, proctalgia Proteinuria, increased serum creatinine Urinary tract infections Increased AST/ALT, fatigue, weight loss, decreased appetite, asthenia, dehydration

that augment, modulate, or restore the immune response of the host; agents that have direct **anticancer** activity (antiproliferation or cytotoxic effect on cancer cells); agents that increase the vulnerability of cancer cells to the body's immune system; agents that change the pathway that transforms normal cells to cancer cells; those agents that enhance the repair of normal cells damaged by therapy; agents that prevent metastasis; and lastly, agents that change the behavior of cancer cells to normal cells (Polovich et al., 2009).

Biologic agents are proteins derived from and/or copied from proteins that exist naturally in the human body. These agents fall into several categories: cytokines (interferons [IFNs], interleukins, and hematopoietic growth factors) and monoclonal antibodies (mAbs). Promising new therapies target cancer cells at a molecular level and hence are called molecular-targeted therapy. These agents aim their antineoplastic activity at cell membrane receptors, signaling pathways and proteins, enzymatic activity, and regulatory cell growth controls that are more aberrant and abundant in cancer cells than in normal cells. Because of this specificity, the therapeutic efficacy is enhanced, while the toxicity to normal cells is decreased (DeVita et al., 2011). Cytokines are hormone-like messenger molecules that cells use to communicate. T lymphocytes produce IFN when in contact with viruses and tumors. The **interferons** are cytokines that initiate immune responses that are antiviral, antitumor (prevent malignant transformation of cells, down-regulate cell division, communicate with other cytotoxic immune cells), and immunomodulatory (enhance natural killer [NK] cell activity).

Interleukins do not possess cytotoxic activity. Their effectiveness is through their influence on the cells of the immune system. Interleukins stimulate the production of cytokines and the migration of active immune cells (T-helper cells, monocytes/macrophages, cytotoxic T cells, and NK cells) to the tumor. Table 19-4 provides an overview of interleukin and IFN dosing, administration, and side effects and major toxicities.

Hematopoietic growth factors represent a milestone in cancer treatment. Because of recombinant DNA technology, these agents are able to mimic the activity of colony-stimulating factors (CSFs). The use of these growth factors has enabled rapid recovery of bone marrow activity, and thus allowing patients to receive frequent, dose-dense therapy. Table 19-5 lists the most common hematopoietic growth factors used with chemotherapy/biotherapy.

Monoclonal Antibodies

Monoclonal antibodies are defined by the Food and Drug Administration as intact immunoglobulins produced by hybridomas, immunoconjugates, immunoglobulin fragments, or recombinant proteins derived from immunoglobulins. The philosophy behind the mAbs used in oncology is to facilitate antitumor effects directly on a specific target associated with cancer cells. The antitumor effect can be demonstrated by apoptosis, antibody-dependent cell cytotoxicity, complement-mediated cytolysis, or by delivery of radiation or cellular toxins. This target specificity facilitates more direct attack on the cancer cells and less toxicity.

The specific targets are usually expressed on the cell surface of cancer cells. Targets identified in current FDA-approved mAbs include cluster of differentiation (CD) markers and growth factor receptors (epidermal growth factors [EGRF], vascular endothelial growth factors [VEGF], etc.). When the antibodies bind to these targets, it activates the immune system and mediates the process of cell destruction.

There are four types of mAbs, dependent on the hybridoma technique used to produce Abs. The antigen that stimulates antibody-forming immune cells is derived from one of four sources: murine (mouse), chimeric (combination of mouse and human antibodies),

TABLE 19	BIOTHERAPY AGENTS		
Drug	**Usual Dose**	**Administration/ Precautions**	**Common and Major Toxicities**
Aldesleukin (inter-leukin-2, Proleukin) Biologic response modifier: cytokine production, prolif-eration of lympho-cytes, enhanced cell cytotoxicity	High dose: 600,000–720,000 units/kg IV every 8 h for 5 consecu-tive days for 2 cycles, separated by 7–10 d 9 million units/m²/d continuous infusion for 4 d, every 3 wk for 6 cycles Premedications: anti-pyretic to reduce fever, H₂ antagonist for pro-phylaxis of gastrointesti-nal irritation/bleeding	IVPB over 15 min Do not use in-line filters 24-h infusion. Subcutaneous Do not mix with NS or bacteriostatic water Do not mix with other meds	Capillary leak syndrome: hypotension, edema, pulmonary congestion, renal insufficiency, arrhythmias, diarrhea, and possibly CNS and hepatic toxicity (dose limiting) Transient myelosuppression, prolonged anemia, transient hyperbilirubinemia, elevated transaminase, electrolyte imbalances Fever, chills, malaise, headache, nasal stuffiness, myalgia, arthralgia, erythroedema, nausea, vomiting (common) Lethargy, delirium, angina pectoris, CHF, frank respiratory failure, infections (uncommon)
Denileukin difitox (Ontak) Recombinant cyto-toxic protein from diphtheria toxin and interleukin-2	9–18 mcg/kg/d × 5 d every 21 d × 8 cycles Premedication: antihistamine and diphenhydramine	IVPB (NS) in 25 mL or 50 mL to keep the concentration ≥15 mcg/mL over 30–60 min Do not filter	Serious and fatal infusion reactions. Monitor weight, edema, blood pressure, and serum albumin prior to and during treatment; hold if albumin levels are < 3 g/dL Capillary leak syndrome, loss of visual acuity Nausea, vomiting, diarrhea, anorexia Pyrexia, rigors, fatigue, headache, peripheral edema, rash, cough, dyspnea, pruritus
IFN-α-2B (Intron-A) Biologic response modifier, antiviral, immunostimulant	2 to 30 million units/m² from 3 times per week to daily Adjustments made based on the patient tolerance and lab values	Subcutaneous, IM, IVP, IV Infusion over 20 min	Acute: fever, chills, nasal congestion, diarrhea, malaise Chronic: fatigue, anorexia, weight loss, depression, anemia Neutropenia, thrombocytopenia: transient (can be dose limiting at higher doses) Cardiovascular toxicity: CHF, arrhythmias: reversible (rare) CNS toxicity: delirium, psychosis, peripheral neuropathy reversible (rare) Hyperglycemia, hypocalcemia (rare)

TABLE 19-5	**HEMOPOIETIC GROWTH FACTORS**		

Drug	Usual Dose	Administration/ Precautions	Common and Major Toxicities
Darbepoetin (Aranesp) Erythropoiesis-stimulating agent	Chemotherapy-induced anemia (required REMS program): (Initial) 2.25 mcg/kg SC weekly or 500 mcg SC every 3 wk Chronic kidney disease: Initial: 0.45 mcg/kg IV or SC weekly or 0.75 mcg/kg IV or SC every 2 wk Myelodysplastic syndrome: 150–300 mcg SC weekly	Subcutaneous (SC) IV Should not be used in the following conditions: With myelosuppressive chemotherapy with curative intent As a substitute for RBC transfusions in patients requiring immediate correction of anemia	FDA warning: increased risk of serious cardiovascular and thromboembolic events, stroke, and death. Cancer patients may also have increased risk of shortened overall survival Allergic reactions, pain at the injection site, dyspnea, cough, hypertension Nausea, vomiting, diarrhea, headache, edema
Epoetin alfa (Procrit, Epogen) Erythropoiesis-stimulating agent	Chemotherapy-induced anemia (required REMS program): Initial: 150 units/kg SC 3 times weekly or 40,000 units SC weekly Chronic kidney disease: Initial: 50–100 units/kg IV or SC 3 times weekly Myelodysplastic syndrome: 40,000–60,000 units SC 1–3 times weekly Anemia due to zidovudine in HIV-infected patients: Initial: 100 units/kg IV or SC 3 times weekly Surgery patients: 300–600 units/kg SC	Subcutaneous IV	FDA warning: increased risk of serious cardiovascular and thromboembolic events, stroke, and death. Cancer patients may also have increased risk of shortened overall survival Hypertension, pain at the injection site, cough, arthralgia Nausea, vomiting, headache, pruritus, rash, fever
Filgrastim (Neupogen) Colony-stimulating factor	5 mcg/kg/d no earlier than 24 h after the end of chemotherapy	Subcutaneous IV Discontinue when postnadir ANC > 10,000/mm^3	Transient bone pain (20%), fever, petechiae, rash, LDH/uric acid/alkaline phosphatase elevation, epistaxis, splenomegaly Headache, nausea, vomiting Splenic rupture, acute respiratory distress syndrome (ARDS), precipitation of sickle cell crises (rare)
Oprelvekin (Neumega) Thrombopoietic growth factor	50 mcg/kg/d beginning 6–24 h after the end of chemotherapy. Discontinue at least 48 h prior to next chemotherapy cycle	Subcutaneous Administer until postnadir platelet count is ≥50,000/mm^3	Fluid retention that may result in peripheral edema, capillary leak syndrome, arrhythmias, or exacerbation of pleural effusion. Use cautiously in patients in which plasma volume expansion should be avoided (e.g., left ventricular dysfunction, heart failure, hypertension) Dilutional anemia (reversible, responds to diuretics) Atrial arrhythmias, visual blurring

TABLE 19-	HEMOPOIETIC GROWTH FACTORS (Continued)		
Drug	**Usual Dose**	**Administration/ Precautions**	**Common and Major Toxicities**
Pegfilgrastim (Neulasta) Colony-stimulating factor	6 mg administered once per chemotherapy cycle	Subcutaneous Do not administer in the period from 14 d prior and 24 h after chemotherapy administration	Transient bone pain (31%–57%), peripheral edema, headache, vomiting, myalgia, arthralgia, weakness, allergic reaction, constipation Splenic rupture, ARDS, precipitation of sickle cell crises (rare)
Plerixafor (Mozobil) Hematopoietic stem cell mobilizer	0.24 mg/kg once daily to 11 h prior to apheresis for up to 4 consecutive days; maximum dose 40 mg/d Dosing based on actual weight	Subcutaneous	Fatigue, headache, dizziness Diarrhea, nausea Injection site reactions, arthralgias, insomnia, vomiting, flatulence
Sargramostim (Leukine) Colony-stimulating factor	250 mcg/kg/d *Acute leukemia*: start 11 d after induction chemotherapy when the marrow is hypoplastic *Mobilization of progenitor cells*: immediately after infusion of progenitor cells *Bone marrow transplant*: given 2–4 h after infusion of bone marrow infusion	2-h IV infusion	Fever, flu-like symptoms (common). Hypersensitivity reactions (greater with filgrastim) Diarrhea, asthenia, rash, malaise, fluid retention (peripheral edema, effusions; occasional) With transplant doses: capillary leak syndrome

humanized (small part mouse fused with human), and human. The effectiveness of the mAbs is limited by the immune response to the source of the antibody.

Specific cell surface proteins function as targets for mAbs, for example, rituximab that binds with CD20 antigen on B cells. mAbs are classified as unconjugated or conjugated. Unconjugated mAbs have direct effects in producing programmed cell death and indirect effects of activating host defense systems to create antitumor activity. There is no attached drug or radioisotope attached, referred to as "naked." With a conjugated mAb, a radioisotope conjugate or a drug-activating enzyme conjugate is attached to produce additional cytotoxic effects.

The future of mAbs is promising as discoveries are made to develop more potential targets and pathways. Combination treatments with mAbs are attractive owing to the potential enhancement of antitumor responses without increases in toxicities. Table 19-6 identifies the currently approved mAbs, their indications, dosing, method of administration, side effects, and nursing considerations.

Goals of Antineoplastic Therapy

The goal of all anticancer therapy is the eradication of all cancer cells. A *cure* is described as a prolonged absence of detectable disease. When cure is unrealistic, *control* (therapy that extends life) can be the goal of therapy. *Palliation* is a legitimate goal for patients with

TABLE 19-6 MONOCLONAL ANTIBODIES

Drug	Dose	Method of Administration	Complications	Considerations
Ado-Trastuzumab Emtansine (Kadcyla) Monoclonal antibody + DM1 cytotoxin microtubule inhibitor Drug specificity: binds to HER2 receptor	Dose is 3.6 mg/kg IV every 3 wk Maximum dose 3.6 mg/kg	IV infusion Do not administer as an IV push or bolus Infuse over 90 min (first infusion) or 30 min (subsequent infusions, if tolerated) Do not mix with dextrose solution Use a 0.22-μm polyethersulfone (PES) filter	Infusion-related reaction, fatigue, nausea, musculoskeletal, pain, thrombocytopenia, headache, increased transaminases, constipation Cardiotoxicity, peripheral neuropathy, pulmonary toxicity, local skin reactions, epistaxis, cough, dyspnea	Not interchangeable with trastuzumab Assess LVEF Perform HER2 testing
Alemtuzumab (Campath) Drug specificity: binds to CD52-positive B and T cells	Usual initial dose: 3 mg over 2 h daily If tolerated, slowly escalate daily to a maintenance dose of 30 mg 3 times per week (i.e., Monday, Wednesday, Friday) for ≤12 wk Requires maintenance dose. Do not exceed recommended maintenance dose of 30 mg 3 times per week	Do not administer as an IV push or bolus Use a 5-μm filter Premedicate with acetaminophen 650 mg orally and diphenhydramine 50 mg orally	*Common:* Severe pancytopenia/marrow hypoplasia, autoimmune idiopathic thrombocytopenia, and autoimmune hemolytic anemia. Can result in opportunistic infections *Dose-limiting effects:* Single doses >30 mg or cumulative doses >90 mg per week have been associated with higher incidence of pancytopenia	Dose escalation to the recommended maintenance dose of 30 mg 3 times per week is required. If alemtuzumab is withheld for ≥7 d, dose escalation must begin at 3 mg again Monitor the patient closely for infusion-related reactions Hypersensitivity/anaphylactic medications should be available during infusion
Bevacizumab (Avastin) Drug specificity: binds to vascular endothelial growth factor (VEGF) receptors	Loading dose: 5 mg/m² over 10 min every 14 d	IV infusion Do not administer as an IV push or bolus Loading dose given over 120 min. If tolerated well, may infuse the maintenance dose over 60 min Use a 0.22-μm filter	*Common:* Gastrointestinal perforations/wound-healing complications. Can be serious or fatal. Symptoms included abdominal pain, which has been seen with constipation and vomiting *System specific:* Proteinuria, nephrotic syndrome, congestive heart failure, and hypertensive crises	Bevacizumab should not be administered at least 28 d following major surgery, and surgical incision should be fully healed. The bevacizumab half-life of 20 d should be considered when determining the length that bevacizumab should be suspended prior to elective surgery Monitor the patient closely for infusion-related reactions Premedications can be considered for infusion-related reactions

Drug	Dose	Method of Administration	Complications	Considerations
			Other: Hemorrhage. Fatal or serious hemoptysis in patients with non–small cell lung cancer. If recent hemoptysis, the patient should not receive bevacizumab	Hypersensitivity/anaphylactic medications should be available during infusion Do not mix with dextrose solutions Gently invert the bag to mix
Brentuximab vedotin (Adcetris) Drug specificity: binds to CD30 cells	1.8 mg/kg IV every 3 wk × 16 cycles	IV infusion over 30 min	Myelosuppression Peripheral sensory neuropathy Headache, dizziness Nausea, vomiting, diarrhea Fatigue, fever, chills, rash, itching, arthralgia, myalgia Insomnia, cough, respiratory infection, Stevens-Johnson syndrome	Maximum 100 kg weight to calculate the dose
Cetuximab (Erbitux) Drug specificity: binds to epidermal growth factor receptors (EGFR)	Loading dose: 400 mg/m^2 over 120 min, maintenance dose 250 mg/m^2 over 60 min weekly Maximum rate: 5 mL/min	IV infusion Do not administer as an IV push or bolus Loading dose given over 120 min. If tolerated well, may infuse a maintenance dose over 60 min Use a 0.22-μm filter Premedication with diphenhydramine 50 mg IV is recommended 1-h observation period is recommended	*Common:* Acneform rash seen in about 90% of patients. Described as skin drying and fissuring, multiple follicular- or pustular-appearing lesions. Most commonly located on the face, upper chest, and back but could also be located on the extremities. Occurs within the first 2 wk of therapy, and most cases resolved with cessation of cetuximab. Events did continue beyond 28 d in nearly half of the cases	

TABLE 19- **MONOCLONAL ANTIBODIES** *(Continued)*

(Continued)

TABLE 19-	MONOCLONAL ANTIBODIES	*(Continued)*		
Drug	**Dose**	**Method of Administration**	**Complications**	**Considerations**
Gemtuzumab (Mylotarg) Monoclonal antibody + calicheamicin (cytotoxic antitumor antibiotic) Drug specificity: binds to CD33-positive antigens As of June 2010, withdrawn from the US market and not available to new patients; only available in the United States under an Investigational New Drug (IND) protocol	9 mg/m^2 IV and repeat dose after 2 wk. Hematologic recovery is not required prior to the second dose	IV infusion over 2 h Chemotherapy precautions should be exercised owing to the chemotherapy component of gemtuzumab Do not administer as an IV push or bolus Premedicate with acetaminophen 650–1,000 mg orally and diphenhydramine 50 mg orally; thereafter, continue prophylaxis with two additional doses of acetaminophen 650–1,000 mg orally, one every 4 h as needed Premedication with methylprednisolone may also be considered Vital signs should be monitored during infusion and for the 4 h following Use a low–protein binding 1.2-μm filter Gently invert the bag to mix and protect from light Monitor the patient closely for infusion-related reactions Infusion	*Common:* Myelosuppression and severe infections may result. Can occur at recommended doses *System specific:* Fatal hepatotoxicity has been reported such as hepatic venoocclusive disease. Symptoms include rapid weight gain, right upper quadrant pain, hepatomegaly, ascites, elevations in bilirubin, and/or liver enzymes. Use with extra caution if bilirubin > 2 mg/dL System specific: Patients with WBC counts ≥ 30,000 cells/μL or symptomatic intrinsic lung disease may be at an increased risk for pulmonary events such as dyspnea, pulmonary infiltrates, pleural effusions, noncardiogenic pulmonary edema, pulmonary insufficiency and hypoxia, and ARDS	Monitor the patient closely for infusion-related reactions such as dyspnea or clinically significant hypotension. Consider discontinuation if anaphylaxis, pulmonary edema, or ARDS occurs Most symptoms occurred after the end of the 2-h infusion and resolved after 2–4 h with supportive treatment with acetaminophen, diphenhydramine, and IV fluids Fewer infusion-related reactions occurred with the second dose Hypersensitivity/ anaphylactic medications should be available during infusion Preparation should be done within a biologic safety hood with the fluorescent light turned off. Use immediately Use chemotherapy checking, handling, and disposal procedures Hypersensitivity/ anaphylactic medications should be available during infusion Gently invert the bag to mix Instruct the patient to wear sunscreen and hats and limit sun exposure

		MONOCLONAL ANTIBODIES	*(Continued)*	

Drug	Dose	Method of Administration	Complications	Considerations
Ipilimumab (Yervoy) Drug specificity: binds to cytotoxic T-lymphocyte–associated antigen 4 (CTLA-4)	3 mg/kg IV every 3 wk for a total of 4 doses	IVPB over 90 min. Keep the concentration between 1 and 2 mg/mL		Can result in severe and fatal immune-mediated adverse reactions due to T-cell activation and proliferation Permanently discontinue with severe enterocolitis and initiate systemic corticosteroids
Ofatumumab (Arzerra) Drug specificity: binds to extracellular loops of CD20-positive B lymphocytes	300 mg, and then 1,000–2,000 mg Administer with inline filter supplied with product	IVPB (NS 1,000 mL, remove drug volume and overfill) at varying rates: Doses 1 and 2: Start at 12 mL/h and double every 30 min (25 mL/h, 50 mL/h, 100 mL/h) to a maximum of 200 mL/h after first 2 h Subsequent doses: start at 25 mL/h and double every 30 min (50 mL/h, 100 mL/h, 200 mL/h) to a maximum of 400 mL/h after first 2 h	Infusion-related reactions Neutropenia, anemia Headache, insomnia Nausea, diarrhea Pneumonia, fever, cough, fatigue, dyspnea, rash, bronchitis	Premedicate with acetaminophen 1,000 mg PO, diphenhydramine 25–50 mg IV/PO, and steroid equivalent to prednisolone 100 mg IV (e.g., methylprednisolone 80 mg or dexamethasone 15 mg IV)
Panitumumab (Vectibix) Drug specificity: binds to epidermal growth factor receptors (EGFR)	6 mg/kg IV every 14 d	IV diluted to a total volume of 100 mL NS over 60 min Doses >1,000 mg IV, dilute to 150 mL over 90 min Use a 0.2- to 0.22-μm filter Do not shake Do not give an IV push or bolus	Infusion-related reaction (4%, severe 1%) (anaphylactoid reactions, bronchospasm, hypotension) Abdominal pain, diarrhea, fatigue, hypomagnesemia, nausea, paronychia, and skin rash, mucositis, eye-related toxicities Constipation, hypomagnesemia, nausea, pulmonary embolism, pulmonary fibrosis, severe dermatologic toxicity	Premedication is not required

(Continued)

TABLE 19-6	MONOCLONAL ANTIBODIES *(Continued)*			
Drug	**Dose**	**Method of Administration**	**Complications**	**Considerations**
Pertuzumab (Perjeta) Drug specificity: binds to human epidermal growth factor receptor 2 protein (HER2)	Initial dose is 840 mg IV then subsequent dose is 420 mg IV every 3 wk	Do not administer as an IV push or bolus Infuse over 60 min (first infusion) or 30–60 min (subsequent infusions, if tolerated)	Infusion-related reaction, fatigue, headache, rash, diarrhea, decreased appetite, mucosal inflammation, nausea, neutropenia, anemia	Binds to a different HER2 epitope than trastuzumab so when combined, a more complete inhibition of HER2 occurs Perform HER2 testing Monitor LVEF
Rituximab (Rituxan) Drug specificity: binds to CD20-positive B lymphocytes	375 mg/m² weekly × 4–8 doses	IV infusion through recommended infusion guidelines Do not administer as an IV push or bolus For first infusions, initiate at 50 mg/h. If no symptoms, increase the rate in 50 mg/h increments every 30 min to a maximum of 400 mg/h as tolerated For second infusion, initiate at 100 mg/h If no symptoms, increase the rate in 100 mg/h increments every 30 min to maximum of 400 mg/h as tolerated	*Common:* Infusion-related reactions or hypersensitivity reactions. Symptoms include hypotension, angioedema, hypoxia, and bronchospasm Fatal reactions have been reported, especially with the first infusions. Symptoms have included hypoxia, pulmonary infiltrates, ARDS, myocardial infarction, ventricular fibrillation, or cardiogenic shock *System specific: Tumor lysis syndrome and severe mucocutaneous reactions (e.g., paraneoplastic pemphigus, Stevens-Johnson syndrome, lichenoid dermatitis, vesiculobullous dermatitis, and toxic epidermal necrolysis)*	Monitor the patient closely for infusion-related reactions. If symptoms occur, slow or stop infusion and administer medical treatment as indicated (i.e., acetaminophen, diphenhydramine, bronchodilators, or IV saline). When symptoms are completely resolved, resuming infusion at 50% of rate (e.g., from 100 mg/h to 50 mg/h) can be considered Premedications such as diphenhydramine and acetaminophen can be considered to prevent infusion-related reactions Hypersensitivity/anaphylactic medications such as epinephrine, antihistamines, and corticosteroids should be available during infusion Antihypertensive medications may need to be held at least 12 h prior to rituximab administration owing to the potential rituximab infusion-related hypotension Gently invert the bag to mix

Drug	Dose	Method of Administration	Complications	Considerations
TABLE 19 MONOCLONAL ANTIBODIES *(Continued)*				
Trastuzumab (Herceptin) Drug specificity: binds to human epidermal growth factor receptor 2 (HER2)	Loading dose (LD) 4 mg/kg over 90 min. Maintenance dose (MD) 2 mg/kg over 30 min weekly (experimental dosing: LD 8 mg/kg, MD 6 mg/kg every 3 wk)	Do not administer as an IV push or bolus Loading dose given over 90 min. If tolerated well, may infuse maintenance dose over 30 min Dextrose solutions should not be used with trastuzumab	*Common and system specific:* Cardiotoxicity including congestive heart failure, disabling cardiac failure, death, and mural thrombosis leading to stroke. Symptoms include dyspnea, increased cough, paroxysmal nocturnal dyspnea, peripheral edema, S3 gallop, or reduced ejection fraction	Obtain baseline cardiac assessment including history and physical exam and one or more of the following: EKG, echocardiogram, and MUGA scan. Extreme caution should be practiced in patients with preexisting cardiac dysfunction Monitor the patient closely for infusion-related reactions such as chills and fever. This was observed in about 40% of patients in clinical trials Treatment can consist of acetaminophen, diphenhydramine, and meperidine, with or without reduction in the trastuzumab infusion rate Hypersensitivity/anaphylactic medications such as epinephrine, antihistamines, and corticosteroids should be available during infusion If known hypersensitivity to benzyl alcohol, reconstitute with sterile water for injection instead of the supplied diluent, which contains 1.1% benzyl alcohol Gently invert the bag to mix

The information here is provided as guidance only. Nurses should always consult the manufacturer's current prescribing information before administering drugs. A pharmacist should be consulted for information on compatibilities, concentrations, and stability.

ALT, alanine aminotransferase; AML, acute myelocytic leukemia; AST, aspartate aminotransferase; AUC, area under the curve; BID, twice daily; BSA, body surface area; CHF, cardiac heart failure; CNS, central nervous system; CYP, cytochrome P450 enzymes; D_5W, 5% dextrose in water; dL, deciliter; EKG, electrocardiogram; FDA, Food and Drug Administration; g, gram; GFR, glomerular filtration rate; IM, intramuscular; I/O, intake/output; IV, intravenous; IVP, intravenous push; IT, intrathecal; IVPB, intravenous piggyback; kg, kilograms; LDH, lactate dehydrogenase; LFT, liver function tests; LVEF, left ventricular ejection fraction; m^2, square meter; mcg, microgram; mg, milligrams; mL, milliliters; min, minute; mm^3, millimeter cubed; NS, normal saline; NYHA, New York Heart Association; PVC, polyvinyl chloride; SC, subcutaneous.

(From Fischer, D. S., Knobf, T. M., Durivage, H.J., & Beaulieu, N. J. (2003). *The cancer chemotherapy handbook* (6th ed., pp. 48–239). Chicago, IL: Mosby; Perry, C., Anderson, C. M., & Donehower, R. C. (2004). Chemotherapy. In M. Abeloff, J. Armitage, J. Niederhuber, & M. Keaton, *Clinical oncology* (3rd ed.). Elsevier.)

advanced or incurable disease. Even when there is no real hope of complete cure, cancer cells often remain somewhat sensitive to antineoplastic agents, so disease progression can be slowed. Agents often can control pain caused by tumor pressure, ease fluid obstruction, and edema and control hypercalcemia and other organic carcinoid processes (Polovich et al., 2009).

The American Cancer Society report shows that the decline in cancer mortality has reached 20%, translating to the avoidance of about 1.2 million deaths from cancer since 1991. That is more than 400 lives saved per day! (Seigel, 2013).

A total of 1,660,290 new cancer cases and 580,350 deaths from cancer are projected to occur in the United States in 2013. Between 1990/1991 and 2009, the most recent year for which data are available, overall death rates decreased by 24% in men, 16% in women, and 20% overall. This translates to almost 1.2 million deaths from cancer that was avoided. Death rates continue to decline for lung, colon, breast, and prostate cancers, which are responsible for the most cancer deaths. Since 1991, death rates have decreased by more than 40% for prostate cancer and by more than 30% for colon cancer, breast cancer in women, and lung cancer in men (Seigel, 2013).

Tumors vary in their responsiveness to chemotherapy. While great strides have been made in childhood cancers in terms of cure, other tumors have responded to chemotherapy, and patients have experienced longer survival times. In some tumor types, chemotherapy has afforded patients improved quality of life through palliation. Remaining cancers are less responsive to chemotherapeutic intervention. Biotherapy agents (IFNs and interleukins) are commonly used in advanced cancers where other treatment methods do not offer positive outcomes. Generally, they have been found to provide longer survival times, longer times to disease progression, and higher response rates than more traditional chemotherapy given for the same malignancy, for example, melanoma and renal cell carcinoma. Although not currently approved as antitumor therapy, hematopoietic growth factors are often used for alleviation of both the symptoms related to malignancy and the side effects of chemotherapy.

Combined Modality Therapy

Although any treatment modality can be used alone, usually antineoplastic regimens rely on drug combinations. In addition, combining the available treatment modalities aims to optimize cancer cell killing while minimizing associated toxicities. One of the important roles of chemotherapy is as **adjuvant** treatment, following surgery and/or radiation therapy, to reduce the incidence of both local and systemic recurrence and to improve the overall survival of patients. A good example of this is in women with breast cancer, where adjuvant chemotherapy is particularly effective in decreasing the rate of recurrence following surgery and radiation therapy. **Neoadjuvant** chemotherapy is the use of chemotherapy prior to treatment for localized cancer when the local therapy is less than completely effective. In this case, vital normal organs are spared, while the tumor is reduced in size and rendered easier to treat by local therapy, that is, surgery. This has led to less extensive surgery and sparing of the larynx, the anal sphincter, and the bladder and better quality of life for patients.

With the exception of oral alkylating agents used for chronic leukemias, single-agent chemotherapy regimens are rare in contemporary practice. *Combination chemotherapy* involves simultaneous multiagent use that capitalizes on synergistic drug actions to maximize their antitumor effects. Chemotherapy drugs can also be combined with biotherapy agents. Combining agents also modifies dose-limiting toxicities. Box 19-5 lists common

BOX 19-5   ANTICANCER DRUG COMBINATIONS

ABVD	Doxorubicin + bleomycin + vinblastine + dacarbazine
AC-T	Doxorubicin + cyclophosphamide followed by paclitaxel
BEP	bleomycin + etoposide + cisplatin
CHOP-R	Cyclophosphamide + doxorubicin + vincristine + prednisone + rituximab
CAF	Cyclophosphamide + doxorubicin + fluorouracil
CVD	Cisplatin + vinblastine + dacarbazine
DCF	Docetaxel + cisplatin + fluorouracil
EC	Etoposide + carboplatin
FOLFOX	Fluorouracil + leucovorin + oxaliplatin
ICE	Ifosfamide + carboplatin + etoposide
IFN + DTIC	Interferon-α-2b + dacarbazine
MAID	Mesna + doxorubicin + ifosfamide + dacarbazine
MP	Melphalan + prednisone
MVAC	Methotrexate + vinblastine + doxorubicin + cisplatin
TIP	Paclitaxel + ifosfamide + cisplatin
XELOX	Capecitabine + oxaliplatin

combinations of antineoplastic agents. A classic example of combination chemotherapy is the MOPP regimen—mechlorethamine (Mustargen), vincristine (Oncovin), procarbazine, and prednisone—used to treat Hodgkin disease. The CHOP-Rituxan protocol is an example of combination chemotherapy with an mAb to treat non-Hodgkin lymphoma. The use of chemotherapy combined with biotherapy is well illustrated in the IFN-DTIC regimen to treat metastatic melanoma.

The specific and fixed sequence in which drugs are administered yields specific and predictable toxicities. Figure 19-1 illustrates a chemotherapy regimen's depletion of bone marrow, which results in neutropenia. The nadir refers to the lowest drop of the blood count between chemotherapy cycles. Chemotherapy regimens that are usually repeated every 21 to 28 days, allow for recovery of the bone marrow. Dose-dense therapy is a standard chemotherapy given with less time between cycles to minimize tumor regrowth between cycles. Hematopoietic growth factors reduce the morbidity associated with myelosuppression and allow the time between cycles to be reduced. Dose intensity (the amount of drug given over a period of time) facilitates optimal exposure of the tumor to chemotherapy agents (Polovich et al., 2009).

Combining antineoplastic agents potentially provides the greatest collective benefit of each therapy and thus the greatest likelihood of cure. A combination of therapies, either for cure or for control, may expose a patient to significant toxicity. Most patients (especially those who have been cured) report that the discomfort caused by these toxicities was well worthwhile (DeVita et al., 2011).

The importance of the nurse's own positive attitude when educating patients about the dramatic potential benefits of chemotherapy and biotherapy in balance with its toxicities and side effects cannot be overemphasized. The nurse offers hope to patients and their families and helps to relieve anxiety related to therapy by reassuring the patient that every effort will be made to control side effects.

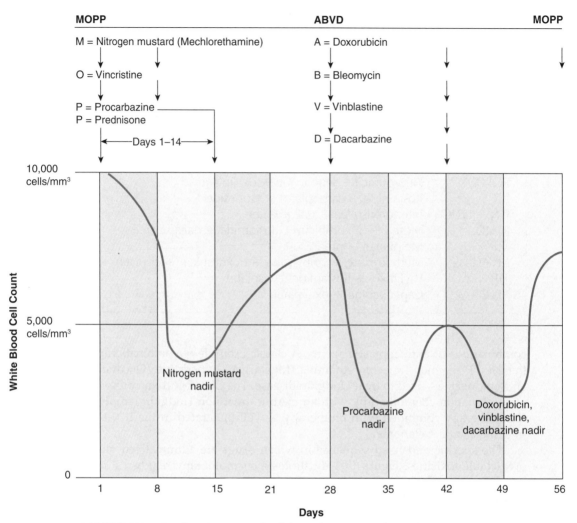

FIGURE 19-1 MOPP/ABV ± D administration schedule and corresponding white blood cell count nadirs. (From Goodman, M. S. (1986). *Cancer: Chemotherapy and care.* Evansville, IN: Bristol-Myers-Squibb.)

SYSTEMIC DRUG DELIVERY TECHNIQUE

Proper pretreatment evaluation can have an enormous impact on the efficacy of the nurse's care plan and on the patient's chemotherapy experience. This evaluation includes a nursing assessment and a review of the treatment plan and orders from a physician/LIP. Before proceeding with treatment, the nurse must review the following:

- Assure that there is a therapy protocol and a written (electronic or paper) and signed order that specifies
  - Patient name
  - Drug name(s)

- Dosage (may be straight dose, mg/kg, or mg/m^2)
- Total dose
- Frequency
- Route of administration
- Rate if IV
- Assure that the physician/LIP has completed informed consent with the patient.
- If the patient has been treated with chemotherapy previously, review documentation regarding previous chemotherapy experience, physical and emotional response, experience with and management of side effects, and successful or unsuccessful intervention(s).
- Assure that the patient has resources to assist with care at home and information regarding community resources.
- Complete an assessment and review the patient's physical history before administering treatment. Assure that any compromised organ systems have been considered in dose calculation, especially the liver and kidneys, which metabolize and clear the agents.
- Assess for and/or review coping mechanisms the patient employs. Make any necessary referrals.
- Identify any hydration and electrolyte replacements that have been ordered.
- Identify any premedications for the drugs the patient is to receive, for example, cimetidine, diphenhydramine, and/or dexamethasone.
- Assure recent laboratory values have been obtained to include appropriate studies of complete blood counts, creatinine, liver function studies, and/or any values pertinent to agents being administered. If abnormal, notify the physician/LIP.
- Assure that the patient is aware of the specific side effects for the drugs being administered, for example, hair loss and nausea/vomiting. Explain to the patient how the treatment team is going to mitigate or assist with these side effects.
- If needed, assure an antiemetic regimen, including both medical and dietary strategies, has been explained and initiated.
- Assure that the patient has patent, adequate venous access.
- Obtain all necessary treatment supplies, such as safe handling equipment, IV therapy materials, and hazardous waste containment. Assure lighting is adequate to facilitate venipuncture and patient observation.
- Be prepared for anaphylaxis or extravasation with the proper emergency equipment readily available. Assure that necessary professional staff and supplies are available in the event of patient emergency.
- Assure that the patient is as physically comfortable as possible, with easy access to a nurse call light.

Successful chemotherapy treatment relies on proper preparation. Some patients require extended pretreatment evaluations for special needs, such as those who are exceptionally anxious, lack family or social support, are cognitively challenged, or are scheduled to receive investigational antineoplastic agents. When chemotherapeutic protocols change, these steps must be repeated or modified to ensure safety, nurse knowledge, and patient education. When the nurse and patient partner to assure the points above have been completed, administration of chemotherapy may begin.

Routes and Modes of Administration

Although chemotherapy can be administered through a variety of routes (Table 19-7), the oral and IV continue to be most common. Antineoplastic agents are delivered orally (Box 19-6) if they can be tolerated and absorbed by the gastrointestinal tract. Many new, oral drugs are currently in development and new indications are being identified for existing drugs. Advantages of oral antineoplastics include convenience for patients, portability, and increased sense of control for patients. Disadvantages of oral cytotoxic medications

TABLE 19-7	**ROUTES OF ADMINISTRATION OF ANTINEOPLASTIC AGENTS**			
Route	**Advantages**	**Disadvantages**	**Complications**	**Nursing Implications**
Oral	Ease of administration Provides feeling of control for the patient Increased patient independence	Inconsistency of absorption Adherence/safety issues Potential drug/herb/diet interactions Cost	Drug-specific complications Swallowing difficulties	Teach compliance with the medication schedule. Connect patients with medication assistance programs.
Subcutaneous/ intramuscular	Ease of administration Decreased side effects	Adequate muscle mass and tissue required for absorption Inconsistent absorption	Infection Bleeding Pain/discomfort	Evaluate platelet count before administration. Use a smallest gauge needle if possible. Prepare the injection site with an antiseptic solution. Assess the injection site for signs and symptoms of infection.
Intravenous	Consistent absorption Required for vesicants	Sclerosing of veins over time	Infection Phlebitis Extravasation Infiltration	Check for blood return before, during, and after drug administration.
Intra-arterial	Increased doses to tumor with decreased systemic side effects Local treatment	Requires a surgical procedure or special radiography for catheter and/or port placement May limit the patient mobility during infusion	Bleeding Embolism Pain Arterial injury Arterial catheter leak, break migration Pump malfunction	Monitor for signs and symptoms of bleeding. Monitor prothrombin time, activated partial thromboplastin time (aPTT). Monitor the catheter site.

TABLE 19	ROUTES OF ADMINISTRATION OF ANTINEOPLASTIC AGENTS (*Continued*)			
Route	**Advantages**	**Disadvantages**	**Complications**	**Nursing Implications**
Intrathecal/ intraventricular	More consistent drug levels in the CSF	Requires lumbar puncture or surgical placement of the reservoir or implanted pump	Increased intracranial pressure Headaches Confusion	Observe for signs of infection. Monitor reservoir or pump functioning.
	Bypasses the blood–brain barrier	Pump occlusion/ malfunction Requires additional education for the nurse, patient, family	Lethargy Nausea/vomiting Seizures Infection	Monitor the patient for headache or signs of increased intracranial pressure.
Intraperitoneal (IP)	Direct exposure of intra-abdominal surfaces to the drug	Requires placement of a peritoneal catheter or IP port	Abdominal pain Abdominal distention Bleeding Paralytic ileus Intestinal perforation Infection Nausea	Warm the chemotherapy solution to the body temperature. Check patency of a catheter or port. Instill the drug/solution according to the protocol—infuse, dwell, and drain or continuous infusion. Reposition the patient according to the protocol to allow for IP distribution.
Intrapleural	Sclerosing of pleural lining	Requires insertion of a thoracotomy tube Physicians/LIPs must administer intrapleural agents	Pain Infection Urinary tract infection Cystitis Bladder contracture	Monitor for complete drainage from pleural space before instillation of the drug. Following instillation, clamp tubing and reposition the patient every 10–15 min for 2 h for adequate distribution of the drug. Attach tubing to suction according to the protocol. Assess the client for pain; provide analgesia. Assess the client for anxiety; provide emotional support. Maintain sterile technique when inserting an indwelling catheter.
Intravesicular	Direct exposure of bladder surfaces to the drug	Requires insertion of an indwelling catheter	Urinary urgency Allergic drug reactions	Instill the solution, clamp the catheter for specified time, and unclamp to drain according to the protocol.

Adapted from Polovich, M., Whitford, J. M., & Olsen, M. (Eds.). (2009). *Chemotherapy and biotherapy guidelines and recommendations for practice* (3rd ed.). Pittsburgh, PA: Oncology Nursing Society; and Temple, S.V., & Poniatowski, B. C. Nursing implications of antineoplastic therapy. In J. K. Itano, & K. N. Taoka (Eds.) (2005). *Core curriculum for oncology nursing* (pp. 793–794). St. Louis, MO: Elsevier Saunders.

BOX 19-6 ORAL ANTINEOPLASTIC AGENTS

Abiraterone acetate (Zytiga)
Altretamine (Hexalen)
Axitinib (Inlyta)
Bexarotene (Targretin)
Bosutinib (Bosulif)
Capecitabine (Xeloda)
Chlorambucil (Leukeran)
Crizotinib (Xalkori)
Cyclophosphamide (Cytoxan)
Dasatinib (Sprycel)
Enzalutamide (Xtandi)
Erlotinib (Tarceva)
Estramustine (Emcyt)
Etoposide (VePesid, Etopophos)
Everolimus (Afinitor)
Hydroxyurea (Hydrea, Mylocel)
Imatinib (Gleevec)
Lapatinib (Tykerb)
Lenalidomide (Revlimid)

Levamisole (Ergamisol)
Lomustine (CeeNU)
Melphalan (Alkeran)
Mercaptopurine (6-MP, Purinethol)
Methotrexate (Trexall)
Mitotane (Lysodren)
Nilotinib (Tasigna)
Pazopanib (Votrient)
Procarbazine (Matulane)
Sorafenib (Nexavar)
Sunitinib (Sutent)
Temozolomide (Temodar)
Thalidomide (Thalomid)
Thioguanine (TG, Tabloid)
Tretinoin (Vesanoid)
Vandetanib (Caprelsa)
Vemurafenib (Zelboraf)
Vismodegib (Erivedge)

---

include adherence issues, inconsistency of absorption, potential for diet/medication inter-actions, and cost/reimbursement issues. All of these issues are taken into consideration when determining a treatment plan (Polovich, et al., 2009). Regardless of the patient preference, drugs (including choice of route) and regimen are dictated by disease type and validated studies.

INTRAVENOUS ADMINISTRATION

Successful IV administration demands careful line selection, site selection, and venipuncture. Line decisions should be based on the planned length of treatment, vascular integrity of the patient, regimen/drug-specific properties, patient preference, and the patient's ability to care for the device. The most noninvasive, smallest gauge device with the fewest number of lumens needed to accommodate the prescribed therapy should be used (INS, 2011).

PERIPHERAL IV

For peripheral venous access, patients should be positioned comfortably in a chair with extended armrests and hand and arm stabilizers or utilize pillows to elevate upper extremities if in bed. Successful IV nurses allow ample and unhurried time to assess both arms and hands to avoid areas of compromise (sclerosis, thrombosis, hematoma, or phlebitis), flexion, pain on palpation, vascular valves, and areas of planned procedures (INS, 2011). In addition, upper extremity veins should be avoided on the side affected by of breast surgery with node dissection, radiation, lymphedema, or stroke (INS, 2011).

The examination of both arms also gives the nurse a baseline reference should changes occur during treatment.

If veins are obscure, comfortably warm, moist compresses may be applied to the patient's hands and forearms. Clothing should be loosened to allow full view of the IV site. Watches and tight jewelry should be removed if they constrict the venous pathway or impede the smooth flow of blood along the venous network. Elderly, poorly nourished, and debilitated patients often have fragile veins. Nurses may attempt to catheterize fragile veins with a loose tourniquet or with no tourniquet because distention and rapid engorgement may cause the vein wall to rupture when the tourniquet is released. A second nurse may also apply gentle hand pressure directly above the venipuncture site to distend it. Other distention techniques include application of moderate heat or asking the patient to clench or pump the fist. Gravity flow may be maximized if the patient dangles the extremity. The nurse may lightly finger-tap the site to distend the vein.

Alternating sites from treatment to treatment may help minimize vascular irritation and phlebitis associated with IV administration of chemotherapy drugs; it also allows time for healing. Documentation should specify which arm and location were used for each treatment.

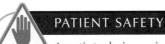

PATIENT SAFETY

Aseptic techniques, including sterile venipuncture procedures, standard precautions, and safe handling of antineoplastics, require a nurse's constant vigilance, especially because of the susceptibility of these patients to systemic infection resulting from neutropenia.

A nurse should employ vein mapping for all venipuncture attempts, using the most distal veins first and moving proximally (INS, 2011). For example, if a forearm venipuncture was unsuccessful, cytotoxic agents administered into a distal site might leak into tissue surrounding the recent proximal puncture. With vesicant therapy, necrosis could result. Thus, if the first venipuncture is unsuccessful, the opposite arm should be used for the next attempt. If the opposite arm is not appropriate, use a site proximal to the original attempt (Polovich et al., 2009).

Large veins along the distal forearm (cephalic, median, and basilic) are easy to access and provide safe, convenient venipuncture sites (INS, 2011). Using these larger veins diminishes the risk of chemical phlebitis from the irritant/vesicant properties of antineoplastic drugs, especially with bolus (IV push) administration. Several factors contraindicate the use of the antecubital fossa. This area includes the important anatomic structures of the median nerve and brachial artery. Serious complications—tissue damage and later, necrosis—may occur. Extensive tissue necrosis could require complicated, costly, and psychologically difficult reconstructive efforts. Moreover, prolonged infusions restrict arm mobility because elbow function is limited during infusion and the area's fat and tissue volume make it difficult to visualize and detect early infiltration. Ventral and lateral wrist veins should also be avoided to prevent nerve damage (INS, 2011).

When considering a peripheral IV, also consider the therapy being delivered. Continuous vesicants (infusing for ≥60 minutes) should be administered through a central line (Polovich et al., 2009). Despite the nurse's technical competence, usable veins sometimes are difficult to locate and access. A limit of two unsuccessful venipunctures is suggested before a nurse seeks assistance from a coworker. Repeated venipunctures increase anxiety levels for both the patient and the nurse and may decrease the likelihood of successful vein catheterization. An angiocatheter is preferred given its stability in the vein. The gauge of the angiocatheter may vary, dependent on the size of the cannulated vein and the length of treatment. Select the smallest gauge and the shortest length catheter to accommodate the prescribed therapy. Steel needles should not be used (Polovich et al., 2009). Once the venipuncture is complete, an occlusive dressing/tape should be applied so that the needle insertion site and immediate surrounding area are clearly visible. Tubing should be taped independently and then looped so that blood return can be checked during administration.

PATIENT SAFETY

Perform a thorough examination of the extremity before inserting the catheter into the vein. Avoid using phlebitic, bruised, inflamed, or sclerotic areas. A useful and often overlooked peripheral infusion site is the basilic vein on the medial aspect of the forearm.

CENTRAL VASCULAR ACCESS DEVICE (CVAD)

A CVAD may be required for patients with a vesicant or known irritant in their treatment programs or with impaired peripheral venous vasculature. Tunneled, nontunneled, or implanted SQ devices can be used for either long- or short-term treatment plans. They can be percutaneously inserted, either centrally or peripherally, with the tip terminating in the central vasculature (superior vena cava, inferior vena cava, or above the junction of the right atrium). Central lines can be manufactured as single or multilumen, of various sizes and lengths, of different materials, as power injectable, with open or closed ends, and with anti-infective properties (INS, 2011). CVADs have become common in antineoplastic administration because of their ease of placement, convenience, and safety benefits. CVADs eliminate most peripheral venipunctures for drawing blood specimens and dramatically enhance patient security and comfort. Some of the other advantages of a central line are that it:

- Preserves the peripheral venous system
- Serves as a line for blood and nutritional products, antibiotics, analgesics, and antiemetics, as well as antineoplastic agents
- Allows home infusion of vesicants and multiple-drug therapies that otherwise can be administered safely only in acute care or outpatient clinic settings
- Is cost-effective

Potential disadvantages include costs of insertion and maintenance, thrombus, infection or sepsis, air embolism, and catheter severance or migration.

Implanted ports offer an alternative to percutaneously inserted central catheters. Advantages include reduced the infection risk and no care requirements for external catheters. Implantable devices are available from a variety of manufacturers. Implanted ports carry a risk of needle dislodgment and consequent extravasation when long-term infusions of vesicant drugs are administered. Proper noncoring needle placement must be assessed and documented at least every 8 hours with these vesicants (INS, 2011).

Vascular access devices afford dramatic quality-of-life advantages, but they demand extraordinary patient and/or caregiver responsibility with maintenance activities. It is imperative that the nurse ensures that the patient and caregiver have learned mainte-nance of the central line. Proper instruction can prevent catheter occlusions caused by inadequate irrigation, infections, or air embolism caused by line mismanagement, or damage caused by poor stabilization, improper connections, or mishandled clamps. If the patient or caregiver cannot properly care for the access device, the device may be compromised and may need to be removed. Before discharge, patients and families need training in meticulous device maintenance and should be able to return demonstrate skills required as well as receive written instructions for later reference. Alternative sup-port for home maintenance of these devices may need to be sought and arranged.

These venous access devices are often so reliable that there is a real risk of complacency for nurses treating these patients. Individual manufacturer recommendations for care and maintenance must be followed strictly, particularly because specific diameters, volumes, lumen sizes, and clamping procedures vary among models. Complications are rare and usually avoidable when professional standards and chemotherapy administration prac-tices are observed. When complications do occur, however, they are severe and often life threatening.

Although IV therapy is the primary use of these devices, these or similar ones can also be placed intra-arterially for organ perfusion, intrathecally for CNS access, or intraperitone-ally for chemotherapy administration into the abdominal cavity.

Box 19-7 lists various devices for long-term venous access. Device selection depends on frequency of access, treatment, duration, administration mode, venous integrity, and patient preference. Criteria for the patient assessment are featured in Box 19-8. Common placement sites are discussed in Chapter 14.

ADMINISTRATION OF INTRAVENOUS ANTINEOPLASTIC THERAPIES

Before, during, and after cytotoxic drug administration, blood return must be checked to ensure line patency. If a fragile vein bursts, or if an IV catheter has perforated its wall, conventional IV fluids are absorbed without damaging surrounding tissue. Also, since IV solutions often contain admixtures incompatible with cytotoxic drugs, there is a potential for precipitates to develop resulting in vein irritation and phlebitis. Compatibility issues are imperative to consider, not only with antineoplastics but with adjunctive drug thera-pies, such as those involving antiemetics or corticosteroids. A flush of compatible IV fluid between drugs avoids inopportune chemical interactions. When administering IV cytotoxic agents, PPE needs to be worn and safe handling techniques need to be employed (Polovich et al., 2009).

Bolus (IV push) administration calls for slow, even pressure. Small-gauge IV catheters offer greater resistance than larger IV catheters. Bolus administration can be accomplished by either the free-flow method or the direct push method, depending upon the agent being delivered. Any unusual resistance calls for cessation of infusion to investigate the cause. If the tip of the IV catheter is resting against the vein wall, careful repositioning may resolve

---

BOX 19-7 SELECTED CENTRAL VASCULAR ACCESS DEVICES AND THEIR USES

Tunneled Central Venous Catheters

Frequent venous access for blood sampling, delivery of blood products, and therapy
Bone marrow transplantation
Multiple transfusions, such as for treating patients with leukemia
Single-bolus injections of chemotherapy
Infusion of total parenteral nutrition, fluids, pain management, and antibiotic therapy
Short- or long-term, inpatient or outpatient chemotherapy infusions, vesicant or nonvesicant
Note: The patient or responsible caregiver must be capable of caring for this device.

Small-Gauge, Peripherally Inserted Central Catheters

Short-term infusion of chemotherapy or vesicant or nonvesicant chemotherapy, total parenteral nutrition, blood, fluids, pain management, and antibiotic therapy
Inpatient or outpatient infusion therapy
Single-bolus injections of chemotherapy
Frequent venous access needed for chemotherapy
Frequent blood sampling
Brief life expectancy
Note: The patient or responsible caregiver must be capable of caring for this device.

Implanted Ports

Infrequent venous access
Single-bolus injections of chemotherapy
Inpatient or outpatient infusion of chemotherapeutic agents
Short- or long-term chemotherapy
Total parenteral nutrition, blood sampling, blood transfusions, fluid replacement, antibiotic therapy, pain management
Alternative for patients physically unable to care for other access device
Young children (when frequent venous access is not required)
Cosmetic concerns or the patient preference

---

the problem. If the nurse applies too much force, the patient may experience pain or venous spasm. Blood return during bolus infusion of a vesicant must be checked every 2 to 5 mL by gently pulling back on the syringe plunger (Polovich et al., 2009). Most adverse reactions can be avoided when there is even push pressure, appropriate blood return checks, and constant supervision of all administration processes.

Short-term chemotherapy may also be delivered with a conventional piggyback approach. When infusing vesicants, IV catheter stability and adequate blood return must be checked every 5 to 10 minutes. Do not pinch the IV tubing to determine blood return and patency. Instead use either a suction check (gently aspirate the line using a syringe at the Y site closest to the patient while clamping off the fluid from the IV bag) or the gravity

---

BOX 19-8   THE PATIENT ASSESSMENT CRITERIA FOR A CENTRAL VASCULAR ACCESS DEVICE

General assessment guidelines for assessing whether a CVAD is appropriate for the patient include the frequency of venous access, longevity of treatment, mode of drug administration, venous integrity, and the patient's preferences. Priorities for central CVAD placement are compared below.

Low Priority	High Priority
Infrequent venous access	Frequent venous access
Short-term therapy	Long-term, indefinite treatment period
Intermittent single injections	Continuous infusion of chemotherapy
Administration of nonvesicant, nonirritating drugs	Administration of a vesicant, irritating drugs
No previous IV therapy	Venous thrombosis or sclerosis from previous IV therapy
Both extremities available	Venous access limited to one extremity
Venous access with two or fewer venipunctures	More than two venipunctures to secure venous access
The patient does not prefer CVAD	The patient prefers CVAD
	Home infusion of chemotherapy
	Prior tissue damage owing to extravasation

---

check (free the IV bag and tubing and gently lower it to a point below the patient's IV site) (Polovich et al., 2009). Immediate cessation of drug administration is required if there is any doubt about venous patency. With vesicants, the compromised site should be treated as an extravasation; with nonvesicants, treatment can be resumed with a new catheter site. Continuous infusion (lasting longer than 60 minutes) also needs to be monitored closely by the chemotherapy-credentialed nurse. When administering a vesicant via continuous administration, peripheral IVs should not be used and blood return should be checked periodically to assure vein patency (Polovich et al., 2009).

After chemotherapy/biotherapy, blood return is checked again to assure catheter patency, and the catheter tubing is flushed with an appropriate, compatible flush solution. If a peripheral line is used, the catheter is removed with a dry sterile sponge. The extremity is elevated and pressure until bleeding stops. A dressing is applied to the site. If a CVAD is used, the line should be flushed with an appropriate capping solution.

Home Infusion Systems

CVADs provide another key benefit to patients requiring continuous or intermittent chemotherapy; they allow treatment at home. External ambulatory infusion systems for antineoplastic agents reduce inpatient admissions and costs and allow patient autonomy and comfort in familiar home surroundings.

All external ambulatory infusion systems are self-powered independent of household electrical current. They are battery powered, lightweight, and reusable. They infuse through either a piston valve (AutoSyringe) or a peristaltic mechanism. The administration rate is controllable. Mechanically powered pumps feature alarm systems that detect any back pressure that might occur with occlusion or infiltration. These pumps also detect air in the line, and an alarm sounds when the fluid reservoir is empty.

The list of ambulatory infusion system products and technologies continually changes as new improvements are made. IV nurses are better served to keep abreast of manufacturer-provided instructional materials, patient education information, and troubleshooting support services of the devices currently favored in their own clinical setting. Nurses also must be familiar with system operations to educate patients and families in early detection of complications, including line occlusion, thrombosis, infiltration or extravasation, and system failure. The following is a list of factors to consider when recommending use of an ambulatory infusion system:

- Level of patient and family understanding of pump and alarm features and functions; degree of patient and family compliance, reliability, dexterity, and comfort with the device; the patient or family visual acuity keen enough to see pump function clearly
- Twenty-four–hour availability or proximity to a health care provider in the event of pump failure or occlusion
- Drug regimen that matches device capacities and features
- Insurance coverage of rental unit.

Infusion systems can be attached by belt or shoulder strap to ease patient movement. Mechanical systems usually call for hands-on programming and reprogramming, requiring an on-site visit from a nurse when changes are needed. The same is true for replenishing fluid and drug reservoirs. Developments to ease ambulatory infusions (such as pump reprogramming by computer or over phone lines, without hands-on human intervention) are potentials for the future.

Regional Drug Delivery

Although systemic IV administration of chemotherapy is most common, there is evidence that supports some tumors respond to local exposure of antineoplastics. Alternative methods of drug administration have been established to deliver high concentrations of chemotherapeutic agents locally, into a body cavity or into the organ site of the tumor. A drug can be directed into the area of known disease, such as intraperitoneally to treat malignant ascites or metastatic seeding of the peritoneum from ovarian cancer. Intravesical administration of chemotherapy and biologic response modifiers is frequently used to treat bladder cancer. Intrathecal or intraventricular administration is used for cancers known to have invaded the CNS, intrapleural is beneficial for malignant effusions and sclerosing purposes, and topical application can be used for early malignancies of the integumentary system. Intra-arterial administration provides higher concentrations for the regional delivery of chemotherapy. Regional delivery of these infusions results in increased exposure of the tumor to the drug, whereas less systemic circulation and exposure to the antineoplastic agent decreases the risk of systemic side effects (Camp-Sorrell, 2011).

Intra-arterial Delivery

Intra-arterial administration delivers antineoplastic drugs directly into the organ or tumor via the main artery supply. Although metastatic hepatic disease is the most common indication for intra-arterial chemotherapy, other organs, such as the brain, head and neck region, and pelvic area can also be perfusion sites for arterial delivery of chemotherapy (Camp-Sorrell, 2011).

The most likely alternative route of antineoplastic administration involving the IV nurse is the intra-arterial infusion, which may use either an arterial catheter or an arterial port. Arterial catheters are percutaneously inserted and can be used for short-term and long-term therapy.

An intra-arterial pump is designed to deliver a constant flow of the drug for hepatic arterial infusion therapy. The arterial catheter and implanted pump are surgically placed. The pump's reservoir is filled, and the catheter access port is flushed after assembly in the OR. The catheter tip position and perfusion of the intended region are confirmed postoperatively before the drug therapy is started. The drug is placed in the pump reservoir and is subsequently forced through a flow-restrictive tubing by pressurized gas. The pump flow rate can be altered by fluctuations in pump temperature. Patients must agree to report any fever so that pump refill schedules can be assessed and adjusted. Potential complications include bleeding, embolism, pain, pump or catheter malfunction, and hepatic artery injury (Camp-Sorrell, 2011), so patients need to be aware of these and be able to verbalize what to report to the nurse. About every 1 to 4 weeks, the pump is refilled by percutaneous injection with either active antineoplastics or a heparin solution to maintain constant perfusion to the area and patency of the catheter. The device's side port may be used for direct intra-arterial access. The nurse who is competent in the use of intra-arterial pumps must be intimately familiar with techniques and risks of this route of drug delivery, adhere strictly to details available from the manufacturer data, and demonstrate competency accessing and filling the pump.

Intrathecal Delivery

Intrathecal therapy is another alternative route of cancer chemotherapy that might call for the IV nurse involvement. A cerebrospinal access device, such as the Ommaya reservoir, is subcutaneously implanted into the lateral ventricle of the brain to avoid repeated lumbar punctures in treating meningeal carcinomatosis, the infiltration by cancer of the cerebral leptomeninges. The reservoir provides access to the cerebrospinal fluid through a burr hole in the skull. Administration of intrathecal chemotherapy is limited to a physician/LIP or specially trained registered nurse (Polovich et al., 2009).

First, the reservoir is pumped several times to fill the device with cerebrospinal fluid (CSF). Then, the skin is prepared and the reservoir is punctured at a 45-degree angle, using sterile technique, with a 25- to 27-gauge scalp vein needle. Sufficient CSF is removed for laboratory studies and to keep exchanges isovolumetric; that is, enough CSF is withdrawn to equal the amount of the drugs to be infused while reserving 3 mL to use as flush following the procedure. Then, a chemotherapeutic agent, such as methotrexate or cytarabine, which is admixed with a preservative-free solution, is injected slowly over 5 to 10 minutes through a scalp vein needle into the reservoir. Following the drug, the device is flushed with the reserved CSF. Remove the needle, and pump the reservoir to distribute the drugs into the intraventricular space. Preservative-free morphine sulfate also can be administered into an Ommaya reservoir for prolonged pain relief (Camp-Sorrell, 2011). The Vinca alkaloid classification of chemotherapies is never given intrathecally due to their high potential for lethal neurotoxicity (Polovich et al., 2009).

COMPLICATIONS OF CHEMOTHERAPY ADMINISTRATION

Regardless of the nurse's skills and implementation of standards, sometimes patients experience problems unique to the administration of cytotoxic agents.

Localized Reactions

The nurse should be prepared for localized reactions whenever any antineoplastic agent is administered IV. A flare reaction is a localized reaction a patient may experience while receiving chemotherapy. The first manifestation may be erythema along the venous pathway at the site of the IV. Blotchiness, hive-like urticaria, or the rapid appearance of welts also may occur. The patient may report itchiness. Nursing assessment parameters to differentiate among a flare, local irritation, and extravasation are outlined (Table 19-8). Preventive measures include additional drug dilution, either by adding the drug to 100 to 200 mL solution

TABLE 19-8	NURSING ASSESSMENT OF EXTRAVASATION VERSUS OTHER REACTIONS			
	Extravasation			
Assessment Parameter	Immediate Manifestations of Extravasation	Delayed Manifestations of Extravasation	Irritation of the Vein	Flare Reaction
Pain	Often described as stinging or burning. Not all patients experience pain with extravasation	Pain intensity increases over time	Aching and tightness along the vein	No pain
Redness	Blotchy redness around the needle site, not always present at the time of extravasation or may be difficult to detect if extravasation occurs in deep tissue	Redness intensifies over time	The full length of the vein may be reddened or darkened	Immediate blotches or streaks along the vein, usually subsides within a few minutes. Wheals may be present
Ulceration	Skin remains intact	If untreated, skin may slough within 1–2 wk followed by tissue necrosis	No ulcerations	No ulcerations
Swelling	Severe swelling usually occurs immediately but may be difficult to detect if extravasation occurs in deep tissue	Swelling tends to increase over time	No swelling	No swelling
Blood return	Inability to obtain blood return	—	Present	Present

Adapted from Polovich, M., Whitford, J. M., & Olsen, M. (Eds.). (2009). *Chemotherapy and biotherapy guidelines and recommendations for practice* (3rd ed., p. 107). Pittsburgh, PA: Oncology Nursing Society.

or by administering the drug slowly. The nurse should always consult and follow the manufacturer's recommendations.

At the beginning of symptoms of a flare reaction, it is critical to distinguish a flare reaction from a drug extravasation. A flare reaction is distinguishable from an extravasation by the absence of pain or swelling and by the presence of blood return from the IV. When suspecting a flare reaction, first verify blood return. If an extravasation is suspected by the lack of blood return, stop the drug and follow extravasation procedures. If a flare reaction seems evident, stop the drug, flush the line with saline, and watch for flare resolution. A flare reaction lasts <45 minutes. In the case of an unresolved flare reaction, a physician/LIP's order can be obtained to administer the following medications to treat the localized reaction:

- Hydrocortisone sodium succinate (Solu-Cortef), slow IV push, 25 to 50 mg; anti-inflammatory agent
- Diphenhydramine (Benadryl) IV push, 25 to 50 mg; antihistamine

Follow medications with a saline flush until the flare has resolved. Resume infusion of the drug. Document the reaction and treatment in the medical record. Premedication with an antihistamine and/or corticosteroid may prevent another episode when the drug is administered again (Polovich et al., 2009).

Irritation

Some antineoplastic agents are known to produce pain or irritation along the venous pathway. These agents include bleomycin, carboplatin, carmustine, dacarbazine, etoposide, fluorouracil, gemcitabine, ifosfamide, irinotecan, liposomal doxorubicin, liposomal daunorubicin, and melphalan (Ener, Meglathery, & Styler, 2004). Patients may complain of pain, tightness, or aching just above the IV site as the medication infuses. The vein may appear darkened, but blood return is present.

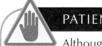 PATIENT SAFETY

Although there are many special cautions for special drugs, it is important to remember that any agent can cause venous pain, in any patient, at any time.

Risk factors for irritation include previous treatment with sclerosing or irritating medications, small veins, low pH of drug infusing, and concentrated solutions. Management of venous irritation may be alleviated with the following measures:

- Restarting the IV in a larger vein in another location
- Diluting the antineoplastic agent
- Applying warm compresses above the catheter insertion site during infusion. Care must be taken to avoid first- or second-degree burns.

Patients should be instructed to report any discomfort during the infusion and any development of a hard cord along the vein after the infusion has completed (Polovich et al., 2009).

Phlebitis

The risk for *chemical phlebitis* (inflammation of the vein due to an irritating drug or solution) exists with most IV anticancer agents, but the risk increases when two or more antineoplastics are combined. Contributing factors to chemical phlebitis are high acid pH, hyperosmolar solutions, rapid infusion rates, drug–drug interactions where precipitate is formed, and incomplete dissolution of medication particles (Perucca, 2010). Chemotherapeutic drugs associated with phlebitis include actinomycin, carmustine, cisplatin, dacarbazine, daunorubicin, doxorubicin hydrochloride, mechlorethamine hydrochloride, mitomycin C, streptozocin, vinblastine, vincristine, and vinorelbine.

Early symptoms of phlebitis may include pain, erythema, occasional limb edema, and a sensation of warmth in the affected extremity. As acute symptoms subside, venous pathways may retain dark-bluish to brown discoloration for some time while arm use is restricted. Acute phlebitis reactions are diagnosed by palpating the tip of the IV catheter along the vein course, using slight pressure to detect tenderness. The best indicator of phlebitis is a feeling of warmth at the IV catheter site associated with inflammatory swelling.

Nurses must exercise utmost caution to prevent phlebitis because treatment may be jeopardized if there is compromised peripheral venous access. Occasionally, a patient with a history of phlebitic treatment sites manifests reactions to any IV drug administration. Evaluate the patient to determine if he or she is a candidate for a central line. To diminish the threat of phlebitis, the nurse may implement various preventive measures, including the following:

- Use a filter when admixing medication to eliminate particulates.
- Use recommended solutions when mixing drugs.
- Reduce the concentration of the cytotoxic agent with further dilution, if able.
- Administer medications at the prescribed rate.
- Rotate the peripheral IV catheter sites.
- Access large veins and use the smallest IV catheter gauge that will deliver the drug infusion to promote hemodilution.
- Administer hydrocortisone sodium succinate (Solu-Cortef), 25 to 50 mg, slow IV push. A medication order is required before this drug can be administered. After ensuring vein patency, the nurse may administer half the dose before antineoplastic administration and the other half after the final flush, immediately before the catheter is removed.

Repetitive needle insertions for blood sampling and antineoplastic administrations increase the likelihood of both phlebitis and thrombosis. In fact, phlebitis develops in some patients despite the most meticulous clinical efforts to avoid it. Once phlebitis has occurred, elevation of the affected extremity, application of topical heat, and administration of systemic analgesics may be indicated.

HYPERSENSITIVITY AND GENERALIZED ANAPHYLACTIC REACTION

A nurse should be prepared for a hypersensitivity or anaphylactic reaction at any time, with any drug, in any patient. Hypersensitivity is an excessive immune system response to an allergen, and anaphylaxis is an exaggerated hypersensitivity response. Anaphylaxis is a medical emergency that may result in respiratory failure, cardiovascular collapse, and possibly death. Hypersensitivity and anaphylactic reactions are allergic reactions mediated by the immune system, often immunoglobulin E. This allergic response can be to the drug itself, the diluent, or the solution and usually occurs within 5 to 30 minutes of drug initiation (Gobel, 2005). Before initiating any treatment, the nurse should be aware of the institution's policies regarding emergencies arising from administration of antineoplastic agents and the location of emergency supplies and equipment.

Taxanes (paclitaxel, docetaxel), platinum compounds (cisplatin, carboplatin, oxaliplatin), L-asparaginase, and epipodophyllotoxins (etoposide, teniposide) are chemotherapy agents that have a high possibility of provoking a hypersensitivity reaction (Gobel, 2005).

When preparing to administer a medication with a potential for hypersensitivity, the nurse must:

- Obtain baseline vital signs
- Complete a physical assessment
- Obtain the patient's allergy history
- Ensure that emergency equipment and medications are readily accessible
- Administer premedications as ordered
- Administer test dose if ordered
- Instruct the patient on hypersensitivity symptoms to report

Signs and symptoms may include flushing, sudden agitation or anxiety, headache, nausea, vomiting, hypotension, cramping abdominal pain, urticaria, generalized pruritus, chest tightness or pain, respiratory distress, wheezing, hives, facial edema, shortness of breath, or an asthma-type reaction. Failure to respond appropriately can result in a generalized anaphylactic reaction, seizures, or cardiopulmonary arrest. Some facilities call for standing orders for hypersensitivity management signed by the responsible physician/LIP before antineoplastic treatment. This time-saving and prudent procedure allows the nurse to begin emergency treatment even before the physician/LIP arrives.

Regardless of whether a patient displays a mild reaction, generalized pruritus, or complete cardiovascular collapse, the nurse should be prepared to do the following:

- Stop the infusion immediately
- Remain with the patient and maintain an IV line with normal saline
- Have another staff member notify the physician/LIP and/or call a local emergency medical service, depending upon the setting
- Monitor vital signs, maintain the patient's airway, and administer oxygen if needed
- Provide calm reassurance to the patient and family
- Administer appropriate drugs, as ordered, based on symptoms
- Monitor the patient until the reaction subsides

Any hypersensitivity reaction and its treatment (Table 19-9) should be documented so the offending drug can be avoided, the patient can be premedicated, or medication desensitization can be considered (Polovich et al., 2009).

TABLE 19-9	EMERGENCY DRUGS FOR HYPERSENSITIVITY OR ANAPHYLAXIS TO ANTINEOPLASTICS OR BIOTHERAPY
Drugs	**Strength or Dose**
Epinephrine	1:1,000 (1 mg = 1 mL)
	1:10,000 (1 mg = 10 mL)
Cimetidine	300 mg in 2 mL
Diphenhydramine	25 mg to 50 mg
Hydrocortisone	100 to 500 mg
Dexamethasone	20 mg
Dopamine	Variable
Methylprednisolone	125 mg
Sodium bicarbonate	8.4% (50 mEq/50 mL)
Lidocaine	100 mg
Nitroglycerin (Sublingual)	0.15 mg

Cytokine Release Syndrome

Another reaction that may occur in the patient receiving biotherapies is cytokine release syndrome. Cytokine release syndrome occurs mainly with the administration of mAbs and is related to the release of cytokines such as interleukin-2 (IL-2), IFN, and tumor necrosis factor (Breslin, 2007). Risk factors for cytokine release syndrome include first infusion of mAbs, patients with high lymphocyte counts, diagnoses of leukemia or lymphoma, and patients receiving mAbs who have not received chemotherapy. The same preparations and precautions should be taken for potential cytokine release syndrome as those for hypersensitivity, as noted above. Signs and symptoms of cytokine release syndrome include fever, chills, nausea, hypotension, tachycardia, headache, rash, tongue/throat swelling, and dyspnea (Breslin, 2007).

If the patient experiences cytokine release syndrome, the nurse should

- Stop the infusion
- Observe the patient until symptoms resolve, most often within 30 minutes
- Administer medications (often diphenhydramine and/or corticosteroids) as ordered if the symptoms do not resolve
- Resume the infusion at a slower rate, once the symptoms have resolved

Any cytokine release syndrome reaction and its treatment should be documented. The nurse should also document the rate at which the reaction occurred, and the rate at which the infusion was restarted and maintained without further symptoms. Future reactions can often be prevented by titrating the medication only to the rate at which the infusion was finally maintained without reaction.

Extravasation

Extravasation is the leakage of a tissue-damaging drug, known as a vesicant, into the tissue surrounding the IV site. A vesicant causes generalized tissue injury through cell death and may cause blistering. Tissue injury may lead to tissue necrosis and possibly severe injury. Table 19-8 outlines venous reactions compared with extravasations. Tissue incurs damage as a result of vesicant extravasation secondary to one of two mechanisms: DNA binding or non–DNA binding. In vesicants where DNA binding occurs (anthracyclines, nitrogen mustard, mitomycin), the drug binds directly to the cell's DNA when it moves into the surrounding tissue. When the cell dies, the DNA complexes are absorbed by the adjacent healthy cells. This allows for a continuous progression of tissue damage since the mutated DNA remains in the body and continues to circulate. In vesicants where DNA binding does not occur (paclitaxel, plant alkaloids), the vesicant has more of an indirect effect on the tissue and is eventually metabolized by the body. There is no continuous cycle of damage, since the DNA is not involved.

Vesicant extravasation can occur in patients receiving vesicants via peripheral and central catheters. Extravasation due to peripheral administration of vesicants can occur by trauma to the vascular wall, movement of the catheter to outside the vein, or administering a vesicant in a vessel distal to a recent venipuncture or recently extravasated site (Sauerland, Engelking, Wickham, & Corbi, 2006). Risk factors for peripheral vesicant extravasation include

- Small fragile veins
- Multiple previous venipunctures
- Sensory deficits such as neuropathies
- Altered mental status or impaired cognition
- Previous therapy with irritating or sclerosing agents
- Improperly secured IV catheter
- Limited vein selection
- Probing while inserting the IV catheter
- Use of steel needles

Extravasation of vesicant drugs can also occur with CVADs, so the nurse must be vigilant in monitoring the patient regardless of the type of line. Extravasations with central line administration can occur because of catheter leakage/rupture, backflow from fibrin sheath or thrombosis, a dislodged Huber needle from port, catheter damage, and migration and dislodgement of the catheter from the vein (Polovich et al., 2009).

PREVENTION

Experience in treating patients with antineoplastic drugs perfects the nurse's technique and is a good patient safeguard. It is important to keep in mind, however, that extravasation of vesicant agents can occur despite the nurse's skill. The nurse's focus should be on perfecting safe IV technique, being prepared (Table 19-10), preventing extravasation (Table 19-11), and implementing prudent preparatory measures should an extravasation occur. Although there are no guarantees, the nurse can be reasonably confident that the impact of extravasation can be mitigated with early detection and treatment.

TABLE 19-10	EXTRAVASATION KIT: ITEMS AND QUANTITIES
Needles	19 gauge (4)
	25 gauge (4)
	Filter needle (1)
Tape	1 inch-paper
Telfa pads	4 × 4 inch (4)
Sterile gauze dressing	4 × 4 inch (2)
Alcohol wipes	(4)
Syringes	Tuberculin: 3 mL, 5 mL, 10 mL, 20 mL
Diluent	Sterile saline solution: 10 mL (1)
	Sterile water: 10 mL (1)
Steroid cream	1% topical lotion (optional)
Antidotes	Sodium thiosulfate (for mechlorethamine and concentrated cisplatin)
Latex or nitrile gloves	Several
Hot pack/cold pack	
Policy and procedure for extravasation management	
Extravasation record	
Camera	(1)

Note: *Restock the kit after each use.* The kit should be available wherever vesicant drugs are being administered.

PATIENT EDUCATION

The patient must be informed of possible consequences when chemotherapeutic agents are administered so that informed consent is comprehensive. A sensitive nurse conveys the risks in such a way that the patient can react to the information appropriately and without unnecessary fear. Signs and symptoms of extravasation may include pain/stinging/burning, swelling, redness, slowing of IV fluids, leaking around IV, and absence of blood return (Polovich et al., 2009).

Constant surveillance by the nurse is required for patients who are confused, unconscious, or in some way unable to perceive or report early signs of extravasation such as the patient with peripheral neuropathies. Alert and cooperative patients may report stinging, burning, and pain or an unusual sensation at the catheter insertion site. Nevertheless, extravasation can occur even without perceptible symptoms.

BEING PREPARED FOR EXTRAVASATION

Before any treatment, the nurse should be familiar with the agents known to produce tissue damage (Table 19-12) and anticipate the possibility of extravasation. When administering any antineoplastic drug, nurses should be prepared for potential extravasation, have antidotes available, ensure venous patency, anticipate insidious infiltration, and monitor the patient. A reference of vesicants and irritants, recommended antidotes, and use of hot or cold compresses should be housed in a convenient place. Antidotes should be kept readily

TABLE 19-11   EXTRAVASATION OF VESICANT ANTINEOPLASTIC AGENTS: PREVENTIVE STRATEGIES

Risk Factor	Preventive Strategy	Rationale
Skill of the Practitioner	Chemotherapy administration is done only by registered nurses who are specifically trained and supervised	Procedures for management of extravasation vary according to the drug infiltrated
		Certain drugs (streptozocin or BCNU) may cause a burning sensation during infusion, which is normal. However, it is abnormal and indicative of a problem if burning occurs during infusion of drugs such as doxorubicin and mitomycin
	No attempts are made by the practitioner to do procedures beyond his or her expertise	Procedures change rapidly. Techniques need to be learned and mastered before assuming the responsibility for administration of chemotherapy.
	Practitioners are skillful in venipuncture	
	Practice is based on institutional policies and procedures that are routinely updated to meet the changing standards and methods of practice.	The definition of customary care in the community helps dictate standard of practice.
	Practitioners are knowledgeable of the signs and symptoms of extravasation and drug therapy.	
Condition of the Veins		
Small fragile veins	Use conventional methods for venous distention, such as heat and percussion.	The risk of vesicant drug seepage exists with repeated venipuncture.
Access limited owing to axillary surgery, vein thrombosis, prior extravasation	Assess all available arm veins. Assess veins in a methodical fashion, taking time to select the most appropriate vein.	
Long-term drug therapy Multiple vein punctures	If practitioners do not feel confident in their ability to catheterize a person's veins successfully, they should seek the assistance of a colleague.	
	After attempting one or two injections without success, the practitioner should seek the assistance of a colleague before trying again.	Multiple vein injections lead to thrombosis and limited availability.
	A patient who consistently needs two or more attempts to secure venous access should be considered a candidate for a venous access device (VAD). The time to place a VAD is before an extravasation, not after.	Treatment should be delayed until a VAD can be placed. Most VADs can be used immediately or within 24–48 h, so delay in drug therapy is not usually an issue.
Drug Administration Technique	Vesicant agents are never given as continuous infusions into a peripheral vein.	The risk of infiltration of a vesicant from a peripheral vein infusion is great owing to the following:

(Continued)

TABLE 19-11	EXTRAVASATION OF VESICANT ANTINEOPLASTIC AGENTS: PREVENTIVE STRATEGIES (*Continued*)	
Risk Factor	**Preventive Strategy**	**Rationale**
	Use a central VAD to administer any vesicant infusing for longer than 30–60 min.	Blood return is not assessed frequently. The longer the infusion, the greater the possibility of IV catheter dislodgment. The patient can move the extremity, which could dislodge the IV catheter. Even a small amount of vesicant can cause tissue damage. Infiltration can be subtle and difficult to detect until a large volume has infiltrated. The patient may be sedated from an anti-emetic and be unable to report sensations associated with extravasation.
	If peripheral line is on an infusion pump, disconnect the pump before administration of chemotherapy. Administer short infusion vesicants by gravity.	The pump forces the drug into tissues.
	When a vesicant is to be given as a continuous infusion, the drug should be infused through an external-based central venous catheter whenever possible.	When an implanted port already exists, the Huber needle should be secured in place and checked at least 3 times a day to ensure placement during continuous infusion of a vesicant.
	Vesicant agents are most commonly administered through the side port of a free-flowing peripheral IV line or through a VAD.	The incidence of vesicant drug extravasation from ports used for continuous infusion is well documented and presents a risk to be avoided, if possible.
	Side-arm Technique Ensure a proper venous access site. The IV fluid should be additive free. A catheter used to access the vein should be at least a 20 gauge to ensure an adequate blood return and fluid flow. Secure the catheter but do not obstruct the entrance site. Assess for blood return. Test the vein with 50–100 mL to ensure an adequate and swift drip of infusion. With IV fluid continuing to drip, slowly inject the vesicant into the IV line. Do not allow the vesicant to flow backward. Do not pinch off tubing except to assess for blood return. Assess for blood return in every 2- to 5-mL injection. Flush the IV catheter with saline at the completion of injection.	The rationale for the side-arm technique is the added dilution of the drug by the continuous drip of the IV fluid. Common pitfalls: Not using a large enough catheter for a brisk infusion of infusate. The vesicant backs up the into IV line. The IV line has to be pinched off to inject the vesicant, which defeats the purpose.

TABLE 19-11	EXTRAVASATION OF VESICANT ANTINEOPLASTIC AGENTS: PREVENTIVE STRATEGIES *(Continued)*	
Risk Factor	Preventive Strategy	Rationale
The site of Venous Access: Choosing the Best Vein	VADs, including tunneled catheters, implanted ports, and nontunneled central venous catheters, are indicated when patients have small, frail veins and are in need of long-term indefinite chemotherapy, continuous infusion of vesicant drugs, or both.	VADs are important options for patients with poor venous access. Externally based catheters are ideal for continuous infusion of vesicant chemotherapeutic agents because the risk of extravasation is very minimal.
	Although a VAD is a good way to prevent extravasation, it is not indicated just because someone is receiving a vesicant drug.	Expert technique and a knowledgeable clinician are the most cost-effective and safe means of administering vesicant drugs.
	Peripheral access is optimal in the large veins of the forearm, especially the posterior basilic vein. The veins in the hand and over the wrist are risky because of potential damage to tendons and nerves should extravasation occur.	Veins in the forearm are large and adequately supporting by surrounding tissue. Adequate tissue exists around veins to provide coverage and promote healing should a problem occur.
	Note: A large, straight vein over the dorsum of the hand is preferable to a smaller vein of the forearm.	
	The antecubital fossa is to be avoided for vesicant drug administration.	The area is dense with tendons and nerves. Seepage of a vesicant can be subtle and go unnoticed. Damage here can result in loss of structure and function.
	If the antecubital fossa appears to be the only vein available for access, the patient needs an access device.	Risking extravasation and subsequent tissue damage is not worth the temptation to give "just one more treatment" before considering other options.
	Hold chemotherapy—insert VAD.	There is no evidence that delayed chemotherapy for 24 h in selected cases is detrimental to the overall outcome.
	Avoid administering chemotherapy in lower extremities.	The risk for thrombosis is increased when chemotherapy is given in lower extremities.
Using a Preexisting IV Line	Do not use a preexisting peripheral IV line if any of the following are true: The IV catheter was placed >24 h earlier. The site is reddened, swollen, or sore, or there is evidence of infiltration. The site is over or around the wrist. Evidence of blood return is sluggish or absent. The IV fluid runs erratically, and the IV seems positional. Consider the patient's stents.	It is unreasonable to disregard the potential for a perfectly adequate venous access line because it was not started by the person administering the vesicant drug. Our ability to assess the vein and evidence of blood return should be adequate to ensure the practitioner of an adequate and safe venous access.

(Continued)

TABLE 19-11	EXTRAVASATION OF VESICANT ANTINEOPLASTIC AGENTS: PREVENTIVE STRATEGIES *(Continued)*	
Risk Factor	**Preventive Strategy**	**Rationale**
	If the IV fluid runs freely; the blood return is brisk and consistent, and the site is without redness, pain, or swelling; then, there is no reason to inflict unnecessary pain by injecting the patient again.	
	Prior dressings must be carefully removed over the catheter insertion site to fully visualize the vein during injection of the vesicant agent.	Dressings and tape can severely impede, both visually and tactilely, an assessment for an extravasation.

Adapted from McCorkle, R., Grant, M., Frank-Stromborg, M., & Baird, S.B. (1996). *Cancer nursing: A comprehensive textbook* (2nd ed.). Philadelphia: W.B. Saunders.

available for administration. A delay in antidote administration may increase the severity of the local tissue damage. If standing emergency orders are available, they should be signed by the responsible physician/LIP and placed in the patient's chart.

CONFIRMING VENOUS PATENCY

A flush of at least 5 to 10 mL normal saline solution may be infused to test venous patency and peripheral IV catheter placement before administering any antineoplastic agents. Do not pinch the IV catheter to determine blood return because of the resulting dramatic change

TABLE 19-12	EXTRAVASATION MANAGEMENT OF VESICANT DRUGS			
Chemotherapeutic Agent	**Vesicant/Irritant**	**Pharmacologic**	**Nonpharmacologic**	**Nursing Considerations**
Mechlorethamine, nitrogen mustard (Mustargen)	Vesicant	Sodium thiosulfate as antidote Prepare a 1/6 molar solution: • Mix 4 mL 10% sodium thiosulfate with 6 mL sterile water for injection • If using sodium thiosulfate 25%, mix 1.6 mL with 8.4 mL sterile water Aspirate the residual drug	Apply ice for 6–12 h post–antidote injection	Sodium thiosulfate neutralizes nitrogen mustard, which is excreted through the kidneys Inject 2 mL of antidote for every 1 mL of drug extravasated Inject subcutaneously using a 25-gauge needle Time is critical to successful treatment of extravasation

TABLE 19-12		EXTRAVASATION MANAGEMENT OF VESICANT DRUGS	*(Continued)*	
Chemotherapeutic Agent	Vesicant/Irritant	Pharmacologic	Nonpharmacologic	Nursing Considerations
Cisplatin (Platinol)	Irritant/vesicant potential	Use 2 mL of antidote for every 1 mg of drug extravasated Remove the needle. Inject the antidote into SQ tissue. Isotonic sodium thiosulfate as antidote Prepare a 1/6 molar solution: • Mix 4 mL 10% sodium thiosulfate with 6 mL sterile water for injection • If using sodium thiosulfate 25%, mix 1.6 mL with 8.4 mL sterile water Aspirate the residual drug Use 2 mL of 10% sodium thiosulfate for every 100 mg of cisplatin extravasated Remove the needle Inject the antidote into SQ tissue		Vesicant potential when concentration of >20 mL of 0.5 mg/mL extravasates If less than this concentration, the drug is an irritant; no treatment is recommended
Anthracyclines: Doxorubicin (Adriamycin), Daunorubicin (Cerubidine), Epirubicin (Ellence), Idarubicin (Idamycin)	Vesicants	Totect is the antidote Dose is based on body weight: • Day 1: 1,000 mg/m^2 • Day 2: 1,000 mg/m^2 • Day 3: 500 mg/m^2 Maximum dose is 2,000 mg on days 1 and 2 and 1,000 mg on day 3	Apply cold pad with circulating ice water, ice pack, or Cryogel pack for 15–20 min at least 4 times/d for the first 24–48 h Remove cold pack 15 min prior to Totect injection	Initiate Totect within 6 h of extravasation Infuse Totect into a different extremity, if possible (or vein if not possible), over 1–2 h Do not apply dimethyl sulfoxide (DMSO) topically Educate the patient about antidote side effects (nausea, vomiting, diarrhea, mucositis, myelosuppression)
Antitumor antibiotics: Mitomycin (Mutamycin), Dactinomycin (actinomycin D, Cosmegen)	Vesicants	No known antidotes available	Apply ice pack to area for 15–20 min 4 times a day for the first 24 h	Monitor for pain, blisters, and skin changes Refer the patient for other services (physical therapy, pain management, rehab) if the physician/LIP agreeable

(Continued)

TABLE 19-12	EXTRAVASATION MANAGEMENT OF VESICANT DRUGS (Continued)			
Chemotherapeutic Agent	Vesicant/Irritant	Pharmacologic	Nonpharmacologic	Nursing Considerations
Plant alkaloids: Vincristine (Oncovin), Vinblastine (Velban), Vindesine, Vinorelbine (Navelbine)	Vesicants	Hyaluronidase is the antidote There are several available preparations of this antidote. They include: • Amphadase [bovine], Hydase, and Hylenex: Vial contains 150 units per 1 mL. Use as prepared. Do not dilute • Vitrase [ovine]: Vial contains 200 units in 2 mL. Dilute 0.75 mL of solution provided with 0.25 mL sodium chloride (concentration after dilution is 150 units/mL)	Warm compresses for 15–20 min at least 4 times/day for the first 24–48 h Elevate the affected extremity	Antidote should be administered as five individual injections (0.2 mL each) directly into the site using a 25-gauge needle. Change the needle with each injection
Taxanes: Docetaxel (Taxotere), Paclitaxel (Taxol)	Vesicants	No known antidotes available	Apply ice pack for 15–20 minutes at least 4 times/d for the first 24 h	Monitor for pain, blisters, and skin changes

Adapted from Polovich, M., Whitford, J. M., & Olsen, M. (Eds.). (2009). *Chemotherapy and biotherapy guidelines and recommendations for practice* (3rd ed., pp. 108–109) Pittsburgh, PA: Oncology Nursing Society.

in pressure within the vein (Polovich et al., 2009). Administration should be postponed until the nurse confirms that fluids are flowing unimpeded into the vein. If an immediate second venipuncture is difficult or ill advised, the nurse may choose to infuse additional normal saline solution into the original site to substantiate the vein competency beyond doubt. Two methods can be used to verify blood return and IV patency prior to hanging an infusion: Using a syringe inserted at the injection port closest to the patient, gently aspirate the line while pinching off fluid from the bag or using a gravity check by removing the bag from the pump, lower it below the patient's IV site, and watch for blood return (Polovich et al., 2009). Only then should the cytotoxic agent be administered. Blood return should be checked at appropriate intervals throughout the agent's infusion. During drug administration, if the nurse suspects the agent is not infusing properly, administration should be interrupted and further assessment of blood return and venous patency should be undertaken. When in doubt, the infusion should be stopped.

MAINTAINING VIGILANT MONITORING

The nurse always must be alert to signs of extravasation, whether apparent or insidious infiltration. If the IV catheter punctures the vein's posterior wall, chemotherapeutic agents can leak into deep SQ tissues. If small-gauge IV catheters are used, particularly where there is a large volume of SQ fat, infiltration is more difficult to detect. This risk underscores the need for early comparison and assessment of the venipuncture site and immediate surrounding skin. Drug and blood flow rates should be monitored frequently. When administering agents using the bolus (IV push) technique, the nurse should pull back on the syringe's plunger approximately every 2 to 5 mL to check blood backflow. In an infusion lasting 30 to 60 minutes, blood return must be checked every 5 to 10 minutes. Blood return is checked periodically for the infusion that is >60 minutes (Polovich et al., 2009). Although a good blood return does not always guarantee that extravasation has not occurred, any changes in blood backflow should be investigated promptly.

Because infiltration is the most frequent complication of IV therapy, when a short-term vesicant infusion is needed, constant nursing attendance is required and the infusion should infuse by gravity. If the vesicant is going to be infused over 60 minutes or longer, a central line for venous access and an electronic infusion device (EID) to regulate the flow rate should be used.

Ensuring Safe Treatment and Care

During chemotherapy infusion, a patient should remain in the treatment area. Nurses in inpatient units should ensure that no diagnostic studies or therapies are scheduled to take a patient with cancer off the unit during infusion of antineoplastic drugs. If it is essential that if a patient must leave the treatment area for any reason, the nurse should accompany the patient to supervise drug infusion while diagnostic or therapeutic interventions are conducted off the treatment unit.

Managing Extravasation

When suspecting an extravasation, nurses should keep in mind the factors that determine the extent of tissue damage.

- DNA-binding vesicants cause more damage than non–DNA-binding agents.
- The higher the drug concentration and the amount of drug extravasated lead to increased damage.
- Locations that have less SQ tissue and important structural/vascular components have an increased risk of damage.
- Patient factors, such as older age, immunocompromise, and/or comorbidities, can lead to more tissue damage.

Some extravasations are difficult to detect in early stages. It bears repeating: If vesicant extravasation is suspected, it should be treated as a presumed extravasation and the infusion should be stopped immediately. The tubing should be disconnected from the IV, but the IV should remain in the patient. Aspirate any residual drug from the IV using a small syringe. The peripheral IV or port needle may then be removed. Ice should be applied 15 to 30 minutes four times daily for most antineoplastic extravasations; the exception are the Vinca alkaloids, which call for local heat application according to the manufacturer's recommendations. More antidotes for extravasation have become available in the somewhat recent past, allowing more opportunity for tissue salvage than ever before. Physicians/LIPs must be notified of suspected/actual extravasations immediately so decisions can be made regarding use of antidotes. Some antidotes also must be used in a certain time period following extravasation, so a timely physician/LIP notification is essential. Table 19-12 reviews

TABLE 19-13	KEY INTERVENTION: TREATING EXTRAVASATION ASSOCIATED WITH CHEMOTHERAPY VESICANTS

Equipment

Infusion apparatus	Sodium thiosulfate
Normal saline solution	Cold packs and heat packs as appropriate

Procedure	*Rationale*
Stop the administration of the vesicant drug and IV infusion	To prevent further drug and fluid leakage into the subcutaneous tissues
Disconnect the IV tubing from the IV device	
Do not remove; in the event of an implanted port, assess the needle site	To determine if the Huber needle is properly placed
Aspirate remaining drug in the IV access device by drawing back on the (1–3 mL) syringe	To remove the drug from tissue if possible
Notify the physician/LIP	To obtain advice and direction
Initiate standing orders, if applicable	To standardize treatment and prevent delay in extravasation management
If indicated, administer sodium thiosulfate subcutaneously with multiple punctures into the suspected extravasation site	Direct infiltration of the antidote into the area of greatest concentration
Remove the IV catheter or Huber needle from port	The site can no longer be used as an IV access
Elevate the extremity before applying a cooling or heat pack and topical antidotes	To minimize swelling, surface (skin) inflammation, and erythematous reactions
Obtain a plastic surgery consult if a large volume is extravasated, patient experiences severe pain after initial injury, or if minimal healing is evident 1–3 wk after initial injury	Early plastic surgery evaluation and treatment may decrease wound severity
Document extravasation in the official patient record and institutional incident report	To enhance later recall and for legal purposes
Obtain photograph of the site and repeat weekly if appropriate	To document extravasation and serial objective evaluations
Provide the patient with written instructions for self-care	To know what symptoms to report immediately, local care of the site and pain management. No medications should be given distal to the extravasation injury
Arrange for the patient follow-up at appropriate intervals	To follow symptomatology and ensure that appropriate interventions are initiated
In the case of a CVAD, collaborate with the physician/LIP to evaluate the need for radiographic flow study to determine the cause of extravasation and the need for future IV access	To determine the cause of extravasation and the need for future IV access

vesicant medications along with their antidotes. Table 19-13 lists key interventions in managing extravasation associated with chemotherapy vesicants.

Nurses should keep in mind that detailed charting of an extravasation should be completed as soon as possible after the patient's emergency needs have been met. This is important not only for medical and legal purposes; comprehensive documentation is important for any incident review activities. Litigation rarely reaches a court until several years after an event. Because a nurse witness is permitted to review medical documents before testimony, records should be as complete and precise as possible. Documentation should include a note in the patient progress notes or nursing notes, completion of an extravasation record, and an adverse event report. Elements of nursing documentation should include the following:

- Date and time
- Type and size of the venous access catheter used
- Insertion site
- Number and location of venipuncture attempts
- Drug(s) and drug administration sequence and administration technique
- Approximate volume of drug (in milliliters) extravasated or suspected of extravasation
- The patient's statements, complaints, reports
- Nursing management of extravasation
- Photographic documentation
- Description of the site
- Time and the physician/LIP notified
- Plastic surgery consultation/notification, if indicated
- Follow-up instructions to the patient and date for return visit
- The nurse's signature

MANAGEMENT OF SIDE EFFECTS

Almost all therapies cause some side effects. Certain drugs or combinations of drugs affect the patient in predictable ways (Polovich et al., 2009). Chemotherapy and biotherapy have known systemic side effects. The oncology nurse can anticipate that the patient who receives multiple therapies such as chemotherapy plus radiation therapy will experience more side effects than if he or she receives either therapy alone. The patient factors, such as physiologic deficits and comorbidities, can enhance the side effects.

Cytotoxic therapy affects the most rapidly growing cells in the body: bone marrow, gastrointestinal (GI) tract, hair follicles, and reproductive organs. The incidence and severity of the side effects of chemotherapy are related to the drug's dose, administration schedule, specific mechanism of action, and specific measures implemented to prevent or minimize side effects. Side effects can be acute, seen in days after drug administration; intermediate, seen in weeks following drug delivery; or chronic, extending from acute into months and years following treatment. Because the number of cancer cells killed is in direct relationship to the dose of the drug, monitoring and minimizing damage to normal cells are critical to the patient receiving the cytotoxic therapy as planned to accomplish the goal of treatment. Some side effects, such as those that affect organ function, can be dose limiting (having side effects that limit or delay treatment).

Biotherapy, like chemotherapy, is dose dependent. The side effects of biotherapy vary based on the specific drug and its action in the body. Management of biotherapy's toxicities is similar or the same as chemotherapy side effect management (Polovich et al., 2009).

Caring for the patient receiving cytotoxic therapy presents many challenges. The focus of interventions is to prevent or minimize side effects to preserve the patient's quality of life. Advances in symptom management have made it easier for the patient undergoing chemotherapy or biotherapy. The key to providing nursing care for the patient undergoing cytotoxic therapy is to assess the patient's status prior to therapy, identify the patient's risk factors, monitor the patient for side effects, noting deviations from baseline, and, last, to evaluate the effectiveness of interventions implemented. Patient education is a vital part of this process. Sharing the findings, plan, and potential interventions with the patient involves the patient in decision making, assists the patient in planning activities, and prepares the patient for self-care and monitoring (Box 19-9).

Myelosuppression

Myelosuppression (suppression of bone marrow activity) is the most common dose-limiting side effect and can affect the intensity of therapy, the quality of life and potentially therapeutic benefit. All chemotherapy affects blood counts, producing a reduction in circulating platelets, white blood cells (WBCs), and red blood cells (RBCs). Myelosuppression that causes infection or bleeding can be life threatening.

Patient education is a critical component in managing myelosuppression. The patient needs to understand that monitoring weekly blood counts is important in determining response to treatment at **nadir** (the point at which the lowest blood count is reached following therapy) and detecting problems early so that appropriate interventions can be instituted. Risk factors for myelosuppression include patient-related factors: age >65 years, female gender, decreased performance status, malnutrition, immunosuppression, drug therapies, or comorbidities, for example, chronic obstructive pulmonary disease (COPD), diabetes, renal impairment, liver disease, and disease and treatment-related factors: metastatic disease, history of chemotherapy, radiation to flat bones, aplastic marrow, malignant bone marrow involvement, prior dose-intensive chemotherapy (Kurtin, 2012).

Neutropenia

Neutropenia (an abnormal decrease in the neutrophil fraction of the WBCs) predisposes the patient to infection. Chemotherapy decreases the neutrophil count as mature neutrophils die and are not replaced. Biotherapy modulates the immune system, so the potential exists for neutropenia (Itano & Taoka, 2005). An absolute neutrophil count (ANC) of 500/mm^3 or less places the patient at severe risk for infection, and neutropenic precautions should be instituted to prevent trauma and infections (Box 19-10).

A fever (>38.1°C or 100.4°F) is often the only reliable sign of infection in the neutropenic patient. Assess the patient for chills (rigors), sore throat, cough, dyspnea, frequency or urgency of voiding, edema, or purulent drainage at sites of skin breaks. A chest radiograph and cultures are obtained. Antipyretics should be avoided as they can mask infection. CSFs are used to manage neutropenia by shortening the duration and/or severity of neutropenia; this facilitates timely chemotherapy treatments with fewer dose reductions. Broad-spectrum antibiotics may be initially ordered to combat infection until a specific organism is isolated from collected cultures.

BOX 19-9 PATIENT EDUCATION: STRATEGIES FOR MANAGING SIDE EFFECTS OF CHEMOTHERAPY

Infection Prevention

- Maintain meticulous hygiene:
  - Wash hands frequently with soap and water or an antiseptic hand rub, especially after using the toilet.
  - Observe good personal hygiene. Bathe daily. Cleanse perineal area after voiding or bowel movements.
  - Practice good oral hygiene before and after meals.
- Avoid injury to the skin or mucous membranes:
  - Use an electric razor to shave.
  - Wear gloves when working in the garden.
  - Use water-soluble lubricant during sexual intercourse. If severely neutropenic, refrain from vaginal intercourse. Avoid anal intercourse.
- Avoid sources of infection:
  - Avoid crowds or people with contagious illnesses.
  - Do not receive live vaccinations. Avoid those vaccinated with a live vaccine within the past 30 days.
  - Do not provide direct care for pets or farm animals, avoiding contact with animal feces, saliva, urine, litter box contents, and barns. Avoid indirect or direct contact with reptiles, fish, and birds.
  - Avoid use of tampons, enemas, or rectal suppositories.
  - Avoid exposure to fresh or dried plants/flowers, areas of construction/renovation, recently plowed fields.
  - Use safe food practices in food preparation, storage, and serving. Eat meat and food that is cooked or washed.
  - Consider influenza and pneumonia vaccination.
- Teach self-administration of hematopoietic growth factors.
- Monitor temperature. Contact the physician/LIP for signs (fever >38°C or 100.4°F) and symptoms of infection (chills, productive cough, shortness of breath, painful urination, sore throat, pain).

Bleeding Precautions

- Be cautious with drugs. Avoid drugs known to affect platelets, for example, aspirin, or increase bleeding; consult your health care provider before taking any unprescribed, herbal, or over-the-counter preparations.
- Avoid injury/trauma to the skin and mucous membranes:
  - Avoid shaving with blade razors; use an electric razor.
  - Use a soft toothbrush and rinse the mouth with a mild saltwater solution. Avoid dental floss.
  - Use caution near sharp objects.
  - Avoid restrictive clothing, tampons.
  - Use water-based lubricant before sexual intercourse; if platelets are <50,000/mm^3, avoid vaginal or anal intercourse.
  - Avoid physically hazardous activity and contact sports. Avoid falls.

(Continued)

> ## BOX 19-9   PATIENT EDUCATION: STRATEGIES FOR MANAGING SIDE EFFECTS OF CHEMOTHERAPY   *(Continued)*
>
> - Contact the physician/LIP for symptoms of bleeding (easy bruising, nosebleeds, bleeding gums, blood in urine or stool, bloody sputum, headache, change in level of consciousness).
>
> ### Fatigue Reduction
>
> - Take short, frequent rest periods.
> - Plan activities around times of increased energy.
> - Engage in regular exercise. Avoid strenuous activities.
> - Change positions slowly to prevent dizziness.
> - Allow family and friends to assist with tasks.
> - Energize self using such activities as meditation, yoga, visualization, listening to music, or relaxing outdoors.
> - Eat a balanced diet with iron-rich foods. Maintain a regular sleep schedule.
> - Report symptoms of fatigue to the physician/LIP to allow diagnosis of causes.
>
> ### Strategies to Reduce Constipation
>
> - Make sure to increase fluid intake to include 2 to 3 L daily.
> - Encourage fruits, vegetables, and high-fiber foods.
> - Avoid constipating foods.
> - Have regular bowel routine.
> - Obtain order for stool softener, laxative, or cathartic.
>
> ### Strategies to Relieve Mucositis
>
> - Practice good oral hygiene. Keep lips moist. Avoid oral irrigators.
> - Drink adequate fluids and eat diet high in calories and protein.
> - Choose bland, soft foods with smooth consistency.
> - Avoid irritants: chemical (citrus, spicy, mouthwashes, tobacco, alcohol) and physical (hot or cold temperatures, poor-fitting dentures).
> - Rinse mouth with baking soda or saline solution after meals and at bedtime. Use antimicrobial solutions as ordered.
> - Use topical protective agents or topical analgesics.

Thrombocytopenia

Thrombocytopenia (decreased platelet count) is a hematologic complication of chemotherapy. The normal platelet count ranges from 150,000 to 400,000/mm^3. Bleeding precautions are instituted when the platelet count drops below 50,000/mm^3. Severe risk of frank bleeding occurs most frequently when the count is <15,000/mm^3. Below a platelet count of 10,000/mm^3, bleeding can be life threatening, and daily counts with platelet transfusion support are needed.

BOX 19-10 CHEMOTHERAPY NADIR

The nadir, which is the lowest point of the WBC count, usually occurs 7 to 10 days from day 1 of chemotherapy. When the marrow starts to recover, there is an increase in the bands, which are immature, segmented neutrophils. The absolute neutrophil count (ANC) consists of both mature and immature neutrophils. The WBC includes all the white blood cells (eosinophils, basophils, and lymphocytes).

The following equation is used to calculate the ANC:

$$(\text{Segs } [segmented\ neutrophils] + \text{bands } [banded\ neutrophils]) \times \text{WBC} \times 10^1 = \text{ANC}$$

$$\text{Example: ([segs] } 45 + [\text{bands}] \ 29) \times (\text{WBC}) \ (1.1 \times 10^1) = 814 \ \text{ANC}$$

The nurse must be alert for thrombocytopenia, signaled by bleeding gums, nosebleeds, petechiae, multiple bruises, presence of blood in the urine and stools, prolonged menstruation, and a headache or change in mentation, which may indicate CNS bleeding. Clinical signs of thrombocytopenia are hypotension, tachycardia, and enlarged liver/spleen.

Anemia

Anemia (decrease in the number and oxygen-carrying capacity of the RBCs) in the patient with cancer should be investigated to determine the cause associated with chronic illness, induced by chemotherapy, as a result of malignant bone marrow involvement or as a consequence of bleeding. The RBC count, hemoglobin (Hgb), and hematocrit (Hct) results provide evidence of anemia and are used to monitor the return of marrow function and the effectiveness of medical treatment. The management of anemia involves iron supplements for iron deficiency anemia if indicated, transfusion of packed RBCs, and the administration of recombinant erythropoietin. In the absence of acute bleeding, many physicians/LIPs will wait to order a transfusion unless the patient is symptomatic or the hemoglobin value is 8 g/dL or lower. Erythropoiesis-stimulating agents (ESAs) can be effective in stimulating RBC production, with elevation in the Hgb and Hct realized in 6 to 8 weeks of therapy. ESAs are not indicated in the patient receiving chemotherapy for curative intent. ESAs require compliance with a Risk Evaluation and Mitigation Strategy (REMS) program and mandates provider training through the ESA APPRISE Oncology program. Informed consent for the patients is required for ESAs. The goal is to administer the lowest dose necessary to avoid PRBD transfusion (Kurtin, 2012). A significant role for nurses is administration of blood products and erythropoietin and monitoring the patient's response.

Signs and symptoms of anemia arise from the diminished oxygen supply tissues and the compensation of the cardiovascular system. Anemic patients present with fatigue, dyspnea, pallor, tinnitus, tachycardia, palpitations, fainting, headaches, and irritability. Patients with anemia are frequently fatigued and should be encouraged to plan frequent rest periods balanced against time for activities to maximize energy. It is important to teach the patient self-care strategies.

Alopecia

Not all chemotherapy causes alopecia (hair loss). Chemotherapy causes damage to the hair at the root resulting in complete hair loss or at the shaft associated with hair thinning. Many patients, especially women, have difficulty dealing with this side effect. The hair loss from chemotherapy is temporary. Hair loss usually occurs approximately 2 to 3 weeks after the administration of the drugs. Hair regrowth can take up to 3 to 5 months after cytotoxic treatment is completed (Polovich et al., 2009).

The patient needs to learn how to minimize trauma to the hair. Mild shampoo and gentle combing and brushing decrease breakage. Short hair is easier to manage and avoids a pulling effect present with long hair. Harsh chemicals, such as hair dyes, and devices, such as curling irons and hair dryers, should be avoided.

Once the hair falls out, lotion or moisturizer can be used on the scalp unless the patient is also receiving radiation to the area of the head. The scalp needs to be protected to avoid burns from the sun and to prevent heat loss in cold weather. Wigs, scarves, and turbans can be worn.

Psychological reassurance and emotional support are important as patients verbalize their feelings about hair loss. Community resources, such as the *Look Good, Feel Better* program, offered by the American Cancer Society, can be especially beneficial as patients cope with alterations in appearance.

Anorexia and Taste Alterations

It is well documented that both cancer and chemotherapeutic agents can cause *anorexia* (loss of appetite resulting in decreased food intake) and changes in taste. This poses a problem for maintaining adequate nutrition. Familiar foods may taste entirely different and in some circumstances may even be perceived as unpleasant. Many patients complain of a metallic or bitter taste, particularly associated with red meats. The patient may be advised to experiment with different spices and flavorings to stimulate the taste buds that have been affected by the chemotherapy. Many patients report smells aggravate anorexia. Patients may minimize odors by cooking away from the dining area. As a general rule, most patients find that cold, rather than hot, foods taste better. Eating small meals frequently may help the patient take in more total calories rather than eating larger but fewer meals. Appetite stimulants (e.g., megestrol acetate) may be ordered.

Dealing with anorexia and taste alterations is an area in which the patient and family education can have a positive impact on patient outcomes. Suggestions should include serving food on glass dishes rather than plastic to help control odors. The use of plastic utensils is helpful for patients who report a metallic taste sensation from silverware. Good oral hygiene and rinsing with nonirritating mouthwash are helpful, especially before meals.

Xerostomia may occur in patients who are taking antiemetics or who have had radiation to the head and neck. For these patients, frequent mouth washing and chewing gum or hard candy can be helpful, and soft, moist foods are more pleasing to the palate.

When all of the usual interventions are unsuccessful, nutritional needs are usually met with supplements, such as liquid protein drinks or protein powder added to food; depending on the severity of symptoms, enteral or parenteral nutrition may be added to the treatment plan.

Cardiotoxicity

Cardiotoxicity (toxicity that affects the heart) from chemotherapy include hypertension, myocardial ischemia, venous thromboembolism, QT prolongation, bradycardia, pericarditis, cardiomyopathy, and heart failure. Hypertension is commonly associated with antiangiogenesis agents, for example, bevacizumab, sorafenib, sunitinib, pazopanib, and vandetanib. Fluorouracil, capecitabine, paclitaxel, docetaxel, and bevacizumab are known to cause myocardial ischemia. Risk factors associated with this cardiac side effect are concurrent radiation therapy, continuous infusions, and preexisting coronary artery disease. Cancer and some cytotoxic agents, such as cisplatin, lenalidomide, and thalidomide, affect the clotting pathways and induces a hypercoagulable state (Fadol & Lech, 2011), which has resulted in thromboembolic events. Dysrhythmias that are found as a result of antineoplastic therapy are QT prolongation (e.g., arsenic, vorinostat, romidepsin) and bradycardia (e.g., paclitaxel and thalidomide). Pericarditis has been reported with cytarabine, doxorubicin, daunorubicin, methotrexate, and bleomycin. Cardiac myopathy can be seen with anthracycline therapy, especially doxorubicin (Adriamycin). When doxorubicin is given before cyclophosphamide, the potential for cardiotoxicity tends to increase, particularly in bone marrow or stem cell transplant patients receiving high-dose cyclophosphamide. The onset of cardiomyopathy can be categorized as acute (occurs within 24 hours), subacute (occurs 4 to 5 weeks following therapy), and chronic (occurs weeks or months following therapy). Attention should be given to the cumulative dose administered and schedule of administration and combined administration of other cardiotoxic therapies, for example, trastuzumab. More than 50% of patients exposed to anthracyclines show signs of cardiac dysfunction 10 to 20 years after treatment with 5% developing overt heart failure (Fadol, 2011).

Patients receiving potentially cardiotoxic drugs should have a baseline MUGA scan or echocardiogram and periodic follow-up testing, so the ejection fraction can be tracked. Serial ECGs are also helpful. Early electrocardiographic changes may show a decrease in voltage of the QRS complex or nonspecific ST-segment and T-wave changes. The damage to the cardiac muscle results in decreased cardiac output with shortness of breath, nonproductive cough, and progression to heart failure.

Patients at greatest risk for development of cardiotoxicity are older adults with a history of hypertension, arteriosclerotic heart disease, or other coronary artery disease. Other contributing factors include prior radiation to the mediastinum or chest wall and a lifetime cumulative dose of doxorubicin >550 mg/m^2. Studies have shown that cardiac damage can be decreased by administering doxorubicin by infusion rather than by IV push.

Strategies employed to prevent heart failure, the end result of cardiotoxicity is to insure patients that VEGF inhibitors have blood pressure control, ongoing monitoring of cardiac function in the face of administration of cardiotoxic antineoplastic drugs, monitor and limit cumulative doses of anthracyclines, add the cardioprotective drug (dexrazoxane) to anthracycline therapy, follow cardiac markers to detect cardiotoxicity early and lastly, institute pharmacological treatment of early heart failure (Fadol, 2011).

Constipation

A patient is considered constipated when evacuation does not occur for 96 hours or when hard, dry stool causes difficulty in defecation. Because individual bowel patterns vary, it is helpful to know the patient's usual habits. Medications (including chemotherapy), anxiety, depression, hypercalcemia, immobility, dehydration, and tumor involvement resulting in intrinsic or extrinsic compression can contribute to constipation.

Intervention depends on the underlying cause. The most common causes are inadequate fluid intake and pain medications. Prophylactic laxatives, lubricants, and cathartics may help move waste through the intestinal system by increasing motility and may be needed if Vinca alkaloids were administered. Rectal exams, suppositories, and rectal enemas should be avoided in patients with neutropenia and thrombocytopenia because they can be irritating to mucous membranes and cause microscopic tears, raising the risk of bleeding and infection. Impaction is best handled with an oil retention or phosphate enema to hydrate the stool.

Teaching patients to adopt various dietary habits, such as increasing intake of fresh fruits and vegetables and fiber, may help treat and prevent constipation. Adequate fluid intake of 2 to 3 L daily is recommended. It is wise to avoid constipating foods such as cheeses, eggs, and refined starches. Physical activity and exercise also help stimulate peristalsis. Rotating opioids may minimize analgesic-induced constipation.

Diarrhea

It is the function of the colon to absorb fluid. When this does not happen, diarrhea (loose or watery stools) is the result. Diarrhea in the oncology patient can have a number of causes. Surgical procedures, such as gastric or intestinal resection, can result in a shortened GI tract or a malabsorption syndrome. Inflammatory bowel syndrome or *Clostridium difficile* and other intestinal infections can also cause diarrhea, as can cancer-related chemotherapy, targeted therapy, radiation therapy, and hematologic transplants.

The nurse needs to know the degree of chemotherapy-induced diarrhea (CID), whether it uncomplicated or complicated (associated with cramping, nausea/vomiting, fever, neutropenia, bleeding, or dehydration). Uncomplicated CID is managed with loperamide and dietary adjustments (Sweed, 2011). Persistent diarrhea with associated symptoms lasting more than 24 hours needs a more aggressive approach so that fluid and electrolyte imbalances can be prevented or treated. Accurate intake and output measurement, weight, and the number and character of the stools provide valuable information for fluid replacement strategies. The major electrolyte lost with diarrhea is potassium. Therefore, potassium-rich foods should be encouraged and fluid intake should consist of at least 2 L daily. In cases of severe diarrhea, IV therapy may be initiated. Pharmacologic intervention should be started as soon as possible.

Fatigue

Fatigue is defined as an overwhelming sense of exhaustion and inability to perform physical or mental work that is not relieved by rest. Chemotherapy-induced fatigue generally peaks in 3 to 4 days following the nadir and can reappear with each cycle. For the biotherapy drugs, like IFN, interleukin-2, and the mAbs, fatigue is common and can be dose limiting. Fatigue can easily be a consequence of anemia or infection. Dehydration, electrolyte imbalances, and compromised nutrition can affect the individual's perception of fatigue. Medications can also contribute to a sense of fatigue, especially if sedation is a side effect. Fatigue is a symptom that can accompany anxiety, depression, stress, pain, or insomnia.

Gonadal Dysfunction

Chemotherapeutic agents, especially the alkylating agents, may affect the function of the ovaries and testicles. The impact of chemotherapy can be felt in three areas: fertility, body image, and sexual functioning. Reduction in the male sperm count can result in temporary or permanent infertility. All men who wish to have children should be counseled on sperm banking prior to the start of chemotherapy. Changes in the menstrual cycle are observed within 6 months of starting antineoplastic therapy. Women can experience amenorrhea and symptoms of medical menopause. When a woman is close to or older than age 40, the chances of permanent menopause and loss of fertility following chemotherapy are more likely than for women in their 20s and 30s. Sometimes the regimen of drugs can be altered in an attempt to preserve ovarian function and ability to bear children or egg retrieval and storage can be pursued.

Roughly 40% to 100% of patients will experience some sexual dysfunction following chemotherapy. The prevalence of sexual dysfunction is unknown as it is often underreported by patients and underassessed by health care providers. Both men and women experience sexual effects of cancer therapy: changes in body and/or appearance, changes in self-image, decreased libido, and difficulty reaching orgasm. For men, erectile dysfunction and premature ejaculation add to sexual changes. For women, menopausal symptoms of sleep disturbances, hot flashes, irritability, and dyspareunia are common. Strategies to improve sexual function may involve pharmaceutical management and counseling, with referral to a specialist if needed.

There is limited information concerning fetal effects of chemotherapy, and therefore it is recommended that birth control should be practiced during chemotherapy and for 1 to 2 months postchemotherapy. Chemotherapy administered to women in the first trimester of pregnancy has resulted in miscarriage. Chemotherapy affects rapidly growing cells, and treatment in the second or third trimester is likely to result in birth anomalies. However, the literature has documented healthy live births without increased birth defects after antineoplastic therapy.

Mucositis

Mucositis (inflammation of the mucosal lining of the gastrointestinal tract, including the oral cavity) is a common side effect of cytotoxic therapy, both chemotherapy (antimetabolites, antitumor antibiotics, alkylating agents, plant alkaloids) and biotherapy (IL-2 and IFNs).

The mucous membranes of the GI tract become red, irritated, and inflamed owing to either the direct effect of the drugs or the indirect result of the myelosuppressive effects of the drugs. Chemotherapy-induced mucositis usually begins 4 to 5 days after treatment and lasts for approximately 10 days and heals spontaneously in 21 days. Pain is a hallmark symptom of oral mucositis. The patient may experience mild irritation and sensitivity to acidic or spicy foods or painful lesions and difficulty swallowing. The specific drug, dose, and patient risk factors determine the degree of mucositis. The nurse should be concerned about patients who have had head and neck radiation or who are receiving steroidal therapy. Patients who are nutritionally compromised and those with high oral flora owing to poor dental hygiene are also at an increased risk.

Preventive measures start with a thorough pretreatment dental evaluation. Assessment of oral cavity for bleeding, erythema, ulceration, and white or yellow plaques is critical to early detection of mucositis. Meticulous attention to the oral cavity with a soft toothbrush or soft swab prevents irritating delicate tissue. Irritating agents such as commercial mouthwashes containing alcohol, tobacco, and elective dental surgery should be avoided.

Application of balm, aloe vera, or a petroleum-based gel to lips prevents cracking and drying. Mouth rinses mixed with baking soda and water or saline solution may soothe the irritated mucous membranes. In addition, several mucositis cocktail formulas are available. Most contain diphenhydramine (Benadryl), an antacid, and a local anesthetic. Though popular, their effectiveness over saline or baking soda solution is unsubstantiated (Daly & Quinn, 2011). Cultures of mouth sores may reveal a need to treat the patient with antifungal and/or antiviral agents. Soft foods with a smooth consistency and cold, wet foods are more soothing to irritated mucous membranes (Box 19-9).

Nausea and Vomiting

Nausea and vomiting (emesis) are among the most common side effects of chemotherapy. For the patient, these distressing symptoms can significantly interfere with quality of life, leading to poor compliance with further chemotherapy treatment. Approximately 70% to 80% of all cancer patients receiving chemotherapy experience vomiting, whereas 10% to 44% experience anticipatory emesis (NCCN, 2013a, 2013b). Chemotherapy-induced nausea and vomiting are classified as acute, delayed, and anticipatory. Acute symptoms occur minutes to hours following chemotherapy and can last 24 to 48 hours. Many chemotherapeutic agents have the potential for delayed nausea and vomiting with onset after 24 hours and lasting for several days. Anticipatory nausea and vomiting occur before chemotherapy and are a result of inadequately controlled symptoms over several cycles of chemotherapy. Uncontrolled nausea and vomiting can be life threatening. It can result in nutritional deficits, fluid and electrolyte imbalances, impaired wound healing, and deterioration of self-care and functional ability. As a general rule, it is easier to control nausea than to stop vomiting.

Predisposing factors for nausea or vomiting include gender (females > males), age (young > old), non–drug user, and a prior history of poor emetic control such as motion sickness, morning sickness, or prior exposure to chemotherapy. Obtaining a history may reveal other causes for nausea and vomiting, such as anxiety, pain, or constipation. The frequency of chemotherapy-induced emesis depends on the emetic potential of the specific chemotherapeutic agents used. Emetic risk of drugs/regimens is identified as high, moderate, low, and minimal. Successful management of nausea and vomiting depends on keen assessment of the patient's risk factors, knowledge of the expected level of emetogenicity of the drugs administered, and a plan for prevention and early treatment to ensure nausea and vomiting control.

The ideal plan to ameliorate nausea and vomiting is an approach that combines pharmacologic interventions with nonpharmacologic strategies. Antiemetics should be initiated prior to chemotherapy and continued throughout the duration of the emetic activity of the chemotherapy drug used. The best antiemetic regimen is one that uses the lowest, maximally effective dose via an appropriate route. The oral and IV antiemetics are equally effective. The 5-HT3 receptor antagonists combined with steroids and the new NK-1 receptor antagonist have demonstrated effectiveness (NCCN, 2013a, 2013b). Practice guidelines from national oncology groups have provided direction for antiemetic use. Although studies and guidelines provide recommendations for practice in preventing and treating nausea and vomiting, drug options must be tailored to what is most effective for the patient.

Nonpharmacologic interventions provide nurses with some latitude and an opportunity for creativity while giving the patient a sense of control. Regulating the environment to eliminate strong food, perfume, and other odors helps reduce nausea. Soft music, low lights, a quiet atmosphere, and relaxation tapes help reduce anxiety and hence nausea. Diversional activities such as cards, movies, or crafts provide distraction from chemotherapy. Some behavioral strategies include hypnosis, progressive muscle relaxation, guided imagery, biofeedback, and acupressure or acupuncture.

Suggestions for dietary adjustment include serving foods cold or at room temperature, and bland foods rather than spicy, fried and fatty, strong-flavored, sour, or tart foods. Clear liquids, gelatin, juice, ginger ale or other carbonated drinks, herbal teas, and sport drinks may help settle the stomach, provide hydration, and furnish electrolytes. It is advisable to avoid foods with strong odors.

Neurotoxicity

Some chemotherapeutic drugs, such as plant alkaloids and taxanes, are neurotoxic. They affect the CNS, peripheral nervous system, and/or cranial nerves. CNS toxicity can be manifest as acute or chronic encephalopathies. Biotherapies, such as IFN and aldesleukin, can result in changes in mentation. Cognitive impairment (changes to ability to think, concentrate, formulate ideas, reason, and remember) has also been noted by breast cancer patients. Peripheral nerve toxicity can affect sensory or motor function. Cranial nerve impairment depends on which nerve is involved. The signs and symptoms of peripheral neuropathy are indicated by patient complaints of numbness and tingling of hands and feet, muscle pain, weakness, and disturbances in position sense, particularly with ambulation. Clinically, deep tendon reflexes disappear. The decreased perception and sensation that the patient experiences can result in accidents. Constipation with or without a paralytic ileus is another problem related to autonomic neurotoxicity, especially from the Vinca alkaloids.

Risk factors associated with neurotoxicity are the following: age (the elderly and pediatric populations), chemotherapy regimens that contain neurotoxic drugs (platinum drugs, taxanes, epothilones, Vinca alkaloids, and newer agents such as bortezomib and lenalidomide) or involve high-dose therapy, chemotherapy that crosses the blood–brain barrier, intrathecal chemotherapy (methotrexate), cranial irradiation, renal impairment, diabetes with existing neuropathy, excessive alcohol consumption, and concomitant drug therapy such as mood-altering drugs.

The first signs of neurotoxicity can be seen as early as during drug administration, in the case of oxaliplatin (Eloxatin) or as late as after five or more treatments with a neurotoxic drug like cisplatin (Platinol). Paclitaxel (Taxol), however, can produce paresthesia within 5 days of administration. When cisplatin is used concurrently with paclitaxel, the potential for neurotoxicity increases. It is recommended that paclitaxel be administered before cisplatin to reduce the potential of toxicity.

Calcium and magnesium infusions have been well studied in the prevention of oxaliplatin-associated peripheral neuropathy. Pharmacologic treatment recommendations include anticonvulsants and tricyclic antidepressants, and topical analgesics can help with neuropathic pain (Lee & Westcarth, 2012). Strategies for coping with cognitive impairment include writing things down, receiving support and validation from family, friends and coworkers, volunteering their time to "give back," depending on others to help remember things, exercise to help with mental clarity, rest at night and short naps to sharpen mental acuity, and activities to stimulate the mind, for example, puzzles. Referrals to occupational and physical therapy can assist with impaired walking and prevention of injury.

Pulmonary Toxicity

The pulmonary effects of chemotherapy/biotherapy are related to the direct damage to the alveoli and the capillary endothelium. The most common types of pulmonary toxicity are interstitial lung disease (ILD), which includes pneumonitis and fibrosis, and pulmonary edema, for example; the capillary leak syndrome seen with IL-2. Additional pulmonary toxicities are emerging such as acute promyelocytic leukemia differentiation syndrome/retinoic acid syndrome, pulmonary venoocclusive disease (VOD), and the newer target therapies that inhibit the tyrosine kinase pathway impacting alveoli and lung pneumocytes (Polovich et al., 2009). Patients receiving bleomycin in doses >250 units/m^2 or 400 units/m^2 total dose, or carmustine in a total dose of 1,400 mg/m^2, are at risk for development of pulmonary toxicity. Patients at a higher risk for this complication are the elderly and those with a smoking history or a preexisting pulmonary condition, history of autoimmune disease, and impaired renal function. In addition to the two previously mentioned drugs, several other drugs can cause pulmonary toxicity, including cyclophosphamide, methotrexate, oxaliplatin, cytarabine, busulfan, bevacizumab, cetuximab, docetaxel, temsirolimus, and gefitinib.

A baseline PFT and ongoing monitoring are helpful in detecting early changes, such as abnormal breath sounds, dry hacking cough, and dyspnea. Steroids may play a role in prevention and have provided symptomatic relief of cough and dyspnea. With increasing symptoms, the chemotherapy/biotherapy is postponed. Antibiotics and oxygen administration may be helpful in combating infection and maintaining adequate tissue perfusion.

Renal Toxicity

Baseline renal function tests (BUN, creatinine and creatinine clearance, urinalysis, and uric acid) should be done before administering chemotherapeutic agents known to affect renal function. The drugs most frequently associated with renal toxicity are cisplatin, methotrexate, iphosphamide, mitomycin, bevacizumab, and interleukin-2. When the patient demonstrates renal insufficiency (elevated blood urea nitrogen and creatinine levels associated with oliguria, proteinuria, and hematuria), consideration needs to be given to reducing the dose to protect the kidneys from further damage and compensate for the longer half-life of the drug—a consequence of poor renal function.

Strategies used to protect the kidneys include vigorous hydration, hypertonic saline solutions, mannitol, and furosemide (Lasix). The patient needs to be monitored for renal compromise. Early intervention can avert the need for dialysis. The patient's urine pH is monitored during high-dose methotrexate to maintain an alkaline environment and to prevent precipitation of the drug in the renal tubules with renal damage.

Tumor lysis syndrome (TLS) is another disorder that can cause renal damage. In patients with a large tumor burden who are receiving chemotherapy where a rapid cell kill is expected, TLS should be anticipated and prevented using allopurinol to reduce uric acid. Additionally, the use of concurrent nephrotoxic drugs increases the patient's risk for renal toxicity. General nursing strategies are to monitor renal function by following renal functions and electrolyte laboratory tests, assessing intake/output and weight, to administer hydration, force diuresis, and administer chemoprotectants including amifostine, mesna, allopurinol or rasburicase, and leucovorin rescue to prevent renal toxicity.

Skin Toxicities

Treatment of tumors has evolved to include drugs that target receptors associated with the cancer cell. Two types of these targeted therapies can cause skin toxicities: epidermal growth factor receptor (EGFR) inhibitors and multikinase inhibitors. The most commonly seen dermatologic side effect associated with EGRF inhibitors, for example, cetuximab (Erbitux), is a mild to moderate papulopustular rash found on the face, scalp, neck, upper chest, and back. Although it resembles acne, it differs in that it lacks the classic acne comedones. The rash associated with cetuximab, panitumumab, and erlotinib has correlated with a higher tumor response rate and longer survival (Eaby-Sandy, Grande, & Viale, 2012). Treatment of the rash includes avoidance of acne OTC medications, use of perfume- and alcohol-free emollients, and avoidance of sun exposure, use of antihistamine for pruritus, antibiotic use if skin rash is infected, and use of analgesics for pain (Polovich et al., 2009). The multikinase inhibitors, generally oral therapies, have side effects involving the skin, hair, nail beds, and mucosa. Topical or systemic steroids can be helpful. The papulopustular rash is the same as with EGRF inhibitors. The hand-foot skin reaction (HFSR) develops within the first 2 to 4 weeks of multikinase inhibitor treatment and manifests itself as a halo of erythema, blisters on pressure areas of the feet and palms of the hands including the fingers. Calluses surrounded by reddened areas are typical for HFSR. Management strategies include avoidance of friction/trauma to the hands and feet, use of thick cotton gloves and socks to protect against injury, urea cream to soften epidermal thickness, topical steroids, topical lidocaine, and other systemic NSAID and analgesics for pain. Dose reduction, interruption, and discontinuation of treatment can be considered if toxicities are unresponsive to symptomatic measures.

Review Questions   *Note: Questions below may have more than one right answer.*

1. If a second venipuncture site is needed, and the patient's other arm is not an option, the second site should be located
   A. Distal to the original site
   B. Proximal to the original site
   C. In the lower extremity
   D. Alongside the original site

2. All of the following drugs are classified as vesicants *except*
   A. Dactinomycin
   B. Daunorubicin hydrochloride
   C. Doxorubicin
   D. Dacarbazine

3. The risk of allergic reactions occurs when administering which one of the following biotherapy agents
   A. Hematopoietic growth factors
   B. Monoclonal antibodies
   C. Interferons
   D. Interleukins

4. All of the following elements of documentation of an extravasation are essential *except*
   A. Mentation of the patient
   B. Date and time of the treatment
   C. Antineoplastic agents given and their sequence
   D. Approximate quantity of drug extravasated

5. Patient education and understanding of antineoplastic treatment is enhanced when
   A. The environment is new
   B. The patient has received sedation for anxiety
   C. The patient is ready to learn
   D. The patient is bilingual

6. Precautions taken when preparing and handling antineoplastic agents include all of the following *except*
   A. Wear personal protective equipment consistent with Occupational Safety and Health Administration (OSHA) guidelines
   B. Prepare drugs under a Class II biologic safety cabinet
   C. Use a nonaerosol needle
   D. Clip or recap all needles after reconstitution of drugs

7. After chemotherapy administration, body fluids are considered to be contaminated for
   A. 12 hours
   B. 24 hours
   C. 48 hours
   D. 72 hours

8. The maximum lifetime dose of doxorubicin, if the patient has had radiation, is usually considered to be
   A. 150 to 175 mg/m^2
   B. 550 mg/m^2
   C. 4,500 to 5,500 mg
   D. 450 mg/m^2

9. The side effect most likely to affect body image is
   A. Diarrhea
   B. Red-tinged urine
   C. Alopecia
   D. Fatigue

10. A reversible side effect of chemotherapy is
   A. Pulmonary fibrosis
   B. Amenorrhea
   C. Myelosuppression
   D. Sterility

References and Selected Readings   *Asterisks indicate references cited in text.*

Alexander, M., Corrigan, A., Gorski, L., Hankins, J., Perucca, R. (Eds.). (2010). *Infusion nursing: An evidence-based approach*. Infusion Nurses Society (3rd ed.). St. Louis, MO: Saunders Elsevier.

*American Society of Health-System Pharmacists. (2006). ASHP guidelines on handling hazardous drugs. *American Journal of Health-System Pharmacy*, 63(12), 1172–1193.

*Blecher, C.S. (Ed.). (2004). *Standards of oncology education: Patient/significant other and public* (3rd ed.). Pittsburgh, PA: Oncology Nursing Society.

*Brant, J.M., & Wickham, R.S. (Eds.). (2004). *Statement on the scope and standards of oncology nursing practice*. Pittsburgh, PA: Oncology Nursing Society.

*Breslin, S. (2007). Cytokine-release syndrome: Overview and nursing implications. *Clinical Journal of Oncology Nursing*, 11(Suppl 1), 37–42.

*Camp-Sorrell, D. (Ed.). (2011). *Access device guidelines: Recommendations for nursing practice and education*. (3rd ed.). Pittsburgh, PA: Oncology Nursing Society.

Casciato, D. (Ed.). (2012). *Manual of clinical oncology* (7th ed.). Philadelphia, PA: Lippincott Williams & Wilkins.

*Daly, C.F., & Quinn, A.M. (2011). Oral Mucositis: Addressing the causes, challenges and clinical management. *Journal of the Advanced Practitioner in Oncology*, 2(1), 4–13.

*DeVita, V.T., Lawrence, T.S., & Rosenberg, S.A. (Eds.). (2011). *DeVita, Hellman, and Rosenberg's cancer: Principles and practice of oncology* (9th ed.). Philadelphia, PA: Lippincott Williams & Wilkins.

*Eaby-Sandy, B., Grande, C., Viale, P.H. (2012). Dermatological toxicities in epidermal growth factor and multikinase inhibitors. *Journal of the Advanced Practitioner in Oncology, 3*(3), 138–150.

*Ener, R.A., Meglathery, S.B. & Styler, M. (2004). Extravasation of systemic hemato-oncological therapies. *Annals of Oncology, 15*(6), 858–862.

*Fadol, A., & Lech, T. (2011). Cardiovascular adverse events associated with cancer therapy. *Journal of the Advanced Practitioner in Oncology, 2*(4), 229–242.

*Gobel, B.H. (2005). Chemotherapy-induced hypersensitivity reactions. *Oncology Nursing Forum, 32*(5), 1027–1035.

*Infusion Nurses Society (INS). (2011). Infusion nursing standards of practice. *Journal of Infusion Nursing, 34*(1S), S1–S110.

*INS/INCC. (2009). The value of certification in infusion nursing. *Journal of Infusion Nursing, 32*(5), 248–50.

*Itano, J.K., & Taoka, K.N. (Eds.). (2005). *Core curriculum for oncology nursing* (4th ed.). St. Louis, MO: Elsevier Saunders.

Jacobs, L.A. (Ed.). (2003). *Standards of oncology nursing education: Generalist and advanced levels* (3rd ed.). Pittsburgh, PA: Oncology Nursing Society.

*Jacobson, J.O., Polovich, M., McNiff, K.K., LeFebvre, K.B., Cummings, C., Galioto, M., et al. (2009). American society of Clinical Oncology/Oncology Nursing Society Chemotherapy Administration Safety Standards. *Oncology Nursing Forum, 36*(6), 1–8.

*Jacobson, J.O. Polovich, M., Gilmore, T.R., Schulmeister, L., Esper, P., LeFebvre, K.B., et al. (2012). Revisions to the 2009 American Society of Clinical Oncology/Oncology Nursing Society Chemotherapy Administration Safety Standards: Expanding the Scope to Include Inpatient Settings. *Oncology Nursing Forum, 39*(1), 31–38.

*Kurtin, S. (2012). Myeloid toxicity of cancer treatment. *Journal of the Advanced Practitioner in Oncology, 3*(4), 209–224.

*Lee, E.L., & Westcarth, L. (2012). Neurotoxicity associated with cancer therapy. *Journal of the Advanced Practitioner in Oncology, 3*(1)11–21.

*National Comprehensive Cancer Network (NCCN). (2013a). *NCCN practice guidelines in oncology: Antiemesis.* www.nccn.org

*National Comprehensive Cancer Network (NCCN). (2013b). *NCCN practice guidelines in oncology: Cancer-related fatigue.* www.nccn.org

*National Institute for Occupational Safety and Health. (2004). *Preventing occupational exposure to antineoplastic and other hazardous drugs in health care settings.* http://www.cdc.gov/niosh/docs/2004-165/pdfs/2004-165

*National Institute for Occupational Safety and Health. (2012) *NIOSH List of Antineoplastic and Other Hazardous Drugs in Health care Settings 2012.* http://www.cdc.gov/niosh/docs/2012-150/pdfs/2012-150.pdf

*Occupational Safety and Health Administration (OSHA). (1986). *Guidelines for cytotoxic (antineoplastic) drugs.* Publication No. 8-1.1. Washington, DC: Department of Labor, Occupational Safety and Health Administration, Office of Occupational Medicine.

*Oncology Nursing Certification Corporation (ONCC). (2013). http://www.oncc.org/

*Oncology Nursing Society (ONS). (2011). *Education of the professional RN who administers and cares for the individual receiving chemotherapy and biotherapy.* Pittsburgh, PA: Author. http://ons.org/about-ons/ons-position-statements/education-certification-and-role-delineation/education-rn-who

*Oncology Nursing Society (ONS). (2013a). *Cancer basics online course.* Pittsburgh, PA: Author. http://www.ons.org/CourseDetail.aspx?course_id=20.

*Oncology Nursing Society (ONS). (2013b). *Oncology Certification for Nurses.* http://www.ons.org/Publications/Positions/Certification

*Perucca, R. (2010). Peripheral venous access devices. In M. Alexander, A. Corrigan, L. Gorski, J. Hankins, R. Perucca (Eds.), *Infusion nursing: An evidence-based approach* (3rd ed., pp. 456–479). Infusion Nurses Society. St. Louis, MO: Saunders Elsevier.

*Polovich, M., Whitford, J.M., & Olsen, M. (Eds.). (2009). *Chemotherapy and biotherapy guidelines and recommendations for practice* (3rd ed.). Pittsburgh, PA: Oncology Nursing Society.

*Sauerland, C., Engelking, C., Wickham, R., & Corbi, D. (2006). Vesicant extravasation part I: Mechanisms, pathogenesis, and nursing care to reduce risk. *Oncology Nursing Forum, 33*(6), 1134–1141.

*Siegel, R., Naishadham, D., & Jemal, A. (2013). Cancer statistics, 2013. *Ca, A Cancer Journal for Clinicians, 63*(1), 11–30.

Skeel, R.T., & Khlief, S.N. (Eds.). (2011). *Handbook of cancer chemotherapy* (8th ed.). Philadelphia, PA: Lippincott Williams & Wilkins.

Sweed, M. (2011). Gastrointestinal and hepatobiliary toxicities of cancer treatments. *Journal of the Advanced Practitioner in Oncology, 2*(5), 293–304.

Wilkes, G.M. (2011). Chemotherapy: Principles of administration. In C. H. Yarbro, D. Wujcik, & B.H. Gobel (Eds.), *Cancer Nursing: Principles and practice* (7th ed., pp. 391–457). Sudbury, MA: Jones and Bartlett.

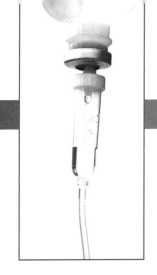

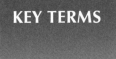

CHAPTER 20

Pain Management

Deborah L. Gentile
Barbara St. Marie

KEY TERMS	Dermatomes	Multimodal
	Epidural	Analgesia
	Intraspinal	Persistent Pain
	Intrathecal	Range Orders
	Lock-Out Interval	Titration to Effect

ROLE OF NURSES IN PAIN MANAGEMENT

The prevalence of pain, the disparities in treatment, the increase of vulnerable populations with pain, as well as understanding that when pain is persistent, it becomes a chronic disease, all relate to the importance of prevention or management of pain for individuals and populations. Pain has been deemed a public health challenge (Institute of Medicine, 2011). Nurses across all clinical settings are in a unique position to impact pain management. As a discipline, nurses have a tremendous opportunity to engage in the practice of pain management. The nurse's role in pain management is broad, and the nursing process—assessment, diagnosis, outcomes identification, planning, implementation, and evaluation—is well suited for this patient population. Furthermore, the capacity of nurses to be an advocate, educator, change agent, and interprofessional collaborator gives nurses a noticeable advantage as they care for the patient in pain.

In addition to the skill sets mentioned above, a number of influencing factors shape the role of the nurse in pain management. Regulatory bodies, standards of care, practice guidelines, and institutional policies and procedures all impact the extent and manner in which nurses provide pain management. The responsibilities of all disciplines involved in

651

pain management are delineated in The Joint Commission (TJC) standards. TJC standards focus on health care provider orientation, education, patient rights, patient education, and postoperative care and contain wording specific to pain management (TJC, 2012). In recent years, evidence-based recommendations, guidelines, and position statements for pain management have been developed by such groups as the American Society of Anesthesiologists Task Force on Acute Pain Management (Horlocker et al., 2010), the American Society for Pain Management Nursing (ASPMN), and the Institute of Medicine (IOM, 2011). Additionally, the scope and standards of practice for pain management nursing were developed in a joint venture involving ASPMN and the American Nurses Association (ANA) and apply to both the nurse generalist and the nurse specialist in pain management. Institutional policies and procedures guide nurses through definitions, responsibilities, assessment and management expectations, and educational requirements for pain management. Influencing factors change as pain management practice evolves and new knowledge becomes available.

Change Management and Quality Improvement

Even with the many advances in pain management strategies, pharmacology, technology, and techniques, pain continues to be poorly managed. Nurses play a key role in making and maintaining pain management as a strategic priority across all health care venues. The need to improve the quality of patient pain outcomes is imperative for the patient's overall health. Box 20-1 identifies select physical and physiological harmful effects of unrelieved pain.

EVIDENCE FOR PRACTICE

What are the effects of unrelieved pain on patient mobility, postsurgical complications, hospital performance, and the cost of care?

BOX 20-1   EXAMPLES OF PHYSICAL AND PHYSIOLOGICAL EFFECTS OF UNRELIEVED PAIN

Cardiovascular *Sympathetic nervous system activation*: hypercoagulation, increased heart rate, blood pressure, cardiac workload, oxygen demand

Gastrointestinal *Stress response causes increase in sympathetic nervous system activity*: intestinal secretions, smooth muscle sphincter tone increase, decreased gastric emptying and intestinal motility

Endocrine *Excessive hormone release*: carbohydrate, protein, and fat catabolism, poor glucose use, decreased insulin, decreased testosterone

Adapted from Wells, N., Pasero, C., & McCaffery, M. (2008). Improving the quality of care through pain assessment and management. In R. G. Hughes (Ed.), *Patient safety and quality: An evidence-based handbook for nurses* (Chapter 17). Rockville, MD: Agency for Healthcare Research and Quality (US). http://www.ncbi.nlm.nih.gov/books/NBK2658/

Furthermore, the quality of pain management impacts the public assessment of health care organizations. To that end, the nurse's role as a change agent cannot be underestimated. Innovations in pain management have transformed the practice. It is important for nurses to understand basic change management strategies and the use of quality improvement methods in all practice settings.

The Centers for Medicare & Medicaid (CMS) are a driving force for institutions to redesign pain management models of care. In the 1940s, Kurt Lewin developed a model for organizational change that remains relevant and widely used. He described three stages of change: (a) unfreeze, (b) change, and (c) refreeze (Burnes, 2004). If nurses understand and use these stages, they can develop a plan to manage each step of the pain management change process in their respective facilities. The first stage is vital to success in any change effort. It involves generating motivation for the change. It may seem obvious that a problem with effective pain management is the reason enough for change, but there are other factors that influence the stakeholders of any organization struggling with this issue.

The following steps will be valuable to "unfreeze" the way pain management is performed. First, the change should be data driven. The most convincing and least threatening motivator for change to occur in practice is accurate data. Second, align the change with organizational values and strategic goals. And third, identify resistance to change and take time to engage in discussion about fears while recognizing elements of past and current practices that are positive. A comprehensive communication plan about an improvement project or practice change is vital to success.

During Lewin's second stage, "change," health care providers begin to embrace the practice change. During this stage, the health care team learns new skills, understands principles around these new skills, and begins to see the positive impact on their patient outcomes and satisfaction. They recognize the personal and organizational benefit of the newly introduced practice. Some of these changes will be time sensitive, but also be aware that each person moves at his or her own pace in adopting practice change.

Lewin's third stage or "refreezing" reflects adoption of the practice change and its maintenance. The data may begin to improve and provide evidence that supports the change. At this point, it is important that all components of the practice change are carried out in a consistent manner. Consistency will create a sense of stability around the change. A celebration of success is recommended to thank everyone involved in the change for their dedication in improving pain management (Bridges, 2009). Well-planned, clear communication throughout the change process is essential to the success of the change effort.

Quality improvement methods provide an operational model to guide improvement processes. One of the most widely used models is the Plan, Do, Study, Act (PDSA) framework developed by Langley, Nolan, and Nolan (1994). The PDSA cycle mirrors the stages of change described above (Figure 20-1). When the cycle is applied to pain management quality improvement projects, it provides a framework to guide design, measurement, implementation, and improvement of a change process. If the improvement project has multiple phases, a PDSA cycle is used to guide each phase. Batalden and Stoltz (1993) developed a worksheet of useful questions to consider when creating a PDSA cycle (Table 20-1).

Measurement and the need for data are identified in the processes of change and quality improvement. Quality measures or indicators related to pain and its management are a source of improvement opportunities. Pain management and the patient's perceptions of pain management are some of the categories of quality indicators recommended for organizations to monitor. One quality indicator is a time indicator, such as the "median time to

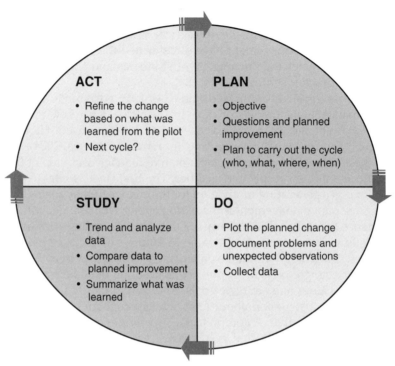

FIGURE 20-1 Plan, Do, Study, Act Cycle. (Adapted from Langley, G., Nolan, K. M., & Nolan, T. W. (1994). The foundation of improvement. *Quality Progress*, *27*, 81.)

TABLE 20-1	QUESTIONS TO CONSIDER FOR PLAN-DO-STUDY-ACT (PDSA) OR QUALITY IMPROVEMENT PROCESS
Plan	• Who is going to do what, by when, where, and how? • Is the "owner" of the process involved? • Which measures are needed to answer our questions and to identify there was an improvement?
Do	• What have we learned from our planned pilot change and data collection? • What have we learned from unplanned information we collected? • Was the pilot change congruent with the plan?
Study	• Was there an improvement? • Did the pilot change work better for all stakeholders or just some of them? • What did we learn about planning for our next change?
Act	• Do we adapt the change? And repeat the PDSA? • Do we abandon this pilot change and try something else? And repeat the PDSA? • If the pilot change efforts are abandoned, what has been learned? • Do we keep this change? • If so, what should be standardized? • What training is needed to provide continuity? • How should continued monitoring be done?

Adapted from Batalden, P. B., & Stoltz, P. K. (1993). A Framework for the continual improvement of health care: Building and applying professional and improvement knowledge to test changes in daily work. *Joint Commission Journal on Quality Improvement*, *19*, 446–447.

pain management for long bone fracture" (Agency for Healthcare Research and Quality, 2011). Another example is the time in minutes that it takes from the moment that a patient enters the emergency department until the patient receives an oral or parenteral pain medication. Patient satisfaction with pain management is an example of another outcome quality indicator. Two questions that all acute care patients are asked after discharge are illustrated in Figure 20-2. These originated from the Hospital Consumer Assessment of Healthcare Providers and Systems (HCAHPS) survey, initiated as a requirement for hospitals receiving Medicare reimbursement. These questions and others are publicly available for use. The results from patient surveys are also available and grouped at the hospital level. Reviewing results for the hospital or unit may provide opportunities for improvement.

Staff Education

Interprofessional staff education encompasses all levels of licensed independent practitioners (LIPs), nursing, advanced practice nurses, and physician's assistants. Throughout this chapter, we refer to this group of professionals collectively as physician/LIP, emphasizing the key requirements for quality pain management (Box 20-2). The term *licensed independent practitioner* originated with TJC and is used in standards for privileging and credentialing. According to TJC, an LIP is "any individual permitted by law and by the organization to provide care and services, without direction or supervision, within the scope of the individual's license and consistent with individually granted clinical privileges." When standards reference the term "licensed independent practitioner," this language is not to be construed to limit the authority of a LIP to delegate tasks to other qualified health care personnel (e.g., physician/LIP's assistants [PAs] and advanced practice registered nurses [APRNs]) to the

During this hospital stay, how often was your pain well controlled?

1 ☐   Never

2 ☐   Sometimes

3 ☐   Usually

4 ☐   Always

During this hospital stay, how often did the hospital staff do everything they could to help you with your pain?

1 ☐   Never

2 ☐   Sometimes

3 ☐   Usually

4 ☐   Always

FIGURE 20-2 Examples of pain management questions to assess patient perceptions of pain management from the HCAHPS survey. (From Centers for Medicare & Medicaid Services. (2013). HCAHPS: Patients' Perspectives of Care Survey. http://www.hcahpsonline.org/files/HCAHPS%20V8.0%20Appendix%20A%20-%20HCAHPS%20Mail%20Survey%20Materials%20(English)%20March%202013.pdf)

BOX 20-2   KEY REQUIREMENTS FOR EFFECTIVE PAIN CONTROL

- Assessment
- Intervention
- Reassessment

---

extent authorized by the state law or a state's regulatory mechanism or federal guidelines and organizational policy" (Medscape, 2013).

To educate only nurses leads to frustration due to the inability to initiate change without challenging the health care team responsible for prescribing treatment. Such conflicts can become unpleasant. Education is an expensive process for institutions with limited resources. Developing self-learning packets for the interprofessional team may expedite access to necessary information involved with change. Interdisciplinary health care team education may also be accomplished through lectures, newsletters, or blogs accessed through e-mail.

To move pain management forward as a profession, a collaborative approach is needed. Pre- and postevaluation of the knowledge and attitudes of all disciplines regarding pain should be implemented within a predetermined time frame. Often, the projection of negative attitudes toward people in pain or with coexisting substance use disorder and pain can be changed through mentoring in real time. Patient education should coincide with staff education so that everyone has consistent and clear expectations of the options available.

Interprofessional Pain Management Teams

The multidimensional nature of pain requires an interprofessional approach to pain management. Many acute care facilities have a team of pain experts to consult and provide recommendations for challenging problems with pain. Team members represent a number of disciplines and may include such roles as pain resource nurses, pain clinical nurse specialists, nurse practitioners, physicians/LIPs who are pain specialists, LIPs, pharmacists, pain psychologists, and addiction specialists. Patients with complex pain syndromes that involve pain with underlying pathophysiology comprise a combination of pain caused by tissue damage (nociceptive) and nerve damage (neuropathic) and may require the advanced knowledge and skills in pain management provided by an interprofessional pain team (Portenoy et al., 2006; Webster, 2008). Consultation by a pain team is also appropriate for treatment of refractory pain, comorbidities, high risk for complications, substance use disorder, or concurrent mental health conditions such as untreated depression or anxiety that pose barriers to effective pain management. There is consensus among pain management professionals that pain and mental health disorders cannot be treated as separate entities (ASPMN, 2012). The integration of a variety of pain management options requires the involvement of the interprofessional health care team (Box 20-3).

DEFINITIONS OF PAIN

The classic definition of pain that nurses have embraced for years is, "Pain is whatever the experiencing person says it is, existing whenever he says it does" (McCaffery, 1968, p. 95). This definition captures the subjectivity of the pain experience and reminds health

---

BOX 20-3 OPTIONS FOR PAIN CONTROL

- Systemic analgesics and adjuvant medications (administered orally, rectally, transdermally, intramuscularly, IV, subcutaneously, by continuous infusion, or by patient-controlled analgesia [PCA])
- Intraspinal opioids, including epidural and intrathecal
- Regional analgesia using local anesthetic agents
- Topical anesthetic agents
- Nonsteroidal anti-inflammatory drugs
- Electrical analgesia through transcutaneous electrical stimulation or electroacupuncture
- Psychological analgesia in the form of hypnosis, relaxation techniques

---

care providers of the importance of listening to our patients and partnering as we design a pain management plan. The definition of pain from the International Association for the Study of Pain (IASP) recognizes the sensory and emotional components of pain as well as the fact that pain may exist without evidence of tissue injury. "Pain is an unpleasant sensory and emotional experience associated with actual or potential tissue damage or described in terms of such damage" (IASP Task Force on Taxonomy, 1994). These definitions lay the groundwork for insight into the phenomenon of pain and may serve to guide our treatments.

Types of Pain

Historically, we classify pain according to location, intensity, duration, or underlying mechanism (Arnstein, 2010). The location of the pain may help the clinician determine the etiology of pain and if there is a fixable solution, for example, a fracture or infection. Pain intensity ratings are widely used in practice and allow the patient to rank pain on a numeric rating scale ranging from 0 to 10, with 10 representing the most intense pain. When using the numeric rating scale, 0 to 3 corresponds to mild pain, 4 to 6 corresponds to moderate pain, and 7 to 10 corresponds with severe pain. Helping patients maintain lower pain intensity scores is always considered successful treatment. Duration and underlying mechanism are closely aligned because the duration of pain may change the underlying mechanism. This is the case with acute pain and chronic/persistent pain.

ACUTE PAIN

Acute pain, such as that caused by surgery, childbirth, and trauma, adds to the overall health care burden. The IASP designated October 2010 through October 2011 as the *Global Year against Acute Pain*. An estimated 100 million surgeries take place annually with 80% of surgical patients reporting postoperative pain (IASP, 2012).

Nociceptors are sensory receptors that respond to a potentially damaging noxious stimulus and can be thermal, chemical, electrical, or mechanical in nature (Pasero, Quinn, Portenoy, McCaffery, & Rizos, 2011). The duration of acute pain can last seconds to days.

The autonomic nervous system responds to acute pain by increasing the sympathetic drive. When the sympathetic drive is increased, there is an increase in heart rate, respiratory rate, blood pressure, but there is also vasoconstriction, and a decrease in peristaltic action. This response is a protective mechanism that serves to create a flight-or-fight response. The cause of acute pain is usually known and persists until the underlying cause is resolved. Factors that influence postoperative pain may be found in Box 20-4.

Postoperative pain varies with the individual, and the nurse should remain cognizant of variables associated with pain. A relatively minor surgery with little trauma may create high pain intensity scores for an individual. A complex surgical procedure may create minimal to moderate pain intensity for an individual. We cannot assume that we are able to anticipate the level of pain following surgery. Universally, nurses must advocate for the patient by ensuring that their pain rating is valued and everything is being done to manage their pain well.

Practice guidelines for acute pain management in the perioperative setting have been developed for the interprofessional community of providers who deliver care under the supervision of anesthesiologists by the American Society of Anesthesiologists Task Force on Acute Pain Management. A number of position statements addressing acute pain management have been developed by ASPMN. Two examples are "Pain Management in Patients with Substance Abuse Disorders" (Oliver et al., 2012) and "Pain Assessment in the Patient Unable to Self-Report" (Herr, Coyne, McCaffery, Manworren, & Merkel, 2011). It is expected that *all nurses* manage their patients' pain well. Patients benefit when nurses study for and take the Pain Management Nursing examination through the American Nurses Credentialing Center. A Core Curriculum for Pain Management Nursing (St. Marie, 2010) exists to advance nurses' knowledge in pain management.

Chronic (Persistent) Pain

In the United States, it has been estimated that 100 to 130 million people suffer from chronic pain (Fishbain, Johnson, Webster, Greene, & Faysal, 2010; IOM, 2011). This rate is higher than that of diabetes (American Diabetes Association, 2011), heart disease (Roger et al., 2011),

---

BOX 20-4 FACTORS THAT INFLUENCE POSTOPERATIVE PAIN

- Site, nature, and duration of the surgical procedure
- Type of incision location
- Degree of intraoperative trauma
- Physiologic and psychological features characteristic of the patient
- Preoperative education preparation
- Amount of preoperative pain or past pain experiences
- Presence of complications
- Intraoperative management of pain
- Anesthetic management before, during, and after surgery
- Quality of postoperative care

and cancer (American Cancer Society, 2012) combined. In recent years, there has been a shift from the term "chronic" pain to **"persistent" pain**, to relieve patients of the stigmatization associated with chronic pain. Persistent pain may or may not have a known nociceptive input and has no autonomic response (Litwack, 2009; Rosner, 1996). Injury or disease may cause persistent pain, but it is perpetuated by factors that are seemingly unrelated or remote from the original cause (Turk & Okifuji, 2010). Persistent pain has been described using chronological markers of 3 to 6 months duration or it's described as pain that extends beyond the expected period of healing. Recent conceptualizations of persistent pain characterize it as extending for a long period of time and/or represent low levels of underlying pathology that does not explain the presence or extent of the pain (Turk & Okifuji, 2010). Persistent pain is now thought of as a chronic disease and can be a result of central sensitization (Sluka, O'Donnell, Danielson, & Rasmussen, 2012).

INPATIENT

When patients on chronic opioid therapy for treatment of their persistent pain are admitted to the hospital for acute treatment that requires further pain management, they may find opioids used for the acute pain is not as effective with usual expected dosing. They may require two to three times the opioid dose of someone who does not have opioid tolerance.

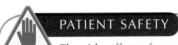

PATIENT SAFETY

The side effect of respiratory depression can remain problematic even in those with opioid tolerance, and safety parameters for closer monitoring need to be implemented.

Multimodal analgesia is a rational approach for managing pain through various pathways and techniques. Preoperative plan for postoperative analgesia would include regional analgesia techniques and opioid and nonopioid analgesics. Knowledge of the amount of opioids used by the patient is gleaned through two methods, medication reconciliation and reviewing the state prescription drug monitoring program. When interviewing the patient, determine the dose and frequency of opioids as accurately as possible (do not accept a vague answer to amount of opioids, this information needs to be accurate) and document the findings in the medical record. A health care provider with a Drug Enforcement Agency (DEA) number and access to this data bank can access records indicating the Scheduled II opioids and benzodiazepines prescribed to the patient within a requested time frame. These databases are updated routinely through community and hospital pharmacies. If the patient is receiving opioids or benzodiazepines from a Veterans Administration Hospital (VAH), or VA-affiliated nursing facilities including assisted living facilities, or methadone clinics, the opioids may or may not be included in this database, depending on the state. This information can be shared with the patient during the medication reconciliation interview to collaboratively determine how much opioid the patient actually consumes. The goal is to accurately understand the baseline use of opioids to estimate the patient's tolerance and probable range of postoperative opioids and nonopioid analgesics. Opioid-tolerant patients continue to require close monitoring on a monitored or unmonitored nursing unit during the early postoperative period (Swenson, Davis, & Johnson, 2005).

OUTPATIENT

There are clinical guidelines for opioid use in chronic noncancer pain that support safe and effective chronic opioid therapy (Chou et al., 2009). One of the most important recommendations addresses patient selection and risk stratification for opioid therapy. Risk stratification can help the prescriber determine the risk involved with prescribing opioid therapy and the monitoring strategies needed for this. In the outpatient setting, there are other strategies used to manage persistent pain problems. These strategies involve various nerve blocks, trigger point injections, implantable spinal cord stimulators, and implantable intraspinal infusion pumps. Patients who may benefit from pain control technology experience pain from spinal cord injuries or have pain that is refractory to conventional methods of pain control.

MECHANISMS OF PAIN

Classifying pain according to its underlying mechanism provides the interprofessional team a means to determine how the pain is transmitted and how to intervene. There are peripheral and central mechanisms of pain that transmit nociceptive and neuropathic pain signals. Nociceptive pain occurs when a normally functioning nervous system is alerted to tissue damage. Nociceptive pain serves as an alarm system to tell us that something is wrong and requires attention. Somatic pain is a type of nociceptive pain that originates in the skin, muscles, bone, or soft tissue. The character, intensity, and location of this type of pain are closely aligned with the type and extent of the injury (Arnstein, 2010). Another type of nociceptive pain is visceral pain. Visceral pain involves hollow and solid organs. It is more diffuse than somatosensory pain and can be referred to distant locations making it difficult for patients to clearly describe the exact pain location.

Neuropathic pain is related to damaged or malfunctioning nerves caused by disease, injury, or unknown reasons (Arnstein, 2010). Neuropathic pain may occur in the peripheral or central nervous systems. Peripheral neuropathy may be experienced by many people with diabetes. Someone with a spinal cord injury may experience central neuropathic pain. Not all patients who suffer nerve damage experience neuropathic pain. The mechanisms involved in this type of pain are very complex, and it is a difficult type of pain to manage.

PAIN MANAGEMENT STRATEGIES FOR THE INFUSION NURSE

Opioids

The term *opioid analgesics* are preferred to other terms such as narcotics or opiates. Opioids are effective when they bind with particular opioid receptors in the body. This section addresses only the mu and kappa receptor agonists. The mu receptor is the most powerful opioid receptor and requires binding with opioids that have an affinity to mu such as morphine sulfate, hydromorphone, and fentanyl citrate. Examples of opioid analgesics with an affinity to the kappa receptor are nalbuphine and buprenorphine HCl (Buprenex®). When a person takes a mu agonist such as morphine and also takes a kappa agonist such as nalbuphine, nalbuphine will compete with morphine so that morphine is no longer able to create analgesia. Furthermore, if the patient is physically dependent on long-term mu agonist opioid therapy, and receives a kappa agonist, he or she may experience physical withdrawal.

Demerol, or meperidine hydrochloride, is an opioid analgesic and has been well documented as problematic by the American Pain Society (2008) and the U.S. Agency for Health

Care Policy and Research Acute Pain Guidelines. When a patient receives meperidine, the body creates a metabolite called normeperidine. As the administration of meperidine continues, the normeperidine accumulates, creating toxicity resulting in seizures (Latta, Ginsberg, & Barkin, 2002).

The route of administration should reflect careful consideration of optimal and timely response. Intramuscular injections are painful, making it necessary for the patient to endure pain before receiving relief. A common misconception is that opioid dosing by the IV route is equal to the IM route (American Pain Society, 2008).

Side Effects

Side effects and complications associated with opioids may be found in Box 20-5. *Opioid-induced sedation and respiratory depression* are two of the most serious opioid-related adverse events. An expert consensus panel, at ASPMN, reviewed the scientific evidence and developed guidelines. Content of these guidelines includes assessment and monitoring practices for adult hospitalized patients receiving opioid analgesics for pain management. Interventions for patient care, education, and system-level changes should focus on promoting quality care and patient safety (Jarzyna et al., 2011).

Sedation is an expected and common adverse effect when beginning opioid therapy and when doses are increased (Pasero et al., 2011). Sedation precedes respiratory depression. The *Pasero Opioid-induced Sedation Scale* (POSS) is a valid and reliable instrument used to assess advancing sedation during opioid therapy. The POSS consists of five levels of sedation from sleep to somnolent with minimal or no response to verbal and physical stimulation. Assessment using the POSS is one element of monitoring patient safety during pain management with opioid analgesics. If the electronic medical record does not have POSS available for assessment, then the organization should explore having it added or devise a cue for nurses to document sedation. The assessment is simple, fast, and vital to the safety of the patient receiving opioids.

Unintended opioid-induced advancing sedation can result in respiratory depression. Respiratory depression has been defined as < 8 respirations per minute (Dahan, Aarts, & Smith, 2010). Clinically significant respiratory depression has been described as a decrease in the rate and depth of respirations from the patient's baseline and not entirely based on

---

BOX 20-5   SIDE EFFECTS AND COMPLICATIONS ASSOCIATED WITH OPIOIDS

- Opioid-induced sedation and, if left untreated, respiratory depression
- Opioid-induced constipation
- Urinary retention
- Nausea, vomiting
- Pruritus
- Mental status changes, including sedation, euphoria, irritability
- Orthostatic hypotension
- Bradycardia

a specific number of respirations per minute (Pasero et al., 2011). Respiratory depression is caused by an accumulation of carbon dioxide in the blood, which communicates with the brain (medulla oblongata) to slow respirations until the carbon dioxide level returns to normal. All opioids can depress brain stem–regulated ventilation, producing a dose-dependent reduction in respiratory rate (Yaney, 1998).

Technology-supported monitoring such as pulse oximetry and capnography in the prevention of adverse events secondary to opioid-induced respiratory depression is an area that requires more study before universal adoption can be recommended. While these monitoring devices are not currently recommended as strategies for all patients receiving opioid therapy, it may be considered for those who are at high risk for respiratory depression (Pasero et al., 2011). Electronic infusion devices (EIDs) and other mechanical technology cannot replace thorough bedside nursing assessment and documentation of level of sedation and respiratory rate, its depth, and quality. Patient attributes or conditions considered risk factors for opioid-induced respiratory depression are identified in Box 20-6.

Constipation is the most frequently reported side effect of opioid therapy. Opioid-induced constipation (OIC) is mediated by the peripheral opioid effect on the mu receptors in the gut wall. OIC results in reduced gastrointestinal motility, increased absorption of fluids from the gut, and decreased epithelial secretion causing stool to remain in the gut lumen for an extended period of time. This allows more fluid to be reabsorbed, and the stool becomes hard and dry (Leppert, 2010). Recently, opioid receptor antagonists such as methylnaltrexone have been used in the successful treatment of OIC. The medication is given

---

BOX 20-6 PATIENT ATTRIBUTES OR CONDITIONS CONSIDERED RISK FACTORS FOR OPIOID-INDUCED RESPIRATORY DEPRESSION

- Male
- Older than 55 years of age
- Body mass index (BMI) >30
- Obstructive sleep apnea
- Neck circumference >17.5 inches
- Mallampati—class 3 and 4 indicate difficulty with intubation
- Retrognathia (a type of malocclusion—maxilla or mandible, which is further posterior than would be expected)
- Witnessed periods of apnea
- Snoring
- Hypertension
- History of respiratory problems
- Renal dysfunction
- Continuous opioid infusion
- Arrivals from postanesthesia care unit (PACU) (medications given in PACU may peak when the patient is transferred from PACU to next unit)

subcutaneously in patients where there are no contraindications such as bowel obstruction. Methylnaltrexone works as a peripheral opioid receptor antagonist, and this peripheral antagonism does not reverse the analgesia (Greenwood-VanMeerveld, 2008).

Urinary retention may be caused by opioid agonists relaxing the detrusor muscle located in the floor of the bladder. The patient may or may not feel the urge to void. Administration of bethanechol can contract the bladder, allowing it to empty. Catheterization is another option for immediate relief of urinary retention; however, risk of hospital-acquired urinary tract infection increases.

Nausea may be reversed either by opioid antagonists, such as nalbuphine HCl (Nubain) or naloxone HCl (Narcan), or by antiemetics. If opioid antagonists are used, the doses should be kept very low to prevent reversal of analgesia. If antiemetics are used, a synergistic effect with the opioid can result in sedation. When reversal of nausea is not accomplished with antiemetics or low-dose opioid antagonists, the physician/LIP should be notified and further evaluation performed. Slow, steady opioid titration in addition to eliminating medications that may contribute to nausea is also preferred (Fine & Portenoy, 2007).

Systemic opioids may cause histamine release resulting in *pruritus*. This may be relieved with antihistamines, with a low-dose opioid antagonist, or by changing the opioid. When opioids are administered through the intraspinal routes such as epidural or intrathecal, pruritus may result and is related to the action of the opioid at the dorsal horn of the spinal cord. Intrathecal morphine-induced pruritus has been reported to be successfully treated with preoperative gabapentin in patients undergoing lower limb surgery (Sheen, Ho, Lee, Tsung, & Chang, 2008).

Technology-Assisted Analgesic Administration

PCA has existed for over 25 years; White (1988) is the classic reference cited in the literature. Systems for self-administering oral analgesics are available, but the term "PCA" is usually used in the context of intravenous, subcutaneous, perineural, and intraspinal (epidural and intrathecal) routes of administration (Arnstein, 2010). The benefit of PCA administration is the elimination of the "analgesic gap" that results when there are delays in the administration of analgesics by health care providers or unanticipated episodes of severe pain (Polomano, Rathmell, Krenzischek, & Dunwoody, 2008). Unfortunately, significant safety concerns about this type of technology-assisted analgesic delivery exist. Infusion pump incident reports are tracked by the U.S. Food and Drug Administration (FDA) and entered into a database known as MAUDE (Manufacturer and User Facility Device Experience). See Box 20-7 for incidents involving PCA infusion devices from 2007 to 2009. Innovations in current technology are aimed at creating a seamless, interoperable system that supports better medication safety strategies. This type of system will link infusion pumps and the people who use them with data systems such as medication orders, drug libraries, electronic health records, bar coding systems, and reporting systems.

PCA delivery of medication includes options for a clinician-delivered bolus dose (an example is an initial loading dose), the patient-delivered dose, and/or a basal rate feature that delivers a continuous infusion without activation by a clinician or patient. Since a basal rate for continuous infusions of opioid is not in the patient's control, there are increases in the risk for sedation and respiratory depression. Box 20-8 highlights those at risk for sedation and respiratory depression. A report by Hagle, Lehr, Brubakken and Shippee (2004) found the incidence of opioid-induced respiratory depression during IV PCA to be 0.19% to

---

BOX 20-7 INCIDENTS INVOLVING INFUSION DEVICES (2007–2009)

- Errors in drug dosing, volume, and concentration
- Rate of infusion
- Decimal point errors while programming
- Designation of an incorrect unit of measurement (mg vs. mL)
- Bolus dosing errors

From Association for the Advancement of Medical Instrumentation. (2010). Infusing patients safely: Priority issues from the AAMI/FDA infusion device summit. http://www.aami.org/publications/summits/AAMI_FDA_Summit_Report.pdf

---

5.2%. As a result, we have evidence that adherence to recent guidelines for prevention and intervention of opioid-induced sedation and respiratory depression is important to promote safe and effective delivery of opioid analgesics (Jarzyna et al., 2011).

When the PCA settings are programmed for bolus-only activation, this allows the patient to control IV delivery of an analgesic and to maintain therapeutic serum medication levels. The patient must be physically able to activate the self-administered dose and be cognitively able to understand the principles of on-demand dosing to be a candidate for PCA therapy. The physician/LIP's order for PCA should include the following:

1. Loading dose, given IV push at initiation of therapy
2. Lock-out interval, during which the PCA bolus device cannot be activated
3. Maintenance dose (basal infusion) (if appropriate, usually not for the opioid niaive patient)
4. Bolus dose
5. Maximum amount the patient may receive within a given time

The loading dose of opioid can be a onetime bolus within safety parameters, or if in a monitored setting, it can be achieved through a technique called titration to effect.

BOX 20-8 PATIENTS AT RISK FOR SEDATION AND RESPIRATORY DEPRESSION

- Known sleep apnea
- Opioid naïve
- BMI > 40
- Thoracic, neck, or upper abdominal surgery or trauma
- Renal insufficiency
- Pediatric or elderly patients
- Those with comorbidities or drugs affecting breathing

From Arnstein, P. (2010). *Clinical coach for effective pain management.* Philadelphia, PA: F.A. Davis Company.

This technique calls for administering small doses of opioid frequently to obtain a level of analgesia. Titration to effect usually occurs within 40 minutes. The patient is monitored during this time through observation of mental status, level of pain relief, respiratory rate, and amount of opioid. The qualified nurse who has received formal education in using this intervention is important for safety. The qualified nurse will understand the pharmacokinetics and pharmacodynamics of the opioid titrated, understand drug-to-drug interactions, as well as assess the metabolism and excretion capabilities of each individual patient in order to keep this intervention safe. Patients cannot be expected to titrate their own opioids when PCA is initiated, and in order for IV PCA to be effective, the loading dose must be nurse administered. Once the loading dose is given and analgesia is increasing, the IV PCA is piggybacked into the proximal port on the IV tubing.

The lock-out interval is another safety feature that prohibits the patient from frequently administering opioid to a point of overmedicating, and it allows adequate time for some effect. The usual interval programmed into the PCA pump is 5 to 10 minutes (White, 1987).

The maintenance dose or basal infusion is the amount of opioid that is infusing continuously. This strategy is used for patients who are opioid tolerant, who are receiving poor analgesia through bolus dose–only capabilities, and who are not on other CNS-depressing medications, such as benzodiazepines. For example, a middle-aged, 70-kg adult with normal renal function would receive morphine sulfate at a rate of 1 mg/h. This maintenance dose usually is administered for the first 12 to 24 hours, after which the rate is reduced or the infusion is stopped and analgesia is maintained through self-administered boluses. The anesthesiologist, surgeon, or primary care physician/LIP determines the maximum amount of opioid the patient may self-administer in a given time based on individual patient attributes, including opioid tolerance. This amount is programmed into the infusion pump and offers another safety system to protect the patient from an overdose of opioid.

PATIENT SAFETY

Family members or friends of the patient must not administer PCA boluses to the patient. Accidental overdose may occur if assessment is incorrect or the opioid starts to accumulate in the bloodstream.

Clinical practice recommendations and standards describe safe practice for PCA use when the patient is unable to actively participate; in this case, an authorized agent (otherwise called "PCA by proxy") for administration of medication via PCA may be appropriate (Infusion Nurses Society, 2011, p. S89–S90; Wuhrman et al., 2007).

A variety of PCA devices are available with diverse features. Refer to Box 20-9 for detailed information.

SUBCUTANEOUS OPIOID INFUSION

The subcutaneous continuous infusion of opioids provides analgesia to patients when IV access is unacceptable or unavailable. The level of analgesia obtained through subcutaneous infusions of opioids is similar to that obtained through IV infusions. The selection of opioid is important to the success of subcutaneous infusions. Morphine sulfate and hydromorphone HCl are the medications of choice. Oxymorphone, fentanyl, and levorphanol have also been

---

BOX 20-9 FACTORS TO CONSIDER IN SELECTING A PCA DEVICE

- Compatibility with currently used IV systems, poles, or conversion to ambulatory system
- Battery life
- Memory retention of pump use
- Display, security, and safety features
- Cost-effective
- Delivery mode (bolus vs. continuous infusion)
- Durability
- Ease of use

---

administered subcutaneously (Pasero et al., 2011). The goal of a subcutaneous infusion is to offer a reduced volume of a more concentrated solution with minimal chemical irritation. The quality of analgesia is limited to the amount of absorption of opioid at the subcutaneous site. The conversion from oral opioid to subcutaneous is equivalent to the conversion from oral opioid to IM. Appropriate conversions are outlined in Table 20-2 (APS, 2008).

The technique for subcutaneous access is simple; however, the use of proper equipment and stabilizing methods enhances patient comfort and compliance. Supplies needed to initiate subcutaneous access and site selection may be found in Box 20-10. A single infusion site can usually receive 2 to 3 mL/h. The most common problems with subcutaneous infusion of opioids are local irritation at the needle insertion site and subcutaneous scarring, which will inhibit absorption of the medication. Frequent site changes (every other day) and reducing the infusion volume can minimize these complications.

INTRASPINAL ADMINISTRATION

Intraspinal analgesia includes both the epidural and intrathecal routes of administration. There are several indications for intraspinal analgesia including (a) pain that is not controlled by analgesics administered by other routes, (b) unacceptable side effects with other modalities or medications, (c) painful conditions or surgical procedures with demonstrated reductions in mortality and morbidity when analgesia is delivered by intraspinal routes (e.g., major thoracic, abdominal, and orthopedic surgery), and (d) confirmed improved

---

TABLE 20-2 EXAMPLES OF CONVERSION TO SUBCUTANEOUS OPIOIDS

Oral to Subcutaneous	Ratio	Example
Oral morphine to SC morphine	2–3:1	Oral morphine 20–30 mg = SC morphine 10 mg
Oral hydromorphone to SC hydromorphone	4:1	Oral hydromorphone 4 mg = SC hydromorphone 1 mg

Adapted from Opioid Conversion Ratios–Guide to Practice. (2010). Eastern Metropolitan Region Palliative Care Consortium. Melbourne. http://www.emrpcc.org.au/wp-content/uploads/2013/03/EMRPCC-Opioid-Conversion2010-Final2.pdf

BOX 20-10   SUBCUTANEOUS ACCESS

Supplies

- Nonsterile gloves
- Analgesic infusion pump that can deliver medication in tenths of a milliliter
- A 27-gauge winged infusion needle or an infusion set that includes a 24-gauge indwelling catheter that is introduced into the subcutaneous tissue by a removable 26-gauge introducer needle
- Transparent dressing or tape and adhesive bandage
- Chlorhexidine 2% + isopropyl alcohol 70% applicator

Process

The site of choice is commonly the subclavicular area, abdomen, or anterior chest wall.

- Prepare the site with chlorhexidine 2% + isopropyl alcohol 70% applicator.
- Insert the needle either at an angle or perpendicular to the skin, depending on the needle used.
- Stabilize the needle consistent with the manufacturer's recommendation.

patient response to epidural analgesia. Patient selection criteria also need to address an absence of contraindications to intraspinal needle/catheter placement such as untreated infection, coagulopathies, or the patient's inability to understand potential side effects (Hayek et al., 2011; Myers et al., 2010; Pasero et al., 2011).

Pain medication delivered through an *epidural* catheter offers safe and effective analgesia at lower opioid dosages and decreased sedation. It also facilitates earlier ambulation and enhances patient comfort. Knowledge of relevant anatomy and physiology ensures a higher level of understanding and subsequent care. *Epi* refers to outside, and *dura* refers to the covering of the spinal cord that encloses the cerebrospinal fluid (CSF). The **epidural** space is a potential space that is part of the spinal canal outside the dura mater, enclosed by protective ligaments. Extending from the base of the skull to the coccyx, the epidural space ends at approximately S1 in many patients (the spinal cord ends at approximately L1) as seen in Figure 20-3.

The epidural space contains a network of large-bore, thin-walled veins. The space also contains fat (in an amount directly proportional to a person's body fat) and extensions for nerves that travel out from the spinal cord. Other terms for the epidural space are the peridural or extradural space.

The **intrathecal** space, containing the CSF, which bathes the spinal cord, runs parallel to the epidural space. The dura and arachnoid mater separate the intrathecal and epidural spaces. Other names for the intrathecal space are subarachnoid space or spinal space. The term *intraspinal* is used to describe both the epidural and intrathecal spaces.

Accessing the epidural or intrathecal space requires specialized training. The anesthesiologist must insert a special needle between the spinous processes and through the ligaments and enter the epidural space with a technique called *loss of resistance*. Loss of

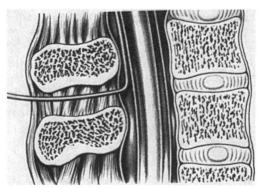

FIGURE 20-3 Close-up of L1 epidural catheter placement.

resistance occurs when the needle enters the epidural space, and the pressure placed on the plunger of the syringe allows the contents to empty into the space. When the needle is properly placed, the catheter is threaded through the needle. If the epidural catheter is used for temporary analgesia, the catheter is taped to the back and connected to the external infusion pump. If the epidural catheter is used for long-term analgesia, the catheter is percutaneously threaded and connected to the implanted pump, port, or external catheter for connection to an external infusion pump (Bennett et al., 2000). When an anesthesiologist accesses the intrathecal space, the needle penetrates through the epidural space, punctures through the dura mater, and enters the intrathecal space. The intrathecal space contains CSF, which can be aspirated by the syringe attached to the accessing needle.

Elimination of opioids from the intraspinal space occurs through two mechanisms: diffusion up the neuraxis in the CSF and vascular uptake in the epidural space. The analgesic action occurs in the spinal cord at the opiate receptors located at the substantia gelatinosa of the dorsal horn. Here, the epidural or intrathecal opioids bind with the opiate receptors, blocking the pain pathway through the dorsal horn to the brain. The lipid solubility of the opioid determines the amount of opioid used, the volume needed, the placement of the epidural catheter tip, the time to produce analgesia, the dermatomal distribution of the analgesia, and the elimination time.

Lipid-soluble opioids (i.e., preservative-free fentanyl citrate) have a more rapid action than water-soluble opioids and create analgesia in a narrow segment, following the **dermatomes** that closely surround the level of opioid injection. Water-soluble opioids (i.e., preservative-free morphine sulfate) create a slower onset but wider spread of analgesia, which in turn is longer lasting because of the increased elimination time. The onset of epidural analgesia with morphine or hydromorphone is 30 to 90 minutes, whereas the onset of analgesia with fentanyl is 5 minutes (Pasero, 2003b).

Epidural analgesia is administered using an epidural catheter. Therapy may consist of bolus dosing, continuous infusion through an external or implanted device, or patient-controlled epidural analgesia (Bader et al., 2010; Mann, 2000; van der Vyver, Halpern, & Joseph, 2002). Local anesthetics can be coadministered with opioids to enhance the analgesia from epidural infusions. By using local anesthetic agents, the pain transmission is blocked at the sympathetic chain ganglion, which lies on either side of and runs parallel to the spinal cord. Local anesthetic agents result in a sympathetic blockade and allows for a reduced the amount of opioid required to create analgesia. There is an increase in the peristaltic action of the bowel, reduce workload on the heart, increase tidal volume of the lung, and increase vascular graft flow, reducing the incidence of deep vein thrombosis when local anesthestics are used. Potential side effects are a significant reduction of blood pressure and numbness along the dermatomal distribution of the catheter tip placement. Commonly used local anesthetic agents are bupivacaine and ropivacaine.

PATIENT SAFETY

If local anesthetics are used in the epidural infusion, caution must be used in raising the patient from a lying to a sitting position and from a sitting to a standing position. Position elevation may cause the blood pressure to decrease, making the patient dizzy or even syncopal.

Prior to placement of the epidural catheter, the patient should be informed of the potential risks involved and informed consent should be obtained. Bleeding can occur in the epidural space and exit out the insertion site of the catheter. Patients who receive anticoagulant therapy or who have liver damage should have a bleeding time determined before catheter placement. The American Society of Regional Anesthesia and Pain Medicine published evidence-based guidelines for regional anesthesia in the patient receiving concurrent antithrombotic or thrombolytic therapy (Horlocker et al., 2010). The recommendations state,

> ...the decision to perform spinal or epidural anesthesia/analgesia and the timing of catheter removal in patient receiving antithrombotic therapy should be made on an individual basis, weighing the small, although definite risk of spinal hematoma with the benefits of regional anesthesia for a specific patient (p. 95).

The recommendation also includes that the patient's coagulation status should be optimized at the time of spinal or epidural needle or catheter placement and that the level of anticoagulation be carefully monitored during the period of epidural catheterization. Catheters should not be removed when the patient is anticoagulated at the therapeutic level due to increased risk of spinal hematoma (Horlocker et al., 2010).

Sterile technique consistent with established standards of practice is used during catheter placement. The physician/LIP should be notified if a patient is febrile before placement or has a known infection. Patients may express concerns related to placement, care, and potential problems. They should be told that the catheter is placed into the tissue around the spinal cord, not into the spinal cord itself. They need to know that their blood pressure may decrease because of muscle relaxation and sympathetic blockade when local anesthetic is injected. Points to cover in obtaining informed consent are found in Box 20-11.

A postdural puncture headache (PDPH) may occur if the needle enters the CSF or intrathecal space and causes the CSF to leave the intrathecal space. Unintentional intrathecal access has been reported to be the most common complication from epidural catheter placement with an incidence of 0.32% to 3% (Grape & Schug, 2008; Maalouf & Liu, 2009). This CSF leak decreases the fluid padding around the brain. Classic PDPH is positional; that is, the patient experiences a headache when upright but not when lying down. The location of the headache varies. PDPH may be relieved with a blood patch as follows: the anesthesiologist aligns the needle in the epidural space close to the dural puncture site.

BOX 20-11   POINTS TO COVER IN OBTAINING INFORMED CONSENT FOR EPIDURAL OR INTRATHECAL ADMINISTRATION

- Bleeding may occur.
- Infection may occur.
- An allergic reaction to the local anesthetic agents may occur.
- Injection is not into the spinal cord but rather into the tissue around the spinal cord.
- During the procedure, the patient may feel a tickle down the leg, which is the catheter coming into contact with the nerve. The patient needs to tell the anesthesiologist about this feeling.
- Blood pressure may decrease because of the medication, and this is why the patient is monitored during this procedure.
- A headache may occur if the needle enters the CSF or intrathecal space.

The anesthesiologist then withdraws 20 to 30 mL of blood from the patient's arm and injects the blood into the epidural needle. The patient lies still for 2 hours after the blood patch and can resume normal activity as tolerated. They are instructed to avoid the Valsalva maneuver, through either lifting or bearing down, for 24 hours. The blood patch is thought to plug the leaking dural membrane and increases pressure in the epidural space, forcing the CSF in the intrathecal space toward the brain to relieve the headache soon after the patch is performed.

 PATIENT SAFETY

Falls Precaution
Determine safety before ambulation. When the patient has an epidural catheter placed in the lumbar region with infusion of local anesthetics, use caution when assisting the patient to a standing position. First, determine the strength in the patient's legs by asking him or her to lift the legs off the bed one at a time (testing for quadriceps strength). Second, determine sensation by touching the patient's thigh. If he or she can feel touch and has the ability to lift the leg off the bed, and then proceed. Third, have the patient stand by the side of the bed and ask her or him to bend the knees slightly and straighten them (again to determine quadriceps strength). If the patient is able to do this, proceed with ambulation. If not, check with the physician/LIP because adjustments can be made in the epidural solution or rate to facilitate ambulation.

EPIDURAL DELIVERY SYSTEMS

A small-lumen, temporary catheter made of nylon or Teflon is placed into the epidural space. Long-term delivery is possible through the use of a long-term epidural catheter or an epidural portal system. Care and management of the catheter should be consistent with Intravenous Nurses Society (INS) Standards of Practice (INS, 2011). The delivery of medications and maintenance of epidural catheters should be established in infusion policies and procedures specific to the Nurse Practice Act. Policies and procedures for obtaining, delivering, administering, documenting, and discarding medication should be in accordance with state and federal regulations (INS, 2011).

All medications administered by epidural catheter should be preservative free. Examples of preservative-free medications include morphine, fentanyl, hydromorphone, ziconotide, clonidine, bupivacaine, and baclofen (INS, 2011). Alcohol, antiseptics containing alcohol, or acetone is contraindicated for preparing the site or accessing the catheter because of the potential for migration of alcohol into the epidural space and risk for nerve destruction. Povidone–iodine may be used; however, it can irritate the nerves if it migrates into the epidural space. A 0.2-μm, surfactant-free, particulate retentive filter should be used in the infusion line for medication administration. Before use, the catheter should be aspirated to determine the absence of CSF and blood (INS, 2011). Epidural catheters may be placed for short- or long-term use.

Mechanical problems may occur with the epidural catheter system, including leaking catheter hub, disconnected catheter, occluded catheter, or leaking at the skin site. Leakage at the catheter hub is common with temporary epidural catheter systems and may be detected if the bedding or clothing is wet. The patient may also experience breakthrough pain from leaking medications not delivered to the patient. The nurse must tighten the hub or replace the hub if it is cracked. Clean technique is appropriate for manipulating the catheter hub. When the catheter becomes disconnected from the medication infusion, the nurse should carefully wrap the end of the catheter with a sterile 4 × 4 and contact the anesthesia provider immediately (Pasero et al., 2011). The anesthesia provider will either opt to repair the catheter or remove it (Figure 20-4).

If occlusion occurs, the EID should stop and alarm. Nursing interventions include ensuring that all clamps are open and checking the tubing for kinks. The hub is loosened and then retightened to secure it to the catheter, and the infusion is restarted. If this is unsuccessful, the anesthesiologist or pain management team should be called. Supplemental pain medication may be given by an alternative route.

The dressing over the catheter exit site may be damp from leaking at the skin site. The nurse needs to assess whether the patient is experiencing pain. If the patient is comfortable, no treatment is necessary other than to replace the wet dressing. If the patient is uncomfortable, the dressing should be removed to see if the catheter has pulled out of the epidural space. The physician/LIP should be notified. Supplemental systemic analgesia should be initiated.

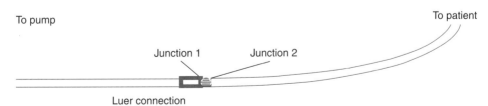

FIGURE 20-4 Epidural catheter and points at which damage may occur. *1*, tighten catheter; *2*, leak may occur:

Aspiration of an epidural catheter by nurses is not universally sanctioned. It should be done only by those who are trained in the procedure and supported by institutional policy and procedure. Aspiration of the epidural catheter is required to determine if the catheter is displaced, either in an epidural vein or in the CSF. Blood or clear fluid aspirated from the catheter, however, does not guarantee either condition and should not be considered conclusive. The anesthesiologist or other physician/LIP should be notified. Assessment of the patient's status should occur and be documented. If the patient is oversedated, the epidural catheter may have migrated into the intrathecal space. If the patient is receiving epidural local anesthetic and feels numbness in the toes only, the catheter may be intrathecal. Aspiration of a small amount of blood (1 to 2 mL) is also inconclusive because the pool of medication in the epidural space may be mixed with a pool of blood in the epidural space that resulted from the trauma of insertion. If the syringe fills with >3 mL of blood and the patient is receiving inadequate analgesia, however, the nurse can conclude that the epidural catheter is in an epidural vein. If so, an anesthesiologist or trained member of the pain management team may want to pull back the epidural catheter. If there is >5 mL clear fluid, the nurse can assume that it is CSF unless there is a high-volume infusion of medication and poor diffusion through the dura, resulting in higher pools of medications in the epidural space. The clear fluid can be tested to determine the glucose level. A higher level of glucose indicates CSF, and the anesthesiologist or other health care provider should be consulted.

When the nurse removes the epidural catheter on completion of postoperative analgesia, the integrity of the removed catheter must be evaluated. If the catheter tip is intact, document "tip intact."

PATIENT SAFETY

There is always the risk of pulling the catheter out of the epidural space. The patient needs to be advised of this risk. The nurse must not allow the patient to suffer in pain while the epidural system is being managed. An alternative form of analgesia is necessary and can be arranged ahead of time to avoid poor pain relief.

Breakthrough pain may indicate that the pump is programmed incorrectly, the epidural catheter is disconnected and leaking, the epidural catheter is no longer epidural, the catheter has migrated into an epidural vein, or the patient is receiving too low a dose. Regardless of the reason for breakthrough pain, intervention must be initiated to provide pain control.

EPIDURAL PORT

The epidural port consists of the portal, catheter, and filter to remove large particulate matter. The catheter portion of the port system is inserted in the epidural space using the technique discussed earlier, and the catheter is then threaded through a percutaneous tunnel. A subcutaneous pocket is prepared for the port. The system is intended for repeated injection or infusion of preservative-free morphine sulfate into the epidural space (Figure 20-5).

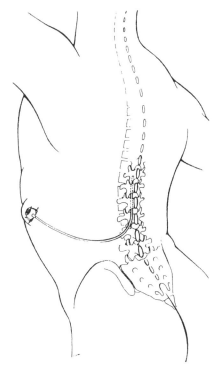

FIGURE 20-5 Epidural port. (Courtesy of Smiths Medical ASD, Inc., St. Paul, MN.)

IMPLANTED PUMPS

In the 1980s and 1990s, advancements in medical technology facilitated convenient alternatives to conventional methods of long-term drug delivery. Systems such as the implanted pump (including pump, catheter, and optional access port) are implanted surgically and require periodic refilling. The pump releases prescribed amounts of medication into the body. Patients with cancer pain or nonmalignant pain may be candidates for implanted pumps. Patient selection criteria differ depending on the cause of pain. If the patient's pain is caused by cancer, the selection criteria include pain severity, inadequate pain relief or unacceptable side effects from other types of pain management, the patient's life expectancy, whether or not the patient has enough body mass to support the weight and bulk of the pump, freedom from infection, and whether or not the patient has a favorable response to a trial. The trial may consist of epidural or intrathecal administration via a single bolus injection or continuous infusion. In the patient with a nonmalignant disease, patient selection criteria are the same with the exception of a life-limiting disease. Additional selection criteria may include a psychological evaluation to determine whether the patient has realistic expectations about pain relief, presence of a psychosomatic component to pain, or if the patient is motivated by secondary gain.

A physician/LIP or nurse may use a portable telemetry computer device during refill and checkup sessions to monitor the pump and to set the prescription as ordered. The pumps have a battery that can last 4 to 7 years. Potential risks include infection at the implant site, catheter plug or kinking, dislodgment, and leaking.

Patients should be instructed to report redness, swelling, and pain near the incision. Changes in pressure or temperature may effect dosing. Blood pressure, concentration, and viscosity of the medication may also affect flow rates. Avoid the pump site during diathermy and ultrasound treatments.

Possible complications include cessation of therapy owing to battery depletion, migration of the catheter access port, pocket seroma, complete or partial catheter occlusion, CSF leak, and drug toxicity. The use of needles larger than 22-gauge may compromise the self-sealing properties of the septum, and noncoring needles are required to minimize the septal damage. The infusion nurse is cautioned to follow procedures for the use of implanted pumps, consistent with the manufacturer's guidelines and institutional policy (Figure 20-6).

When the pump is implanted, the surgeon should complete the patient registration and implantation record. The manufacturer issues the patient a wallet-sized identification card containing information pertinent to the implanted pump. The physician/LIP should fill in the space provided for any medical emergency instructions. The patient should carry this card at all times. Instructions for patients with implanted pumps are listed in Box 20-12.

STAFF EDUCATION

Although information on the safe administration of epidural or intrathecal medication and monitoring of potential side effects is available, little has been written about preparing the registered professional nurse for administering and monitoring epidural or intrathecal analgesia. The initial step is to establish the rationale and criteria on which the policy and procedure for administration of epidural or intrathecal analgesia will be based, as outlined in Table 20-3.

An epidural module is available through the American Society for Pain Management Nursing (Pasero, 2003a). A position paper is also available through the American Society for Pain Management Nursing (2013) (http://www.aspmn.org/Organization/position_papers. htm). These resources can help with developing a clinical education program intensive and facilitates outcome measurement of knowledge and skills.

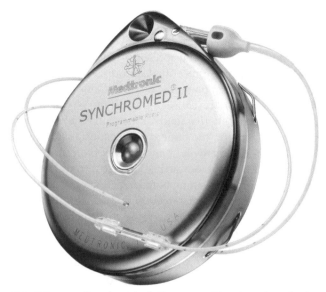

FIGURE 20-6 SynchroMed II pump. (Reprinted with the permission of Medtronic, Inc.© 2012.)

BOX 20-12   INSTRUCTIONS FOR PATIENTS AFTER PUMP IMPLANTATION

- Avoid traumatic physical activity (i.e., contact sports).
- Consult the physician/LIP during febrile illness.
- Report any unusual symptoms or complications relating to the specific medication therapy or the device.
  - ○ Watch for redness, swelling, or pain over the pump site.
  - ○ Avoid heating pad over pump.
  - ○ Avoid hot tub.
  - ○ Avoid other opioids or CNS depressants unless prescribed by your health care provider.
  - ○ If local anesthetics are infused through the pump, take precautions when changing positions from lying to sitting or sitting to standing. Also report numbness to lower extremities and take precautions with ambulating.
- Return at the prescribed time for pump refill.

Perineural Local Anesthetic Infusions

Perineural local anesthetic infusions block nerve conduction and may offer excellent postoperative pain control by achieving uninterrupted pain relief, minimizing opioid requirements, and avoiding the adverse effects of opioids (Pasero et al., 2003). Continuous local anesthetic is delivered through a 16-gauge introducer needle placed under the subcutaneous tissue and above the fascia or muscle adjacent to or in the wound site after surgery. After placing the introducer needle, the surgeon threads a 20-gauge catheter through the needle.

TABLE 20-3   NURSE'S INVOLVEMENT WITH EPIDURAL/INTRATHECAL INFUSIONS

Criteria	Rationale
Complete initial and ongoing institutional and government requirements related to administration of analgesia via catheter	Ensure consistency with guidelines

Educational content includes
  Related anatomy and physiology
  Patient assessment
  Monitoring
  Troubleshooting of devices
  Managing potential side effects
  Emergency interventions
  Legal ramifications
  Patient/family education	

Adopt an interprofessional approach to communicating with all other members of the pain service	An interprofessional approach toward dialogue ensures positive patient outcomes
Participate in quality improvement activities related to pain management	Systematically evaluate safety and effectiveness; document care and response

The surgeon removes the introducer needle and secures the site with a semipermeable transparent dressing. The patient receives a loading dose of local anesthetic before beginning the continuous infusion via disposable infusion pump or EID. Pain intensity is monitored and documented. Breakthrough pain may be managed with oral or IV analgesics.

Toxic effects of continuous local anesthesia include dizziness, ringing in the ears, a metallic taste, perioral anesthesia, and slowed speech. If signs of toxicity are recognized early, decreasing the infusion rate may alleviate the problem. Elderly patients may be at a higher risk for toxicity owing to a decreased ability to eliminate local anesthetics. If patients are discharged from the hospital or Same Day Surgery Center, the nurse should instruct the patient and family about what to do and whom to call about unrelieved pain, symptoms of infection, determining when the infusion is complete, removing the catheter, and dressing the site (Pasero et al., 2007).

Postoperative Range Orders

Whether pain management is by systemic infusion therapy or more locally, the most current and best evidence should support pain control measures. For postoperative pain, the goal of pain management is to keep the patient's pain score low enough to allow for deep breathing and coughing, early ambulation, decreased complication rates, and improved overall quality of life. A critical review of **range orders** or "as-needed" orders for opioid analgesics was done by the American Pain Society and the American Society for Pain Management Nursing (ASPMN, 2004). A consensus statement was developed to clarify protocol and enhance safety and effectiveness of orders for opioid analgesic agents. This consensus statement recommends that institutions allow PRN range opioid orders in order to meet safe and effective pain management. The prescriber should construct orders that contain a dosage range with a fixed time interval. The dosage range should be large enough to permit appropriate and safe dose titration with the maximum dose within the range not greater than four times the minimum dose. The nurses should base decisions about the implementation of range orders following a thorough assessment of pain and knowledge of the opioid to be given (American Society for Pain Management Nursing, 2004). Although range orders are often misunderstood or can be confusing, they are an effective method for pain management when properly written and implemented (Glassford, 2008; Rosier, 2012).

DOCUMENTATION OF PAIN: THE FIFTH VITAL SIGN

Documentation should follow the concept that pain intensity is recorded to reflect assessment, intervention, and reassessment. If blood pressure, pulse, respirations, and temperature are documented on a graphic sheet, the pain intensity rating also should be on the same graphic sheet. A single graphic facilitates documentation and ensures that all members of the health care team who view the graphic sheet see pain information. If the pain rating is poor (per the institution's definition or by the patient's definition) and pain medications are given, then pain evaluation needs to follow at the appropriate interval based on the route of administration and anticipated medication effects. Policies and procedures should define pain ratings and interventions as well as methods for providing PCA and epidural, intrathecal, and other forms of pain management in as safe and effective manner as possible.

Documentation should include the type of pain management provided, route of administration, methods used, IV or other access route, site care and maintenance, assessment of pain and degree of pain relief, and problems encountered with medication side effects or device used. Flow sheets facilitate the accuracy of documentation and provide a guideline for all areas of concern, including pain rating (intensity) and sedation scale (Figures 20-7 and 20-8). When PCA systems are implemented, the nurse records the date, time, medication, patient's name and room number, physician/LIP's name, and his or her own name on an appropriate flow sheet. Many facilities have developed individualized flow sheets specifically for PCA or epidural management. The American Pain Society has developed quality assurance standards for pain relief (Box 20-13).

Preanalgesia intervention	Postanalgesia intervention
Pain intensity score	Pain intensity score
Mental status	Mental status
Respiratory status History of sleep apnea	Respiratory status
Functional status	Functional status
Current pain medications Past pain medications History of addiction or treatment, including alcohol abuse or street drugs History of or current renal or liver dysfunction Medication reconciliation including Prescription Drug Monitoring Program	Medication intervention (include multimodal analgesia)
Patient's pain management expectations Partner with patient on their expectations Understand any history of anxiety, depression, or insomnia	When next intervention will take place. Intervention may need to occur before the next designated intervention time. Plan how you would intervene if this occurred.
Determine patient's experience with or desire for: Nonpharmacological intervention for pain Complementary intervention for pain	Nonpharmacological intervention for pain Complementary intervention for pain

Determine the patient's ability to manage their own pain upon discharge	Ensure safe medication use upon discharge through patient education. Explain the following:
	  a. What "prn" means, explain the pattern of opioid use prior to discharge.
	  b. Locking opioids in a safe in their home to keep family and friends safe. Do not store opioids in a medicine cabinet.
	  c. Not to share opioids or take opioids of others.
	  d. Do not use alcohol or street drugs while managing pain with opioids.

FIGURE 20-7 Pain assessment parameters—electronic medical record (EMR). The impact of the EMR on assessment of pain, intervention, and reassessment of pain is unknown. Evaluating a patient's pain is not a simple "yes/no" type of assessment. The evaluation has to be comprehensive if it is to protect the patient from medication harm and must allow the nurse a full perspective of the patient's condition. Some of the features of inpatient care with pain assessment and items for documentation are found here. In some institutions, the EMR can be adapted to accommodate the needs of the patient in pain. These items are not an exhaustive list and would best serve the patient if the information pertaining to his or her pain could be located in one place within the EMR. (Editorial comment by Barbara St. Marie.)

PATIENT-CONTROLLED ANALGESIA
Sample Flow Sheet

HOSPITAL I.D.	PATIENT I.D.

DATE _____

MEDICATION _____

LOADING DOSE _____
(IF APPLICABLE)

TIME	12MN	2A	4A	6A	8A	10A	12N	2P	4P	6P	8P	10P
DOSE VOLUME (ML)												
LOCK-OUT												
4-HR LIMIT (ML)												
# DOSE DEL.												
TOTAL VOL. DEL.												
SEDATION (1–5)												
PAIN (1–5)												
RESP.RATE												
NURSE'S SIG.												
ADMIN.SET CHANGE												
NEW PCA UNIT												
CONDITION I.V. SITE												

SCALES

SEDATION
1 = WIDE AWAKE
2 = DROWSY
3 = DOZING INTERMITTENTLY
4 = MOSTLY SLEEPING
5 = AWAKENS ONLY WHEN AROUSED

PAIN
1 = COMFORTABLE
2 = IN MILD DISCOMFORT
3 = IN PAIN
4 = IN BAD PAIN
5 = IN VERY BAD PAIN

FIGURE 20-8 Sample flow sheet for patient-controlled analgesia.

In more than 75% of hospitals in the United States, nursing documentation is entered into an electronic health record (Jha et al., 2009). Each entry is time-stamped allowing for extraction of patient-level data and provides time-specific data for analyzing pain management practices. Systems also provide the ability to create customized reports to facilitate "real-time" pain management. For example, a report may be created to target patients in severe pain. Components for monitoring quality of care include the patient's comfort goal while at rest or with activity, pain intensity rating, time of initial assessment, medication

---

BOX 20-13   AMERICAN PAIN SOCIETY QUALITY ASSURANCE PAIN RELIEF STANDARDS

- Recognize and treat pain promptly.
  - Chart and display pain and relief (Process).
  - Define pain and relief levels to initiate review (Process).
  - Survey patient satisfaction (Outcome).
- Make information about analgesics readily available (Process).
- Promise patients attentive analgesic care (Process).
- Define explicit policies for use of advanced analgesic technologies (Process).
- Monitor adherence to standards (Process).

---

time and medication information, time of reassessment, pain intensity at time of reassessment, and how much time elapsed between intervention and reassessment. When reports like this are available to the health care team, decisions can be made based on identified gaps in pain management care and safety matters.

Review Questions   *Note: Questions below may have more than one right answer.*

1. Aspiration of > 5 mL of clear fluid from an epidural catheter is indicative of which of the following?
   A. Catheter migration
   B. The aspirant may be medication
   C. The aspirant is CSF
   D. The catheter is positioned in the epidural vein

2. When a patient experiences breakthrough pain with an epidural infusion, nursing interventions would include which of the following?
   A. Believe the patient and record the level of pain, and medicate through another route and medication
   B. Check the catheter hub for leakage
   C. Increase the medication dose consistent with nursing judgment
   D. Verify the physician/LIP's order in the clinical record

3. Which of the following opioid agonist/antagonists may be administered to reverse nausea?
   A. Nalbuphine (Nubain)
   B. Nortriptyline
   C. Neupogen (Filgrastim)
   D. Tramadol (Ultram)

4. Epidural morphine has been associated with a high incidence of pruritus thought to be related to which of the following?
   A. An allergic reaction causing histamine release
   B. Action of the opioid at the dorsal horn
   C. Activity of the opioid at the chemoreceptor sites
   D. Rostral spread of the opioid in the CSF

5. Alcohol is contraindicated for site preparation or when accessing an epidural catheter because of the potential for
   A. Migration into the epidural space
   B. Possible nerve damage
   C. Obliterating the catheter
   D. Damage to the silastic

6. Temporary epidural catheters are typically used for
   A. Postoperative pain management
   B. Trial of epidural analgesia for patient response
   C. Long-term use for patients with intractable cancer pain
   D. A and B only

7. Nursing standards of practice for pain management have been established by which of the following organizations?
   A. American Pain Society
   B. American Epidural Society
   C. American Academy of Pain Medicine
   D. American Society for Pain Management Nursing

8. What is the most important factor in pain assessment?
   A. The patient's self-report of pain intensity
   B. The nurse's report of the patient's pain intensity
   C. The physician/LIP's report of the patient's pain intensity
   D. All of the above

9. Options for pain control include which of the following:
   A. Systemic analgesics
   B. Intraspinal opioids
   C. Subcutaneous opioids
   D. Perineural local anesthetic agents
   E. All the above

10. Pain can be classified according to its
    A. Underlying mechanism
    B. Nerve penetration
    C. Intensity
    D. Duration

References and Selected Readings   *Asterisks indicate references cited in text.*

*Agency for Healthcare Research and Quality. (2011). *Section 3. Measuring Emergency Department performance.* Rockville, MD. http://www.ahrq.gov/research/findings/final-reports/ptflow/section3.html

*American Cancer Society. (2012). Cancer prevalence: How many people have cancer? http://www.cancer.org/cancer/cancerbasics/cancer-prevalence

*American Diabetes Association. (2011). Diabetes statistics. http://www.diabetes.org/diabetes-basics/diabetes-statistics/

*American Pain Society. (2008). *Principles of analgesic use in the treatment of acute pain and cancer pain* (6th ed.). Glenview, IL: Author.

*American Society for Pain Management Nursing. (2004). *The use of "as-needed" range orders for opioid analgesics in the management of acute pain.* A consensus statement of the American Society for Pain Management Nursing and the American Pain Society. Pensacola, FL: Author.

American Society for Pain Management Nursing. (2010). A joint statement from 21 Health Organizations and the Drug Enforcement Administration. Promoting pain relief and preventing abuse of pain medications: A critical balancing act. http://www.aspmn.org/pdfs/A_JOINT_STATEMENT_FROM_21_HEALTH_ORGANIZATIONS.pdf

American Society for Pain Management Nursing. (2013). Position papers. http://www.aspmn.org/Organization/position_papers.htm

American Society of Anesthesiologists Task Force on Acute Pain Management. (2012). Practice guidelines for acute pain management in the perioperative setting. *Anesthesiology, 116*(2), 248–273.

Arkoosh, V.A., Palmer, C.M., Yun, E.M., Sharma, S.K., Bates, J.N., Wissler, R.N., et al. (2008). A randomized, double-masked, multicenter comparison of the safety of continuous intrathecal labor analgesia using a 28-gauge catheter versus continuous epidural labor analgesia. *Anesthesiology, 108*(2), 286–298.

*Arnstein, P. (2010). *Clinical coach for effective pain management*. Philadelphia, PA: F.A. Davis Company.

Association for the Advancement of Medical Instrumentation (AAMI). (2010). Infusing patients safely: Priority issues from the AAMI/FDA infusion device summit. http://www.aami.org/publications/summits/AAMI_FDA_Summit_Report.pdf

*Bader, P., Echtle, D., Fonteyne, V., Livadas, K., De Meerleer, G., & Vranken, J.H. (2010). *Guidelines on pain management: Post-operative pain management* (pp. 61–82). Arnhem, The Netherlands: European Association of Urology. http://guideline.gov/content.aspx?id=23897

*Batalden, P.B., & Stoltz, P.K. (1993). A Framework for the continual improvement of health care: Building and applying professional and improvement knowledge to test changes in daily work. *Joint Commission Journal on Quality Improvement, 19*, 446–447.

Belverud, S., Mogilner, A., & Schulder, M. (2008). Intrathecal pumps. *Neurotherapeutics, 5*(1), 114–122.

*Bennett, G., Burchiel, K., Buchser, E., Classen, A., Deer, T., Du Pen, S., et al. (2000). Clinical guidelines for intraspinal infusion: Report of an expert panel. *Journal of Pain and Symptom Management, 20*(2), S37–S43.

Bozimowski, G. (2012). Patient perceptions of pain management therapy: A comparison of real-time assessment of patient education and satisfaction and registered nurse perceptions. *Pain Management Nursing, 13*(4), 186–193.

*Bridges, W. (2009). *Managing transitions: Making the most of change* (3rd ed.). Philadelphia, PA: Da Capo Lifelong Books.

Bruehl, S., Apkarian, A.V., Ballantyne, J.C., Berger, A., Borsook, D., Chen, W.G., et al. (2013). Personalized medicine and opioid analgesic prescribing for chronic pain: Opportunities and challenges. *The Journal of Pain, 14*(2), 103–113.

*Burnes, B. (2004). Kurt Lewin and the planned approach to change: A re-appraisal. *Journal of Management Studies, 41*(6), 977–1002.

Centers for Disease Control and Prevention (CDC). (2011). *Guidelines for the prevention of intravascular catheter-related infections*. http://www.cdc.gov/hicpac/pdf/guidelines/bsi-guidelines-2011.pdf

*Chou, R., Fanciullo, G.J., Fine, P.G., Adler, J.A., Ballantyne, J.C., & Miaskowski, C. (2009). Clinical guidelines for the use of chronic opioid therapy in chronic noncancer pain. *The Journal of Pain, 10*, 113–130.

*Dahan, A., Aarts, L., & Smith, T.W. (2010). Incidence, reversal, and prevention of opioid-induced respiratory depression. *Anesthesiology, 112*(1), 226–238.

Deer, T.R., Smith, H.S., Burton, A.W., Pope, J.E., Doleys, D.M., Levy, R.M., et al. (2011). Comprehensive consensus based guidelines on intrathecal drug delivery systems in the treatment of pain caused by cancer pain. *Pain Physician, 14*(3), E283–E312.

Dougherty, P.M., Palecek, J., Paleckova, V., Sorkin, L.S., & Willis, W.D. (1992). The role of NMDA and non-NMDA excitatory amino acid receptors in the excitation of primate spinothalamic tract neurons by mechanical, chemical, thermal, and electrical stimuli. *The Journal of Neuroscience, 12*(8), 3025–3041.

*Fine, P.G., & Portenoy, R.K. (2007). *A clinical guide to opioid analgesia*. New York, NY: Vendome Group, LLC.

*Fishbain, D., Johnson, S., Webster, L., Greene, L., & Faysal, J. (2010). Review of regulatory programs and new opioid technologies in chronic pain management: Balancing the risk of medication abuse with medical need. *Journal of Managed Care Pharmacy, 16*(4), 276–287.

*Glassford, B. (2008). Range orders for pain medication. *Critical Care Nurse, 28*(4), 66–67.

*Grape, S., & Schug, S.A. (2008). Epidural and spinal analgesia. In P. E. Macintyre, S. M. Walker, & D. J. Rowbotham (Eds.), *Clinical pain management: Acute pain* (pp. 255–270). London, UK: Hodder Arnold.

*Greenwood-VanMeerveld, B. (2008). Methylnaltrexone in the treatment of opioid-induced constipation. *Clinical and Experimental Gastroenterology, 1*, 49–58.

*Hagle, M.E., Lehr, V.T., Brubakken, K., & Shippee, A. (2004). Respiratory depression in adult patients with intravenous patient-controlled analgesia. *Orthopedic Nursing, 23*(1), 18–27.

*Hayek, S.M., Deer, T.R., Pope, J.E., Panchel, S.J., & Patel, V.B. (2011). Intrathecal therapy for cancer and noncancer pain. *Pain Physician, 14*(3), 219–248.

*Herr, K., Coyne, P.J., McCaffery, M., Manworren, R., & Merkel, S. (2011). *Pain assessment in the patient unable to self-report*. http://www.aspmn.org/Organization/documents/UPDATED_NonverbalRevisionFinalWEB.pdf

*Horlocker, T.T., Wedel, D.J., Rowlingson, J.C., Enneking, F.K., Kopp, S.L., Benzon, H.T., et al. (2010). Regional anesthesia in the patient receiving antithrombotic or thrombolytic therapy: American Society of Regional

Anesthesia and Pain Medicine evidence-based guidelines (third edition). *Regional Anesthesia and Pain Medicine, 35,* 64–101.

Hughes, R.G. (Ed.). (2008). *Patient safety and quality: An evidence-based handbook for nurses.* Rockville, MD: Agency for Healthcare Research and Quality (US). http://www.ncbi.nlm.nih.gov/books/NBK2651/

*Infusion Nurses Society. (2011). Infusion nursing standards of practice. *Journal of Infusion Nursing, 34*(1 Suppl.), S1–S108.

*Institute of Medicine. (2011). *Relieving pain in America: A blueprint for transforming prevention, care, education, and research.* Washington, DC: The National Academies Press.

*International Association for the Study of Pain (IASP). (2012). Why acute pain? http://www.iasppain.org/Content/NavigationMenu/GlobalYearAgainstPain/GlobalYearAgainstAcutePain/default.htm

*International Association for the Study of Pain Task Force on Taxonomy. (1994). *Classification of chronic pain* (2nd ed.). http://www.iasppain.org/Content/NavigationMenu/Publications/FreeBooks/Classification_of_Chronic_Pain/default.htm

Jamison, R.N., & Edwards, R.R. (2012). Integrating pain management in clinical practice. *Journal of Clinical Psychology Medicine Settings, 19*(1), 49–64.

*Jarzyna, D., Jungquist, C.R., Pasero, C., Willens, J.S., Nisbet, A., Oakes, L., et al. (2011). American Society for Pain Management Nursing guidelines for opioid-induced sedation and respiratory depression. *Pain Management Nursing, 12*(3), 118–145.

*Jha, A.K., DesRoches, C.M., Campbell, E.G., Donelan, K., Rao, S.R., Ferris, T.G., et al. (2009). Use of electronic health records in U.S. hospitals. *The New England Journal of Medicine, 360,* 1628–1638.

*Langley, G.J., Nolan, K.M., & Nolan, T.W. (1994). The foundation of improvement. *Quality Progress, 27,* 81–86.

*Latta, K.S., Ginsberg, B., & Barkin, R.L. (2002). Meperidine: A critical review. *American Journal of Therapeutics, 9,* 53–68.

*Leppert, W. (2010). The role of opioid receptor antagonists in the treatment of opioid-induced constipation: A review. *Advances in Therapy, 27,* 714–730.

*Litwack, K. (2009). Somatosensory function, pain, and headache. In C.M. Porth & G. Matfin (Eds.), *Pathophysiology: Concepts of altered health states* (pp. 1225–1259). Philadelphia, PA: Wolters Kluwer Health/Lippincott Williams & Wilkins.

*Maalouf, D.B., & Liu, S.S. (2009). Clinical application of epidural analgesia. In S.R. Sinatra, O.A. de Leon-Casaola, B. Ginsberg., & E.R. Viscusi (Eds.), *Acute pain management* (pp. 221–229). Cambridge, NY: Cambridge University Press.

*Mann, C. (2000). Comparison of intravenous or epidural patient-controlled analgesia in the elderly after major abdominal surgery. *Anesthesiology, 92*(2), 433–441.

Martin, T.J., & Ewan, E. (2008). Chronic pain alters drug self-administration: Implications for addiction and pain mechanisms. *Experimental and Clinical Psychopharmacology, 16*(5), 357.

*McCaffery, M. (1968). *Nursing practice theories relate to cognition, bodily pain and man-environment interactions.* Los Angeles, CA: University of California at Los Angeles Students' Store.

McCaffery, M., & Pasero, C. (1999). *Pain: Clinical manual* (2nd ed.). St. Louis, MO: Mosby.

*Medscape. (2013). Is an NP a licensed independent practitioner? http://www.medscape.com/viewarticle/777639_3

*Myers, J., Chan, V., Jarvis, V., & Walker-Dilks, C. (2010). Intraspinal techniques for pain management in cancer patients: A systematic review. *Supportive Care in Cancer, 18,* 137–149.

*Oliver, J., Coggins, C., Compton, P., Hagan, S., Matteliano, D., Stanton, M., St. Marie, B., Strobbe, S., & Turner, H. (2012). Pain management in patients with substance use disorders. *Pain Management Nursing, 13*(3), 169–183.

Pasero, C. (2000). Pain control: Continuous local anesthetics. *American Journal of Nursing, 100*(8), 22.

*Pasero, C. (2003a). *Epidural analgesia for acute pain management self-directed learning program.* Lenexa, KS: American Society for Pain Management Nursing.

*Pasero, C. (2003b). Epidural analgesia for postoperative pain. *American Journal of Nursing, 103*(10), 62–64.

*Pasero, C., Quinn, T.E., Portenoy, R.K., McCaffery, M., & Rizos, A. (2011). Opioid analgesics. In C. Pasero & M. McCaffery (Eds.), *Pain assessment and pharmacologic management* (pp. 277–622). St. Louis, MO: Elsevier Mosby.

*Polomano, R.C., Rathmell, J.P., Krenzischek, D.A., & Dunwoody, C.J. (2008). Emerging trends and new approaches to acute pain management. *Pain Management Nursing, 9*(1), S33–S41.

*Portenoy, R.K., Bennett, D.S., Rauck, R., Simon, S., Taylor, D., Brennan, M., et al. (2006). Prevalence and characteristics of breakthrough pain in opioid-treated patients with chronic noncancer pain. *The Journal of Pain, 7*(8), 585–591.

Ritter, H.T.M. (2011). Making patient-controlled analgesia safer for patients. ECRI Institute and Institute for Safe Medication Practice. http://patientsafetyauthority.org/ADVISORIES/AdvisoryLibrary/2011/sep8(3)/Pages/94.aspx

*Roger, V.L., Go, A.S., Lloyd-Jones, D.M., Adams, R.J., Berry, J.D., Brown, T.M., et al. (2011). Heart disease and stroke statistics—2011 update: A report from the American Heart Association. *Circulation, 123,* e18–e209.

*Rosier, P.K. (2012). Facing up to the challenge of range orders. *Nursing, 42*(12), 64–65.

*Rosner, H.L. (1996). *A practical approach to pain management* (pp. 6–7). Boston, MA: Little, Brown.

Samuels, J.G., & Bliss, R.L. (2012). Analyzing variability in pain management using electronic healthy record data. *Journal of Nursing Care Quality, 27*(4), 316–324.

Shane, R. (2009). Current status of administration of medicines. *American Journal of Health-System Pharmacy, 66*(5 Suppl. 3), S42–S48.

*Sheen, M.J., Ho, S.T., Lee, C.H., Tsung, Y.C., & Chang, F.L. (2008). Preoperative gabapentin prevents intrathecal morphine-induced pruritus after orthopedic surgery. *Anesthesia and Analgesia, 106*(6), 1868–1872.

*Sluka, K.A., O'Donnell, J.M., Danielson, J., & Rasmussen, L.A. (2012). Regular physical activity prevents development of chronic pain and activation of central neurons. *Journal of Applied Psychology, 114*(6), 725–733.

*St. Marie, B.J. (2010). *Core curriculum for pain management nursing* (2nd ed.). Lenexa, KS: ASPMN.

*Swenson, J., Davis, J., & Johnson, K. (2005). Postoperative care of the chronic opioid-consuming patient. *Anesthesiology Clinics of North America, 23*(1), 37–48.

*The Joint Commission. (2012). *2013 Hospital accreditation standards.* Oakbrook Terrace, IL: Joint Commission Resources.

*Turk, D.C., & Okifuji, A. (2010). Pain terms and taxonomies of pain. In S.M. Fishman, J.C. Ballantyne, & J.P. Rathmell (Eds.), *Bonica's management of pain* (4th ed., pp. 13–23). Philadelphia, PA: Lippincott Williams & Wilkins.

*van der Vyver, M., Halpern, S., & Joseph, G. (2002). Patient-controlled epidural analgesia *versus* continuous infusion for labour analgesia: A meta-analysis. *British Journal of Anaesthesia, 89,* 459–465.

Watanabe, S., Pereira, J., Hanson, J., & Bruera, E. (1998). Fentanyl by continuous subcutaneous infusion for the management of cancer pain: A retrospective study. *Journal of Pain and Symptom Management, 16,* 323–326.

*Webster, L.R. (2008). Breakthrough pain in the management of chronic persistent pain syndromes. *The American Journal of Managed Care, 14*(4 Suppl.), 116–122.

Wells, N., Pasero, C., & McCaffery, M. (2008). Improving the quality of care through pain assessment and management. In R.G. Hughes (Ed.), *Patient safety and quality: An evidence-based handbook for nurses* (Chapter 17). Rockville, MD: Agency for Healthcare Research and Quality (US). http://www.ncbi.nlm.nih.gov/books/NBK2658/

*White, P.F. (1987). Mishaps with patient-controlled analgesia. *Anesthesiology, 66,* 81–83.

*White, P.F. (1988). Use of patient-controlled analgesia for management of acute pain. *Journal of the American Medical Association, 259*(2), 243–247.

*Wuhrman, E., Cooney, M.F., Dunwoody, C.J., Eksterowicz, N., Merkel, S., & Oakes, L.L. (2007). Authorized and unauthorized (PCA by proxy) dosing of analgesic infusion pumps: Position statement with clinical practice recommendations. *Pain Management Nursing, 8*(1), 4–11.

*Yaney, L.L. (1998). Intravenous conscious sedation: Physiologic, pharmacologic, and legal implications for nurses. *Journal of Intravenous Nursing, 21,* 9–19.

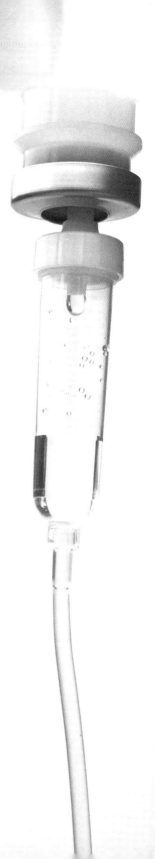

PART 5

SPECIAL POPULATIONS

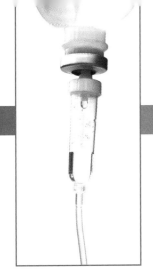

CHAPTER 21

Pediatric Infusion Therapy

Wendi S. Redfern
Jeanne E. Braby

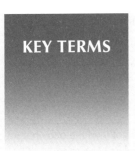

KEY TERMS	Developmental Stage	Thermoregulation
	Maintenance Fluids	Total Nutrient
	Methemoglobinemia	Admixture
	Pain management:	Umbilical access
	BSPECLD	

INFUSION THERAPY IN INFANTS AND CHILDREN

This chapter focuses on aspects of infusion therapy specific to neonatal and pediatric patients. It highlights developmental considerations, disorders, and disease processes unique to this population, intravenous (IV) therapies commonly used in children and adolescents, and necessary adaptations and adjustments to vascular access techniques and devices for the neonatal and pediatric population. Two ongoing considerations in the administration of pediatric infusion therapy are emotional preparation of the child and initiation of vascular access. This chapter examines these topics in detail, along with special nursing considerations and specific intravascular therapeutic modalities.

PSYCHOSOCIAL STAGES OF DEVELOPMENT

Children are not small adults. An area of concern is the child's emotional needs, which require patience, education, and understanding from infusion nurses. Psychosocial age and ability, as well as each child's particular developmental stage, exert major influences on emotional needs. When hospitalized, some children regress and exhibit behaviors more common in a younger age group (e.g., a child who is toilet trained may regress to the diaper stage). These children resume developmental landmarks once treatment ends or the child's condition stabilizes. Thus, even though children of varied ages and intellectual capacities receive similar infusion therapies, they require education before, during, and after infusion therapy that considers their particular emotional and developmental variables.

Developmental Stages

A full understanding of each developmental stage enables the health care team to provide individualized care that focuses on each child's physical functioning and emotional coping skills. This level of care is appropriate and nonthreatening. It enhances the ability of staff to recognize that a child's needs vary markedly, according to stress levels as well as by growth and developmental levels.

A significant difference between children and adults is in the preparation for the procedure. A developmentally tailored approach is essential when working with children. Table 21-1 reviews growth, development, and useful approaches when working with children of different developmental stages.

This chapter cannot cover all the principles and theories of growth and development. Instead, important principles are highlighted. Erikson is credited with the development of

TABLE 21-1	**GROWTH AND DEVELOPMENT: INTRAVENOUS INSERTION STRATEGIES FOR PEDIATRIC PATIENTS**		
Age	Growth	Development	IV Tips
Infancy (birth to 12 mo) (includes neonatal period from birth to 28 d)	• Rapid • Maturation of body systems • Birth weight doubles at 6 mo/triples by 1 y	• Social affective play • Attachment to caregivers • Separation anxiety begins at approximately age 6 mo.	• Do not feed the baby before IV placement or aspiration may occur. • Provide comfort during and after the procedure, using a pacifier and distraction, such as a mobile.
Toddler (12–36 mo)	• Weight gain slows • Birth weight quadruples by 30 mo • Height at 3 is half adult height • Head circumference growth slows • Chest circumference larger than the head/abdomen	• Cause-and-effect thinking • Exploratory phase • Imaginative play	• Require short, concrete explanations immediately before treatment • Give simple choices • Assistant required for positioning
Preschool/early childhood (36 mo to 6 y)	• Growth stabilizes • Annual weight gain is 2.2 kg (5 lb) • Height increase ranges from 6.4–7.6 cm (2.5–3 inches) • Most growth in legs	• New gross motor skills • Fantasy vs. reality • Follows simple commands • Fear blood loss/invasive procedures	• Need preparation before procedure • Distracted with age-appropriate toys • Play therapy with medical toys • May need help to hold the child still

TABLE 21-	GROWTH AND DEVELOPMENT: INTRAVENOUS INSERTION STRATEGIES FOR PEDIATRIC PATIENTS *(Continued)*		
Age	Growth	Development	IV Tips
School-age (6–12 y)	• Growth/development gradual • Annual weight gain is 2–3 kg (4.5–6.5 lb) • Height increase is 5 cm annually (2 inch)	• Solitary, interactive play • Superhero fascination • Fantasy about procedures based on the level of understanding	• Can be told about IV a short time in advance • Allow to assist with tasks like tearing tape and counting I/O • Allow for privacy • Allow the child to cry
Adolescence		• Logic, reasoning, and concept of permanence • Develop skills • Dramatize • Identify role models	• Approach using adult terms • Prepare teens in advance, allowing them to participate in care
• Early (11–13)	• Little size difference between sexes • Growth spurt at the end of early stage	• Seek independence • Peers are important	
• Middle (13–15)	• Girls surpass boys in height and weight; then boys surpass girls	• Sexual identify and body image • Mortality is a concern	
• Late (15+)	• Body proportions similar to adult parameters	• Career planning • High idealism • Favor close, intimate relationships • Seek significant other	

the most widely accepted theory of personality development (Erikson, 1963). Each stage has two components, the desirable and undesirable aspect (Table 21-2). There are five stages that relate to childhood: trust versus mistrust, autonomy versus shame and doubt, initiative versus guilt, industry versus inferiority, and identity versus role confusion. Successful completion of each stage is ideal. Hospitalization can cause children to regress to an earlier stage. Parents need to know that this is a normal response.

The Newborn and Infant

The newborn stage is from birth to 28 days, while the infant stage is from 29 days to 12 months. For the purpose of this review, the neonate and premature infant will be included in the infant stage. Unique considerations will be delineated when necessary. Neonates, and in particular low birth weight and premature infants, have a low tolerance for physiologic stress, including changes in environmental temperature, bright lights, and loud noises. When performing a procedure, it is important to keep those factors in mind. Temperature regulation becomes more efficient as the infant matures.

TABLE 21-2	ERIKSON'S STAGES OF PSYCHOSOCIAL DEVELOPMENT: INFANCY TO 18 YEARS		
Stage	Basic Conflict	Important Events	Outcome
Infancy (birth to 18 mo)	Trust vs. mistrust	Feeding	Reliable, affectionate care instills a sense of trust
Early Childhood (2–3 y)	Autonomy vs. shame/doubt	Toilet training	Control over physical skills and a sense of independence lead to feelings of autonomy
Preschool (3–5 y)	Initiative vs. guilt	Exploration	A sense of purpose is created when children assert control and power over their environments
School-Age (6–11 y)	Industry vs. inferiority	School	New social and academic demands require new coping skills; success ensures competence
Adolescence (12–18 y)	Identity vs. role confusion	Social relationships	Teens need to develop a sense of self and personal identity. Success leads to an ability to remain true to oneself

 PATIENT SAFETY

All infants breathe through their nose instead of their mouth; awareness of this concept will help to enhance patient safety.

While a pacifier is useful to comfort an infant, it is essential to be mindful of the infant's breathing and assure that the nares remain patent. In some cases, it may be necessary to stop a procedure to suction the infant and ensure that the infant is able to breathe comfortably and effectively. Lengthy procedures may also require that the procedure be halted; allowing the infant to recover from physiological stress.

The psychosocial need of the infant is to begin to develop trust. The infant learns trust when his or her primary needs are met. Along with the basic need of nourishment, the infant needs to feel secure. Caregivers can help the infants feel secure by quickly responding to their cries, talking to them in a soft, soothing voice, keeping them warm and dry, and provide comfort during holding whenever possible.

Communication with the infant depends on his or her developmental age. Younger infants usually respond best to a soft soothing voice prior to and during procedures. As the infant grows, developing trust may mean playing a game of "peek-a-boo" to begin establishing rapport.

Crib side rails should always remain up unless a caregiver physically has a hand on the infant. By 4 to 5 months of age, infants begin to put things in their mouths; therefore, safe care dictates keeping all small objects out of reach.

 PATIENT SAFETY

Medical equipment is a choking hazard. All small objects should remain out of reach of infants and toddlers.

In addition, all infants under 1 year of age should be in a safe sleep environment. The components of safe sleep are a firm mattress and no toys or loose blankets in the crib (Flook & Vincze, 2012). Band-aids or adhesive dressings that could be "chewed off" are considered a choking hazard and should be avoided. By 4 to 8 months, infants may begin to exhibit "stranger anxiety." Postprocedure, infants should be cuddled and allowed to play.

THE TODDLER

The toddler stage is from 1 to 3 years of age. Toddlers are beginning to use and develop language. Although they have a short attention span, toddlers are able to understand simple directions. The toddler's psychosocial developmental task is developing autonomy. They should be allowed choices when possible. Pain should be assessed and managed using toddler language (hurt, owie, boo-boo). Toddlers often have a favorite toy, blanket, or sleep friend. Parents should be encouraged to remain with their toddler.

The toddler should be given age-appropriate information just prior to any procedure. Communication should be done by speaking slowly and using short simple explanations. Directions should be given one at a time. It is important to use words the toddler understands to describe what the toddler will see, hear, and smell. Dolls and toys to demonstrate the medical equipment will aid in the toddler's ability to understand. For example, the toddler can first be shown how the doll will get an IV. Similar to the infant, it is important to keep small objects out of reach and not leave the toddler unsupervised.

THE PRESCHOOLER

The preschool stage is from 3 to 6 years, and at this phase of psychosocial development, the child's task is to develop initiative. The preschool child should be offered reasonable choices (e.g., site for injection) to help foster independence and a sense of control. They are starting to socialize with groups. They fear being left alone and bodily harm. Preschool-aged children need clear rules and boundaries to develop their sense of security. By this stage, the preschool child has physically improved coordination, balance, and muscular strength.

An infusion therapy–teaching tool with pictures and large-print words in simple language can help preschoolers understand the procedure. Distraction using age-appropriate toys is an effective intervention. These items can include a Slinky, a clear sealed acrylic "magic wand" with floating sparkles, a kaleidoscope, and a bottle of bubbles for blowing. Medical play therapy, consisting of practicing IV therapy on a doll, is an ideal teaching strategy that enhances emotional preparation through acting out.

Similar to the toddler, explanations should be honest using terms of sensation (i.e., feel, hear, see, or smell). Usually, it is best to tell the child that the venipuncture will hurt but only for a short time. Define the term "time" by comparison with other procedures. For example, say, "The actual IV start takes about the same time it takes you to say the alphabet or count to 50." It is important to assure the child that any procedure is not a punishment. Rewards such as stickers, given for cooperation, are well received.

THE SCHOOL-AGE CHILD

The school-age child (6 to 12 years) is physically maturing at a fast rate, although, emotional and social maturity does not always occur at the same rate. This is the stage of competence; the psychosocial task of the school-age child is developing industry. They are able to take on responsibilities, including home chores and schoolwork. School-agers have increased attention spans and are eager learners. The school-age child understands cause and effect and logical reasoning. They are able to describe pain and continue to fear bodily harm. The school-ager desires privacy and enjoys a sense of control. Allow children to participate by tearing tape, opening alcohol swabs, or holding tubing. Family is still very important, but they may begin to prefer friends.

Explanations about procedures should be in language the school-ager understands. Written instructions are also an option. The child should be encouraged to ask questions and talk about his or her feelings. School-agers can handle longer teaching sessions and respond well to praise. Rewards are useful in recognizing their achievements. They also need to be reassured that procedures are not punishments. Behavior limits may need reinforcement. Parents need to be included in decisions, but the school-age child should be given opportunities for decision making.

THE 12- TO 18-YEAR-OLDS

The psychosocial task for the 12- to 18-year-olds is the development of identity. The adolescent is struggling to obtain a sense of self. They are preoccupied with their body appearance and the need to fit in with their peers. Separation from their peers can be difficult. They may have wide mood swings, and risk-taking behavior is common. The adolescent may challenge authority but still need adult support. Their rapid growth spurts may cause them to be easily fatigued, and their sleep patterns may change.

The appropriate approach for the adolescent is similar to that of the adult. Procedures should be explained and instructions given in writing. They should be encouraged to ask questions and talk about their feelings. Keep privacy as a priority during procedures and recognize concerns about body image. Decision making and involvement in self-care are essential for the adolescent.

DEVELOPMENT APPROACH FOR ALL AGES

Always be honest with children. Specifically, do not promise a certain number of IV attempts or "only one stick" because a child will lose trust if several attempts turn out to be necessary. Language used is important. Nurses may be able to assuage a child's fear of needles by telling the child that once the IV is in place, the needle is no longer there and only a small "straw" is in the vein.

Safety is always the primary concern for all hospitalized children. Their hospital bed should remain a safe place (Hockenberry et al., 2011). Invasive procedures should be performed in a treatment room whenever possible, and parents should be encouraged to stay with their child.

PATIENT SAFETY

When parents speak up, health care professionals should perceive and reflect their actions in a manner that fosters true collaboration and empowerment and should encourage and reinforce the parents' role in making queries by providing thoughtful and complete answers.

Parents are often permitted around-the-clock visiting hours to stay with their hospitalized children, even in neonatal and pediatric intensive care units. For ill children, this can be comforting and provides an emotional support system. Frey, Ersch, Bernet, and Baenziger

(2009) suggested that parents who stay with their hospitalized children are inevitably involved in safety issues and may help detect critical (harmful or potentially harmful) events precipitated by health care professionals.

> **PATIENT SAFETY**
>
> Provide parents with timely and comprehensive updates regarding their children in language they understand. Some children's hospitals encourage parents to be part of "family-centered" rounds, allowing them to gain a better understanding of their child's total treatment plan and current status since the entire medical team is available to answer questions and address concerns.

During the procedure, parents/caregivers may provide emotional support and represent security during an actual procedure, but they should not be used to restrain a child unless no other assistance is available (i.e., in-home care). Parents/caregivers can be instructed to use positioning for comfort techniques to hold a child still for venipuncture while still helping a child feel secure (Sparks, Setlik, & Luhman, 2007; Figure 21-1).

If a parent chooses not to accompany a child into the treatment room for IV insertion, the infusion nurse should honor this decision and not make parents feel guilty. Providing comfort and praise after the IV insertion is an ideal means of parental involvement.

Knowledge of the expected developmental stage is important; however, the health care team must remember to assess each child individually, not just according to age or physiologic maturity. In some cases, children have disease processes, such as renal disease, that can result in growth delays, causing staff to mistake the child's actual age. When teaching parents and children, it is best to ask, "What questions do you have?" as opposed to asking, "Do you have any questions?" This simple change in wording gives the learner permission to ask questions of the health care team without feeling intimidated. Child and family education is addressed in Box 21-1.

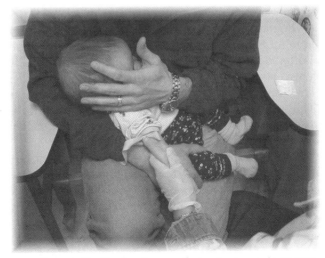

FIGURE 21-1 Positioning for comfort prior to venipuncture. (Courtesy of A. M. Frey.)

BOX 21-1   CHILD AND FAMILY EDUCATION
• Follow developmental principles when providing education to patients and families • Provide instruction in clear, simple language • Verify understanding with demonstration using teach-back principles (Wilson, Baker, Nordstrom, & Legwand, 2008) • Think about health literacy and supply teaching materials written at elementary level

Pain Assessment and Reduction

Studies indicate that infants and children respond to noxious stimuli and experience pain (Leahy et al., 2008; Walco, 2008; Walden & Gibbins, 2008; Zempsky, 2008a, 2008b). In one study, pediatric inpatients reported IV line placement as the leading cause of procedure-related pain, on the same level of pain as postsurgical pain (Cummings, Reid, Finley, McGrath, & Ritchie, 1996). The memory of previous painful events, including venipuncture, can have both psychological and physiological impact on later painful episodes (Leahy et al., 2008). Evidence suggests that repeated painful procedures may have cumulative effects on the developing brain (Walden & Gibbins, 2008).

Assessment of pain in children requires the use of different pain scales (Jacob, 2009). Self-report is the most reliable indicator of pain; however, this is not possible in the preverbal child. Behavioral observations are used in some neonatal and pediatric pain scale tools. The FLACC Pain Assessment Tool is an example of a behavioral tool comprised of an interval scale that measures pain from 0 (no pain behaviors) to 10 (highest pain behaviors). The behaviors observed using the FLACC scale are: Facial expression, Leg movement, Activity, Cry, and Consolability (Table 21-3).

There are also pain scales that evaluate the neonate using physiologic indicators along with behaviors. The premature infant pain profile (PIPP) scale is used for infants 28 to 40 weeks of gestational age. The variables assessed are gestational age, eye squeeze, behavioral state, nasolabial furrow, heart rate, oxygen saturation, and brow bulge (Jacob, 2009) (Table 21-4).

Everyone who starts IVs in children should be knowledgeable in techniques to maximize comfort and minimize pain. An easy acronym to remember these techniques is BSPECLD (Table 21-5). Buffered lidocaine can be administered intradermally or with needleless injection. This can be very effective in reducing the pain from a needlestick.

Sucrose has been very effective in reducing pain response in infants during invasive procedures. The sucrose is administered orally or via a syringe at least 2 minutes prior to the procedure, preferably with a pacifier since nonnutritive sucking has been shown to be a nonpharmacological pain-relieving method (Cohen, 2008).

Pain Ease is a vapocoolant (topical skin refrigerant) with rapid onset (Farion, Splinter, Newhook, Gaboury, & Splinter, 2008). Spray continuously for 4 to 7 seconds from a distance of 3 to 7 inches, or a cotton ball can be saturated and held over the site for 4 to 7 seconds. Avoid using vapocoolant on patients with poor circulation, on children < 4 years old, or on broken skin.

Frequently, topical anesthetic creams are a choice in the pediatric population. EMLA is a topical anesthetic made of lidocaine 2.5% and prilocaine 2.5%. It requires a minimum of 60 minutes to provide effective pain relief. Liposomal lidocaine LMX4 is another topical anesthetic cream containing 4% lidocaine. The onset of action is quicker than that of EMLA

TABLE 21-	FLACC PAIN SCALE		
	Scoring		
Category	**0**	**1**	**2**
Face	No particular expression or smile	Occasional frown, withdrawn	Frequent to constant quivering chin, clenched jaw
Legs	Normal or relaxes	Uneasy, restless, tense	Kicking, or legs drawn up on the abdomen
Activity	Lying quietly, normal position, moves easily	Squirming, shifting, tense	Arched, rigid, or jerking
Cry	No cry (awake or asleep)	Moans or whimpers	Crying steadily, screams, or sobs
Consolability	Content, relaxed	Reassured by occasional touching, hugging, or being talked to	Difficult to console or comfort

(30 minutes). Both creams may be associated with the development of **methemoglobinemia** in susceptible children, particularly in young infants (Zempsky, 2008a, 2008b). Table 21-6 provides a summary of some medications for pain reduction.

Distraction can be one of the greatest skills to develop for use in pediatric care for non-pharmacologic pain control (Cohen, 2008). Have the child blow bubbles or take a deep

TABLE 21-	PIPP PAIN ASSESSMENT TOOL					
Observe	**Indicator**	**0**	**1**	**2**	**3**	**Score**
Chart	Gestational	>36 wk	32–35 wk, 6 d	28–31 wk, 6 d	<28 wk	
15 s	Behavior	Active, awake, eyes open, facial movement	Quiet, awake, eyes open, no facial movement	Active sleep, eyes closed, facial movement	Quiet sleep, eyes closed, no facial movement	
Baseline heart rate and oxygen saturations for 30 s	Heart rate maximum	0 beats/min increase	5–15 beats/min increase	15–24 beats/min increase	25 beats/min increase	
	Oxygen saturation minimum	92%–100%	89%–91%	85%–88%	<85%	
Facial actions for 30 s	Brow bulge	None	Minimum	Moderate	Maximum	
	Eye squeeze	None	Minimum	Moderate	Maximum	
	Nasolabial furrow	None	Minimum	Moderate	Maximum	

Evaluation of pain
Score 0–6 No action
Score 7–12 Nonpharmacological intervention, for example, swaddling, sucking (reassess in 30 min)
Score > 12 Pharmacological intervention (reassess in 15–30 min)

TABLE 21-5	BSPECLD TECHNIQUES
B	Buffered lidocaine
S	Sucrose
P	Pain ease
E	EMLA
C	Child life
L	Liposomal lidocaine LMX
D	Distraction

breath when you puncture the vein to "blow the hurt away." Counting and singing are other good distractors for a preschool or school-age child. Tell them to sing or count louder if they have any pain. For the older child, distraction may include asking about school, teachers, pets, and favorite places.

Guided imagery can also be helpful to reduce the anxiety and pain associated with IV insertion. Guided imagery encourages children to employ pleasant imagery as a distraction to pain. The child is encouraged to describe the details of the pleasant experience using different senses (e.g., see, hear, and feel). Instruct the child to concentrate on the pleasurable event. Guided imagery when combined with other nonpharmacologic techniques such as relaxation and deep breathing can be an effective approach to pain reduction (Phipps et al., 2010). Other techniques include rocking/holding, reduced light, swaddling/nesting, touch/massage, and positioning for comfort.

Nurses can become proficient in the use of nonpharmacological pain techniques or they may seek assistance from a certified child life specialist, a professional who has studied child development and the reactions of children to health care settings (Leahy et al., 2008). The child life specialist is available to help the child's fear and anxiety by helping them understand and cope with the hospital stay through preparation, support, and play.

A combination of age-appropriate pharmacological and nonpharmacological pain techniques used with children prior to IV insertion helps to maximize comfort and minimize pain. In some cases, IV conscious sedation may be necessary to provide a more generalized sedation for insertion of a peripherally inserted central catheter (PICC).

TABLE 21-6	NUMBING AGENTS
Product	**Method**
EMLA cream (topical)	Place on the potential insertion site and cover with transparent dressing >1 h before procedure.
LMS-4 cream (topical)	Place on the potential insertion site 30 min or more before procedure. May cover with transparent dressing to avoid disturbance or ingestion by a child
Lidocaine hydrochloride 0.5%, 1% without epinephrine (intradermal) or needless injection device	Create an intradermal wheal 0.05–0.1 mL near the insertion site with a 26- or 29-gauge insulin needle.

PHYSIOLOGIC STAGES OF DEVELOPMENT

Physiologic Considerations

Human beings change both physically and emotionally throughout childhood, whereas parameter characteristics remain relatively constant after adulthood. For example, body circumference increases more than threefold in length and approximately 20-fold in weight from birth through adolescence (Hesselgrave, 2009). The body circumference of the adult, however, changes relatively little throughout the remainder of life. Thus, the stress levels and basal metabolic rates of the child are much higher than in an adult patient.

In the premature baby and term infant, renal function is immature, with inability to concentrate and excrete effectively, acidify urine, or maintain fluid and sodium balance. In the term infant, renal immaturity results in excretion of larger volumes of solute-free water than is seen in older pediatric patients (Blayney, 2013) by the end of the 2nd year, renal function reaches full maturity.

The immature hepatic system in the neonate and infant can affect intravenous medication and/or solution administration. Throughout the first year of life, the liver function remains immature. Digestive and metabolic processes are usually complete by the beginning of toddlerhood (Wilson, 2009).

THE SKIN

Skin color, turgor, temperature, moisture, and texture all reflect the child's state of hydration and nutrition. Knowledge of the condition of the integumentary system particularly that of premature infants, is of extreme importance to the infusion specialist. The skin of the premature infant requires special precautions due to underdevelopment of the stratum corneum, with resultant thin, fragile skin. This dermal fragility can lead to dermal stripping, loss of water, and increased absorption and possible toxicity of agents, such as solvents and bonding agents that are applied to the skin. Neonatal skin care is a special skill. Because there is less cohesion between the dermis and epidermis, tape removal can strip epidermis, so as little tape as possible and tape padded with gauze or cotton fibers is used.

For skin disinfection in premature neonates, the Association of Women's Health, Obstetric and Neonatal Nurses (AWOHNN) (Beauman & Swanson, 2006) recommends using chlorhexidine or povidone iodine and allowing it to dry, removing these products with sterile water or saline after the procedure is complete to avoid the risk of chemical burns. Evidence is currently inconclusive for chlorhexidine use in low birth weight infants. The use of isopropyl alcohol and alcohol-based disinfectants should be avoided in preterm infants. Except for specific congenital or acquired skin conditions, such as dystrophic epidermolysis bullosa, eczema, and other disorders, the barrier function of the integumentary system of the full-term neonate and older child is intact.

FONTANELS

The infant's anterior fontanel remains open until the child is nearly 2 years of age. This provides an additional tool by which to assess hydration. The anterior fontanel is either completely flat or slightly sunken in a normal state. It is depressed in fluid deficit and bulging with increased pressure indicative of cerebral edema, hemorrhage, or fluid volume excess.

Urinary Output

Accurate measurements allow the practitioner to manage fluid balance. Fluid restriction or deficit is reflected by a high specific gravity; a low measurement reflects fluid retention or overload. If the child is in diapers, the weight of the dry diaper is subtracted from that of the wet diaper; the weight in grams equals the volume voided in milliliters.

Hypoglycemia

There are multiple etiologies of hypoglycemia in infants; however, hyperinsulinemia is often the cause of persistent hypoglycemia in the neonate (Fraser Askin, 2009). Other causes include abrupt discontinuation of IV dextrose solutions and high glucose demand that is not met, such as in a septic infant. Infants and children who are hypoglycemic display blood glucose levels of <45 mg/dL, have poor oral intake, and exhibit neurologic symptoms, such as lethargy, hypotonia, tremors or twitching, irritability, and eye rolling (Fraser Askin, 2009). An older child may complain of headache or display hallucinations or mental confusion. The mechanisms of hypoglycemia remain incompletely understood. Treatment involves oral or IV glucose, depending on the severity of the hypoglycemia.

Thermoregulation

Thermoregulation, the maintenance of normal body temperature, is a challenge to the premature neonate owing to large surface area, dermal immaturity, and thin layer of subcutaneous fat. Physiologic stress and increased metabolism, in response to hypothermia, will result in higher oxygen and caloric requirements. This process of thermoregulation continues throughout the infant's first several months of life. Neonates do not shiver to maintain heat as adults do, and during infancy, the child's ability to shiver increases. The older infant usually has acquired the benefit of insulation by the gradual growth of adipose tissue. By early childhood, the skin is thicker and the body has a higher percentage of fat and a decreased surface area–to-volume ratio; these factors enable children to cope with environmental cold stresses much better than the young infant.

When performing procedures such as IV insertion and dressing changes, the nurse must maintain a neutral thermal environment for the infant to prevent the possibility of cold stress, thus permitting the infant to maintain a normal core temperature with minimum oxygen consumption and calorie expenditure. Maintain temperature control by carefully exposing only the necessary extremity during a procedure and bundling the infant in a blanket. It is especially important to keep the infant's head covered to minimize heat loss. If the room is cold, warming lights can be used to help keep the baby warm. Low birth weight and premature infants should remain in an incubator whenever possible since incubators are designed to maintain both temperature and humidity. A warm environment can be maintained using a variety of tools, including the following: warmer beds, incubators, cotton blankets, head coverings, heat lamps kept a safe distance from the skin, and hot packs for infant use; thereby ensuring that only the extremity of the IV insertion site is exposed.

Vessel Size

Venous and arterial vessels in the infant and child are smaller than those in the adult. Anatomically positioned in the same locations throughout one's life, the small size and presence of subcutaneous fat may contribute to difficulty in locating those vessels. Vasodilation prior to venipuncture is helpful, along with other location measures including transillumination and infrared or near-infrared technologies (Frey & Pettit, 2010).

BLOOD VOLUME

The major differences from neonate to adult include a gradual decrease in blood volume, maturation of the immune system with regard to blood typing, changes in blood counts, and changes in requirements. Circulating blood volume changes throughout development with neonates ranging from 80 to 85 mL/kg versus the adolescent and adult at 60 to 65 mL/kg (Table 21-1) (Hazinski, 2013). The higher proportion of blood volume to lower body weight of the neonate and infant means that blood loss percentage is much higher in this group, even with small losses. The following is an example comparing blood volume loss between a 5-kg infant and a 75-kg adult.

$$25 \text{ mL blood loss from } 75\text{-kg adult} = <0.4\% \text{ of total circulating blood volume } (5,250 \text{ mL})$$

$$25 \text{ mL blood loss from } 5\text{-kg infant} = 6\% \text{ of total circulating blood volume } (400 \text{ mL})$$

Owing to smaller body surface area (BSA) and large circulating blood volume, the same amount of blood loss could be devastating to an infant, whereas it would not harm an adult.

Specific physical assessment areas indicative of hematologic function in children include color changes in the skin, lips, conjunctivae, mucous membranes, and nails, such as blue for cyanosis, pale for anemia, or yellow for jaundice. Examination of the fingernails and toenails for clubbing, the skin for petechiae, and the mucous membranes for bleeding are key assessment findings for the practitioner. Blood oozing from old venipuncture sites is often an indicator of a bleeding disorder or disseminated intravascular coagulation. When the application of a tourniquet on an extremity promotes evidence of petechiae distal to the tourniquet site, idiopathic thrombocytopenic purpura (ITP) or other platelet disorders may be of concern. Evidence of a bleeding disorder warrants analysis of specific clotting studies. Laboratory values as simple as the complete blood count, which includes hemoglobin, hematocrit, white cell count, platelet levels, and cell differential, can provide a very good picture of the child's hematologic status. These values vary among age groups. In the newborn, neutropenia rather than neutrophilia is a more common indicator of sepsis (Burke & Salani, 2013).

FLUID BALANCE

Physiologic differences in children make them more vulnerable to changes in their fluid status. Water and electrolyte distribution varies drastically from infancy to adulthood. In general, the amount of water content decreases with age and changes in areas of distribution. The BSA is proportionately much greater in infants and children than in adults. This leads to increased loss of insensible fluid through perspiration through the skin. The preterm neonate is estimated to have a BSA that is five times greater than that of an older child or adult (Ellett, 2009).

The newborn has the largest proportion of free water in the extracellular spaces. At a rate of exchange seven times greater than that of the adult, the infant exchanges approximately half of its total extracellular fluid daily. The basal metabolism rate is also twice as great in relation to body weight in the infant as it is in the adult.

PATIENT SAFETY

An awareness of dehydration is a safety imperative. Dehydration or contraction of the body fluid compartments will occur whenever the loss of water and salt exceeds the intake. Fever, sweating and diarrhea produce losses in excess of normal.

As the child matures, there is a fluid shift from the extracellular fluid compartment. After the first year, total body water content decreases and distribution gradually changes to less fluid in the extracellular fluid compartments and more fluid in the intracellular fluid compartments. By the age of 2, 24% of body water is in the extracellular fluid, approximately equal to that of an adult.

ELECTROLYTES

Infants and children are especially prone to fluid and electrolyte imbalances because their bodies consist of more water in proportion to surface area than those of adults. Moreover, their immature body organs compromise their ability to handle imbalances.

Laboratory values to monitor in children include sodium, potassium, chloride, calcium, and glucose. In particular, plasma sodium concentration does not vary greatly from infancy to adulthood. In the premature neonate and full-term neonate, potassium and chloride concentrations are higher than any other time, whereas magnesium and calcium levels in the infant are lower than in older children and adults. Phosphate levels remain slightly higher than adult levels until about 5 years of age, at which time electrolyte parameters are within normal adult ranges.

Gastrointestinal disturbances, such as diarrhea, most often alter potassium levels. Children usually do not experience cardiac symptoms until the serum potassium falls below 3 mEq/L. Hyperkalemia is more common, especially in premature infants. The hallmarks of hyperkalemia in children are similar to those in adults—peaked T waves and widening of the QRS complex and ST segment depression on the electrocardiogram (Blayney, 2013).

Other common electrolyte imbalances in children include hypocalcemia, hyponatremia or hypernatremia (as seen with dehydration), and chloride disturbances. Infants are especially prone to hypocalcemia due to the increase of calcium deposition in the bones during times of stress and growth hormone secretion. Hypocalcemia is also attributed to blood transfusion with citrate preservative, pancreatitis, newborn intake of cow's milk, vitamin D deficiency, and malabsorption. Conversely, lower calcium can result from excessive use of diuretics, tumor lysis syndrome during the initiation of chemotherapy, and immobilization (Roberts, 2013; Secola & Reid, 2008).

ASSESSING FLUID NEEDS

The amount of fluid required for maintenance levels depends on insensible water losses from the lungs, skin, urine, and stool output. Metabolic expenditures are an additional consideration when computing fluid requirements. Younger children have a higher fluid requirement due to a higher percentage of total body water. Requirements vary among term, low birth weight, and premature, high-risk infants. Adolescent fluid requirements are similar to those for adults.

A precise record of intake and output is the most valuable assessment tool for determining fluid requirements. To ensure accuracy in judging fluid needs, strict monitoring of intake and output, including diaper weights, for children receiving infusion therapy is essential. Infants have a greater urine volume per kilogram of body weight and a smaller bladder volume capacity than older children. Expected urine output with adequate intake should be 2 to 3 mL/kg/h for infants, 2 mL/kg/h for toddlers, 1 to 2 mL/kg/h for school-age children, and 0.5 to 1 mL/kg/h for adolescents (Hazinski, 2013).

MAINTENANCE REQUIREMENTS

Maintenance fluid requirements for neonates and children differ in terms of the volume allowed over 24 hours, but all fluid need calculations are in milliliters per kilogram of weight (Hazinski, 2013). There are multiple methods of assessing 24-hour maintenance fluids based on weight or meters squared (Ellett, 2009; Hazinski, 2013). These methods address only maintenance requirements for normal metabolism; they do not address insensible losses or additional metabolic expenditures that require further replacement therapy.

> In the weight method, the most commonly used fluid estimates are based on the child's weight in kilograms. The advantage of this method is its simplicity (Table 21-7).
>
> In the meters-squared method, the child's height and weight are plotted on a nomogram to obtain a surface area in meters squared (m^2). This method uses an arbitrary estimated requirement of 1,500 to 1,800 mL of fluid per square meter.

Alterations in Fluid Needs

The most common cause of altered fluid and caloric needs is changes in temperature. In the neonate, the use of radiant warmers and single-walled incubators may effectively maintain the newborn's temperature, but this temperature elevation in turn increases the infant's insensible fluid losses. Phototherapy, although effectively used to treat newborn hyperbilirubinemia, increases insensible fluid losses and water requirements. These various losses must be included when determining fluid replacement needs. Other conditions that affect fluid requirements include diarrhea and nasogastric tube output.

TABLE 21	CALCULATING MAINTENANCE FLUID REQUIREMENTS
Newborn	60–100 mL/kg/24 h (up to 72 h of age)
0–10 kg	100 mL/kg/24 h for the first 10 kg
11–20 kg	100 mL/kg/24 h for the first 10 kg, plus 50 mL/kg/24 h for each kg >10 kg
21–30 kg	100 mL/kg/24 h for the second 10 kg, plus 50 mL/kg/24 h for each kg >10 kg, plus 20 mL/kg/24 h for each kg >20 kg

TABLE 21-8	ASSESSMENT: PARAMETERS FOR DETERMINING THE LEVEL OF DEHYDRATION		
	Level of Dehydration		
Parameter	**Mild**	**Moderate**	**Severe**
Alertness	Normal	Normal to listless	Normal to lethargic or comatose
Blood pressure	Normal	Normal	Normal to reduced
Eyes	Normal	Sunken orbits	Deeply sunken orbits
Extremities	Warm, normal capillary refill	Delayed capillary refill	Cook and mottled
Fontanel	n/a	Sunken	Sunken
Heart rate	Normal	Increased	Increased; bradycardia may be present
Mucous membranes	Slightly dry	Dry	Dry
Pulse	Normal	Normal or slightly decreased	Moderately decreased
Skin turgor	Normal	Decreased	Decreased
Urine output	Slightly decreased	<1 mL/kg/h	<0.5–1 mL/kg/h
Weight loss	3%–5%	6%–9%	≥10%

DEHYDRATION

Dehydration can occur rapidly in children who lose more water than they receive. Being alert for signs of dehydration is an important aspect of caring for pediatric patients. Physical assessment parameters for dehydration are outlined in Table 21-8.

The classifications of dehydration are type, depending on the level of serum sodium, and by degree, depending on the weight loss, patient history, and physical assessment. The three types of dehydration are as follows:

- Isotonic—sodium is within normal limits and electrolyte and water deficits are equal (e.g., mild vomiting and diarrhea).
- Hypertonic—sodium is elevated and water losses are greater than electrolyte losses (e.g., too concentrated formula intake).
- Hypotonic—sodium is low and electrolyte losses are greater than water losses or water intake is large (e.g., diabetes insipidus, drowning in fresh water) (Ellett, 2009).

To determine the degree of dehydration, nurses must calculate the percentage of weight lost. For each 1% of weight loss, the patient has a loss of 10 mL/kg of fluid, requiring replacement in addition to maintenance and ongoing losses. If a child presents with severe dehydration, administration of a fluid bolus of normal saline or lactated Ringer's at a dosage of 20 to 40 mL/kg is necessary. Oral rehydration is initiated at a rate of 50 to 100 mL/kg if the child is mildly to moderately dehydrated. Infusion therapy continues if the child does not tolerate oral rehydration therapy or the child's condition warrants IV correction.

Fluid Overload

Fluid overload and intoxication are less common than dehydration but can occur more readily in infants, whose immature kidneys are unable to excrete excess fluid. A serum sodium <130 mEq/L in an infant that is not associated with dehydration is a sign of water intoxication (Perkin, deCaen, Berg, Schexnayder, & Hazinski, 2013). Treatment includes reducing fluid delivery and administering IV furosemide.

Acid–Base Balance

Acid–base balance is part of the overall picture of fluid balance. In the neonate and infant, higher BSA equals increased metabolism and more production of waste products requiring excretion. Buffering mechanisms are less mature, resulting in a deficit of bicarbonate. Combined with increased production of waste and an immature renal system, metabolic acidosis is more common in this age group (Hazinski, 2013). As the infant matures, pH ranges approach normal parameters of 7.35 to 7.45.

When a child has diarrhea, he or she loses bicarbonate in the stool resulting in a metabolic acidosis. Conversely, when a child is vomiting or has a nasogastric tube, metabolic alkalosis can result from the large amount of acid lost in gastric secretions. When replacing electrolytes, frequent monitoring of laboratory values and fluid balance is necessary to prevent acid–base imbalances.

Parenteral Nutrition

Parenteral nutrition (PN) is the intravenous administration of nutrients, including sterile water, carbohydrate in the form of dextrose, fat, protein in the form of amino acids, electrolytes, vitamins, minerals, trace elements, and medications. PN support should only be used when feeding into the gastrointestinal tract is contraindicated or inadequate. PN has become one of the most important therapeutic parameters in the successful management of certain pediatric diseases, but it does not come without its risks, and close monitoring is necessary. Specific guidelines have not been determined, but in general, PN is started if it is anticipated that an undernourished infant will not be able to receive enteral feeds for 1 to 2 days, if a well-nourished infant will not be able to receive enteral feeds for 3 to 5 days, and if a well-nourished child will not be able to receive enteral feeds for 5 to 7 days. Infants born prematurely typically start on PN support within 24 hours of birth due to low nutrient stores (Davis, 1998; Koletzko, Goulet, Hunt, Krohn, & Shamir, 2005).

PN can be supplied via a peripheral access or central access depending on the strength of the solution. Peripheral access limits the amount of calories that can be provided because the osmolarity maximum for a peripheral line is 900 mOsm/L. Given the density of certain PN additives, this means a very large volume would have to be supplied to meet the patient's calorie needs, which are usually not possible due to fluid restrictions. Therefore, peripheral PN is used for short-term benefit; usually <2 weeks. If full nutrition support is needed, PN needs to be administered through a form of central access. Some examples of conditions that may need full PN support are prematurity, diaphragmatic hernia, gastroschisis, malrotation/volvulus, necrotizing enterocolitis, abdominal trauma, and chylothorax (Samour & King, 2012).

With the addition of PN to their therapy, affected children can be expected to gain weight normally with only parenteral nutrients. In addition, PN supplies enough calories to maintain the positive nitrogen balance required for normal growth and development. The parameters used to determine caloric needs are age, resting energy requirements, level of physical activity, and severity of illness.

Constituents of Parental Nutrition

Usually, hospital or home IV agency pharmacy staff formulate PN solutions and perform admixture of solutions under a laminar-airflow hood. As stated previously, the general constituents for PN are protein, carbohydrates, fat, electrolytes, minerals, trace elements, vitamins, and medications. Pediatric requirements for IV nutrition follow general guidelines and are based on protein, calorie, and fluid needs per kilogram of body weight.

Protein for PN solutions is provided in the form of crystalline amino acids, which deliver 4 cal/g. Amino acid solutions for infants contain similar amino acids that are found in the plasma of breast-fed infants. The type of amino acids used to make the solution cause the pH to be lower, which is excellent for the neonate because this allows more calcium and phosphate to be added without precipitating, which is imperative for bone development. Protein may be limited in patients with cirrhosis with encephalopathy, in patients with chronic kidney disease who are not on dialysis, and in patients who have protein metabolism or urea cycle disorders. Conversely, examples of instances when protein needs may be increased are in patients with burns, sepsis, large wounds, and after trauma (Corkins et al., 2010).

Carbohydrates are provided as dextrose, which provides energy for body tissue function. If carbohydrate supply is inadequate, the body breaks down protein or fat to provide metabolic needs. Dextrose, administered in milligram per kilogram per minute increments, provides the main calorie source and typically provides 40% to 60% of the total calorie goal (6 to 14 mg/kg/min infusion rates). Dextrose in PN is in monohydrate form, so it provides not 4 kcal/g but 3.4 kcal/g. For example, 100 mL of 5% dextrose in water solution contains 5 g dextrose, or 17 kcal, and 100 mL of 10% dextrose in water solution contains 10 g dextrose, or 34 kcal. The strength of dextrose that can be administered peripherally in a child is 12.5%. Greater concentrations given through a peripheral IV can cause sclerosis, phlebitis, and extravasation injury if infiltration occurs. Although concentrated dextrose is needed to provide calories, the volume of fluid needed to dilute very concentrated dextrose is often deleterious to fluid balance in children, especially neonates. Higher concentrations of dextrose (up to 25%) in less volume of fluid may be delivered by a central catheter (Corkins et al., 2010).

The other source of nonprotein calories is lipids, delivered as a fat emulsion used to supply essential fatty acids that are needed for brain and somatic growth, immune system function, skin integrity, and wound healing. IV fat emulsions in the United States contain egg phospholipids as an emulsifier, water, and soybean or safflower oil as a source of polyunsaturated fats. Originally, fat infusion was kept to a minimum (only 2% to 10% of daily calorie intake) because it was thought that a higher fat intake resulted in pulmonary changes. This hyperlipidemia is now thought to have been brought on by rapid infusion rates, so a slower infusion rate over longer period is now the rule. Fat emulsions come in strengths of 10%, with 1.1 kcal/mL, and 20%, with 2 kcal/mL. Both may be infused peripherally or centrally, but the 20% solution is used most often. The typical lipid dosage for infants is between 2.5 and 3 g/kg/d, which equals 25% to 30% of total energy needs. Children over 2 years of age should also receive approximately 30% of their total calorie goal from lipids (Finberg et al., 1986). Fat should not provide more than 60% of total calories in any patient because ketotic acidosis may occur (Sapsford, 1994).

EVIDENCE FOR PRACTICE

Do the nutritional benefits of lipid emulsions outweigh the potential risks of adverse effects on the immune system?

Micronutrients, minerals, vitamins, and trace elements are added to the PN solution in amounts established for IV maintenance requirements, based on recommended dietary allowances. Because calcium, phosphorus, and magnesium are incompletely absorbed from the gastrointestinal tract, IV dosages are much lower than the recommendations for oral intake. Calcium and phosphorous may precipitate in the PN solution when higher levels are prescribed; adjustment of the protein and pH level of the solution may assist in solubility. The yellow color of the total peripheral nutrition (TPN) solution results from the addition of multivitamins. Because multivitamins limit the shelf life of TPN, patients on home TPN are taught to add vitamins and other medication additives such as heparin immediately prior to infusion.

In some cases, **total nutrient admixtures** (TNA), in which all the nutrients are added to one bag, have been used in children. One major disadvantage of these three-in-one solutions is that the opacity of the lipids prevents the patient or caregiver from visually examining the bag for calcium–phosphate precipitates. The more common practice is to infuse the dextrose/amino acid solution separately in one bag, using a 0.22-µm filter into one arm of a Y set, and to infuse the fat, unfiltered, into the other arm of the Y. These smaller positively charged filters are able to remove microorganisms, gram-negative endotoxins, and reduce the risk of air embolism. If a TNA solution is used, a larger 1.2-µm filter must be used to allow for the lipid droplet to pass through. These filters can prevent particulate matter and larger organisms from passing through but are not able to filter out the smaller bacterial contaminants. Two-in-one infusion sets should be changed out at a minimum of every 72 hours and three-in-one (TNA) and lipid infusion sets should be changed out as soon as the infusion is done, or if the patient needs additional infusions, at least every 24 hours (Koletzko et al., 2005; Mirtallo, Canada, & Johnson, 2004).

Nursing Assessment and Management

Once the child has been deemed a candidate for PN, a complete physical assessment including height, weight, head circumference, and nutrition and laboratory evaluations is completed by the physician/licensed independent practitioner (LIP), dietitian, and other members of the nutrition support team. Duration and route of PN are determined, and the appropriate catheter is placed. Initiation, advancement, and goals vary depending on age groups.

Infusions may run over 24 hours for the very sick hospitalized child or may be cycled down gradually by 4-hour increments daily, maintaining the same volume of infusion over less time. Cycling down to between 12 and 16 hours of daily infusion allows the child far more freedom. This is particularly true for children on home PN, who may infuse at night while asleep and still follow a fairly normal lifestyle of school and activities. Cycling the PN also may prevent or delay the onset of liver dysfunction (Btaiche & Khalidi, 2002). To prevent wide variations in serum glucose, the PN rate can be run at half the rate for the first and last hours of the cycle to lessen the likelihood of hypo-/hyperglycemia. Most infusion pumps can be programmed to taper up and down at the start and end of PN infusion for ease of delivery (Kirby, Corrigan, & Emery, 2012).

TABLE 21-9	SIGNIFICANT LABORATORY VALUES FOR THE PATIENT RECEIVING PARENTERAL NUTRITION		
Parameter	Interpretation	High Value	Low Value
Prealbumin	Preterm: 9–33 mg/dL Term: 11–34 mg/dL Older children: 20–50 mg/dL	Dehydration	Acute protein malnutrition Infection Aggressive hydration
Transferrin	Preterm: 140–370 mg/dL Term: 200–370 mg/dL Older children: 180–260 mg/dL	Iron deficiency Hypoxia Chronic blood loss Stress	Impaired synthesis Protein malnutrition Chronic infection Chronic liver disease
Albumin	Preterm: 2.5–4.5 g/dL Term: 2.5–5.0 g/dL 1–3 mo: 3.0–4.2 g/dL 3–12 mo: 2.7–5.0 g/dL >1 y: 3.2–5.0 g/dL	Dehydration	Protein malnutrition Impaired digestion Excessive protein loss Chronic liver disease Advanced malignancy Hypervolumic dilution Chronic infection Nephrotic syndrome

The nurse frequently monitors the patient's physical status and screens, intervenes for, and reports abnormal findings: temperature spikes, inappropriate glucose spills, chills, rashes, irritability, decreased level of consciousness, and any change in growth or clinical picture. The nurse immediately reports any observable abnormality to the nutrition team. Results of various serum chemistry and hematology tests are assessed daily for the first week and then weekly for the stable patient in the hospital or at home. Significant laboratory values are listed in Table 21-9.

Another major area of nursing intervention in the child receiving PN is psychological support. Most such patients are acutely ill infants. Even though a child on central PN may be NPO (*nil per os* or *nothing by mouth*), cuddling and holding the child should assist in meeting maternal needs. Also, allowing parents and caregivers every opportunity to participate in their child's care is extremely important. First, the nurse should assess the family's level of comprehension about PN and intervene by offering support to decrease parental anxiety. As soon as the decision is made to place the child on PN, it is best to use the preoperative teaching methodology of explaining purpose, procedure, and potential complications. Of course, all further questions can be handled daily. Permitting this open channel of communication not only supplies parents with the knowledge they need to become involved, but also assists them in comprehending the purpose of PN and why adherence to protocols is so important.

COMPLICATIONS

Disadvantages of PN are its potential complications. Every nurse must fully understand the possible complications of PN, including the specific symptoms of each. Complications are subdivided into two categories: catheter related and metabolic.

Catheter-related complications have been previously addressed. Metabolic complications include the following:

- Glucose disturbances
- Electrolyte imbalances

- Mineral disturbances
- Acid–base imbalance
- Hepatic disorders
- Metabolic bone disease
- Refeeding syndrome
- Vitamin and mineral status for patients on long-term PN support

Close attention to detail during the initial assessment and ongoing monitoring can treat or even prevent most of these complications. Some predisposing metabolic abnormalities, however, may require immediate medical intervention. With the incremental advances in technology and the formation of nutrition support teams, the incidences of even the more common complications have decreased to acceptable rates.

INFUSION THERAPIES FOR NEONATES AND CHILDREN

Transfusion Therapy

This section provides an overview of the therapeutics unique to pediatric patients. Transfusions of blood and blood components may be administered to a child through a peripheral IV for one-time or infrequent transfusion or through a central device for chronic transfusions. Because transfusion carries the risk of iron buildup, children with prescribed chronic transfusion therapy are often on IV chelating agents in addition to transfusion therapy.

INDICATIONS FOR TRANSFUSION THERAPY

In general, indications for transfusion therapy in children include acute hemorrhage, anemia, abnormal component function or component deficiency, and removal of harmful substances, such as bilirubin, during exchange transfusion. An acute reduction in blood volume of a child can produce clinical evidence of shock. When 5% to 10% of the child's circulating blood volume is lost and/or additional blood loss is expected, transfusion is indicated (Hazinski, 2013). Decreased production or altered function of platelets usually results from a maternal problem or disorder (e.g., prenatal aspirin intake), congenital disorder, acquired disorder (e.g., ITP), or chemotherapy-induced thrombocytopenia.

The most common blood components given to children are packed red blood cells (PRBCs). The volume of PRBCs to be administered is weight based and typically 10 to 15 mL/kg unless significant blood loss has occurred.

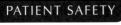

PATIENT SAFETY

Pediatricians request blood and blood products in milliliters per kilogram increments instead of units because a single unit of PRBCs may equal the entire blood volume of several infants.

Platelets, fresh frozen plasma (FFP), and plasma derivatives given for congenital or acquired lack of dysfunction of that component are dosed on volume, and replacement needs are titrated to desired therapeutic effect. Blood products may be modified before transfusion through several methods to reduce the risk of complications in at-risk children. These modifications include irradiation, leukocyte depletion, and warming.

Irradiation reduces the ability of leukocytes to engraft in the patient and reduces the risk of graft versus host disease in an immunocompromised recipient (Conte, 2008). Irradiation should occur just prior to administration to limit the adverse effects of processing. Recipients of irradiated blood include transplant recipients, children with lymphoma or leukemia, and neonates. Leukocyte depletion, by one of several methods, reduces the risk of febrile, nonhemolytic reactions, especially in patients who have had multiple prior transfusions. Leukocyte-depleted red cells and platelets also are given to prevent alloimmunization in children who receive platelets frequently or transmission of cytomegalovirus (CMV) when CMV-negative blood products are not available.

Warmed blood products, heated in a controlled system, are used in exchange transfusions, patients with cold agglutinin disease, hypothermic patients, and in those receiving large amounts of blood quickly. Although not indicated for routine transfusion therapy, warming reduces the chance of hypothermia, dysrhythmias, and cardiac arrest in these situations.

Indications for transfusion of platelets, plasma, and plasma components are similar to those in adults. Table 21-10 lists some parameters for blood component therapy in children.

For the first several days of life, the mother's serum is used for compatibility testing. In infants older than 1 week and those previously transfused, compatibility testing is done on the child's blood. Group O red blood cells that are Rh negative or the same Rh as the infant's are used frequently. In addition, red blood cells are tested for CMV and are given to neonates only if CMV negative. The freshest cells possible are used to avoid potassium loading in infants.

Blood and blood products in children may be administered by a 24-gauge peripheral catheter in neonates and by a 24- or 22-gauge catheter in older children. As stated by Keller (1995), "A review of the literature revealed that red blood cells could safely be transfused through needles smaller than 18 to 20 gauge at relatively high infusion rates without increasing the risk of hemolysis." A pump capable of infusing blood is recommended for

TABLE 21-10	PARAMETERS FOR BLOOD COMPONENT THERAPY	
Product	Indication	Dosage/Rate of Administration
RBC	Anemia without volume expansion	10 mL/kg, not to exceed 15 mL/kg at 2–5 mL/kg/h
Albumin	Hypovolemia	5%: 10–20 mL/kg as fast as tolerated 25%: 2–4 mL/kg over 30–60 min via pump
Cryoprecipitate	Factor replacement due to congenital disease	1 unit/5 kg not faster than 1 mL/kg/min; IV push or drip
FFP	Volume expansion; increase levels of plasma coagulation factors in children with deficiency	Acute hemorrhage: 15–30 mL/kg as indicated Clotting deficiency: 10–15 mL/kg at 1–2 mL/min IV push or drip
Platelets	Control bleeding associated with deficiency in number or function (count <20,000 or <50,000 in presence of active bleeding)	1 unit (50–70 mL)/7–10-kg body weight Administer over 30 min to maximum of 4 h; IV push or drip

transfusion therapy in children; in neonates, blood may be prefiltered by the blood bank and then infused from a syringe on a syringe pump. In children, volume and fluid balance considerations negate the simultaneous infusion of saline, particularly in neonates; instead, the peripheral or central IV device must be flushed with 1 to 3 mL saline before and after the transfusion. The rate of blood transfusion may be very slow or even staggered with boluses of dextrose in neonates. A total volume of 50 mL or 20% ordered: whichever is smallest, should be administered slowly over the first 15 minutes, and then the rate is increased to an hourly IV rate tolerated by the child (Bryant, 2009).

NURSING ASSESSMENT AND MANAGEMENT

Central venous pressure (CVP) is the best indicator for restoration of blood volume to normal; the pulse rate is less reliable, and 24 to 36 hours may pass before hemoglobin reflects the true extent of blood loss. A red blood cell mass deficit occurs with chronic anemia; transfusion with packed cells is not indicated until the hemoglobin level drops below 7 g/dL (Carson et al., 2012). The patient's cardiopulmonary status, activity level, and hemoglobin should be assessed before transfusion because an unstressed child can tolerate hemoglobin values quite low without showing signs of heart failure. The most common form of anemia seen in children is iron deficiency anemia (which rarely is treated with transfusion); other treatments may be indicated, including iron therapy, folic acid, or vitamin B_{12} (Bryant, 2009).

EXCHANGE TRANSFUSION

Exchange transfusion is a procedure in which most or all of the blood volume is replaced with compatible red blood cells and plasma from one or several donors. Exchange transfusion was first used in the early 1950s for management of hemolytic disease of the newborn. Other indications include hyperbilirubinemia, sickle cell vasoocclusive crisis, and polycythemia. Exchange transfusions optimally are undertaken using two IV sites or an IV and an intra-arterial site. A combination of peripheral, central, or umbilical access devices can be used.

Various types of exchange transfusion exist with the disease state and desired volume of blood exchanged determining the approach: single, double, or partial exchange. A double-volume or two-volume exchange usually is performed when exchange transfusion equals twice the patient's blood volume. Ideally, two vascular access sites are used to allow simultaneous withdrawal and infusion. Common sites include the umbilical vessels and peripheral or central veins. If only one access is available, the push–pull method is used. Calcium and dextrose levels are monitored closely during the exchange because blood preservatives may cause levels to decrease. Complications can include those similar to volume overload, catheter complications, and transfusion therapy (Bryant, 2009).

POSSIBLE COMPLICATIONS

As with other therapies, transfusion therapy is not without risks. Potential complications include acute hemolytic reactions, nonhemolytic reactions (e.g., febrile and allergic reactions), alloimmunization, circulatory overload, infectious disease transmission, and coagulopathy (Bryant, 2009). The type of reaction may be difficult to ascertain initially.

Pharmacology and Pharmacokinetics

Children respond differently to medications than adults. There are age-related differences that occur secondary to physiologic changes affecting the absorption, distribution, metabolism, and excretion of drugs. Illness and disease states also affect the child's ability to properly metabolize and excrete medications.

Oral absorption depends on a number of age-related variables, including pH, gastric emptying time, gastric transit time, surface area of the small intestine, and pancreatic enzymes. Infants and children have an immature, thinner layer of epidermis and increased skin hydration that increases the percutaneous absorption of medication. In addition, infants have a larger body surface area–to-weight ratio, increasing the relative amount of medication being absorbed. Intramuscular and subcutaneous absorption is variable and unpredictable in neonates and infants because they have less muscle mass and subcutaneous fat, with a higher proportion of total body water (Gostisha & Braby, 1999).

Intravenous administration usually guarantees proper delivery of medications; however, physical growth and development affects the distribution of drugs. The volume of distribution changes with both the drug and with the age of the patient. Neonates and infants have decreased levels of plasma protein, serum albumin, and altered plasma protein binding; therefore, some drugs that bind with plasma proteins will not bind in the neonate and infant. This results in higher amounts of circulating unbound drugs that can increase adverse effects (Yaffe & Aranda, 2011).

Neonates and infants have a higher proportion of body fluid for weight, which results in the volume of distribution being greatest for neonates. It decreases as the child matures and children achieve adult levels by the age of 12. Lipid-soluble drugs have a decreased distribution volume due to the lower percentage of fat tissue in neonates and infants. Reaching levels equivalent to that of adults by puberty, boys have an average of 12% body fat, with girls averaging 25% body fat.

Drug metabolism primarily occurs in the liver and is determined by age. The newborn infant has a prolonged half-life of some drugs due to the immature drug metabolic degradation system. Liver function reaches adult levels between 1 and 2 years of age. Pediatric patients may need more frequent dosage intervals of many drugs, due to their increased metabolism. Drug metabolism reaches adult levels at puberty (Gostisha & Braby, 1999).

Drug excretion occurs mainly in the renal system. Less efficient renal function due to immaturity in the neonate or disease process in the older child may decrease excretion of drugs, causing longer half-life and possible toxicity. Neonates have decreased renal blood flow, glomerular filtration rate (GFR), and tubular function. Renal blood flow reaches adult levels at 5 to 12 months of age, GFR at 3 to 5 months of age, and renal tubular function at 7 to 8 months of age (Blayney, 2013). Children 2 to 6 years of age generally excrete drugs very rapidly; this process gradually slows down as they approach puberty.

Pediatric medications are dosed by weight; however, many physiologic functions that affect drug clearance do not scale directly to weight (Yaffe & Aranda, 2011). Therapeutic drug monitoring can prevent serious toxic problems. While there are reference books available, as well as online information, appropriate pediatric drug dosing is best done with a consultation by a pediatric registered pharmacist who is skilled in kinetics and can monitor the patient's clinical status and response to drug therapy (Bradley & Nelson, 2010; Yaffe & Aranda, 2011). Drug serum levels are useful for monitoring the effectiveness of drug therapy in children.

PATIENT SAFETY

If at all possible, manipulation of medications should be performed by a pharmacist to ensure appropriate dilution and sterility.

Remember to practice the five rights of medication administration (right person, right medication, right dose, right route, and right time) with all pediatric patients. Dosing is weight and renal function dependent.

Monitoring of aminoglycosides can prevent ototoxicity and nephrotoxicity in neonates and infants who often have impaired renal function. Drug monitoring is especially important when any age child presents with renal and/or hepatic failure. A free drug level (rather than serum concentration) is diagnostic for highly protein bound drugs in neonates who have low albumin concentrations.

Obtaining trough levels, or the lowest drug level, just before a scheduled drug administration, will guide in therapeutic drug management. Trough levels are appropriate for antiseizure medications and for medications such as digoxin, which takes considerable time to distribute to the tissue receptors. A peak drug level, or highest drug level, is drawn 30 minutes after the drug and postflush have infused. Peak concentrations monitor drugs with short half-lives and for determining toxicity.

In many cases, drugs are not FDA approved for pediatric IV administration but are used based on the ongoing and published research studies, experience with adults, and the emergency status of the child. For this reason, children are often referred to as therapeutic orphans, indicating the lack of information about interactions between medications and children's body processes (Anderson, 2011).

CONDITIONS AND DISEASE STATES

Certain conditions are diagnosed early in life and require a basic understanding so that holistic treatment plans incorporating developmental considerations can be formulated. Primary indications for pediatric infusion include fluid therapy, medication administration, antineoplastic therapy, nutritional support, and transfusion therapy. While certainly not all encompassing, included below is a summary of a few key conditions that commonly require infusion therapy.

Blood Disorders

SICKLE CELL DISEASE

Sickle cell disease (SCD), a chronic and potentially life-threatening disorder, is caused by inheriting an autosomal recessive gene that causes a group of blood disorders. In the United States, SCD is the most commonly inherited disorder with 8,000 new cases identified, by way of newborn screening, annually (Savage, 2008). One in every 500 African American births and 1 in every 36,000 Hispanic American births are diagnosed with sickle cell anemia. Sickle cell trait is a genetic marker that does not cause SCD in carriers, and children with the trait are generally healthy. However, when two individuals with sickle trait have children together, the risk of a child being born with SCD is 25% (http://www.nhlbi.nih.gov/health/health-topics/topics/sca/atrisk.html).

There are several types of SCD, with the most common in the United States being sickle cell anemia, sickle-hemoglobin C disease, and sickle β-plus thalassemia. Sickle cell anemia is the formation of abnormally shaped, typically described as sickle shaped, red blood cells that do not flow through blood vessels easily and obstruct normal flow along the bloodstream leading to organ ischemia if not treated. Normal red blood cells are smooth and flow with ease. Sickle-shaped cells are stiff and sticky and cause vasoocclusion of the microcirculation. Vasoocclusion of the microcirculation results in pain episodes, tissue damage, organ ischemia, stroke, and eventually organ death (Bryant, 2009).

Stressful conditions, such as illness, acidosis, dehydration, and temperature elevation, can enhance sickling. As red blood cells "sickle" from a lack of oxygen, they clump and slow blood flow, resulting in hemolytic anemia and acute and chronic tissue damage secondary to vasoocclusion. These painful episodes, which are unpredictable and vary in severity, are commonly referred to as sickle cell crises. Blockage of blood flow through vessels results in lung tissue damage (acute chest syndrome), pain episodes (arms, legs, chest, and abdomen), stroke, and priapism (painful prolonged erection). Damage to the spleen makes SCD patients, especially young children, easily overwhelmed by certain bacterial infections. Anemia is usually present, and chronic ischemia can damage liver, kidneys, bone, brain, and tissue.

Early treatment is essential to prevent worsening of pain and major complications such as progressive organ failure. Most pain episodes are treated at home with medications, such as ibuprofen, acetaminophen with codeine, or morphine for severe pain. Increased oral fluids, a heating pad applied to the affected area (cold should be avoided as it increases sickling), deep breathing exercises, and distraction methods such as music, videotapes, and imagery, as well as alternative medicine treatments, may help with pain relief. If patients become febrile or if oral **pain management** is inadequate, many pediatric centers treating sickle cell crises provide fast track admission and treatment with IV fluids, electrolytes, blood/exchange transfusions, antibiotics, and pain management, incorporating an age-appropriate pain assessment tool. Sickle cell centers use an effective team approach to manage the sickle cell patient, including a physician/ LIP, nurse practitioner, nurses, psychologists, social worker, child life therapist, nutrition counselor, and pain management team. SCD is not yet curable, although hydroxyurea, erythropoietin, and bone marrow transplants do offer hope in specific cases (Bryant, 2009; Savage, 2008).

Hemophilia

The term hemophilia describes a group of inherited coagulation disorders that occur when one or more coagulation proteins are missing or malfunction. Deficiency of factor VIII, often called hemophilia A or classic hemophilia, is the most common factor deficiency, followed by hemophilia B (Christmas disease or factor IX deficiency) and hemophilia C, or factor XI deficiency. Hemophilia, transmitted as an X-linked recessive disorder, commonly appears in males and is transmitted by females (Bryant, 2009).

Diagnosis is often made after an unusual bleeding episode and by eliciting a history of bleeding disorders or prolonged bleeding. Laboratory testing includes tests for hemostasis as well as specific clotting factor assays. In hemophilia, platelet function tests such as platelet counts and bleeding time will be normal, whereas factor assays may be abnormal.

Malfunction or absence of these coagulation factors result in a tendency to have excessive bruising and prolonged bleeding, especially following tooth loss, trauma or surgery, and menstruation. Bleeding can manifest itself as subcutaneous, intramuscular, hemarthrosis, hematuria, and epistaxis (Bryant, 2009).

Primary therapy for treating hemophilia is IV replacement of the missing clotting factors (recombinant factors VIII or IX) or the administration of drugs that stimulate release of clotting factors (desmopressin acetate) or prevent clot destruction (aminocaproic acid [Amicar]) (Bryant, 2009). Treatment may also involve applying local and topical therapies to the affected area, such as ice, elevation, rest, splinting, and pressure bandage wrapping. For therapy, patients may require long-term IV access, such as an implanted central port (Figure 21-2). Parents often give therapies at home when an episode of bleeding occurs. Immediate treatment allows for quick resolution of bleeding and decreases the likeliness of complications. In addition, patients will receive prophylactic treatment prior to dental work and surgical procedures.

Other goals of treatment include the prevention of bleeding, recognizing and controlling bleeding, and maintaining mobility and physical fitness while preventing long-term injuries. Engaging families in the treatment plan is essential for long-term health. Clinical research trials for gene therapy hold promise for the future (http://www.nhlbi.nih.gov/health/health-topics/topics/hemophilia/treatment.html).

IMMUNODEFICIENCIES

The infant acquires circulating antibodies from the mother during the last several prenatal weeks; therefore, premature infants have a less efficient humoral immunity. With exposure to outside antigens, the infant's antibody production begins. Children with primary or secondary immune compromise often receive immunoglobulin replacement therapy or bone marrow–stimulating colony factors. Infusion of IV gamma globulin or IV IgG (IVIG) warrants specific mention because the use of this plasma derivative in children has grown substantially since the 1980s, when safe, effective IV preparations became licensed in the United States. IVIG is used as an adjunctive therapy for those with a severe bacterial infection who require a boost in passive immunity as well as supportive therapy for those patients with deficiencies of the humoral immune system, such as, severe combined immunodeficiency syndrome (SCIDS), common variable immune deficiency, and idiopathic thrombocytopenic purpura.

SEVERE COMBINED IMMUNODEFICIENCY SYNDROME

SCIDS is a primary genetic immunodeficiency in where there is a lack of humoral and cell-mediated immunity. The absence of functioning T cells and B cells leaves the infant at risk for severe if not fatal infections. Diagnosis is often made early in infancy with a history of recurrent or rare infections. Hematopoietic stem cell transplant is the definitive treatment; however, supportive care until transplant includes infusion of IVIG and bacterial and fungal prophylaxis. Preventing infection and providing support to the family are the priorities of care for these patients (Bryant, 2009).

Childhood Cancer

Because of research, new drug combinations, and aggressive therapy, the mortality rate for children with cancer has decreased greatly since the 1960s with an overall survival rate of >80%. Still, cancer remains the primary cause of death from disease in children (Hockenberry, 2008). Common cancers in children include leukemias, central nervous system tumors, lymphoma, neuroblastoma, Wilms tumor, rhabdomyosarcoma, lymphoma, and osteosarcoma. The suspected causes of cancers in children remain unknown and continue to challenge

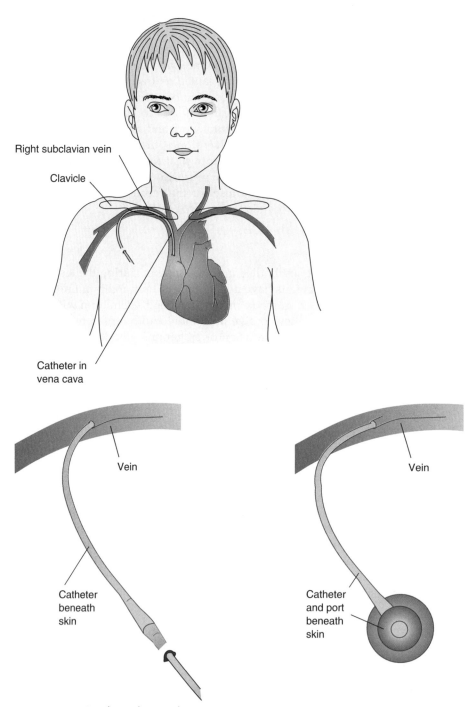

FIGURE 21-2 Implanted central port.

epidemiologists. Specialists continue to look for associations between genetic factors, environmental (toxins, chemical agents), and infectious agents.

LEUKEMIAS

Leukemia, specifically acute lymphoblastic leukemia is the most common malignancy in children. Immature white blood cells proliferate in the bone marrow, spleen, and lymphatic tissue, causing symptoms such as anemia, bone or joint pain, anorexia, fever, abdominal pain, hepatosplenomegaly, tachycardia, heat and exercise intolerance, ecchymosis, and other signs of abnormal clotting, general malaise, and pallor. Subtypes of leukemias are recognized and are related to prognosis (McCarthy, 2008).

History and physical manifestations, along with a blood count containing immature leukocytes, are the most common suspicious hallmarks of leukemia. The child is often referred to a tertiary oncology center after these initial findings. Subsequent bone marrow aspiration or biopsy confirms diagnosis.

Treatment of leukemia involves chemotherapy intravenously and by other routes, with or without radiation therapy. Other options include bone marrow transplantation. Owing to the intense therapy requiring reliable IV access for infusion of chemotherapy and blood sampling, a central catheter, such as a tunneled central line or an implanted port, is usually inserted in patients with leukemia.

TYPES OF ACCESS

Emergency Intravenous Medication Administration

Of great concern to many practitioners is correct administration of IV medications given to a child during advanced life support. These medications are administered by weight, age, or both; patient length, with the use of a Broselow tape, has also been used to determine weight with a high degree of accuracy (Lubitz et al., 1988). Some institutions, particularly in pediatric critical care areas, use bedside charts that list the individual doses of emergency drugs for the weight of that particular child. In addition, large multidose charts listing doses of drugs and sizes of equipment used in a pediatric code may be posted in the emergency or treatment room areas. This information is extremely helpful to nursing and medical personnel who work with adult patients and are not familiar with these dosages from experience.

Although most medications are administered by peripheral or central IV, emergency medications and fluids to treat respiratory and cardiac arrest may be administered by the intraosseous (IO) route if IV access cannot be obtained.

Intraosseous Access

During a resuscitation effort, it is imperative to obtain intravenous access as quickly as possible. Unless a central venous catheter is already in place, do not delay resuscitative efforts to obtain central access. If peripheral access is not obtained within 2 minutes or 2 attempts, IO access should be initiated (Kleinman et al., 2010).

IO access is usually reserved for the critically ill child and can be a fast and reliable method for the delivery of medications, fluids, and blood products into the bone marrow cavity. Figure 21-3 medication delivery and onset into the bone marrow is comparable to

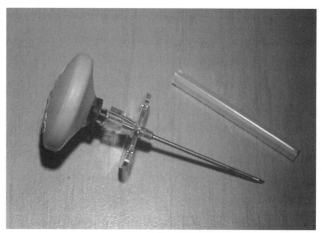

FIGURE 21-3 Intraosseous administration.

the intravenous route (Tobias & Ross, 2010). In the semiconscious child, administration of analgesia is imperative, as the procedure is painful.

The tibia and femur are the preferred sites for IO administration because the limbs are readily accessible during resuscitation efforts and the marrow cavity is well developed, even in neonates (Tocantins & O'Neil, 1945). Access should be attempted 1 to 2 cm below the tibial tuberosity, thus avoiding the growth plate at the end of the bone (Hawkins, 2008; Figure 21-3). The tibial sites are preferred because less subcutaneous tissue over the bone enhances ease of access, as opposed to the femur, where subcutaneous tissue may make IO access difficult. Other sites include the distal medial tibia, midanterior distal femur, iliac crest, and humerus. The sternum in children older than 3 years of age is an additional site but is not an option in younger children because the sternum is too thin to support the IO needle. Contraindications to IO access include site infections, fractures, an extremity with vascular injury, burns, and bone disorders, such as osteogenesis imperfecta (brittle bone disease) and osteopetrosis (marble bone disease), in which bones may fracture easily (Hawkins, 2008).

A short, rigid needle with a stylet is used to obtain IO access; alternatively, a lumbar puncture needle may be used for infants, although this needle can bend easily and is awkward to insert. Disposable bone marrow aspiration needles are now manufactured for IO access; 12, 15, or 18 is the recommended gauge because a small-lumen needle can become blocked with bone fragments or bend on insertion (Hawkins, 2008).

After antimicrobial cleansing of the desired site, the IO needle is inserted perpendicular to the bone surface at a slight angle away from the epiphyseal plate. Using a small power driver specifically designed for IO placement or using a screwing motion, insert the needle into the bone until decreased resistance is noted and the needle stands without support, usually at a depth of 1 cm in an infant or a child (Miller, Montez, Puga, & Philbeck, 2012). Further advancement may cause penetration of the opposite wall of the bone and result in extravasation into soft tissue. Some manufactures are now marking the shaft of the IO needle to indicate depth. After insertion, remove the stylet and attempt to aspirate bone marrow content. Similar to blood, this sample may be used for important laboratory studies to indicate success of resuscitative efforts (Hawkins, 2008).

A short connector tubing and flush solution, similar to that used with IV catheters, is connected to the hub of the IO needle, and a split sterile gauze dressing and tape are placed

TABLE 21-?	TYPES OF INFUSIONS ADMINISTERED FOR THE IO ROUTE	
Fluids	Medications	Blood Products
5%, 10%, and 50% dextrose	Analgesics	Albumin
Saline	Anesthetics	Dextran
Lactated Ringer's	Antibiotics	PRBC
Parenteral nutrition	Anticonvulsants	Plasma
	Antisera	Whole blood
	Catecholamines	
	Contrast media	
	Miscellaneous (e.g., atropine, calcium, dobutamine, dopamine, epinephrine, heparin, insulin, levarterenol, lidocaine, phenytoin, sodium bicarbonate)	

to secure the site. The site should be observed for infiltration into surrounding tissues; the same bone should not be used for repeated access if infiltration occurs. Types of infusions given by the IO route are listed in Table 21-11. Gravity flow, manual pressure, or infusion pump are acceptable means of administering fluids, blood, or medications.

Complications are relatively rare with the most common complication being osteomyelitis and can be associated with the infusion of hypertonic solutions or long-term therapy. Other complications can include the following:

- Cellulitis
- Compartment syndrome
- Abscess
- Local necrosis
- Fat embolism (although a possibility, this has not been reported in children, probably because of the low fat content of bone marrow in children, especially those younger than 4 years of age)
- Bilateral tibial fractures

To prevent complications, the site should be monitored closely, especially during infusion of potential vesicants (Hawkins, 2008). Replacement of the IO needle with IV access is recommended as soon as conventional IV access is feasible.

Peripheral Infusion Devices

Until the late 1970s, the winged infusion needle was the device of choice for short-term IV therapy and withdrawal of blood samples for laboratory analysis in pediatric patients. Then, 22-gauge catheter-over-needle devices made of plastic, and later Teflon, became available and could be used for longer-lasting IV access in pediatric patients (Weinstein, 2007). Many pediatric institutions still use winged infusion needles for blood sampling because the vacuum withdrawal method used in adults is often too aggressive for tiny pediatric veins.

Catheter-over-the-needle device design has advanced to include thin-wall safety catheters for greater flow rates, smaller gauge (24 and 22), shorter length, and nonkinking material.

Small-gauge safety catheters such as the 24 for neonates and the 24 and 22 for children and adolescents are the choice when <6 days of IV therapy is prescribed (Centers for Disease Control and Prevention [CDC], 2011; INS, 2011). After 2 weeks, peripheral access sites become increasingly unavailable, and the use of a longer-lasting or central device may be warranted.

Peripheral Access

EQUIPMENT

Equipment and supplies are set up before venipuncture, usually in a treatment room, if possible, thus preserving the child's room and bed as a safe place where invasive procedures are not performed (Hockenberry et al., 2011). If a treatment room is not available or if the patient's condition prohibits relocating, supplies may be prepared away from the bedside so as not to cause undue anxiety before the actual venipuncture. In the home, supplies usually are set up in an area where lighting is maximized and a flat surface, such as a kitchen table, can be used as a work area. The nurse will need the following:

- A peripheral IV safety catheter in 24- or 22-gauge size
- Luer-locking microbore connector tubing
- Needleless cap
- 1 to 2 mL of flush solution in a syringe
- Padded arm board
- ½- and 1-inch tape or securement device (Figure 21-4)

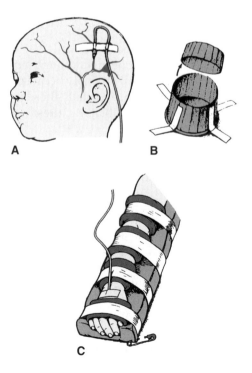

FIGURE 21-4 Infant taping and securement. **A:** Scalp vein IV site. **B:** Paper cup taped over the IV site for protection. **C:** Arm board used to secure the IV site is in the hand.

- Semipermeable transparent dressing
- Gauze pads
- Alcohol or chlorhexidine gluconate scrub to clean the site
- Nonsterile gloves
- Latex-free tourniquet or rubber band
- Site protector (optional)
- Warm packs (optional)

IV INSERTION

Peripheral IVs are used to administer fluids, medications, and PN and drawing of occasional blood samples. Although the standards of the Intravenous Nurses Society state that indwelling peripheral IV catheters should not be used routinely to acquire blood samples in children, the frequency of venous sampling for certain diagnostic tests makes necessary the use of peripheral IV devices (INS, 2011). Examples include short-duration blood tests that require blood sampling every 15 minutes (e.g., growth hormone) to every 4 to 6 hours (e.g., clotting studies or blood glucose levels). In such cases, the IV is used only for that purpose to avoid skewing results of the laboratory tests (INS, 2011).

Depending on the child's age, identifying a site for administering IV therapy typically is more difficult than in the adult. Both hydration status and previous infusion therapy may be used as predictors of obtaining venous access. In the child, the site selected for IV therapy should involve minimal risk and allow maximum efficacy and safety.

PATIENT SAFETY

To reduce the risk of tubing disconnections, establish guidelines for safe handling of infants and children with lines and drains, teach these guidelines to parents, and monitor adherence to the guidelines.

General IV insertion techniques have been described previously and are not discussed in this chapter; however, some special techniques for achieving venous access in children are highlighted. To dilate veins in children, a smaller tourniquet may be necessary. In neonates, a latex-free rubber band with a tape tab provides an easily removable tourniquet for scalp IVs (Figure 21-5). In some cases, especially when placing an IV in a premature neonate, no tourniquet is used. Additional aids to locate and dilate veins may include warm soaks or transillumination; however, a recent study indicated a decrease in successful peripheral cannulation with the use of transillumination (Peterson, Phillips, Truemper, & Agarwal, 2012), while another study indicated that ultrasound-guided placement led to less attempts and quicker cannulation on pediatric patients with a history of difficult access (Donniger, Ishimine, Fox, & Kanegaye, 2009). Further nursing research is warranted for the feasibility and success rates associated with the use of technological devices during intravenous insertion.

EVIDENCE FOR PRACTICE

What studies are needed to determine feasibility of technological devices during IV insertion?

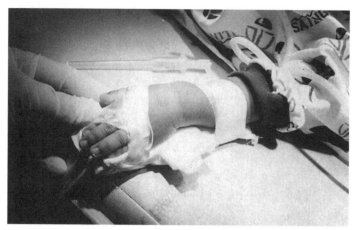

FIGURE 21-5 Latex-free rubber band. (Courtesy of A. M. Frey.)

Insertion of IVs in children requires stabilization of the extremity before venipuncture so that movement of the child does not dislodge the newly inserted device, making necessary subsequent sticks. An arm board is usually adequate for stabilization (Figure 21-4). Successful cannulation is dependent on developmental preparation of the patient, through preparation of required supplies, and ensuring that support personnel are available to assist with stabilization of the patient and the IV after insertion.

PATIENT SAFETY

Wrapping an IV site with a compression wrap should be avoided.
Covering the IV site limits site assessment and early detection of IV infiltrate.

PERIPHERAL INTRAVENOUS SITES

When selecting the optimal site for IV therapy, nurses should follow certain basic strategies. These include using veins distally to proximally and inserting the IV device in line with venous flow—for example, facing down or toward the heart in a scalp vein or facing up in an arm or a leg vein. A vein in the nondominant extremity should be chosen when possible. The thumb should be left untaped or another extremity used if the child sucks his or her thumb. In addition, the nurse always closely monitors an infusing IV, at least every hour, depending on the type of infusate, size of the patient, and location of the IV access device.

Traditionally, the head was frequently used in the neonate and young infant because the scalp has an abundant supply of superficial veins (Figure 21-6). The bilateral superficial temporal veins just in front of the pinna of the ear and the frontal vein, which runs down the middle of the forehead, are usually easy to find and involve minimal risk to the patient. Scalp veins are readily available until approximately 12 to 18 months of age, when hair follicles mature and superficial layers of skin thicken, making venous access difficult. The scalp as an IV site, however, can be distressing to parents, who may believe that the IV is in the brain. Moreover, a scalp IV can restrict mobility and be easily dislodged. With the

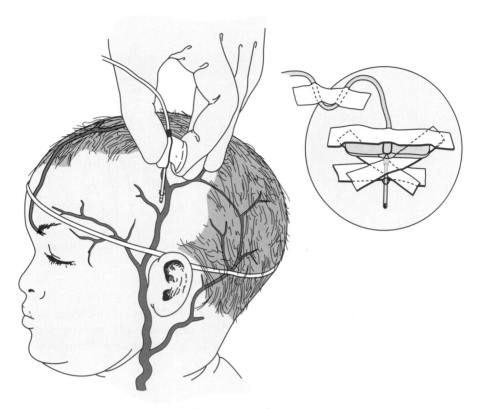

FIGURE 21-6 Insertion of the catheter into scalp veins.

advent of small IV catheters for peripheral access, scalp veins are no longer the first choice for IV access in infants.

If the scalp is chosen as the IV site and the head must be shaved, the smallest area possible should be shaved or clipped, saving the hair for the parents as the child's first haircut, which should help alleviate some distress at the use of this site. When inserting an IV in the scalp, the nurse should be aware of artery location, because distinguishing veins from arteries in this area is difficult. Use of an arterial IV could damage the artery and the area to which oxygenated blood is delivered. Inadvertent arterial puncture reveals bright red blood, pulsation, and blanching of the skin caused by arteriospasm when the IV device is flushed (Briening, 2008). Should arterial puncture occur, the IV device should be removed and pressure held on the site until bleeding stops.

Other favorable peripheral IV sites, moving from distal to proximal locations, include upper extremity sites (hand, forearm, upper arm, and antecubital fossa) and lower extremity sites (toes, foot, and ankle). Some unusual sites such as the axilla, abdomen, and popliteal area also have been used when chronically ill infants and children exhibit greatly diminished peripheral venous access from long use.

Foot veins are used up to walking age and occasionally in older children when other usual sites are not available, such as in patients with burns or multiple traumas (Figure 21-7). Depending on the regulations of the state's Board of Nursing and institutional policy, the

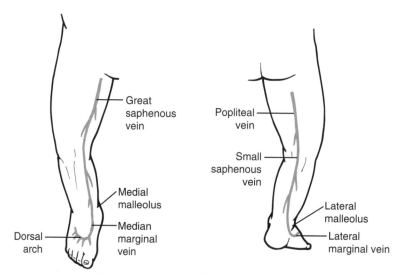

FIGURE 21-7 Veins of the foot and leg.

external jugular and femoral veins may be used for IV access and blood samples, although these last two sites usually are accessed by a physician/LIP, nurse practitioner, or emergency personnel. Follow the guidelines for LIPs in your area. Peripheral access sites for pediatric patients are highlighted in Table 21-12.

TECHNIQUE

Intravenous insertion in children requires patience and practice until the learning curve is diminished and skill level increases. No more than two attempts at IV access should

TABLE 21-12 COMMONLY USED PERIPHERAL SITES	
	Vein
Preferred Site	
• Hand	Metacarpal, dorsal venous arch, tributaries of cephalic and basilic
• Forearm	Accessory cephalic, basilic, median antebrachial
• Antecubital fossa	Cephalic, basilic, median antebrachial
• Upper arm	Basilic, cephalic
• Foot	Saphenous, median marginal, dorsal arch
• Scalp	Frontal, temporal, posterior auricular, occipital, supraorbital
• Lower leg	Greater saphenous, lesser saphenous
Auxiliary Site	
• Wrist	Superficial veins on ventral surface[a]
• Knee	Popliteal vein—usually limited to neonates due to mobility
• Axilla	Axillary vein: usually limited to neonates
• Abdomen	Superficial veins: rarely used

[a]Infiltration in this area may result in pressure on the radial nerve

be made. Veins should be located by anatomy and palpation prior to venipuncture. If unsuccessful, the nurse should consult a more experienced person or consider alternate access. Limiting the number of venipuncture attempts decreases physical and emotional trauma to the child and can preserve venous integrity. Consideration should be given to using an IV specialty nursing team for IV procedures in children because such teams have a higher rate of success when placing IVs and can be quite cost-effective (CDC, 2011).

A firm but gentle insertion technique is necessary for a successful venipuncture in a child because blood return may not appear as readily as in the adult, and the nurse may not feel the characteristic pop of entering a vein. With certain brands of safety catheters, the blood return is first evidenced in the catheter immediately after the vein is punctured. Threading the IV catheter can occasionally be difficult in children. After initial flashback of blood, but before threading the catheter into the vein, the nurse verifies that the catheter tip and the stylet have entered the vein lumen by advancing the IV device slightly. Other measures include attaching a small connector tubing with flush solution and flushing gently as the catheter is advanced. Sometimes, just waiting a few seconds until the child has calmed down can decrease the incidence of venous spasm and facilitate catheter threading.

Maintaining Access

Site monitoring is of the utmost importance in pediatric patients because infiltration can occur quickly and effects can be devastating if the infiltrated infusate has caustic properties. Infants and children are at increased risk for an infiltration and extravasation injury secondary to fragile veins, activity level, and limited communication skills (Tofani et al., 2012). Additionally, children are at risk if the catheter has been in place >72 hours or if they are receiving medications with an extreme pH, hypotonic and hypertonic solutions, and vasoactive, or cytotoxic medications (Clark et al., 2013). IV sites in those areas with very little superficial tissue, particularly the dorsum of the foot in infants, are more prone to extravasation injury. Infiltration injuries can be a reason for litigation if the injury is extensive or limits function. Recommended frequency for peripheral IV site assessment ranges from every 1 to 2 hours, or, more often, if the infusate is a known irritant or vesicant. Peripheral IV sites used as saline locks, without an infusate running, should be assessed at least once per shift (every 8 to 12 hours). Regardless of the clinical setting in which care is being given, patients and caregivers are taught how to recognize signs of IV complications and to take corrective actions. Peripheral IV access should not be used for continuous infusions in alternative settings, such as the home, unless the site can be monitored. For this reason, central venous access is often used in the home and alternative setting.

Postinsertion Care of the Peripheral Intravenous Site

Frequent assessment of the site must be done; dressing changes usually are done only when the IV site is changed, as recommended by infection control research (CDC, 2011). Peripheral and central catheter care is summarized in Table 21-13.

Stabilization is essential, primarily in the younger child whose comprehension of the importance of not manipulating the IV site is minimal. The use of a sutureless securement device is preferred for stabilization and tends to extend the life of the peripheral IV (Brown, 2009). Taping the IV in a U-shaped chevron or H pattern with a tension loop, so that if the child pulls on the IV, it affects the loop, not the IV site, is also an acceptable method of securement (Figure 21-8). Sites requiring stabilization include those over joints, such as

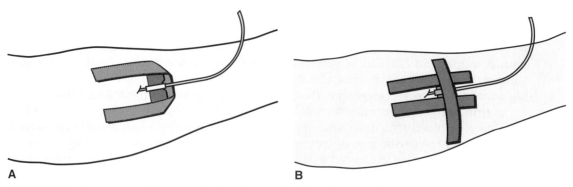

A   **B**

FIGURE 21-8 Securing an IV site (taping). **A:** U method. **B:** H method.

the dorsum of the hand near the wrist. The advantage of using a padded arm board for stabilization is that it restricts the child's range of movement, thereby decreasing the risk of dislodging the IV needle. The foot also demands stabilization, primarily when using the large saphenous vein. An important aspect of IV access in the foot involves maintaining normal joint configuration by placing padding under the foot, thus preserving the natural bend at the ankle and preventing foot drop or contracture injuries.

In younger children, especially toddlers, great care must be taken to protect the IV site. Coverings such as transparent dressings, a clear plastic IV protector, and an easily removable wrap secured with Velcro or stretch netting may keep little fingers away from the IV site while providing easy visualization. Stretch netting slipped over the IV can serve to protect the site as well, especially for home IV access. A roller bandage should not be used to cover an IV site because it is time consuming to unravel and makes site assessments difficult (INS, 2011). In general, children's medical centers rarely use restraints because restraints not only are confining but foster a sense of frustration and mistrust in the child. Restraints should be used only with an extremely uncooperative child or a child who may injure himself or herself or remove the IV. In those cases, alternate resources, such as parental monitoring, should be considered.

SITE ROTATION

A 1992 study in a pediatric critical care unit demonstrated that peripheral IV sites could remain in place safely for up to 144 hours (6 days), after which the incidence of bacterial colonization increased threefold. In fact, this same study demonstrated that newer sites had an increased chance of complications over those sites left in place (Garland, Dunne, Havens, & Hintermeyer, 1992). The 2011 INS guidelines recommend not rotating IV sites in pediatric patients unless a complication occurs (INS, 2011). Removal of the IV should be done carefully, without using scissors near the site.

MANAGING COMPLICATIONS

Complications of IV therapy in children are similar to those of adults. The most common peripheral IV complication is infiltration, which can lead to an extravasation injury. The use of a pediatric infiltration grading tool can be helpful in early identification and reduction in tissue injury (Pop, 2012). Risk for extravasation can be linked to the infusate and the child's activity (Tofani et al., 2012). Current pediatric treatment modalities include immediately stopping the infusion, application of cold or warm depending on the infusate, elevation of the extremity, and local pharmaceutical intervention specific to the infusate (Madsen, 2008).

Young children very rarely exhibit a phlebitic response to peripheral IV access, which differs from the much higher rates of phlebitis found in adults. Phlebitis rates reported in children hospitalized in intensive care units were 13%, whereas for those children on general units, phlebitis rates were 10%. In children older than 10 years, phlebitis rates reported (21%) approached those of adults (Nelson, 1987; Tully, Friedland, Baldini, & Goldman, 1981). Risk factors for the development of phlebitis include catheter location, infusion of hyperalimentation fluids with continuous IV lipid emulsions, and length of intensive care stay before catheter insertion (Garland et al., 1992).

Intermediate-Term Midline Intravenous Access

A midline catheter, longer than the peripheral IV, reaches the larger vessels of the upper arm and in neonates and children, the upper thigh. These larger blood vessels are presumed to provide greater blood flow and better hemodilution of infusions. Midline catheters are available in 24- and 22-gauge sizes, with lengths of 3 to 6 inches for children. Midline catheters are still considered peripheral IV access devices as the tip ends before entering the larger vessels, however, should be considered for treatment durations of 1 to 4 weeks (INS, 2011).

As in PICC placement, caution should be taken when choosing site location particularly in children with congenital cardiac defects involving decreased blood flow to the right extremity (INS, 2011).

Ideally, assistance from vessel visualization technology would be used during placement to guide in appropriate site location and success in placement (Hadaway, 2010). The tip of a midline catheter does not extend beyond the extremity in which it is placed; therefore, radiographic confirmation of tip placement is optional and recommended only when there is difficulty in catheter insertion or flushing. As with most medical equipment, adult-sized versions of these devices are tested initially and then studies in children are undertaken. Although very few research studies or outcome data have been published regarding midlines in neonates and children, these catheters have been used to administer IV fluids, medications, and blood products (Rosenthal, 2008). Some limited success with midline catheters has been reported. In one neonatal report, midlines lasted an average of 6.3 days, surpassing the peripheral IV duration average of 24 to 48 hours in neonates (Dawson, 2002). Further research is indicated to address the maximum dwell time of a functioning midline catheters (Pettit & Wyckoff, 2007). Complications reported in children include phlebitis, pain, and erythema at the insertion site, occlusion, and dislodgment (Rosenthal, 2008). Varying degrees of success have been reported with the use of these devices in children; more research, particularly in the pediatric population, is certainly a mission for the infusion nurse.

Central Venous Access

The use of central venous access has been widely accepted for infusion therapy in pediatrics when multiple attempts for peripheral access have failed or the child requires a long-term, hyperosmolar, or vesicant therapy (Spagrud et al., 2008). Many types of central access devices exist, including nontunneled catheters, PICCs, surgically placed cuffed tunneled catheters, and totally implanted devices (port). In the neonate, umbilical catheters (venous and arterial) are considered a central access device. Choice of device and insertion site

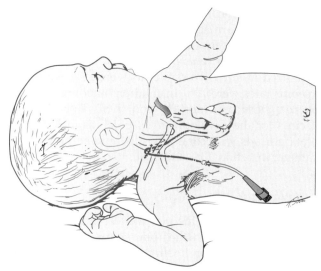

FIGURE 21-9 Broviac catheter.

depends on the child's age, duration and type of therapy prescribed, input from the patient and family, and disease process, taking into consideration the risk for catheter-associated bloodstream infection rates associated with certain sites (Baskin et al., 2009).

> ### PATIENT SAFETY
> Infants and children with congenital cardiac defects should not have central venous access devices placed in the right arm as certain cardiac surgical procedures utilize the subclavian artery for palliation of the cardiac defect (INS, 2011).

Parents and children are concerned about catheter care, safety, cost, and body image. For instance, an infant may bite through the catheter during the teething period or a toddler may easily dislodge the catheter. A child who is extremely afraid of needles may not do well with an implanted port, which has to be accessed with a needle periodically. Conversely, an older child or adolescent may choose an implanted port over a tunneled catheter to avoid disturbance of body image. If the central device is to be used for continuous infusions or cycled daily therapies, such as TPN, a tunneled catheter, such as a Broviac, may be the best choice (Figure 21-9). Pediatric hospitals often use clinical nurse specialists who can demonstrate pros and cons of each device, assist families in their choice of venous access, introduce children with similar devices, and help decrease anxiety about insertion and care.

VASCULAR ACCESS DEVICES

PERIPHERALLY INSERTED CENTRAL CATHETERS

A PICC is defined as a central vascular access device inserted into a peripheral vein, usually of the arm or leg, with the tip residing in the superior or inferior vena cava (INS, 2011). Infants have additional site choices involving the scalp, leg, and foot. Before reports of PICC use in neonates and children, central venous access was accomplished using a medical or surgical procedure to place a nontunneled, tunneled, or implanted device or an umbilical catheter in neonates. The development of smaller, easier to insert, more biocompatible catheters resulted in a renewed interest in the PICC as a central access device choice in neonates and children.

Pediatric-sized PICCs are manufactured of polyurethane, or softer Silastic material shown to have low incidence of irritation and thrombus formation, allowing PICCs to remain in place for months to years (CDC, 2011).

If a PICC is in place for an extended period of time, a child's growth may require that the catheter be replaced to ensure correct tip location. Appropriate PICC sizes for infants and children range from neonatal sizes as small as 1.1 French (28 gauge) to typical adult sizes. Catheter size should be determined so that the smallest catheter can be placed while still meeting infusion needs (Pettit & Wyckoff, 2007). Care should be taken and manufactures' recommendations should be followed for smaller French catheters with blood sampling and flushing to avoid occlusion or catheter destruction.

PICCs are typically inserted in children in the hospital or outpatient setting with maximum sterile barrier precautions (CDC, 2011). Insertion does not necessarily require general anesthesia; however, the use of a local anesthetic or conscious sedation will provide for easier insertion and patient comfort (Hockenberry et al., 2011). Ultrasound, once a tool used only by radiologists, now has become smaller and more portable and is being used increasingly by nurses, as well as radiologists, to locate veins suitable for PICC placement in pediatric and neonatal patients (Nichols & Doellman, 2007). Aside from the developmental approach necessary to prepare children and possible sedation requirement, the technique of insertion is similar in adults and children. If the vein is difficult to locate, the additional use of a transilluminator or warming packs may enhance the likelihood of successful PICC placement.

In neonates, PICC site location may include the veins of the antecubital fossa, as well as the axillary, saphenous, popliteal, and external jugular veins (Pettit & Wyckoff, 2007). In older children, the median cubital basilic, basilic, and cephalic veins in the antecubital fossa, or slightly above or below this site, are ideal.

Maintenance of PICC catheters in pediatric patients includes dressing care, maintenance of patency, changing of end caps, site protection, and avoidance of complications (Table 21-13).

Blood pressure measurement over the PICC catheter should be avoided; however, it can be obtained distal to the insertion site. Care must be taken to avoid undue pressures when flushing these small catheters. Smaller syringe sizes lead to increased pressure and catheter rupture or embolization could occur (Pettit & Wyckoff, 2007). In addition, rapid injectors used in radiology are avoided unless the placement of a catheter specific for power injectors is evident (INS, 2011).

Although PICCs are associated with fewer complications than surgically placed catheters, PICC use in neonates and children is not without complications; some of which can be severe or fatal (Pettit & Wyckoff, 2007). Major complications in neonates with PICCs include mechanical complications such as occlusion (due to smaller catheter sizes) and catheter-related bloodstream infection (Doellman et al., 2010). Infants are at increasing risk for infection due to their immature immune system. Other reported complications include pain/phlebitis, dislodgment, and catheter migration or fracture. The validity of catheter-related bloodstream infection rates are complex due to inconsistent definitions and reporting (Pettit & Wyckoff, 2007).

NONTUNNELED CENTRAL VENOUS ACCESS DEVICE

For the purposes of this chapter, nontunneled catheters include percutaneously placed femoral, jugular, and subclavian catheters. These catheters are referred to as nontunneled

TABLE 21-1	ROUTINE CARE AND MAINTENANCE OF THE INFUSION SITE
Device	**Patency**
Peripheral	• 1–3 mL saline flush q8h or after each medication administration if no fluids infusing
PICC	• 2 mL of 10–100 units/mL heparinized saline q12–24h • For any age child with one or more medication doses daily, use 10 units/mL • If more than one lumen, flush each lumen as needed
Nontunneled catheter • Jugular • Subclavian • Femoral	• 2 mL of 10–100 units/mL heparinized saline q12–24h • For a child of any age with one or more medication doses daily; use 10 units/mL • If more than one lumen, flush each lumen as needed
Tunneled catheter (Broviac)	• 2 mL of 10–100 units/mL heparinized saline q12–24h • For a child of any age with one or more medication doses daily, use 10 units/mL
Implanted port	• 2 mL of 10 units/mL heparinized saline for a child of any age with one or more medication doses daily • At discharge and monthly: use 5 mL of 100 units/mL heparinized saline flush

to distinguish them from longer-dwelling cuffed Silastic catheters that are surgically tunneled under the skin. In children, as well as in adults, nontunneled catheters often are used for IV access in critical situations, such as in a patient with multiple trauma or in children in the pediatric intensive care unit who need several weeks of IV access and possibly PN.

Nontunneled percutaneously placed catheters usually are short and may have from one to four lumens (Figure 21-10). They usually are made of a stiffer material such as polyurethane for easier insertion by percutaneous skin puncture. In children, these catheters may be inserted nonsurgically using a local anesthetic and mild sedation.

Although venous anatomy is similar in all age groups, some differences in children necessitate choosing specific sites over others. The preferred sites for percutaneous placement of nontunneled central lines in children are femoral veins, internal and external jugular veins, and subclavian veins. For anatomic reasons, the right side is preferred when catheterizing the internal jugular or subclavian veins.

The femoral site has easily identifiable landmarks for catheter placement, is easy to apply pressure to the site if needed, and its location will not hinder any cardiopulmonary resuscitation efforts. The internal and external jugular veins also have the advantage of ease of identification of landmarks and accessibility along with a larger diameter and present fewer technical difficulties with catheterization. The right internal jugular vein runs an almost straight course to the superior vena cava, whereas the left is more angled.

The subclavian vein is the least common site because of anatomic considerations. In infants younger than 1 year of age, higher arching of the subclavian vein causes acute angles that can obstruct placement (Doellman et al., 2010). After 1 year of age, the subclavian arch assumes the horizontal position similar to that of the adult. Curvature and softness of the chest and clavicles make landmarks difficult to identify, and the apices of the lungs are higher in children. Subclavian catheter insertion in neonates is technically difficult and can

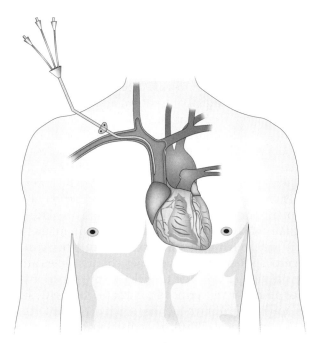

FIGURE 21-10 Nontunneled PICC.

result in life-threatening complications such as pneumothorax, hydrothorax, hemothorax, and massive hemorrhage.

Maintenance includes, site assessment and assurance of an intact and occlusive dressing. Dressing changes should be done weekly or more often, and as needed. Catheter stiffness, high incidence of thrombus, and easy dislodgment limit the use of these catheters to a relatively short period. Catheters placed in jugular and femoral locations may be occluded because infants tend to have a shortened neck and frequently adduct their legs, causing kinking in the catheter placed in the neck or groin. The femoral location is also the diaper area, and the dressing may become soiled frequently and exposed to infective organisms prevalent in this region. These factors, in addition to potential for air embolism, also limit the use of this device for home infusion, particularly in younger children. Contraindications to percutaneous insertion of a nontunneled central venous access device include vascular abnormality or disease in the involved extremity, skin compromise or injury at the proposed entry site, or a treatment plan requiring a different type of device.

TUNNELED CENTRAL VENOUS CATHETERS

Tunneled catheters are most often chosen for long-term venous access, as are implanted ports, which are discussed in the next section. In the early 1970s, Broviac developed the first tunneled catheter for patients who required long-term TPN (Broviac, Cole, & Schribner, 1973). Broviac catheters have since become a popular choice when long-term central venous access is needed, such as with children who have cancer.

Single- and double-lumen devices are used in children; the triple-lumen devices tend to be somewhat large for pediatric use. A tunneled catheter is passed through a subcutaneous "tunnel" between the insertion site and exit site and contains a Dacron polyester cuff that anchors the catheter in place several weeks after the insertion (Doellman et al., 2010; INS, 2011).

Tunneled catheter insertion in children requires the expertise of a surgeon or interventional radiologist dictating placement in the operating room or radiology suite (Doellman et al., 2010). Often, several procedures are coordinated with catheter insertion to avoid multiple episodes of sedation. For example, a patient newly diagnosed with leukemia may have one visit to the operating room for Broviac insertion, bone marrow biopsy, and lumbar puncture.

Vein selection and site insertion are dependent on the child's age, activity level, and anatomy (Doellman et al., 2010). In some children, chest access sites are not available because of many previous central lines, vein thromboses, or other surgery or complications. An alternate site for catheter placement is the femoral vein to the inferior vena cava, particularly in children younger than walking age. The proximal portion of the catheter is then tunneled under the skin of the abdomen or out onto the thigh. In older children, the catheter usually is inserted percutaneously into the subclavian vein. In infants and neonates, because of the small size of the subclavian vein and proximity of other structures, this approach can be extremely dangerous. Therefore, in younger children, the catheter is inserted through the external or internal jugular vein and tunneled to the superior vena cava.

After proper placement is verified by chest radiography, subcutaneous tunneling of the catheter occurs down the chest wall to the fourth or fifth intercostal space, depending on the catheter type (Doellman et al., 2010). This distal exit site from the original phlebotomy site provides a barrier against infection, facilitates catheter maintenance, and provides the child with full-range neck mobility (CDC, 2011).

Care of tunneled catheters includes dressing changes; flushing to maintain patency; prevention of infection, occlusion, and dislodgment; as well as patient and family education addressing care required at home. Dislodgment may be prevented by carefully looping the external "tail" of the catheter under the dressing or taping it to the chest. Children of all age groups who have tunneled catheters should wear T shirts to prevent inadvertent catheter trauma. If breakage of the catheter occurs, a permanent splicing procedure can be accomplished using a manufacturer's repair kit that matches the broken segment of the tunneled catheter. Tunneled catheter removal is a surgical procedure, and because of adherence of the Dacron cuff to tissue in the subcutaneous tunnel, it usually is done using local anesthesia and conscious sedation.

Care of tunneled catheters is continually researched, and procedures for children are based on the manufacturer's guidelines, catheter volume, experience with adults, and ongoing and previously published research studies. In the past, institutional practices varied; however, recently collaboratives such as National Association of Children's Hospitals and Related Institutions (NACHRI) and Solutions for Patient Safety (SPS) have joined forces to share knowledge and minimize variations in practice leading the way for evidence-based bundles (Box 21-2).

Umbilical Catheterization

Most sites for neonatal IV therapy are similar to those used for infants and older children. A site unique to the newborn population is the umbilicus, which contains two arteries and one vein. Umbilical catheterization is common practice in many neonatal intensive care units for the treatment of acutely ill infants. This mode of therapy provides an easy route for vascular administration of transfusions, medications, fluids, PN, and blood withdrawal. Unique catheters are designed specifically for umbilical arteries and veins. These catheters are available as single or double lumen in sizes ranging from 3.5 to 5 French.

BOX 21-2   INNOVATIVE COLLABORATION

Over the past several years, health care has been challenged by various payers to improve quality and outcomes in several areas. Organizations around the country have joined forces to share knowledge concerning hospital-acquired conditions and quality improvement strategies. Child Health Corporation of America (CHCA), National Association of Children's Hospitals and Related Institutions (NACHRI), and National Association of Children's Hospitals (NACH) have combined and formed Children's Hospital Association (CHA) and are composed of 220 children's hospitals with a mission to advocate for children's health. Additionally, the Ohio-originated SPS is a nationally known pediatric collaborative with a focus on transparent sharing of process improvement strategies, development and sustainability of evidence-based bundles, practice compliance, and outcomes aimed at preventing harm and reducing hospital-acquired infections.

   Children's Hospital Association (CHA) http://www.childrenshospitals.org

   Solutions for Patient Safety http://solutionsforpatientsafety.org

PROCEDURE

Within minutes of birth, the umbilical arteries normally constrict; delays in the process, however, occur in states of hypoxia and acidosis. Most infants are catheterized in the 1st day of life because umbilical catheterization is more difficult or impossible past the 4th day of life. The procedure for umbilical catheterization begins with aseptic technique, including hand washing, gloving, masking, and gowning. Equipment is set up using a cut down tray and recommended catheter size. All IV tubings must be purged of air. The infant is restrained temporarily using leg/arm restraints and an assistant. Cleanse the umbilical stump with a povidone–iodine solution; excess should not be allowed to pool at the infant's side or skin irritation or blistering may occur (Furdon, Horgan, Bradshaw, & Clark, 2006). The sterile field is set up around the umbilicus, using a fenestrated drape that exposes the umbilical area. Dissection begins at the umbilical cord approximately 1.5 cm from the skin until the umbilical vessels are identified. Two thick-walled, pinpoint-sized arteries are easily distinguishable from a large, thin-walled vein. The heparinized catheter is passed through either the umbilical artery or vein, depending on the type of therapy desired.

   There are important differences between arterial and venous umbilical catheterization. Umbilical artery catheters (UACs) are used primarily for the purpose of continuous invasive arterial blood pressure monitoring and/or arterial blood sampling. In situations in which venous access cannot be obtained, certain medications, peripheral concentration TPN (<12.5% and <900 mOsm/L), or blood products may be administered via the umbilical artery catheter. This should be a short-term solution until venous access can be obtained. Umbilical venous catheters (UVCs) are commonly used to administer fluids, medications, and blood products. UVCs provide a mechanism for measuring CVP, the pressure in the right atrium, and can also be used to obtain venous blood samples (Bradshaw & Furdon, 2006).

   Placement differs between the umbilical arterial and venous routes (INS, 2011). The UAC is located in the descending aorta, and its position is usually referred to as "low" or "high." The tip of a low catheter is between the third and fourth lumbar vertebrae, while high catheter tips are located between the sixth and ninth thoracic vertebrae (Furdon et al., 2006). These positions avoid the arteries that branch off the aorta to provide blood flow to major organs. A 2004 Cochrane systemic review of evidence concluded that high UAC tip placement was associated with fewer ischemic and thrombotic complications and longer duration of the catheter use. The tip of the UVC should be positioned in the inferior vena cava above the level of the diaphragm near the right atrium, and intracardiac placement should be avoided (Bradshaw & Furdon, 2006).

Once the catheter is placed correctly and position is confirmed radiographically, a suture may be placed superficially through the stump and tied firmly to the catheter for anchorage. The umbilical catheter may be taped to the infant's abdomen using goalpost taping, or tape bridge, with a commercially available securing device, or with a transparent nonocclusive dressing (Helton Rapoport & Salazar Young, 2008). If an infant has both a UAC and a UVC, it is important that they be identified correctly either by labeling or by using a consistently different method of taping each catheter. Additional maintenance care involves a clear occlusive dressing without the use of ointments, which have been linked to an increase in fungal infections (CDC, 2011).

The UAC usually is connected to a three-way stopcock for pressure monitoring, blood drawing, and fluid administration. For safety, all UACs are continuously transduced with alarms set on a cardiorespiratory monitor that will alert the caregiver if the line becomes disconnected. It is of the utmost importance to maintain patency of the indwelling catheter because blood clots can otherwise form. When fluids are not infusing, the catheters require flushing with heparin (1 to 10 units/mL preservative-free normal saline).

Risks and complications associated with umbilical catheters include bleeding from the umbilical stump, hemorrhage, perforation of vessels, air embolism, and infection (INS, 2011). Complications in UVCs also include those associated with other central venous lines in infants such as arrhythmias, heart perforation, and cardiac tamponade.

The most frequent complication of UACs is vascular compromise, including thrombosis and arterial vasospasm, resulting is ischemia or infarction to an organ or extremity (Furdon et al., 2006). It is important to assess the distal sites for perfusion (color, temperature, and capillary refill time). Clinical signs of ischemia have been reported in the toes, feet, legs, and buttocks (Furdon et al., 2006). Other complications that may result from vessel thrombosis include necrotizing enterocolitis and renal insufficiency.

Early intervention for any complication can reduce the risk of morbidity and mortality when using umbilical access for IV therapy. Because of the many risks of complications and the short dwell time when using the umbilical vessel for IV therapy, many physicians/LIPs now prefer to use an alternate peripheral or central site as soon as possible.

Implanted Central Venous Access Ports

Low-profile pediatric ports have been available for several years and are made of stainless steel, titanium, plastic, or a combination of these materials. Ports are convenient and comfortable and are the preferred device for children who require intermittent therapy over a long period of time, who can tolerate the needle access, and who do not like the inconvenience of an external catheter (Doellman et al., 2010). When advising patients and family about venous access devices, an important consideration is that the port requires access with a needle at least monthly for flushing to ensure patency (Wallace, 2008). Venous access ports are implanted in the chest, upper abdomen, thigh, or forearm, with the catheter threaded into a central vein (Doellman et al., 2010). An exit site is avoided with the port portion secured in a subcutaneous pocket. Ports are accessed from the top or side, depending on the design, with a small noncoring needle or, in some brands, an IV catheter (Doellman et al., 2010). Needle gauge and length should be decided such that the smallest gauge for infusion is used and the length is sufficient to touch the back of the port.

A hospital or home IV nurse, parents, or patients themselves in some cases may access the port after return demonstration of correct technique.

Needles are changed every 6 to 7 days while the port is being used; dressing changes should be coordinated with needle changes to ensure sterility and effective site cleaning, thereby minimizing the risk of central line infection (Etzel Hardman, 2008). When the port is not being used for infusion of medications, PN, transfusion therapy, or blood sample withdrawal, patency is maintained by flushing the port with heparinized saline (Wallace, 2008).

Complications reported with ports are similar to those identified for tunneled catheters, including infection and occlusion; in most studies, implanted ports had longer survival times and fewer complications than tunneled catheters (Etzel Hardman, 2008). Although risk of port dislodgment is minimal, the noncoring needle may be dislodged and cause infiltration and possible tissue injury if vesicant drugs are being administered. Slight discomfort has been reported with needle access of the port, but this can be mitigated with the use of a topical anesthetic, distraction, and the use of a child life specialist (Wallace, 2008).

Surgical Cut Down

Although alternative choices of access, such as the IO and central venous routes, have diminished the need for venous cut down, this method remains a viable option for emergency vascular access in resuscitation of the pediatric patient. When acute hypovolemia and acidosis cause severe, enough peripheral vasoconstriction that percutaneous placement of venous access is impossible, and if IO access cannot be achieved, venous cut down may be warranted.

The most common cut down sites are the distal saphenous vein at the ankle, the proximal saphenous vein at the groin, the basilic vein at the antecubital, and the axillary vein, which is used in newborns. Because this procedure requires venous laceration or minor surgery, a physician/ LIP or surgeon usually performs it. Meticulous sterile technique is required. Complications reported with venous cut down include local injury of contiguous structures such as an artery or a nerve, hemorrhage, hematoma, extravasation, phlebitis with prolonged use, localized cellulitis, suppurative phlebitis, and catheter-related bloodstream infection. Obtaining successful IV access is essential to provide efficacious pediatric advanced life support. In many cases, during a code situation, peripheral veins have collapsed because of cardiac arrest and poor perfusion.

Complications

CENTRAL LINE–ASSOCIATED BLOODSTREAM INFECTIONS

Of utmost nursing priority is that of central line–associated bloodstream infection prevention. Similarly, to that in adults, nurses must adhere to recommendations from both the CDC and consortiums pertaining to insertion and maintenance bundles that address best practices for central line–associated bloodstream infections (CLABSI) prevention. Key bundle elements are specific to nursing practice and offer the nurse opportunities to put research into practice. Adult literature had revealed the efficacy of chlorhexidine bathing for the prevention of catheter-associated bloodstream infections. In 2013, a multicenter cluster randomized trial by Climo et al. (2013) revealed that daily bathing with chlorhexidine gluconate (CHG) embedded cloths reduced CLABSI by 28% as well as a 23% reduction in the incidence of hospital-acquired multidrug-resistant infections in the adult population. While further research in the pediatric population is warranted, a recent study showed that daily CHG bathing decreased the incidence of bacteremia and was well tolerated by most children (Milestone et al., 2013).

EVIDENCE FOR PRACTICE

Chlorhexidine bathing has been an intervention in the adult population since 2007 aimed at preventing catheter-associated bloodstream infections and has only recently been studied in the pediatric population. A 2013 publication found that critically ill children, >2 months of age, bathed with CHG daily had fewer line infections than those children not bathed with CHG. Initial concerns with introducing CHG bathing in children included the risk of skin breakdown and intolerance; however, there were minimal skin reactions found (Milestone et al., 2013). One percent of children experienced skin irritation and no severe adverse reactions were noted. This is an area that requires further research to duplicate findings and further support interventions to decrease hospital-associated infections.

OCCLUSION

Occlusion may be mechanical, thrombotic, or nonthrombotic. Mechanical occlusions may be evaluated by assessing the catheter for kinking or clamping, repositioning the child, and further assessing as needed using dye studies. Thrombotic occlusions may be corrected with tissue plasminogen activator. Nonthrombotic occlusions are treated with hydrochloric acid, ethanol, or sodium bicarbonate, depending on the cause and pH of the occlusion. Although in a Cochrane review, no studies were found investigating the safety and efficacy of nonthrombotic treatments, both surgical and chemical, in pediatrics (van Miert, Hill, & Jones, 2012).

EVIDENCE FOR PRACTICE

Clearly, further research investing treatment modalities for catheter occlusion in pediatrics is warranted.

INFUSION EQUIPMENT

Options for volume control, delivery of small doses of medication, and assurance of safety in pediatric patients include microdrip administration sets, microbore tubing, Luer-lock connections, volume control chambers, and infusion pumps (Brown, 2009). None of these devices, however, can replace close surveillance of the patient by the health care provider.

When choosing a pump for a pediatric patient, accuracy and safety are of utmost importance.

PATIENT SAFETY

Never rely on infusion pumps to alarm as a warning for an infiltrated IV in a child.

Techniques and Equipment for Administration

One of the most frequently encountered problems with administration of medications to pediatric patients is limiting the amount of fluid used to administer and flush the drug through the IV tubing. When a child receives multiple-drug therapies, the potential to exceed fluid requirements exists. Volumes can be limited by using microbore tubing and minimal dilution volumes. Each method of drug administration is applicable to specific drugs and desired therapeutic outcomes. Methods of IV medication administration in children include direct IV push or bolus, continuous, and intermittent infusion.

Direct IV push or bolus is usually defined as an IV injection given over 5 minutes or less. Examples of IV push or bolus medications include antibiotics (e.g., ampicillin), anticonvulsants (e.g., phenytoin), sedatives (e.g., midazolam), and antineoplastic drugs (e.g., vincristine). The IV push or bolus method is used when therapeutic serum levels are needed quickly to achieve the desired effect, whether it is a high serum level of an antibiotic, cessation of seizure activity, or sedation for a procedure. Not all medications can be given in this manner because of local and systemic effects, such as phlebitis, cardiac dysrhythmias, hypotension, or anaphylaxis. The nurse administering an IV push or bolus dose must administer the drug at a certain rate and/or dilution according to drug references. Monitoring is essential to assess for both the desired and/or adverse effects of the medication.

Continuous infusions are used primarily for maintenance fluids, administration of drugs that require maintenance of a steady blood level, or of potent drugs that must be highly titrated to individual needs. In situations when a large volume infusion pump is not available, there are microdrip administration sets for gravity infusion (60 gtt/min) tailored specifically for infants and children. IV tubing specific for large volume infusion pumps as well as an in-line calibrated volume control chamber (50-, 100-, and 150- mL sizes are available) should be used on all children whose prescribed fluid rate is less than the volume of the chamber. The calibrated chamber also is used to administer intermittent doses of medications (Brown, 2009).

Intermittent infusions are used mainly for antimicrobials. They can be administered by several different methods:

- Large volume infusion pump with or without calibrated chamber
- IV push
- Syringe pump
- Ambulatory infusion pump

The in-line calibrated chamber is used commonly in general pediatric settings. Medication is injected into the in-line calibrated chamber and infused at a prescribed rate. Once the infusion is complete, the usual practice is to flush the chamber and tubing with a volume of IV solution compatible with the medication, such as 5% dextrose in water or 0.9% sodium chloride. The advantage of this method is its simplicity; however, in neonates, the tubing volume may be too large for the child's fluid needs. There is a debate over whether the chambered IV set is required when an electronic infusion device is used. Manufacturers of electronic infusion devices claim that their product is guarded against free flow fluid, and products that are safety tested in proven clinical trials should be chosen for neonatal and pediatric patients.

Considerations for evaluating a pump for pediatric use should include its ability to set variable pressure limits, have low alarm limits, program as low as tenths of milliliters per hour, and have tamper-proof features.

An increasingly popular and accurate method of IV medication administration in children is the syringe pump and invention of smart pump technology. Smart pump technology has increased the safety of medication administration by having a preprogrammed formulary including infusion rates (Aguis, 2012). The syringe pump can be connected by an extension set directly onto a heparin lock or in a piggyback fashion into the primary line. A syringe of diluted medication, prefilled by the pharmacy or by the nurse caring for the patient, is attached to microbore tubing, and the medication can then be infused at a prescribed rate. Devices that electronically control volume, rate, and, sometimes, dose have become the norm rather than the exception in pediatric IV therapy. Electronic infusion devices with a high degree of accuracy, no free flow capacity, ability to infuse rates from tenths of a milliliter to hundreds of milliliters, controlled pressure settings, and microbore tubing sets are available for use in neonatal and pediatric patients. Syringe pumps are often used in intensive care and medical surgical units to deliver small-volume medications accurately.

ALTERNATE-SITE INFUSION THERAPY

Subacute Care

Recovery from a long-term illness or injury may require care in a subacute facility. A plethora of services is available including rehabilitation and development. Nurses and other providers must be educated in ongoing monitoring and care of the access sites.

Home Infusion

Neonates and infants can be sent home safely under the care and supervision of agencies skilled in neonatal and pediatric care. Much routine and some high-acuity stable neonatal and pediatric IV therapy have moved out of the hospital and into the home, subacute care facility, or outpatient infusion center. Home infusion is a more comfortable and economical choice than hospitalization. Occasionally peripheral IVs, but more often, midline, PICC, and tunneled or implanted central devices are chosen for pediatric home or alternate site care. IV therapies administered in the home or at alternate sites include fluids, antibiotics or antifungals, PN, chemotherapy, analgesics, chelating agents, pain control medications, and blood components.

In the home setting, single-use pressurized pumps are convenient for individual doses. Pediatric patients usually receive one or more doses in a controlled environment to verify that there is no adverse reaction. With TPN, the therapy is usually cycled to infuse over several hours before discharge to home or transfer to alternative site care. Small electronic pumps that can be hidden in a backpack are often used for intermittent and continuous doses, and large-volume pumps can be used for such therapies as cycled TPN. Individual dosing systems provide premixed diluted drug doses that are easy for the caregiver or patient to administer. Individual patient doses may be premixed by the home care pharmacy in an elastomeric infusion pump or other single-use device. After administration of the dose, the disposable pumps are either returned to the home care pharmacy or discarded. This system of IV medication infusion is very popular in home care.

Readiness, willingness, and ability of the patient and family and extensive teaching with demonstrated feedback should be documented before patient discharge and be ongoing during the patient's course of treatment until service is discontinued. School-age and older children can participate in their own care. Outcome data on pediatric home care, lacking in the published literature, is another opportunity for nursing research. The pediatric home infusion nurse must be an experienced IV practitioner, indicated by CRNI status, as well as an expert in recognition and treatment of pediatric abnormal states. In 1995, Ringel summarized this concept, "Pediatric infusion has to be done by a company dedicated to pediatrics or that has a pediatrics division. If children are assigned to a provider that does not have the expertise for high-acuity patients, they (children) can end up back in the hospital" (Ringel, 1995).

Infusion care of the infant or child is highly specialized. At all times, best practices should be employed to ensure positive outcomes, regardless of the clinical setting in which care is provided.

ACKNOWLEDGMENTS

The authors acknowledge the contributions of Emily Dix for the section "Parenteral Nutrition" and the original author, Anne Marie Frey.

Review Questions   *Note: Questions below may have more than one right answer.*

1. The appropriate timing for preparing a toddler for a procedure is:
   A. an hour before
   B. as you are performing the procedure
   C. immediately prior to the procedure
   D. the day before the procedure

2. An IV in the frontal vein might be the site of choice in which of the following children?
   A. A 2-month-old with hydrocephalus
   B. A neonate with sepsis on 3 days of antibiotic therapy
   C. A 20-month-old with leukemia
   D. A 16-month-old in respiratory arrest

3. What size peripheral IV catheters are recommended for use in children?
   A. 18 and 20 gauge
   B. 14 and 16 gauge
   C. 5 and 7 French
   D. 24 and 22 gauge

4. The ideal location to place an IV in a hospitalized child is:
   A. At the bedside
   B. In the treatment room
   C. In the playroom
   D. In the home of the patient

5. After two attempts at IV access during resuscitative efforts, which of the following sites should be used?
   A. Intracardiac
   B. Intra-arterial
   C. Intrathecal
   D. Intraosseous

6. The vascular access site unique to the newborn population is the:
   A. Umbilicus
   B. Anterior fontanel
   C. Subclavian area
   D. Antecubital fossa

7. What type of vascular access device would you recommend for an adolescent with a therapy plan longer than 1 year?
   A. Broviac catheter
   B. Subclavian catheter
   C. Implanted port
   D. Hickman catheter

8. The *best* method for calculating maintenance fluid requirements for a child is:
   A. Broselow tape
   B. Weight method
   C. Age method
   D. Meters-squared method

9. In PN solutions, which component provides energy for body tissue function?
   A. Amino acids
   B. Selenium
   C. Dextrose
   D. Fatty acids

10. The most common component given to children is which of the following?
    A. Platelets
    B. PRBCs
    C. Whole blood
    D. Fresh frozen plasma

References and Selected Readings   *Asterisks indicate references cited in text.*

*Aguis, C.R. (2012). Intelligent infusion technologies. *Journal of Infusion Nursing*, 35(6), 364–368.

*Anderson, B.J. (2011). Developmental pharmacology, filling one knowledge gap in pediatric anesthesiology. *Pediatric Anesthesia*, 21(3), 179–182.

Arbeiter, H.I., & Greengard, J. (1944). Tibial bone marrow infusions in infancy. *Journal of Pediatrics*, 25, 1.

*Baskin, J., Pui, C., Reiss, U., Wilimas, J., Metzger, M., Ribeiro, R., et al. (2009). Management of occlusion and thrombosis associated with long term indwelling central venous catheters. *Lancet*, 374, 159–169.

Batton, D.G., Maisels, J., & Applebaum, P. (1982). Use of peripheral intravenous cannulas in premature infants: A controlled study. *Pediatrics*, 70, 488.

*Beauman, S.S., & Swanson, A. (2006). Neonatal infusion therapy: Preventing complications and improving outcomes. *Newborn and Infant Nursing Reviews*, 6(4), 193–201.

*Blayney, F. (2013). Renal disorders. In M. Hazinski (Ed.), *Nursing care of the critically ill child* (pp. 703–772). St. Louis, MO: Elsevier Mosby.

Bossert, E., & Beecroft, P.C. (1994). Peripheral intravenous lock irrigation in children: Current practice. *Pediatric Nursing*, 20, 346–355.

*Bradley, J.S., & Nelson, J.D. (2010). *Nelson's pocket book of pediatric antimicrobial therapy* (18th ed.). Elk Grove Village, IL: American Academy of Pediatrics.

*Bradshaw, W.T., & Furdon, S.A. (2006). A nurses' guide to early detection of umbilical venous catheter complications in infants. *Advances in Neonatal Care*, 6(3), 127–138.

*Briening, E. (2008). Arterial catheter insertion: Perform. In J. Trivits Verger & R.M. Lebet (Eds.), *AACN procedure manual for pediatric acute and critical care* (pp. 1121–1127). St. Louis, MO: Saunders Elsevier.

*Broviac, W., Cole, B., & Schribner, B.H. (1973). A silicone rubber atrial catheter for prolonged parenteral alimentation. *Surgery, Gynecology & Obstetrics*, 136, 602.

*Brown, T.L. (2009). Pediatric variations of nursing interventions. In M.J. Hockenberry & D. Wilson (Eds.), *Wong's essentials of pediatric nursing* (pp. 686–753). St. Louis, MO: Mosby Elsevier.

*Bryant, R. (2009). The child with hematologic or immunologic dysfunction. In M.J. Hockenberry & D. Wilson (Eds.), *Wong's essentials of pediatric nursing* (pp. 911–948). St. Louis, MO: Mosby Elsevier.

*Btaiche, I.F., & Khalidi, N. (2002). Parenteral nutrition associated liver complications in children. *Pharmacotherapy*, 22, 188–211.

*Burke, M.L., & Salani, D. (2013). Hematologic and oncologic emergencies requiring critical care. In M. Hazinski (Ed.), *Nursing care of the critically ill child* (pp. 825–850). St. Louis, MO: Elsevier Mosby.

*Carson, J.L., Grossman, B.J., Klienman, S., Tinmouth, A.T., Marques, M.B., & Fung, M.K. (2012). Red blood cell transfusion: A clinical practice guideline from the AABB. *Annals of Internal Medicine, 157*, 49–58.

*Centers for Disease Control and Prevention. (2011). *Guidelines for the prevention of intravascular catheter-related infections.* http://www.cdc.gov/hicpac/pdf/guidelines/BSI

Chameides, L. (1994). *Textbook of pediatric advanced life support.* Dallas, TX: American Heart Association.

*Clark, E., Giambra, B.K., Hingl, J., Doellman, D., Tofani, B., & Johnson, N. (2013). Reducing risk of harm from extravasation. *The Art and Science of Infusion Nursing, 36*(1), 37–45.

*Climo, M.W., Yokoe, D.S., Warren, D.K., Perl, T.M., Bolon, M., Herwaldt, L.A., et al. (2013). Effect of daily chlorhexidine bathing on hospital acquired infection. *The New England Journal of Medicine, 368*(6), 533–542.

*Cohen, L.L. (2008). Behavioral approaches to anxiety and pain management for pediatric venous access. *Pediatrics, 122*, S134–S139.

*Conte, T.M. (2008). Blood product support. In N. E. Kline (Ed.), *Essentials of pediatric hematology/oncology nursing* (pp. 178–183). Glenview, IL: Association of Pediatric Hematology/Oncology Nurses.

*Corkins, M.R., Balint, J., Bobo, E., Plogsted, S., Yaworksi, J.A., & Seebeck, N.D. (2010). *The ASPEN pediatric nutrition support core curriculum.* Silver Spring, MD: American Society for Parenteral and Enteral Nutrition.

*Cummings, E.A., Reid, G.J., Finley, G.A., McGrath, P.J., & Ritchie, J.A. (1996). Prevalence and source of pain in pediatric inpatients. *Pain, 68*(1), 25–31.

*Davis, A. (1998). Pediatrics. In L.E. Matarese & M.M. Gottschlich (Eds.), *Contemporary nutrition support practice: A clinical guide* (pp. 349–351). Philadelphia, PA: WB Saunders.

*Dawson, D. (2002). Midline catheters in neonatal patients: Evaluating a change in practice. *Journal of Vascular Access Devices, 7*(2), 17–19.

Dieckmann, R. (1997). *Pediatric emergency and critical care procedures.* St. Louis, MO: Mosby-Year Book.

*Doellman, D., Pettit, J., Catudal, J.P., Buckner, J., Burns, D., Frey, A.M., et al. (2010). *Best practice guidelines in the care and maintenance of pediatric central venous catheters.* Draper, UT: Pedivan Association of Vascular Access.

*Donniger, S.J., Ishimine, P., Fox, J.C., & Kanegaye, J.T. (2009). Randomized controlled trial of ultrasound guided peripheral intravenous catheter placement versus traditional techniques in difficult access pediatric patients. *Pediatric Emergency Care, 25*(3), 154–159.

Dumont, D. (2012). Preventing central line-associated bloodstream infections (CLABSI). *Nursing, 42*(6), 41–46.

*Ellett, M.L. (2009). The child with gastrointestinal dysfunction. In M.J. Hockenberry & D. Wilson (Eds.), *Wong's essentials of pediatric nursing* (pp. 813–860). St. Louis, MO: Mosby Elsevier.

*Erikson, E.H. (1963). *Childhood and society* (2nd ed.). Stanford, CA: Stanford University Press.

Erikson, E.H. (1966). Eight ages of man. *Journal of Psychiatry, 2*, 281–307.

*Etzel Hardman, D. (2008). Totally implantable central venous port: Accessing, management, and deaccessing. In J. Trivits Verger & R.M. Lebet (Eds.), *AACN procedure manual for pediatric acute and critical care* (pp. 1107–1115). St. Louis, MO: Saunders Elsevier.

*Farion, K.J., Splinter, K.L., Newhook, K., Gaboury, I., & Splinter, W.M. (2008). The effect of vapocoolant spray on pain due to intravenous cannulation in children: A randomized controlled trial. *Canadian Medical Association Journal, 179*(1), 31–36.

*Finberg, L., Dweck, H.S., Holmes, F., Kretchmer, N., Mauer, A.M., Reynolds, J.W., et al. (1986). Prudent lifestyle for children: Dietary fat and cholesterol. *Pediatrics, 78*(3), 521–525.

*Flook, D.M., & Vincze, D.L. (2012). Infant safe sleep: Efforts to improve education and awareness. *Journal of Pediatric Nursing, 27*(2), 186–188.

*Fraser Askin, D. (2009). Health problems of newborns. In M.J. Hockenberry & D. Wilson (Eds.), *Wong's essentials of pediatric nursing* (pp. 243–321). St. Louis, MO: Mosby Elsevier.

*Frey, A.M., & Pettit, J. (2010). Infusion therapy in children. In M. Alexander, A. Corrigan, L. Gorski, J. Hankins, & R. Perucca (Eds.), *Infusion nursing: An evidence-based approach* (p. 550). St. Louis, MO: Saunders.

*Frey, B., Ersch, J., Bernet, V., & Baenziger, O. (2009). Involvement of parents in critical incidents in a neonatal-paediatric intensive care unit. *Quality and Safety in Health Care, 18*(6), 446–449.

*Furdon, S.A., Horgan, M.J., Bradshaw, W.T., & Clark, D.A. (2006). Nurses' guide to early detection of umbilical arterial catheter complications in infants. *Advances in Neonatal Care, 6*(5), 242–256.

*Garland, J.S., Dunne, W.M., Jr., Havens, P., & Hintermeyer, M. (1992). Peripheral intravenous catheter complications in critically ill children: A prospective study. *Pediatrics, 89,* 1145–1150.

Glaeser, P.N., & Losek, D. (1986). Emergency intraosseous infusions in children. *American Journal of Emergency Medicine, 4,* 35.

*Gostisha, M.L., & Braby, J. (1999). Physiologic principles unique to children. In M.E. Broome & J.A. Rollins (Eds.), *Core curriculum for the nursing care of children and their families* (pp. 17–30). Pitman, NJ: Jannetti Publications.

Guilbeau, J.R., & Broussard, L.P. (2010). Community-associated methicillin-resistant *Staphylococcus aureus* (MRSA). *Nursing for Women's Health, 14*(4), 310–317.

*Hadaway, L. (2010). Infusion therapy equipment. In A.M. Corrigan, L. Gorski, J. Hankins, & R. Perucca (Eds.), *Infusion nursing: Evidence-based approach* (pp. 456–479). St. Louis, MO: Saunders Elsevier.

*Hawkins, H.S. (2008). Intraosseous needle placement: Perform. In J. Trivits Verger & R.M. Lebet (Eds.), *AACN procedure manual for pediatric acute and critical care* (pp. 1143–1149). St. Louis, MO: Saunders Elsevier.

*Hazinski, M. (2013). Children are different. In M. Hazinski (Ed.), *Nursing care of the critically ill child* (pp. 1–18). St. Louis, MO: Elsevier Mosby.

*Helton Rapoport, K., & Salazar Young, C. (2008). Umbilical vessel catheter: Care and management. In J. Trivits Verger & R.M. Lebet (Eds.), *AACN procedure manual for pediatric acute and critical care* (pp. 1414–1423). St. Louis, MO: Saunders Elsevier.

*Hesselgrave, J. (2009). Developmental influences on child health promotion. In M.J. Hockenberry & D. Wilson (Eds.), *Wong's essentials of pediatric nursing* (pp. 71–96). St. Louis, MO: Mosby Elsevier.

*Hockenberry, M.J. (2008). History and philosophy of pediatric oncology nursing. In N.E. Kline (Ed.), *Essentials of pediatric hematology oncology nursing* (pp. 2–3). Glenview, IL: Association of Pediatric Hematology/Oncology Nurses.

*Hockenberry, M.J., McCarthy, K., Taylor, O., Scarberry, M., Franklin, Q., Louis, C.U., et al. (2011). Managing painful procedures in children with cancer. *Journal of Pediatric Hematology Oncology, 33*(2), 119–127.

*Infusion Nurses Society. (2011). Infusion nursing standards of practice [Supplemental material]. *Journal of Infusion Nursing, 34,* 1S.

*Jacob, E. (2009). Pain assessment and management in children. In M.J. Hockenberry & D. Wilson (Eds.), *Wong's essentials of pediatric nursing* (pp. 171–196). St. Louis, MO: Mosby Elsevier.

Kalechstein, S., Permaul, A., & Cameron, B.M. (2012). Evaluation of a new pediatric intraosseous needle insertion device for low-resource setting. *Journal of Pediatric Surgery, 47,* 974–979.

*Keller, S. (1995). Small gauge needles promote safe blood transfusions. *Oncology Nursing Forum, 22,* 718.

Kelly, J.S. (2008). Painless vascular cannulation: Ethyl chloride, vapocoolants and cryoanalgesics. *Canadian Medical Association Journal, 179*(1), 31–36.

Kelly, M.S., Conway, M., Wirth, K.E., Potter-Bynoe, G., Billett, A.L., & Sandora, T.J. (2013). Microbiology and risk factors for central-line associated bloodstream infections among pediatric oncology patients: A single institution experience of 41 cases. *Journal of Pediatric Hematology and Oncology, 35*(2), 71–76.

*Kirby, D.F., Corrigan, M.L., & Emery, D.M. (2012). Home parenteral nutrition tutorial. *Journal of Parenteral Enteral Nutrition, 36,* 632–644.

Klein, C.J., Havranek, T.G., Revenis, M.E., Hassanali, Z., & Scavo, L.M. (2013). Plasma fatty acids in premature infants with hyperbilirubinemia. *Nutrition in Clinical Practice, 28*(1), 87–94.

Kleinman, R.E. (2009). *Pediatric nutrition handbook* (6th ed.). Elk Grove Village, IL: American Academy of Pediatrics.

*Kleinman, M.E., Chameides, L., Schexnayder, S.M., Sampson, R.A., Hazinski, M., & Atkins, D.L. (2010). 2010 American Heart Association guidelines for cardiopulmonary resuscitation and emergency cardiovascular care science. *Circulation, 122,* S876–S908.

*Koletzko, B., Goulet, O., Hunt, J., Krohn, K., & Shamir, R. (2005). Guidelines on paediatric parenteral nutrition of the European Society of Paediatric Gastroenterology, Hepatology, and Nutrition (ESPGHAN) and the European Society for Clinical Nutrition and Metabolism (ESPEN), supported by the European Society of Paediatric Research (ESPR). *Journal of Pediatric Gastroenterology and Nutrition, 41,* S1–S87.

Le, H.D., DeMeijer, V.E., Robinson, E.M., Zurakowski, D., Potemkin, A.K., Arsenault, D.A., et al. (2011). Parenteral fish-oil-based lipid emulsion improves fatty acid profiles and lipids in parenteral nutrition-dependent children. *American Journal of Clinical Nutrition, 94*(3), 749–758.

*Leahy, S., Kennedy, R.M., Hesselgrave, J., Gurwitch, K., Barkey, M., & Millar, T.F. (2008). On the front lines: Lessons learned in implementing multidisciplinary peripheral venous access pain management programs in pediatric hospitals. *Pediatrics, 122*, S161–S170.

*Lubitz, D.S., Siedel, J.S., Chameides, L., Luten, R.C., Zaritsky, A.L., & Campbell, F.W. (1988). A rapid method for estimating weight and resuscitation drug dosages from length in the pediatric age group. *Annals of Emergency Medicine, 17*(6), 576–581.

*Madsen, L. (2008). Administration of vesicants. In N.E. Kline (Ed.), *Essentials of pediatric hematology/oncology nursing* (pp. 90–92). New York, NY: Association of Pediatric Hematology/Oncology Nurses.

*McCarthy, K. (2008). Leukemia. In N.E. Kline (Ed.), *Essentials of pediatric hematology oncology nursing* (pp. 15–20). Glenview, IL: Association of Pediatric Hematology/Oncology Nurses.

Miccolo, M.A. (1990). Intraosseous infusion. *Critical Care Nurse, 10*, 35–47.

*Milestone, A.M., Elward, A., Song, X., Zerr, D.M., Orscheln, R., Speck, K., et al. (2013). Daily chlorhexidine bathing to reduce bacteraemia in critically ill children: A multicentre, cluster-randomised, crossover trial. *Lancet, 381*, 1099–1106.

*Miller, L.J., Montez, D.F., Puga, T.A., & Philbeck, T.E. (2012). Intraosseous vascular access in the 21st century: Improvements further reduce complication rates. *Annals of Emergency Medicine, 60*(4 Suppl.), S112.

*Mirtallo, J., Canada, T., & Johnson, D. (2004). Safe practices for parenteral nutrition formulations. *Journal of Parenteral Enteral Nutrition, 28*(6), S39–S70.

Mofenson, H.C., Tascone, A., & Caraccio, T.R. (1988). Guidelines for intraosseous infusions. *Journal of Emergency Medicine, 6*(2), 143–146.

*National Institute of Health. (2012). http://www.nhlbi.nih.gov/health/health-topics/topics/sca/atrisk.html

*Nelson, D.B., & Garland, J.S. (1987). The natural history of Teflon catheter-associated phlebitis in children. *American Journal of Diseases of Children, 141*, 1090–1092.

*Nichols, I., & Doellman, D. (2007). Pediatric peripherally inserted central catheter placement: Application of ultrasound technology. *Journal of Infusion Nursing, 30*(6), 351–356.

*Perkin, R.M., DeCaen, A.R., Berg, M.D., Schexnayder, S.M., & Hazinski, M.F. (2013). Shock, cardiac arrest, and resuscitation. In M.F. Hazinski (Ed.), *Nursing care of the critically ill child* (pp. 101–154). St. Louis, MO: Elsevier Mosby.

*Peterson, K.A., Phillips, A.L., Truemper, E., & Agarwal, S. (2012). Does the use of an assistive device by nurse impact peripheral intravenous catheter insertion success in children? *Journal of Pediatric Nursing, 27*, 134–143.

*Pettit, J., & Wyckoff, M.M. (2007). *Peripherally inserted central catheters* (2nd ed.). Glenview, IL: National Association of Neonatal Nurses.

*Phipps, S., Barrera, M., Vannatta, K., Xiong, X., Doyle, J.J., & Alderfer, M.A. (2010). Complementary therapies for children undergoing stem cell transplantation. *Cancer, 116*(16), 3924–3933.

*Pop, R.S. (2012). Pediatric peripheral intravenous infiltration assessment tool. *Journal of Infusion Nursing, 35*(4), 243–248.

Powers, R.J., & Wirtschafter, D.W. (2010). Decreasing central line associated bloodstream infection in neonatal intensive care. *Clinics in Perinatology, 37*(1), 247.

*Ringel, M. (1995). Providing pediatric infusion therapies: Putting the pieces together. *Infusion, 2*(2), 20–25.

*Roberts, K.E. (2013). Fluid, electrolyte, and endocrine problems. In M. Hazinski (Ed.), *Nursing care of the critically ill child* (pp. 679–701). St. Louis, MO: Elsevier Mosby.

*Rosenthal, K. (2008). Bridging the IV access gap with midline catheters. *Med/Surg Insider*, Fall, 1–5.

*Samour, P., & King, K. (2012). *Pediatric nutrition* (4th ed.). Sudbury, MA: Jones and Bartlett Learning.

*Sapsford, A. (1994). Energy, carbohydrate, protein, and fat. In S. Groh-Wargo, M. Thompson, & J.H. Cox (Eds.), *Nutrition care for high risk newborns* (p. 83). Chicago, IL: Precept Press.

*Savage, B. (2008). Sickle cell disease. In N.E. Kline (Ed.), *Essentials of pediatric hematology oncology nursing a core curriculum* (pp. 288–292). Glenview, IL: Association of Hematology Oncology Nursing.

Schechter, N.L., Zempsky, W.T., Cohen, L.L., McGrath, P.J., McMurtry, C.M., & Bright, N.S. (2007). Pain reduction during pediatric immunizations: Evidence-based review and recommendations. *Pediatrics, 119*(5), e1184–e1198.

*Secola, R., & Reid, D. (2008). Side effects of treatment: Oncologic emergencies. In N.E. Kline (Ed.), *Essentials of pediatric hematology/oncology nursing* (pp. 154–155). Glenview, IL: Association of Pediatric Hematology/Oncology Nurses.

*Spagrud, L., VonBaeyer, C., Ali, K., Mpofu, C., Fennell, L., Frifen, K., et al. (2008). Pain, distress, and adult child interaction during venipuncture in pediatric oncology: An examination of three types of venous access. *Journal of Pain and Symptom Management, 36,* 173–184.

*Sparks, L.A., Setlik, J., & Luhman, J. (2007). Parental holding and positioning to decrease IV distress in young children: A randomized controlled trial. *Journal of Pediatric Nursing, 22*(6), 440–447.

*Tobias, J.D., & Ross, A.K. (2010). Intraosseous infusions: A review for the anesthesiologist with a focus on pediatric use. *Anesthesia and Analgesia, 110,* 391–401.

*Tocantins, L.M., & O'Neil, J.F. (1945). Complications of intraosseous therapy. *Annals of Surgery, 122,* 266–277.

*Tofani, B.F., Rineair, S.A., Gosdin, C.H., Pilcher, P.M., McGee, S., Varadarajan, K.R., et al. (2012). Quality improvement project to reduce infiltration and extravasation events in a pediatric hospital. *Journal of Pediatric Nursing, 27,* 682–689.

*Tully, J.L., Friedland, G.H., Baldini, L.M., & Goldman, D.A. (1981). Complications of intravenous therapy with steel needles and Teflon catheters: A comparative study. *American Journal of Medicine, 70,* 702–706.

*van Miert, C., Hill, R., & Jones, L. (2012). Interventions for restoring patency of occluded central venous catheter lumens. www.thecochranelibrary.com

Vlaardingerbroek, H., Veldhorst, M., Spronk, S., van den Akker, C., & van Goudoever, J.B. (2012). Parenteral lipid administration to very low-birth-weight infants: Introduction of lipids and use of new lipid emulsion—A systematic review and meta-analysis. *The American Journal of Clinical Nutrition, 96*(2), 255–268.

Voepel-Lewis, T., Zanotti, J., Dammeyer, J., & Merkel, S. (2010). Reliability and validity of the face, legs, activity, cry, consolability behavioral tool in assessing acute pain in critically ill patients. *American Journal of Critical Care, 19*(1), 55–61.

*Walco, G.A. (2008). Needle pain in children: Contextual factors. *Pediatrics, 122,* S125.

*Walden, M., & Gibbins, S. (2008). *Pain assessment and management guideline for practice* (2nd ed.). Glenview, IL: National Association of Neonatal Nurses.

*Wallace, J.D. (2008). Central venous access devices. In N.E. Kline (Ed.), *Essentials of pediatric hematology/oncology nursing* (pp. 165–168). Glenview, IL: Association of Pediatric Hematology/Oncology Nurse.

*Weinstein, S.M. (Ed.). (2007). *Plumer's principles and practice of intravenous therapy* (8th ed.). Philadelphia, PA: Lippincott Williams & Wilkins.

*Wilson, D. (2009). Health promotion of the infant and family. In M.J. Hockenberry & D. Wilson (Eds.), *Wong's essentials of pediatric nursing* (pp. 322–376). St. Louis, MO: Mosby Elsevier.

*Wilson, F.L., Baker, L.M., Nordstrom, C.K., & Legwand, C. (2008). Using the teach back and Orem's self-care deficit nursing theory to increase childhood immunization communication among low income mothers. *Issues in Comprehensive Pediatric Nursing, 31,* 7–22.

*Yaffe, S.J., & Aranda, J.V. (Eds.). (2011). *Neonatal and pediatric pharmacology: Therapeutic principles and practices* (4th ed.). Philadelphia, PA: Lippincott Williams & Wilkins.

*Zempsky, W.T. (2008a). Optimizing the management of peripheral venous access pain in children: Evidence, impact, and implementation. *Pediatrics, 122,* S121.

*Zempsky, W.T. (2008b). Pharmacologic approaches for reducing venous access pain in children. *Pediatrics, 122,* S140–S153.

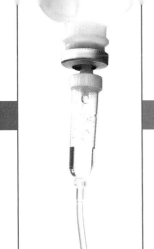

22

Infusion Therapy in an Older Adult

Sherry Cannizzo
Susan Gresser

Functionality
Homeostasis
Hypodermoclysis

Older Adult
Physical Capacity

DEMOGRAPHICS: AN AGING POPULATION

Although people age at different rates, changes to the human body are a hallmark of aging. Normal aging, beyond the effects of disease, is a complex process that involves many different body systems and presents in a wide variety of symptoms and syndromes (Smith & Cotter, 2012). Advances in medical science and technology have resulted in an increased life span. In 2010, older adults comprised approximately 13% of the US population (U.S. Census Bureau, 2011). Along with the growth of the general elderly population has come a remarkable increase in the number of Americans reaching age 100. The segment of the population aged 65 years and older increased most dramatically between 1990 and 2000 by 15.1%. In the same decade, older adults between 85 and 94 years experienced the fastest rate of growth by 29.9% and those over 95 years by 25.9% (U.S. Census Bureau, 2011). By 2030, the older adult population will reach about 72.1 million. Two maps demonstrate the percent of individuals aged 65 years and older and 85 years and older, living in US counties at the time of the 2010 census. This information can be used for planning care requirements for this population and for the numbers of nurses and additional education needed in infusion therapy for the older adult (Figure 22-1).

As the population continues to age, the health care system will need to respond accordingly. Health care professionals will be working with an increasing number of older adults, chronic diseases, and accompanying treatments; the challenges of geriatric syndromes will take on greater importance. Health care professionals' preparation and competence to care

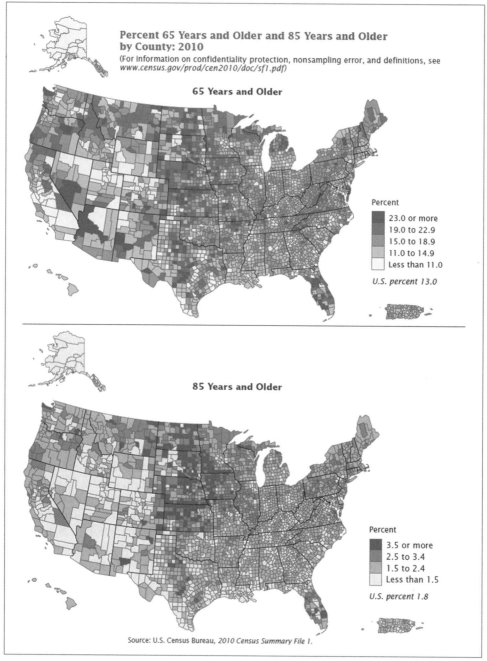

FIGURE 22-1 Individuals (in percentage) aged 65 years and older **(top)** and 85 years and older **(bottom)** by US county in 2010. (From U.S. Census Bureau. (2011). The older population: 2010–2010 Census Briefs. http://www.census.gov/prod/cen2010/briefs/c2010br-09.pdf)

for older adults are of serious concern. Nurses are in a pivotal role to influence the overall quality of care of older adults. Initiatives have been underway for several years to increase the competence of nurses at the point of care to understand the processes of aging and best practices to effectively manage age-related changes as well as the spectrum of diseases and other conditions that often are associated with aging. **Physical capacity**, the body's ability to perform various functions, and **functionality**, the effectiveness of performing activities such as activities of daily living, can both be adversely affected by aging and may require interventions to correct or minimize these effects.

Infusion therapy is one method of delivering various treatments that can be very effective for the older adult. However, there are special considerations that must be taken into account for this therapy to have quality outcomes. This chapter addresses the important considerations in initiating, delivering, and maintaining infusion therapy in the older adult patient. The term **older adult** describes a broad category of individuals who range from 50 to 100 years of age, though the term is generally associated with individuals aged 65 years and older. Many physiologic changes associated with the older adult begin in the sixth decade of life, although variations exist among individuals. Infusion nurses caring for older adults are supported in the need for additional clinical knowledge and technical expertise with the Infusion Nurses Society (INS) (2011) standard on older adult patients (p. S7–S8). The document is a guide to the needs of the older adult patient and organizational resources.

THE OLDER ADULT PATIENT AS A HEALTH CARE CONSUMER

As a consumer of health care, the older adult patient has special needs associated with the aging process that challenge the health care system and health care providers. The older adult patient may require administration of complex infusion therapies to treat a multitude of clinical conditions that may occur simultaneously. Older adults today are educated consumers. For some, adopting healthy lifestyles, such as engaging in regular physical activity and eating a healthy diet has reduced the risk of chronic disease as well as the rate of disability. These same lifestyle behaviors also help older adults better manage their chronic diseases. In the past, patients did not usually question the wisdom of their provider, and took a more passive approach to decision-making. Today, issues of informed consent and self-determination have become more prominent, and most patients, young and older adults alike, are taking a much more active role in planning treatments that are effective and personally acceptable. Many older patients are collaborating with their providers and partnering with them to monitor the decisions that they, as consumers, make. Decisions that are clinically relevant and ethically appropriate are the challenges of the caregiver and older adult; there must be a careful balance of such in light of medical requirements and what resources will be beneficial and available (Mitty & Post, 2012).

EVIDENCE FOR PRACTICE

In 2011, the cost of chronic disease totaled nearly $3 trillion. What will the impact of chronic disease be in the future? How will self-management affect the financial burden?

Physiology of Aging: Homeostasis

The kidneys, heart and blood vessels, lungs, skin, adrenal glands, hypothalamus, pituitary gland, parathyroid gland, and gastrointestinal tract are the regulatory organs associated with maintaining the body's homeostasis. Homeostasis is the ability of the body to maintain a balance of volume and composition of body fluids within normal ranges. The kidneys are a primary force in homeostasis because they work to adjust the amount of water and electrolytes that exit the body in an amount equal to the quantity of solution entering the body, through either parenteral or oral feedings. Circulating blood reaches the kidneys in sufficient volume to regulate water and electrolytes, and the pumping action of the heart provides circulation through the kidneys, which produce and excrete urine.

The lungs are involved in homeostasis through ventilation. Antidiuretic hormone (ADH), which causes fluid retention, is manufactured in the hypothalamus and stored in the pituitary gland. ADH also is involved in controlling blood volume. When blood volume is increased, ADH secretion is decreased and water is excreted through the kidneys. Parathyroid hormone affects calcium and phosphate concentrations and influences reabsorption of calcium, a key factor in maintaining fluid and electrolyte monitoring and replacement. The gastrointestinal tract also plays a major role in homeostasis by absorption and reabsorption through the small intestine. For the body to maintain homeostasis, all these organs must work in synchronicity.

In otherwise healthy adults, physiologic changes may cause reactions related to medication changes—that is, they influence the absorption, distribution, and clearance of medications. Absorption in older adults is complete, yet slower. Age-related changes also affect the rate and extent of absorption. As people age, they lose lean body mass and gain adipose tissue. With less fluid available, water-soluble medications can reach toxic levels more quickly. Vigilant monitoring is needed with potentially nephrotoxic agents, H_2-antagonists, hypoglycemics, and nonsteroidal anti-inflammatory agents. With decreases in kidney and liver function, clearance and excretion of drugs also take longer. Monitoring serum protein and albumin levels, as well as renal and liver functions, is essential to help the older patient avoid toxicity or undertreatment (Amella, 2004).

Normal homeostatic mechanisms in aging become less efficient in the face of external trauma, surgical intervention, disease process, or infection. The older patient is vulnerable to complications associated with routine infusion therapy. An overview of age-related physiologic changes is summarized in Table 22-1.

Physiology of Aging: The Immune System

With aging, the immune system undergoes natural changes and declines. There is a reduced efficiency of the immune response, both from the innate immune system, which is responsible for an immediate response to bacteria or viruses, and the adaptive immune system, which elicits a delayed response and is often more effective once activated (Graham, Christian, & Kiecolt-Glaser, 2006). Because of this natural decrease in function, older adults are at greater risk for impairment and death from infection. They are especially at risk for intravenous catheter–associated infection due to their potentially immunocompromised status.

Physiology of Aging: The Cardiovascular System

Cardiovascular changes are profound, contributing to a slower response to the stress of blood loss, fluid depletion, shock, and acid–base imbalances. Changes in renal and cardiac status have the potential to place the patient at great risk for the development of infusion-related complications.

TABLE 22-	THE AGING OF THE BODY'S SYSTEMS	
Body System	**Physiologic Changes**	**Signs/Symptoms**
Skin	• Loss of subcutaneous tissue and thinning of the dermis	• Underlying tissue more fragile; inability to respond to heat or cold quickly; proneness to heat stroke; loss of moisture; wrinkling
Sensory	• Loss of lid elasticity • Ocular changes in the cornea, iris, pupil, lens	• Eyelids droop or turn inward • Increased astigmatism; need for more light; glare problems; need for eyeglasses • Cataracts
	• Auditory canal narrows • Calcification of ossicles • Changes in the organ of Corti • Olfactory bulb and cells decrease	• Increased cerumen • Hearing loss • Impaired sound transmission; tinnitus • Inability to discriminate odors
Cardiovascular	• Decreased stress response • Stiffer valves • Conductivity altered	• Diminished cardiac output • Diastolic murmurs • More ectopic beats; less ability to respond to changes in blood pressure
	• Vessels less elastic	• Poorer perfusion to vital organs with resulting hypoxia; varicosities; peripheral pulses not always palpable
Pulmonary	• Enlargement and rigidity of the chest wall • Airway collapse	• Poor expansion with less efficient air exchange; shallow breathing; less effective cough • Less efficient oxygen exchange
Gastrointestinal	• Increase in incidence of hiatal hernia • Decrease in abdominal strength • Reduced gastric acid • Slowed neural transmission • Weakened intestinal walls	• Reflux • Peptic ulcers • Vitamin deficiencies • Constipation • Incontinence • Diverticulosis
Renal	• Decrease in renal blood flow, and glomerular filteration rate	• Decreased creatinine clearance • Decreased ability to concentrate urine and conserve water • Poor response to stress
Musculoskeletal	• Shrinkage of vertebral discs • Loss of bone mass • Muscle atrophy	• Loss of height by 1.5–3 inches • Tendency toward fractures • Decreased strength • Decreased stamina
Neurologic	• Diminished REM sleep • Altered pain sensation • Tactile sense decreases • Sleep disorders	• Difficulty with balance and position changes • Decreased perception of pain • Loss of sensation in the extremities

(Continued)

TABLE 22-1	THE AGING OF THE BODY'S SYSTEMS (*Continued*)	
Body System	**Physiologic Changes**	**Signs/Symptoms**
Immune	• Decrease in thymus mass • Increase in immunoglobulins	• Decline in cell-mediated immunity with possible reactivation of herpes, tuberculosis • Autoimmune response not associated with disease
Endocrine	• Loss of sensitivity to insulin • Decrease in sex hormones	• Blood glucose does not return to normal as rapidly • BPH, testicular firmness; vaginal dryness and atrophy • Longer time to orgasm

BPH, benign prostatic hypertrophy; REM, random eye movement.
Adapted from Jett, K. (2012). Chapter 4: Physiological changes. In T. A. Touhy & K. Jett, *Ebersole & Hess' Toward healthy aging: Human needs & nursing response* (8th ed., pp. 44–61). St. Louis, MO: Elsevier/Mosby.

PATIENT SAFETY

Fluid volume excess or hypervolemia, also called fluid overload, is a serious risk in the older adult patient receiving IV fluids. Using an electronic infusion device, monitoring lung sounds, and dividing blood components into smaller amounts, or aliquots, are recommended practices especially for older adult patients.

Physiology of Aging: Skin and Connective Tissue

The skin, the body's first defense against disease, changes in texture, depth, and integrity as the person ages. After age 60, epidermal cell replacement decreases, resulting in a marked thinning of the epidermis and an increased fragility of the skin's surface. The result is dry, transparent, paper-thin tissue that tears easily and heals slowly. Changes in the dermis create a loose, wrinkling effect. The skin becomes pale, and nerve endings are less sensitive. The older adult is at risk for thermal injuries. Subcutaneous fat cells decrease, resulting in changes to the superficial fascia, including decreased production of sebum and sweat. Loss of subcutaneous tissue and resultant thinning of the skin present a venous access challenge. Purpura and ecchymoses may appear because of dermal fragility; minor trauma may inflict bruising.

PATIENT SAFETY

Because of fragile skin and less tissue support, stroking the veins gently to promote venous filling is recommended rather than patting, which may cause bruising and tissue damage.

Physiology of Aging: Fluid Balance

Physiologic changes of aging affect the older adult's fluid balance. Fluid reserves are limited, and total body water is reduced by 6%, creating a potential for fluid volume deficit. Gastrointestinal changes such as decreased volume of saliva and gastric juice and decreased calcium absorption

---

BOX 22-1   FLUID VOLUME ASSESSMENT PARAMETERS IN THE OLDER ADULT PATIENT

Skin turgor of the forehead/sternum

Temperature <98.6°F

Decreased rate/filling of hand veins

Intake and output

Daily weight

Tongue—the center should remain moist

Blood pressure—possibility of orthostatic hypotension

Swallowing function

Functional assessment of the patient's ability to obtain fluids

Adapted from Metheny, N. M. (2012). *Fluid and electrolyte balance: Nursing considerations* (5th ed.). Burlington, MA: Jones & Bartlett Learning.

---

cause the mouth to be drier and increase potential for sodium and potassium deficit during episodes of vomiting and gastric suction. Oral intake may be altered as a result of medications, treatments, advanced cognitive impairment, swallowing impairments, and other functional challenges (Gilmour & Penny, 1991). Assessment guidelines are presented in Box 22-1.

The usual assessment measures to determine fluid balance should be adjusted when providing care to the older adult. For example, testing skin turgor on the forearm is no longer a valid measure because the skin loses elasticity with age. Skin turgor is best assessed in the older patient by tenting the tissue on the forehead or over the sternum. Alterations in skin elasticity are less marked in those sites (Metheny, 2012).

Physiology of Aging: Senses

People use their senses, both consciously and unconsciously to experience the world around them. As people age, changes in the senses (vision, hearing, smell, taste, and touch) can alter that experience (Cacchione, 2012). Changes in sensation may also affect the older adult's response to treatment. After age 50, subtle changes in the hearing process result in difficulty in differentiating sounds. Normal changes in hearing in the older adult are often from decreased function of the hair fibers in the ear canal. Build-up of cerumen can cause distortion and loss of hearing. Presbycusis is the loss of ability to discern high-frequency sounds. Older adults experience normal slowing of the pupils to dilate and contract, which alter the ability to adjust to light and dark. There is a loss of elasticity in the lens and stiffening of muscles, which can lead to decreased ability to change the shape of the lens and focus on fine print. The senses of smell, taste, and touch are also affected by the process of aging and become decreased over time. Because of decreased tactile sensation, infiltration might go unnoticed, contributing to the potential for development of tissue necrosis, infection, or compartment syndrome. Older patients may need assistive devices, such as hearing aids, eyeglasses, and visual aids, to learn the skills associated with infusion therapy.

Physiology of Aging: Vascular System

Chronic disease, such as asthma, chronic obstructive pulmonary disease, and hypertension, and the changes associated with atherosclerosis and arteriosclerosis affect the blood vessels in the older patient. Vessels are fragile, with small, thin-walled surface capillaries easily observed across the extremities and chest of the older patient. Vascular fragility is a potential problem for IV access; a tourniquet sometimes is often not necessary as it can cause constriction and potential for bruising. Use of a blood pressure cuff may offer enough pressure for easier insertion. Consider locations of previous IV insertions as well as what kinds of movement the older adult will require with the use of the limb where the IV is located.

Physiology of Aging: Cognitive Changes

Confusion is not a normal change or occurrence that comes with aging. However, cognitive changes can occur that may have increased prevalence related to advanced age. Cognitive processing slows down with aging. Some thinking abilities will remain relatively stable while others may decline. The ability to concentrate on multiple tasks concurrently decreases, making it more difficult to withstand multiple teaching priorities. If confusion should occur as a part of delirium or dementia, the older adult's ability to process IV therapy treatment will be compromised. Teaching may become complicated because the patient has difficulty in differentiating between recent and remote memory. IV therapy poses risks of infection and phlebitis, thereby increasing the risk of confusion related to delirium. The older adult's risk factors for confusion should be assessed prior to initiation of infusion therapy. Principles of patient teaching in the older adult are listed in Box 22-2.

BOX 22-2   PRINCIPLES OF PATIENT TEACHING FOR THE OLDER ADULT PATIENT RECEIVING INFUSION THERAPY

- Address the patient by his or her proper name.
- Hearing impairment and sensitivity to outside sounds require patience.
- Speak slowly, clearly, and directly to the patient.
- Explain steps in logical order.
- Take steps to decrease anxiety.
- Use familiar terminology.
- Attend to physical needs before and during teaching; for example, offer fluids and toilet breaks.
- Break down psychomotor skills into individual steps.
- For visual changes, use 14- to 16-point font and double spacing on all reading materials.
- For hearing changes, use lower pitch of voice and use pictures, models, and demonstrations.

Adapted from Thomas, M. H. (2011). Chapter 9: Health care delivery settings and older adults. In S. E. Meiner (Ed.), *Gerontologic nursing* (4th ed., pp. 148–175). St. Louis, MO: Elsevier Mosby.

ACCESS AND EQUIPMENT

When providing infusion therapy to older adult patients, careful consideration should be given to the type of treatment ordered, duration of therapy, and availability of IV access. The smallest gauge possible for the therapy being delivered should be used. Consideration must be given to the type of catheter–tubing connection used as some products may be irritating to frail skin. Padding may be necessary underneath parts of the catheter that could be irritating to the skin. A securement device should be applied in order to keep the catheter from being dislodged and to prevent injury to the skin surface and underlying tissue. Fragile skin should be taken into account when removing the securement device and adhesive; a removal agent may be part of the procedure. The patient's skin should be held firmly and the tape removed slowly and carefully in order to prevent trauma to the skin.

When a central venous access device is needed for long-term therapy, the type of device should be carefully considered. Consideration should be given to the patient's living circumstances, availability of family or other support systems, and ability to manipulate the equipment involved and to maintain a secure, intact dressing (Fabian, 2010).

Flow Control

Electronic infusion devices (EIDs) are encouraged for all older adult patients as they are more sensitive to rapid changes in fluid volumes, which can result in fluid and electrolyte imbalance, dyspnea, and heart failure due to IV fluid overload. If available, lockout features on the pump should be used with confused or disoriented individuals. An electronic flow control device should be an accessory to quality patient care and not a substitute for ongoing monitoring. Additionally, the older adult patient using IV tubing and pump is at risk for a fall and fall-related injury; provide education and visual reminders as needed to prevent a fall and/or injury (INS, 2013).

EVIDENCE FOR PRACTICE

Eastwood, G. M., Peck, L., Young, H., Prowle, J., Vasudevan, V., Jones, D., et al. (2012). Intravenous fluid administration and monitoring for adult ward patients in a teaching hospital. *Nursing & Health Sciences, 14,* 265–271.

Ferenczi, E., Datta, S. S., & Chopada, A. (2007). Intravenous fluid administration in elderly patients at a London hospital: a two-part audit encompassing ward-based fluid monitoring and prescribing practice by doctors. *International Journal of Surgery, 5,* 408–412.

In two countries, 5 years apart, by different disciplines, investigators examined the practices of monitoring for fluid volume excess in adult patients as well as only in patients aged 65 years and older. Both research teams found that electrolytes and renal functions were monitored; one team found that intake and output were also monitored. However, daily weights were done in 15% or less of the patients receiving IV therapy. Both research teams recommended that daily weights are a noninvasive yet preventive measure to keep older adult patients safe when receiving IV therapy.

Site Selection

In the older adult, there may be loss of subcutaneous fat, thinning of skin, and lack of supporting tissue, which should be taken into account when considering a site for intravenous access. Use sites with more supporting tissue and not over a joint (INS, 2013). Although it is recommended to begin at the most distal site, the hands should not be the first choice due to the loss of subcutaneous fat and thinning of the skin. Placement of the device should also allow for as much movement as possible. Avoiding bruised, fragile veins and conserving veins for future use are major considerations.

Insertion Technique

Although a tourniquet may be used, it should be snug, not tight; it can also be avoided. If needed, a tourniquet should be removed as soon as possible to avoid excessive distention of the veins, which may contribute to bruising and difficult placement of intravenous catheter. Additionally, if the vein is overly distended, the venipuncture may cause the vein to rupture and be unusable for infusion therapy. The veins should be palpated carefully to determine their state of health and condition. Due to thickening and stiffening of veins in the older adult, it may make catheter insertion and placement more difficult (INS, 2013).

Table 22-2 lists the special insertion techniques required in an older adult. Skin tension is determined by assessing the direction or axis of the vessel. Traction is ensured by placing the thumb directly along the vein axis 2 to 3 inches below the intended venipuncture site. The palm and fingers of the hand are used to apply traction, hold, and stabilize the patient's extremity. Traction is maintained throughout the procedure (Fabian, 2010).

TABLE 22-2   SPECIAL TECHNIQUES FOR IV INSERTION IN THE OLDER ADULT PATIENT

Intervention	Rationale
Avoid tourniquet in patients with fragile veins or who are taking anticoagulants or steroids	Tourniquet may not be needed; use of tourniquet may contribute to hematoma formation
If tourniquet is used, release it quickly	Quick release decreases backflow of blood
Multiple-tourniquet technique may be an option to facilitate venous distention:	
Grasp the patient's mid-upper arm and stroke the arm downward toward the hand. Place a tourniquet on the extremity	Stroking promotes venous filling
Wait 1–2 min and then place a second tourniquet below the antecubital fossa and continue to stroke the lower forearm	Placement of the second tourniquet stimulates venous pressure and forces venous distention to small veins that otherwise would not be visible
A third tourniquet may be placed after an additional 1–2 min at a point just above the wrist	The third tourniquet promotes additional venous distention, particularly in the very small veins of the digits and lower wrist
Release the first tourniquet and evaluate the inner wrist, thumb, knuckle, and fingers for distention	Although not *ideal* for infusion purposes, the veins in this area will fill owing to venous pressure and provide adequate hemodilution for infusion purposes
In the edematous patient, use anatomic landmarks	Facilitates location of appropriate veins
Gently tap the vein to distend; do not slap	Avoids hematoma formation and bruising
Use transillumination	Assists in visualizing veins
Insert the catheter with steady, firm motion	Prevents bruising associated with difficult venipuncture
Consider preflushing the catheter in patients with spidery, capillary-type veins	Avoids trauma associated with sudden flushing
Use a one-handed approach	Allows you to secure the patient's extremity

The directional line of the vessel is determined. If the vein is very small, venous distention may be inadequate and imaging techniques may be used, including ultrasound. A small-gauge IV catheter should be selected and positioned with the bevel up. The catheter should be positioned at a 20- to 30-degree angle to the vein track and brought close to the skin directly above the insertion site. A lower angle decreases vein trauma on insertion (Fabian, 2010).

The direct technique may be used for patients with good or stable veins. This technique involves penetrating the skin and vein simultaneously. However, for patients with small, fragile veins, the clinician may find the indirect, two-step technique more beneficial. This technique involves penetrating the skin, then lowering the angle of the catheter to 10 to 15 degrees, restabilizing the vein, and then penetrating the vein wall (Fabian, 2010). If the veins are extremely fragile and if a tourniquet has been used, it may be helpful to release the tourniquet as soon as blood return is evident. Doing so prevents damage from high-pressure backflow of blood from the catheter insertion point.

The hooded technique also may help reduce vein damage. In this approach, the clinician advances the catheter forward over the bevel tip into the vein. This action retracts the stylet tip inside the catheter. Then, the clinician threads the catheter into the vein by grasping the hub of the catheter and advancing the catheter and stylet as a unit up the vein. This procedure minimizes the possibility of perforating the vein during threading. The clinician must maintain stabilization and skin tension throughout the process, or rebound of the skin and vein being released could cause the catheter to rupture the vein (Fabian, 2010).

IV THERAPY MAINTENANCE AND MONITORING

Securing, dressing, and stabilizing the IV catheter are unique challenges when providing infusion therapy to the elderly patient. Although the catheter should be secure, use of excessive tape is discouraged because of the fragility of the patient's skin. Adaptations to taping technique should be used as needed. The use of additional products such as a protective skin barrier should be considered. The protective skin barrier is best applied in a concentric circle from the center to the periphery and allowed to air dry before the dressing is applied (Fabian, 2010). The elderly patient may be confused owing to physiologic reasons or medications, and the nurse should make every effort to ensure safety with the infusion device.

The IV tubing should be long enough to provide adequate range of motion but not so long as to dangle on the floor or get caught on the bedside or IV pole. A Luer-locking device provides added protection to prevent accidental disconnection. Surgical stretch mesh gauze also may be used to cover the IV site, providing stability and protecting the catheter from snagging bed garments. Roll-type gauze should be avoided as it is not easily removed and decreases ability to observe the site, consistent with institutional guidelines and established practice standards (Fabian, 2010).

The infusion therapy site should be evaluated at regularly established intervals and as needed to ensure patency. For peripheral IV (PIV) catheter sites, specific evidence-based recommendations are available based on the patient's age and condition, type of therapy, and venue of care (Gorski et al., 2012). For patients receiving "nonirritant/nonvesicant infusions *and* who are alert and oriented *and* who are able to notify the nurse of any signs of problems," monitor the PIV site every 4 hours. For "adult patients who have cognitive or sensory deficits or who are receiving sedative-type medications and are unable to notify the nurse of any symptoms," monitor the PIV site at least every 1 to 2 hours (Gorski et al., 2012,

p. 292). For the older adult patient, monitoring the site every 1 to 2 hours may be advisable for early identification of phlebitis or infiltration (Fabian, 2010).

> ### PATIENT SAFETY
>
> Frequent monitoring of infusion therapy sites in older adults is important because of decreased peripheral sensation; monitoring also needs to be individualized—based on the patient's condition, type of therapy, infusion device, and cognitive status.

Recent clinical practice guidelines related to infusion therapy have mixed recommendations for PIV catheter site rotation. The CDC (2011) continued to recommend PIV routine replacement every 72 to 96 hours to reduce the risk of infection and phlebitis in adults; it is an "unresolved issue" for any recommendation to replace PIVs in adults only when clinically indicated (p. S6). However, replacement of PIV catheters when clinically indicated has been recommended by a Cochrane Collaboration systematic review (Webster, Osborne, Rickard, & Hall, 2010) and the Infusion Nurses Society Standards of Practice (2011). Due to limited IV access in the older adult, less frequent site rotation is beneficial to preserve potential sites for future access. For all patients, but particularly for older adults, the frequency of catheter site rotation should be based on the patient's condition and access site, skin and vein integrity, length and type of therapy, and venue of care (INS, 2011).

Hypodermoclysis

Hypodermoclysis, also known as subcutaneous infusion, can be used for fluid replacement, in place of IV therapy, in the older adult who is unable to tolerate an intravenous catheter or has veins that are difficult to access due to dehydration or previous insertion attempts (INS, 2013). The older adult may have decreased subcutaneous fat, which must be taken into consideration when selecting a site. According to Barton and colleagues (as cited by Scales, 2011), recommended sites for subcutaneous catheter insertion in the older adult are the abdomen, thighs, and scapula. Of note, early studies demonstrated there was no difference in absorption after fluid administration by the subcutaneous or intravenous route (Barton, Fuller, & Dudley, 2004). Hypodermoclysis should be considered as an effective alternative for fluid replacement in the older adult in nonemergent situations. Last, hypodermoclysis also can be used to administer pain medication subcutaneously, thus avoiding multiple attempts at intravenous catheter insertion.

SUMMARY

Infusion therapy for older adults offers an additional option for medication administration and management, hydration, and nutritional supplementation. With careful consideration of the unique needs of the older adult and the normal physiologic changes that occur, infusion therapy can be a valuable intervention and best practice in quality care for older adults.

Review Questions *Note: Questions below may have more than one right answer.*

1. Principles of education in the older adult patient include which of the following?
   A. Speak slowly, clearly, and directly
   B. Address the patient by name
   C. Use familiar terminology
   D. All of the above

2. Which of the following skin layers is associated with development of dry, transparent surfaces?
   A. Deep fascia
   B. Dermis
   C. Epidermis
   D. Superficial fascia

3. Skin turgor in the adult patient should be measured at what location?
   A. Forehead
   B. Sternum
   C. Abdomen
   D. Inner aspect of the forearm

4. All the following are true when determining skin tension *except*
   A. Assess direction of vessel
   B. Assess axis of vessel
   C. Eliminate traction
   D. Determine directional line of vessel

5. The technique used to reduce vein damage is referred to as
   A. Retraction
   B. Hooded
   C. Threaded
   D. Advanced

6. Total body water in the older patient is reduced by what percentage?
   A. 2%
   B. 5%
   C. 6%
   D. 8%

7. Which of the following statements is true concerning fluid volume assessment in the older adult patient?
   A. It is difficult to assess.
   B. It is a poor indicator of hydration.
   C. It is corrected only by infusion therapy.
   D. It can be assessed by examining the hand veins.

8. In older adults, a primary cause of change in mental status, particularly confusion, is which of the following?
   A. Stress
   B. The aging process
   C. Infection
   D. Visual changes

9. Frequent monitoring of PIV sites in older adults may be necessary because of
   A. Anticipated change in mental status
   B. Decreased perception of pain
   C. Less subcutaneous tissue
   D. Sleep disorders

10. An older adult's physical capacity is
    A. The body's ability to perform various functions
    B. Related to his or her age and mental status
    C. Related to functional capacity and mental status
    D. The effectiveness of performing various functions

References and Selected Readings *Asterisks indicate references cited in text.*

*Amella, E.J. (2004). Presentation of illness in older adults. *American Journal of Nursing, 104*(10), 40–51.

*Barton, A., Fuller, R., & Dudley, N. (2004). Using subcutaneous fluids to rehydrate older people: Current practices and future challenges. *QJM, 97,* 765–768. doi:10.1093/qjmed/hch119. http://qjmed.oxford-journals.org/content/97/11/765.full.pdf+html

*Cacchione, P.Z. (2012). Sensory changes. In M. Boltz, E. Capezuti, T. Fulmer, & D. Zwicker (Eds.), *Evidence-based geriatric nursing protocols for best practice* (4th ed., p. 48). New York, NY: Springer.

*Centers for Disease Control and Prevention (CDC). (2011). Guidelines for the prevention of intravascular catheter-related infections. http://www.cdc.gov/hicpac/pdf/guidelines/bsi-guidelines-2011.pdf

*Fabian, B. (2010). Chapter 30: Infusion therapy in the older adult. In M. Alexander, A. Corrigan, L. Gorski, et al. (Eds.), *Infusion nursing: An evidence based approach* (3rd ed., pp. 571–582). St. Louis, MO: Elsevier Mosby.

*Gilmour, J., & Penny, S. (1991). Hydration & ageing. *The New Zealand Nursing Journal, 84,* 15–17.

*Gorski, L.A., Hallock, D., Kuehn, S.C., Morris, P., Russell, J.M., & Skala, L.C. (2012). INS position paper: Recommendations for frequency of assessment of the short peripheral catheter site. *Journal of Infusion Nursing, 35,* 290–292.

*Graham, J.E., Christian, L.M., & Kiecolt-Glaser, J.K. (2006). Stress, age, and immune function: Toward a lifespan approach. *Journal of Behavioral Medicine, 29*(4), 389–400.

*Infusion Nurses Society. (2011). Infusion nursing standards of practice. *Journal of Infusion Nursing, 34*(1 Suppl.), S57–S59.

*Infusion Nurses Society. (2013). *Policies and procedures for infusion nursing of the older adult* (2nd ed.). Norwood, MA: Author.

Lopez, J.H., & Reyes-Ortiz, C.A. (2010). Subcutaneous hydration by hypodermoclysis. *Reviews in Clinical Gerontology, 20,* 105–113. http://dx.doi.org/10.1017/S0959259810000109

*Metheny, N.M. (2012). *Fluid and electrolyte balance: Nursing considerations* (5th ed.). Burlington, MA: Jones & Bartlett Learning.

*Mitty, E.L., & Post, L.F. (2012). Health care decision making. In M. Boltz, E. Capezuti, T. Fulmer, & D. Zwicker (Eds.), *Evidence-based geriatric nursing protocols for best practice* (4th ed., p. 562). New York, NY: Springer.

*Smith, C.M., & Cotter, V.T. (2012). Age-related changes in health. In M. Boltz, E. Capezuti, T. Fulmer, & D. Zwicker (Eds.), *Evidence-based geriatric nursing protocols for best practice* (4th ed., p. 23). New York, NY: Springer.

*Thomas, M.H. (2011). Chapter 9: Health care delivery settings and older adults. In S.E. Meiner (Ed.), *Gerontologic nursing* (4th ed., pp. 148–175). St. Louis, MO: Elsevier Mosby.

Thurlow, K.L. (2002). Infections in the elderly, part. 2. *Emergency Medical Services, 31*(4), 44.

*Touhy, T.A., & Jett, K. (2012). Chapter 6: Physical changes that accompany aging (pp. 68–83); Chapter 16: Pain and comfort (pp. 259–271). In *Ebersole & Hess' Toward healthy aging: Human needs & nursing response* (8th ed.). St. Louis, MO: Mosby.

*U.S. Census Bureau. (2011). The older population: 2010–2010 Census Briefs. http://www.census.gov/prod/cen2010/briefs/c2010br-09.pdf

*Webster, J., Osborne, S., Rickard, C., & Hall, J. (2010). Clinically-indicated replacement versus routine replacement of peripheral venous catheters. *Cochrane Database of Systematic Reviews,* Issue 3, Article No. CD007798. doi: 10.1002/14651858.CD007798.pub2.

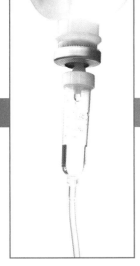

CHAPTER 23

Infusion Therapy across the Continuum of Care

Sharon M. Weinstein

THE EVOLVING HEALTH CARE ENVIRONMENT

In today's complex health care industry, hospitals have strong financial incentives to discharge patients as soon as possible. Hospitals and other health care providers face an increasingly complex dilemma: how to provide the highest quality care at the lowest price. Because of continuing advances in medical science and technology and the influence of managed care insurance contracts, patients discharged from hospitals now can receive complex, high-level services, once available only in hospitals, in alternate care settings. The patient population receiving treatment outside the hospital ranges from critically ill newborns to chronically ill older adults. The nurse needs an array of clinical and critical thinking skills to care for these patients, often while working within an autonomous practice setting.

Cost-cutting measures have enhanced the growth of new ways to provide infusion therapy services. The growth of infusion therapy in the home and alternate clinical settings has created countless opportunities for infusion nurses nationwide. Infusion nurse specialists must assess the level of skills and services currently being provided and determine venues where they can best use their skills, including, but not limited to settings such as the following:

- Hospitals
- The physician/licensed independent practitioner (LIP)'s offices
- Home care
- Long-term care facilities
- Infusion pharmacies
- Subacute settings
- Teaching for other professionals
- Ambulatory infusion centers (AICs)
- Insertion of peripherally inserted central catheters (PICCs) and midline catheters
- Hospice settings

This chapter examines alternate settings for the delivery of infusion therapy. It discusses the influence of managed care and cost-containment efforts. It thoroughly explores home infusion therapy, along with the parameters mandated by The Centers for Medicare & Medicaid Services (CMS), patient selection, the role of various health care team members, and typical infusion therapies provided in the home. It also explores additional sites for infusion therapy delivery, including hospice, subacute care, AICs, and long-term care.

INFLUENCE OF MANAGED CARE

Managed care is a system of controls to manage access, costs, and quality of health care services. The controls may include any or all of the following:

- Preferred provider contracts
- Prior approval/authorization
- Patient education/incentives
- Use review/quality assurance

Two other controls used in managed care include case management and capitation. Case management is a program to manage high-cost health care cases by exploring alternative care options to achieve the same patient outcomes while better controlling costs. Case management requires the insurance company and the provider of services (i.e., home care agency and infusion pharmacy) to discuss the necessary infusion therapy orders for the patient before the initiation of services. Usually, the parties determine and agree on a number of nurse visits necessary for the infusion therapy ordered. Periodic updates and communication continue throughout the duration of the therapy. Patients and caregivers are taught to administer the ordered therapy with limited nursing monitoring, which results in decreased nursing visits and costs.

Capitation is a system of prepayment for health care in which a provider receives a flat monthly fee for agreeing to provide specified services to members of Health Maintenance Organizations (HMOs) assigned to the provider for a contracted time (usually a year). Unlike traditional fee-for-service (FFS) systems, capitated systems pay providers, either individually or collectively, the same amount per member each month, in advance, regardless of how many times the members use their services. Usually, risk sharing is involved, meaning that the HMO and contracted provider share the financial risks and rewards to provide cost-effective care.

Under the auspices of the managed care umbrella

- Payers are changing
- New delivery systems are designed around risk sharing
- Payers/providers are competing for managed care savings (profits)
- Competition is increasing
- Risk is shifting (in both directions)
- Attitudes of providers, payers, and employers are changing

Under the prior system, providers were paid on an FFS basis; they are now paid on a discounted FFS basis or by capitation. The patient base was the local community; now it is covered members/patients. The philosophy of care was to treat the disease and restore health; however, the paradigm has shifted and reflects the chronic disease focus worldwide. Providers globally are also focused on wellness. When providers are reimbursed under bundling or capitated contracts, the incentive is to keep members healthy, provide care in the least costly setting, and decrease total costs. The members are scheduled to have infusion therapy care and procedures performed in alternative clinical settings such as in the home, outpatient clinics, or AICs, rather than in the hospital to avoid the higher costs.

HOME HEALTH CARE

Home health care originally was conceived as a stage in the continuum of care after hospitalization, during which recovery and rehabilitation could continue effectively in the patient's home at a lower cost than if furnished in a hospital. Today, home care services are viewed as low-cost alternatives for inpatient hospital care. Provision of services in the home decreases health care costs across the board and improves access to health care to all age groups in the community. The National Voluntary Consensus Standards for Home Health Care provided by the National Quality Forum (NQF, 2010) defines home health care as:

> any health care services provided to clients in their homes, including but not limited to skilled nursing services, home health aide services, palliative and end-of-life care (e.g., in-home hospice services), therapies (i.e., physical, speech–language, and occupational), homemaker services/ personal care, social services, infusion and pharmacy services, medical supplies, and equipment and in-home physician services (NQF, 2013).

The Federal government uses quality measures to assess how well home health agencies care for patients with certain conditions. By law, any measures reported on the Home Health Compare Web site must reflect accepted standards of health care quality.

The NQF is an independent organization created to develop and implement a strategy for health care quality measurement and public reporting. The NQF brings together stakeholders from throughout the health care industry to jointly decide which quality measures meet certain industry standards. While NQF endorses some of the quality measures reported on Home Health Compare, it does not monitor or review the data that are collected from and about home health agencies.

NQF considers several factors when deciding whether a quality measure should be reported:

- Whether it addresses care or treatment that improves people's health or well-being
- Whether it can be measured accurately and reliably in different home health agencies
- Whether the information can be used to improve the quality of care or to inform patients' decisions about where to go for care (NQF, 2013).

IV therapy in the home care setting has become well-accepted practice with the many advantages including cost saving, decreased length of hospital stays, care of patients surrounded by family and caregivers, and a lower risk of infection (O'Hanlon, 2008). Therapies that are frequently provided in the home setting include antibiotic therapy, chemotherapy, total parenteral nutrition (TPN), rehydration, and pain management. Commonly used diagnoses requiring infusion therapy in the home setting include cellulitis, sepsis, osteomyelitis, urinary tract infections, pneumonia, multiple sclerosis, cancer, gastrointestinal diseases, dehydration, and immune deficiencies (National Home Infusion Association [NHIA], 2013). Home IV therapy allows patients and families to enjoy an increased quality of life, a sense of participation in the therapy, and a feeling of control over illness. Clinicians in the home care setting need to be competent to carry out the skills as well as educate patients and/or caregivers to manage, monitor, and sometimes self-administer therapy. The expanded role of IV therapy in the home setting will only continue to grow, and how agencies and clinicians are prepared to adapt will make the difference in quality outcomes (Martel, 2012).

Quality and Safety

During the past decade, spurred by national initiatives and research, health care has increased its emphasis on safety and competence in practice. The Institute of Medicine (IOM) recommends that all health care agencies offer continuing education programs that impact quality clinical outcomes (Institute of Medicine, 2010).

Although home IV therapy has tremendous benefits, it also carries a high risk to both the patient and clinician if not performed within standards of practice. To protect both the patient and the clinician, IV therapy must only be performed by clinicians who have the specialized educational and technical skills required. Practice that is evidence based is required to meet quality standards and is effective and efficient (INS, 2011a,b). Practice that is based on "how we have always done it" or based on skills picked up "on the job" can lead to misinformation and substandard care. Quality education programs are essential to correct misinformation and teach evidence-based practice.

CLINICAL COMPETENCIES

Competencies are the knowledge and skills required to safely practice. Competency assessment is an evaluation measuring a set of skills and knowledge required to provide care. Key components are technical skills and critical thinking—with the ability to apply these competencies appropriately. Across the continuum of care, Standards of Practice, professional guidelines, and facility policies and procedures are the framework from which competencies are developed.

Competence is defined as the individual's capacity or potential to perform his or her own job (Billings & Halstead, 2009). Accrediting bodies such as The Joint Commission (TJC) look at competence as part of the process of maintaining a high-quality work force (TJC, 2012). Areas that are generally targeted for competency testing include the areas that are considered high risk or low volume. IV therapy is considered a high-risk procedure, and some of the therapy used in the home care setting can also be considered low volume. Risks include infection, thrombosis, hypersensitivity, infiltration/extravasations, and vein inflammation. Clinicians' practice is guided by standards of practice such as those published by the INS as well as infection control practice guidelines such as the Centers for Disease Control and Prevention (CDC) (O'Grady et al., 2011). It is the responsibility of the organization and the practicing clinician to maintain these standards when providing infusion therapy.

Reimbursement for Home Care Services

Third-party payers for home care therapies are diverse. Most home infusion therapy services are paid on a per diem basis, a convention initiated in the 1980s, when these services were first utilized as a cost-effective substitute for inpatient care. Per diem billing allows payers to aggregate all the individual costs within a single line item for each day the patient is on service. This method streamlines claims submission processing and enhances utilization and financial management of infusion therapy services, while facilitating cost comparisons to other IV therapy treatment settings, such as acute and chronic hospitals and skilled nursing facilities (SNFs) (Table 23-1).

In the 1990s, the Health Insurance Portability and Accountability Act (HIPAA) required nationalized coding standards for all health care payers as a means of reducing the administrative costs inherent in allowing each payer to use its own coding system. As part of this process, in 2002, the federal government published a complete set of Health Care Common Procedure Coding System (HCPCS) per diem "S" codes for home infusion

TABLE 23- **MEDICARE PAYMENT RATES FOR INTRAVENOUS DRUG INFUSIONS ACROSS SETTINGS, 2012**

	Inpatient	SNF	Home Care
Drug	Packaged within Diagnostic Related Group (DRG) payment	Packaged within SNF PPS payment	Paid separately to pharmacy
Supplies and equipment	Within DRG	Within PPS	Limited supply coverage for gravity infusion under home health benefit
Drug administration	Within DRG	Within PPS	Within home health PPS payment
Cost sharing	Inpatient hospital deductible of $1,156	None for days 1–20 and $144.50 per day for days 21–100	None for home health

therapy per diem billing. This code set is the only HIPAA-approved, comprehensive code set available to submit home infusion claims that supports the typical per diem contracts present in the commercial marketplace. Consequently, most commercial and some government insurers use the HCPCS per diem "S" codes for home infusion service billing. The codes were modified in 2013 by the Centers for Medicare & Medicaid Services (CMS). The HCPCS per diem "S" codes specifically include administrative services, professional pharmacy services, care coordination, and necessary supplies and equipment. All drugs, enteral formulae, and nursing visits are coded and billed separately on the claim for reimbursement (Table 23-2).

Combined with a working knowledge of precisely what types of therapy that various payer sources cover, it is essential that the written record of care, including the diagnosis, be consistent with the type of therapy provided. As in the tertiary care setting, a series of codes has been developed to reflect procedures (current procedural terminology [CPT]) and diagnoses (International Statistical Classification of Diseases and Related Health Problems

TABLE 23-2   SELECT EXAMPLES OF HOME INFUSION CODES

Description	Interval	HCPCS Code
1. Home infusion therapy, antibiotic, antiviral, or antifungal, once every 3 h; administrative services, pharmacy services, care coordination, and all necessary supplies and equipment (drugs and nursing visits coded separately), per diem	Q 3 h	S9497
2. Home infusion therapy, antibiotic, antiviral, or antifungal, once every 4 h; administrative services, pharmacy services, care coordination, and all necessary supplies and equipment (drugs and nursing visits coded separately), per diem	Q 4 h	S9504
3. Home infusion therapy, antibiotic, antiviral, or antifungal, once every 6 h; administrative services, pharmacy services, care coordination, and all necessary supplies and equipment (drugs and nursing visits coded separately), per diem	Q 6 h	S9503
4. Home infusion therapy, antibiotic, antiviral, or antifungal, once every 8 h; administrative services, pharmacy services, care coordination, and all necessary supplies and equipment (drugs and nursing visits coded separately), per diem	Q 8 h	S9502
5. Home infusion therapy, antibiotic, antiviral, or antifungal, once every 12 h; administrative services, pharmacy services, care coordination, and all necessary supplies and equipment (drugs and nursing visits coded separately), per diem	Q 12 h	S9501
6. Home infusion therapy, antibiotic, antiviral, or antifungal, once every 24 h; administrative services, pharmacy services, care coordination, and all necessary supplies and equipment (drugs and nursing visits coded separately), per diem	Q 24 h	S9500
7. Home infusion therapy, continuous (24 h or more) chemotherapy infusion, administrative services, professional pharmacy services, care coordination, and all necessary supplies and equipment (drugs and nursing visits coded separately), per diem	Continuous—24 h or more	S9330

[ICD10]). ICD is a medical classification list by the World Health Organization (WHO); it codes for diseases, signs and symptoms, abnormal findings, complaints, social circumstances, and external causes of injury or disease.

The CPT code set is maintained by the American Medical Association through the CPT Editorial Panel (AMA, 2013). The CPT code set describes medical, surgical, and diagnostic services and is designed to communicate uniform information about medical services and procedures among physicians/LIPs, coders, patients, accreditation organizations, and payers for administrative, financial, and analytical purposes. New editions are released each October. The current version is the CPT 2013. It is available in both a standard edition and a professional edition.

CPT coding is similar to ICD-9 and ICD-10 coding, except that it identifies the services rendered rather than the diagnosis on the claim ICD-10 (effective October 2013).

CPT is currently identified by the Centers for Medicare & Medicaid Services as level 1 of the Health Care Procedure Coding System.

Pay for Performance (P4P)

Long before the passage of the Patient Protection and Affordable Care Act of 2010, a movement has been in place to alter the practice of medicine. For years, performance in medicine was determined by a patient's outcome; today's focus is on **pay for performance** (P4P) programs. P4P programs are performance-based payment arrangements that align financial rewards with improved outcomes and changed behavior. The impetus behind P4P originated in response to rising medical costs, growth in chronic care conditions, and consumer demands for efficiency and improvements in the quality of care (Baker, 2003).

P4P programs typically include three kinds of performance measures: structural measures, which engage key systems to improve quality of care; process measures, which assess performance against evidence-based guidelines and protocols; and outcome measures, which focus on a patient's progress and condition.

Alternatives to P4P

Many providers and payers are exploring Integrated Provider Performance Incentive Plans (IPPIPs), Alternative Quality Contracts (AQCs), and Accountable Care Organizations (ACOs) as alternatives to traditional P4P programs. While they are similar to P4P, the focus is on the flexibility of their structure, payments, and risk assumption.

An ACO is a network of doctors and hospitals that shares responsibility for providing care to patients. In the Affordable Care Act (ACA), an ACO would agree to manage all of the health care needs of a minimum of 5,000 Medicare beneficiaries for at least 3 years.

Specific Considerations Related to Medicare

Home care has been one of the fastest growing benefits in the Medicare program, which is the largest purchaser of home health services in the United States. The number of Medicare beneficiaries has been expanding by approximately 2% each year (Disbrow) and is expected to accelerate even more rapidly with the enrollment of the baby-boomer generation.

Eligibility for the home care benefit within the Medicare program requires that the following conditions be met:

- The patient must be at least 65 years of age and have received acceptance for Medicare coverage.
- The patient must be homebound. In other words, the patient must be confined to the home in such a way that leaving requires considerable effort and the assistance of another person or an adaptive device such as a cane, walker, or wheelchair. Absences from the home must be infrequent, of short duration, and for the purposes of receiving additional medical care.
- Home care services must be provided under a Plan of Care established and reviewed by a licensed physician/LIP directly involved in the patient's care. Written physician/LIP orders are required for home care.
- The home care services the patient needs must be skilled intermittent nursing, physical therapy, occupational therapy, or speech therapy.
- A certified Medicare program provider who agrees to adhere to the extensive Medicare Conditions of Participation regulations and requirements and accepts Medicare's reimbursement for the provision of those services must provide home care (CMS, 2013).

Services eligible for Medicare reimbursement fall under Part A or B. Implementation of a prospective payment system (PPS) reduced the cost of hospitalization by shifting the end point of care to the home, thereby contributing to the growth of the alternative care delivery system. The home health PPS is composed of six main features, detailed in Box 23-1.

Patient Criteria for Home Care Infusion Therapy

In addition to meeting Medicare criteria for home care, patients must meet other criteria to qualify as candidates for home infusion therapy (Box 23-2). Patients are responsible for specific aspects of their infusion therapy, including administration of the ordered therapy, monitoring, catheter line management, operation of electronic infusion equipment (if necessary), and other duties. The patient, caregiver, or both are taught to identify signs and symptoms of complications that must be reported to the nurse and are also taught how to identify any other situations that require immediate attention. A 24-hour emergency phone number is provided to patients and families should they need help.

Appropriate Diagnosis

The type of drug therapy ordered may determine a patient's appropriateness for home infusion therapy. Many drugs given in the inpatient setting are acceptable for home infusion programs.

The therapy ordered must be consistent with the patient's diagnosis and ability to receive care in the home. Common diagnoses for antibiotic therapy include osteomyelitis, otitis media, sinusitis, cryptococcal meningitis, pneumonia, subacute bacterial endocarditis,

---

BOX 23-1   SIX FEATURES OF THE HOME CARE PPS

1. Payment for the 60-day episode

An agency is paid half of the estimated base payment for the full 60 days as soon as the fiscal intermediary receives the initial claim and the residual at the close of the 60-day episode.

2. Case-mix adjustment—Adjusting payment for a beneficiary's condition and needs

The HHA assesses the patient's condition and likely skilled nursing care, therapy, medical social services, and home health aide service needs, at the beginning of the episode of care. The assessment must be done for each subsequent episode of care a patient receives.

3. Outlier payments—Paying more for the care of the costliest beneficiaries

Additional payments are made to the 60-day case-mix adjusted episode payments for beneficiaries who incur unusually large costs.

4. Adjustments for beneficiaries who require only a few visits during the 60-day episode

The PPS has a low-utilization payment adjustment for those whose episodes consist of four or fewer visits. These episodes will be paid the standardized, service-specific per-visit amount multiplied by the number of visits actually provided during the episode.

5. Adjustments for beneficiaries who change HHAs

The PPS includes a partial episode payment adjustment. A new episode clock will be triggered when a beneficiary elects to transfer to another HHA or when a beneficiary is discharged and readmitted to the same HHA during the 60-day episode.

6. Consolidated billing

Under the PPS, an HHA must bill for all home health services that include nursing and therapy services, routine and nonroutine medical supplies, home health aide, and medical social services, except durable medical equipment (DME).

HHA, home health association; PPS, prospective payment system.

Adapted from Centers for Medicare & Medicaid Services. 2013 Home health PPS. http://www.cms.gov/Medicare/Medicare-Fee-for-Service-Payment/HomeHealthPPS/index.html

---

primary bacteremia, cellulitis, urinary tract infections, pyelonephritis, septic arthritis, histoplasmosis, peritonitis, toxic shock syndrome, Lyme disease, rickettsial infection, opportunistic infections related to acquired immunodeficiency syndrome, and many others. All types of patients with cancer are appropriate candidates for home infusion of antineoplastic agents, especially combination protocols. Fluorouracil (5-FU) is a common antineoplastic agent infused in the home setting. Additional infusion therapies for the oncology patient may include nutritional support, pain management, antiemetics, antibiotics, and leucovorin rescue regimens.

BOX 23-2 CRITERIA FOR THE PATIENT SELECTION FOR HOME INFUSION

1. Appropriate diagnosis
2. Medical stability
3. Appropriate venous access device for ordered therapy
4. Evaluation of drug therapy
5. Laboratory profile
6. Presence of a caregiver
7. Learning ability of the patient/caregiver
8. Appropriate home environment
9. Financial resources

MEDICAL STABILITY

Medical stability is necessary for patients regardless of their ability to perform the ordered therapy including infusions. A family member or other caregiver may assume full responsibility for performing all procedures. Another person may be needed as a backup, depending on the home situation. Ideally, the patient should have a comprehensive assessment before discharge from the hospital. This allows the home health agency/home infusion pharmacy to assess the patient's needs and ability to provide the care. However, last minute referrals make this step difficult. The hospital or referral source needs to assist in this very important step.

VENOUS ACCESS

Appropriate vascular access is essential for home infusion therapy. Some patients may be discharged with an infusion device in place that was used in the hospital, including a jugular vein catheter, subclavian vein catheters (triple lumens), tunneled catheters (Hickman/Broviac, Groshong), implanted ports (chest or arm), PICCs, midline catheters, or peripheral catheters. Other times, the skilled and competent home care nurse initiates the vascular access device placement in the home, such as a peripheral catheter for short-term therapy or a midline catheter for long-term therapy. Teaching protocols for catheter care management and flush procedures for the type of access are required and must be patient specific to address all areas of maintenance for self-care.

Certain drugs and infusions require the insertion of a central venous access device. The Infusion Nurses Society (INS) *Infusion Nursing Standards of Practice* is specific about appropriate venous access. Some of the most common drugs that must be given through a PICC line or other central access device include vancomycin, oxacillin, penicillin, dopamine, and Dilantin, just to name a few. It is very important for the patient to receive the appropriate line prior to the initiation of therapy.

EVALUATION OF DRUG THERAPY

Each drug ordered is evaluated for all aspects of the administration: length of time required for the administration, dosing frequency, duration of therapy, insurer approval of the method of administration, and patient risks. For example, antibiotics may be administered over 30 minutes to 2 hours, depending on the drug and volume of solution. Dosing may be every 4, 6, 8, 12, or 24 hours. Duration may be 4 to 8 weeks or even longer. Certain drugs such as morphine and chemotherapy must be administered with an electronic pump or device. It is common to place a patient on an ambulatory infusion pump when the dosing schedule of the drug is every 4 to 6 hours. Oxacillin and penicillin are common drugs frequently dosed every 4 hours, and the pump allows the patient and caregiver to get some rest. Some drugs require close monitoring and the presence of a nurse in the event of an anaphylactic reaction.

LABORATORY PROFILE

Procedures must be established for routine laboratory studies and transmission of reports to the physician/LIP, home infusion pharmacist, and home care agency. The nurse should report changes in laboratory values immediately to the physician/LIP so that adjustments can be made in the treatment plan consistent with the patient's clinical condition. Laboratory testing of blood levels including complete blood counts (CBC), and metabolic panels may be performed weekly or biweekly for patients receiving TPN, antineoplastic therapy, and antibiotics or antifungal agents. Certain drugs, such as vancomycin, gentamicin, and tobramycin, may require routine peak and trough levels to avoid toxicity. The infusion pharmacist is vital in monitoring the patient and an excellent resource for the physician/LIP and nurse involved in the care of the patient.

PRESENCE OF A SUPPORT SYSTEM

Even if the patient meets the criteria for home care as discussed earlier, many adjustments need to be made in the home. The patient often is very ill and still recovering from whatever condition necessitated the hospitalization. The infusion therapy orders usually are a continuation of the therapy the patient received as an inpatient. Planning is necessary to provide 24-hour support from a family member or other caregiver until the patient can assume the procedures and self-care. The home care nurse/infusion nurse makes the initial visit and teaches the patient and/or caregiver to provide the ordered therapy. In most cases, this can be accomplished on the first visit; sometimes, however, the nurse must make extra visits until the patient and/or caregiver is competent. A nurse is always available on call should any problems arise. A home health aide may be available to help the patient with personal care.

TECHNICAL CRITERIA

The compliant patient or caregiver administers drugs and treatments as ordered, follows aseptic technique, reports signs and symptoms of complications, and monitors and records intake and output, weights, temperature, blood glucose, and other parameters as indicated. The elderly patient must be evaluated for manual dexterity to perform the required procedures. Many patients have arthritis in their fingers and hands and are unable to assemble and manipulate the infusion equipment to participate in their care. Some patients have a limited educational background and are unable to learn the procedures they are taught. Some patients experience dementia, depression, or mental illness and are incapable of assuming responsibility for their care. In addition, the home environment must be evaluated for basic needs (i.e., telephone, electricity, hot and cold water, refrigeration). When these basic needs are unmet, the physician/LIP must be notified so that another plan of care that is safe for the patient can be considered.

FINANCIAL RESOURCES

Before acceptance to home care, the patient's insurance benefits are assessed. Although many patients have outstanding health care benefits for inpatient care, they may have limited or no benefits for home care. Some patients may have insurance coverage for home care services but no prescription coverage. Some patients may be able to pay out of pocket for the cost of the drugs and supplies needed to receive infusion therapy in the home. If the patient is unable to pay, the physician/LIP is notified, and he or she must consider alternate plans or place the patient in a subacute facility paid for by insurance. As we discussed in P4P, the ACA will reshape the provision of home infusion services with the requirement for an ACO. As hospitals identify how to reduce readmission rates and avoid penalties, home infusion may become an even more important post-discharge therapy option for their patients.

Role of Health Care Professionals in Home-Based Infusion Therapy

The home infusion program must be full service, available 24 hours a day, and able to meet the patient's total needs for nursing, supplies, delivery, inventory, and storage. Qualified professional personnel must be responsible for the direction, coordination, and supervision of all professional services. Care should be consistent with the highest standards of the three accrediting organizations that provide guidelines: The Joint Commission (TJC), the Accreditation Commission for Health Care (ACHC), and the Community Health Accreditation Program (CHAP) of the National League for Nursing (NLN). Table 23-3 compares TJC, ACHC, and CHAP.

Policies and procedures for the provision of home infusion services must be consistent with published practice standards. The INS has published Infusion Standards for all patients regardless of their clinical setting (INS, 2011). The procedures must be comprehensive and

TABLE 23-3	COMPARISON OF TJC, ACHC, AND CHAP		
	TJC	ACHC	CHAP
Accredits networks	Yes	Yes	Yes
Accredits ambulatory infusion centers	Yes	Yes	Yes
Year that service began	1988	1985[a]	1965[b]

[a]ACHC was recognized by the CMS as a national accreditation organization for hospices that request participation in the Medicare program.
[b]Through "deeming authority" granted by the CMS; the CHAP has the regulatory authority to survey agencies providing home health, hospice, and home medical equipment services to determine if they meet the Medicare Conditions of Participation and CMS Quality Standards. Before "deemed" status is assigned, one must apply and demonstrate its ability to meet or exceed the Medicare conditions of participation as cited in the Code of Federal Regulations.
ACHC, Accreditation Commission for Health Care; CHAP, Community Health Accreditation Program; TJC, The Joint Commission.

address all the infusion therapies provided. The home infusion therapy program must be consistent with the organization's philosophy and purpose.

Positive outcomes should be the treatment goal for restoring the patient to a functional capacity and enabling the patient and family to return to a level consistent with the stage of disease and its progress. Outcome measurements, based on those developed by TJC, ACHC, and CHAP, enhance the level of care provided and help ensure excellence.

THE DISCHARGE PLANNER/HOME CARE COORDINATOR

Discharge planning begins during hospitalization. The home care coordinator may be involved in identifying appropriate candidates for home infusion therapies. The discharge orders must be consistent with the type of infusion therapy, medication, dose, route, duration, frequency interval, and method of administration. The discharge planner facilitates coordination with the supplier before the patient is discharged from the hospital to ensure the safe and timely arrival of medications and related supplies and equipment. Open lines of communication enable the infusion provider to meet the patient's current and ongoing needs for care and ensure a high degree of confidence.

THE PHYSICIAN/LICENSED INDEPENDENT PRACTITIONER

The physician/LIP orders the referral to the appropriate alternate care setting. He or she writes the plan of treatment for the patient in need of home infusion therapy. In addition to routine infusion orders and other treatments, the individualized plan also should define functional limitations, goals, and duration of treatment. For some modalities, a letter of medical necessity is required. The physician/LIP also maintains the role of "gatekeeper," providing recertification for ongoing care, reviewing progress notes, and coordinating the home care plan.

THE NURSE AS THE HOME CARE INFUSION PROVIDER

The home care infusion nurse maintains ongoing communication with the physician/LIP regarding the patient's status and changes in orders. The nurse continues to assess the patient, and whenever the patient's condition changes or deteriorates, he or she notifies the physician/LIP and may send the patient to the physician/LIP's office or to the hospital.

Once the referral to home care has been completed and insurance coverage or other reimbursement is verified, the nurse should complete a referral checklist (Figure 23-1). The nurse should review the Patient's Bill of Rights, Responsibilities for Participation in the Home Infusion Program, and the assignment of benefits document. Then, the nurse performs an initial patient assessment that includes review of body systems, review of current and past medical history, psychosocial assessment, evaluation of available support systems, and assessment of functional limitations, environment, and cognitive and technical skills. He or she clarifies the orders if needed; develops the patient's plan of care; coordinates interdisciplinary communication for physical therapy, occupational therapy, speech therapy, social worker, or nurse aide as needed; and orients the patient to the services being provided.

A designated nurse case manager must coordinate services for each patient. The infusion therapy nurse case manager is selected for his or her expertise and experience and preferably is a Certified Registered Nurse in Infusion Therapy (CRNI). A list of case manager responsibilities is provided in Box 23-3. This nurse is the home care nurse who is

Home Infusion Referral Checklist

Home Care Provider:

[ ] _____

[ ] _____

INFORMATION TO:	DATE/INITIAL

INFORMATION TO:

    A. DISCHARGE PLANNER INFORMED _____

    B. IV TEAM INFORMED _____

    C. HOME AGENCY INFORMED: _____

        Name of agency_____

        Address _____

        Phone # _____ FAX # _____

        Local contact_____

    D. LOCAL PHYSICIAN/LIP IDENTIFIED (if applicable) _____

        Name_____

        Address _____

        Phone # _____ FAX # _____

TYPE OF REFERRAL:

    A. Parenteral nutrition _____

    B. Enteral nutrition _____

    C. IV antibiotics _____

    D. Pain management _____

    E. Nupogen _____

    F. Chemotherapy _____

    G. Catheter care _____

    H. Other _____ _____

TEACHING COMPLETED:

    A. HOME INFUSION_____ _____

    B. SUBCLAVIAN/CATHETER CARE _____

        [ ] Port   Type_____

        [ ] Hickman/Groshong [ ] Subclavain [ ] Other_____

        # Lumens_____

SUPPLIES NEEDED FROM HOSPITAL ON DISCHARGE:

_____

_____

_____

_____

DELIVERY DATE _____ START OF INFUSION _____

DATE OF REFERRAL FROM PHYSICIAN/LIP_____ DATE OF DISCHARGE_____

SIGNATURE/INITIAL _____ _____ TITLE _____

_____ _____   _____

_____ _____   _____

FIGURE 23-1 Home infusion referral checklist.

BOX 23-3   RESPONSIBILITY OF THE CASE MANAGER

- Initial assessment of the patient, family, and home environment
- Development of a plan of care
- Appropriate referral and follow-up
- Coordination of services
- Implementation of the plan of care
- Ongoing evaluation
- Plan for termination of home care

assigned as a case manager to the patient and is responsible for coordinating care among all disciplines: nursing, physical therapy, occupational therapy, speech therapy, social work, and home health aides. Also, the nurse case manager monitors the patient's progress toward goals, independence, and discharge from home care.

The plan of care should include patient teaching for the ordered therapy, including managing the catheter, using aseptic technique, changing dressings, flushing the IV line and heparin-locking the catheter, connecting and disconnecting continuous or intermittent administration, changing tubings and other devices, handling infusion equipment, performing emergency interventions, observing for signs and symptoms of possible complications, handling inventory, and managing an electronic infusion device, if necessary.

PATIENT SAFETY

The nurse should provide teaching with return demonstrations until the patient or caregiver is confident, independent, and competent. Even then, the nurse provides ongoing support and monitoring. However, some patients may be discharged at this point depending on the insurance.

The nurse should provide specific teaching packets with pictures and individualize the teaching plan to the patient's specific needs. Once therapy is initiated in the home, the nurse must take adequate time to ensure the patient's competence with the therapeutic regimen. Language barriers often inhibit a successful teaching program. Every effort should be made to address the patient in the language he or she best understands. Table 23-4 provides an example of infusion teaching in Spanish.

The nurse should develop, review, and sign the teaching plan for the patient. A copy should become part of the patient's clinical record, with a second copy given to the patient and kept in the place of residence.

Home care providers should offer infusion classes for nurses before patient assignment to enhance skills and learning with verification and documentation of infusion competencies. Ongoing education is necessary to keep abreast of the latest technologies, equipment, and infusion therapy procedures. Competency of infusion skills for nurses should be documented and validated on an annual basis. The resources of professional societies and the role that such organizations play in development of the nurse's knowledge base cannot be overlooked. These societies provide the collegiality and professional camaraderie that

TABLE 23-4 PATIENT EDUCATION: A SPANISH LANGUAGE REFERENCE	
English	**Spanish**
I am here to check your IV.	Vengo a revisarie la aguja del suero intravneso.
Do you have pain at your IV site?	Tiene dolor en el lugar de la inyección.
If pain or swelling begins, please tell your nurse.	Si el dolor o la inflamación comienza, por favor informe a su enfermera.
I am here to start your IV.	Yo estoy aquí para iniciar el intravenosa.
May I check your PICC dressing?	Puedo comprobar su preparación intravenosa PICC.
You will receive your IV at home.	Usted recibirá su intravenosa en su casa.

enable nurses to grow in this rapidly changing field. Infusion nursing professionals should be encouraged to publish case studies about their success stories in home infusion care and to share their knowledge and expertise with others. Box 23-4 lists available resources. Safety is a serious concern for the nurse, and security measures should be taken to ensure that an escort is available as needed and that other measures are taken. See Box 23-5.

EVIDENCE FOR PRACTICE

Home health agencies are implementing the case manager model to create a bridge between the prescriber/gatekeeper and the patient. How does this affect quality and timeliness of service?

BOX 23-4   RESOURCES FOR ONGOING EDUCATION

Accreditation Commission for Health Care (ACHC)
American Association of Blood Banks (AABB)
American Hospital Association (AHA)
American Medical Association (AMA)
American Society of Health-System Pharmacists (ASHP)
American Society for Parenteral and Enteral Nutrition (A.S.P.E.N.)
Association for Practitioners in Infection Control (APIC)
Case Management Society of America (CMSA)
Centers for Disease Control and Prevention (CDC)
Community Health Accreditation Program (CHAP)
Infusion Nurses Society (INS)
The Joint Commission (TJC)
National Association for Home Care (NAHC)
National Home Infusion Association (NHIA)
National Hospice Organization (NHO)
National Subacute Care Association (NSCA)
Oncology Nursing Society (ONS)

BOX 23-5   CAREGIVER SAFETY AND SECURITY DURING HOME VISITS

To ensure safety of the caregiver, security measures should be followed:
- Call for police or security escort as needed.
- Ensure safety when leaving and entering the car and the patient's place of residence.
- Use a navigation system or map the area before making the visit.
- Lock valuables in the trunk of your vehicle.
- If the home situation appears unsafe, leave immediately.
- Have emergency assistance numbers readily available.
- Pay attention to your surroundings.

The Pharmacist

The roles and responsibilities of the pharmacist vary in different parts of the country. In general, the pharmacist is responsible for reviewing medical records for current and past medical history and nutritional and medication history; obtaining and correlating the physician/LIP's orders; checking allergies and drug compatibilities; and facilitating delivery of medications, solutions, supplies, and equipment to the patient's place of residence. The pharmacist also reviews laboratory data and monitors pharmacokinetic dosing with the physician/LIP for certain drugs and therapies.

An infusion therapy provider is usually a state-licensed pharmacy that specializes in provision of infusion therapies to patients in their homes or other sites. Infusion therapy always originates with a prescription order from a qualified physician/LIP who is overseeing the care of the patient.

A nationally-accepted, technical definition of a home infusion therapy pharmacy is a:

Pharmacy-based, decentralized patient care organization with expertise in USP 797-compliant sterile drug compounding that provides care to patients with acute or chronic conditions generally pertaining to parenteral administration of drugs, biologics and nutritional formulae administered through catheters and/or needles in home and alternate sites. Extensive professional pharmacy services, care coordination, infusion nursing services, supplies and equipment are provided to optimize efficacy and compliance (NHIA, 2011).

The Patient

The patient and family are active participants in home infusion therapy; they must be involved in every aspect of care. It is essential to have knowledge of his or her condition, the treatment plan, anticipated outcomes, potential complications, and methods of communicating with the members of the team.

Types of Home Infusion Therapy

Home infusion therapies are diverse and encompass many modalities. Such modalities include antibiotics and anti-infectives, hydration, antiemetics, antineoplastics, nutritional support, pain management, blood and blood component therapy, cardiovascular drugs, drugs to prevent transplant rejection, and venous sampling.

Some health care providers prefer that the first dose of some drugs be administered in a monitored clinical setting, but many first doses are now administered in the patient's residence in the presence of a nurse. This change may be attributed to changes in technology and pharmaceuticals as well as to the increased availability of professional nurses with appropriate IV therapy credentials.

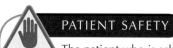

PATIENT SAFETY

The patient who is scheduled to receive the first dose in the home should have a thorough allergy profile and history, including a risk assessment for first dosing.

An appropriate order for emergency anaphylaxis should be provided. The medication should be available immediately and sent to the home before the first administration of the medication. Components of the anaphylactic kit may include epinephrine, diphenhydramine, hydrocortisone, acetaminophen, sodium chloride solution, IV administration set, needles, and syringes. Allergic reactions may occur with subsequent doses of medication as well. The home care infusion nurse must be able to identify and differentiate allergic responses from anaphylactic reactions and teach the patient and caregiver.

In the home care program, provision must be made for handling infectious patient waste. The U.S. Environmental Protection Agency (EPA), a federal regulatory board, has developed many advisories regarding infectious waste. With the passage of the Medical Waste Tracking Act of 1988, Congress mandated to the EPA the investigation and development, if needed, of guidelines for handling home-generated waste.

Although procedures vary on a global level, in the United States, there are three main methods for medical waste generators to dispose of their waste: On-site, truck service, and mail-back disposal. On-site treatment is generally only used by very large hospitals and major universities. Truck service involves hiring a medical waste disposal service whose employees are trained to collect and haul away medical waste in special containers (usually cardboard boxes or reusable plastic bins) for treatment at a facility designed to handle large amounts of medical waste. Mail-back medical waste disposal is similar, except that the waste is shipped through the U.S. postal service instead of by private hauler. Prepackaged kits are available from various manufacturers and include sharps disposal systems and several types of spill kits. Today's emphasis on safety in the workplace has enhanced these efforts.

ANTIBIOTICS AND ANTI-INFECTIVES

The delivery of antibiotics and anti-infective agents in the home is a rapidly growing home care service. To qualify, the patient should be medically stable and compliant, the infection should be treatable in the home, and a reliable venous access should be available. Disease conditions amenable to home care IV antibiotic therapy include long-lasting and deep-seated infections. Awareness of a patient's medication history and allergic reactions allows guided monitoring before, during, and after IV antibiotic administration. Recognition of potential adverse drug reactions associated with each class of antibiotics and anti-infectives is an important part of safe and effective infusion therapy (Barrio, 1998).

NUTRITIONAL SUPPORT

The advent of TPN in the 1960s enabled physicians/LIPs to support intestinally compromised patients indefinitely. Technical barriers have diminished over time. Advanced products, catheters, and technologies have enabled advanced nutritional support to be provided to patients with the appropriate diagnoses. If the patient is under the Medicare program, he or she must require TPN for 90 days or more to qualify. The American Society for Parenteral and Enteral Nutrition (A.S.P.E.N.) has been publishing Standards of Practice and Clinical Guidelines for more than 20 years.

In the home setting, the patient usually receives TPN as a cyclic administration rather than a continuous 24-hour infusion. With the cyclic infusion, the patient receives a full day's prescribed requirement of fluid, glucose, protein (amino acids), lipids, and other additives over 12 to 18 hours. The pharmacist prepares the TPN solution, but the nurse, patient, or caregiver must add some drugs to the solution just before administration. Home monitoring must be done, including weekly to daily weights, temperature, blood glucose monitoring, intake and output, and weekly blood sampling.

Many patients begin their TPN solution in the evening, to be administered while they are sleeping, and disconnect in the morning. The patient, caregiver, or both learn to flush the IV catheter and perform catheter maintenance to keep the line patent. This allows the patient to be free from using the infusion pump during the day. When it is necessary to visit the physician/LIP's office, the patient does not have to deal with TPN administration and equipment, especially when nonambulatory equipment is supplied.

HYDRATION

Elderly patients often become dehydrated, especially during very hot weather, the influenza season, or periods of inadequate fluid intake. The goal for home hydration is to maintain the patient's fluid balance by providing multiple electrolytes, supplemental vitamins, or plain IV solutions (without additives) and also to avoid hospitalization for those people who resist admission for this therapy.

PAIN MANAGEMENT

Continuous or intermittent administration of analgesics in the home allows those in need of pain relief to remain with their families while experiencing a degree of comfort not previously available. Manufacturers have developed sophisticated equipment to ensure safe administration of these drugs in an unmonitored environment. Pain medications may be administered by a patient-controlled analgesia pump through IV, epidural, intrathecal, subcutaneous, or other routes of administration. The most frequently ordered medications are morphine sulfate and hydromorphone. A common concern among patients and families is addiction. Health care providers should assure patients and caregivers that addiction is a minimal concern and that doses should be administered as needed.

ANTIEMETICS

Antiemetic protocols aimed at intermittent infusion facilitate the care of the patient receiving antineoplastic therapy and ensure patient comfort. Protocols may call for antiemetic infusions as a single-agent treatment or combined with TPN therapies. Patients with a diagnosis of hyperemesis gravidarum may also benefit from home IV antiemetic therapy.

ANTINEOPLASTICS

Chemotherapeutic agents are administered by various infusion systems to patients in their homes. Vesicant and nonvesicant agents are administered through centrally placed IV catheters, PICCs, implanted chest or arm ports, tunneled catheters, and implanted pumps. In some patients, the chemotherapeutic agents may be initiated in a chemotherapy clinic or physician/LIP's office. The infusate is connected to an ambulatory infusion pump and sent home. The home care infusion nurse monitors the patient, changes tubings and dressings, and disconnects the equipment at the end of therapy.

BLOOD AND BLOOD COMPONENT THERAPY

Transfusion of blood and blood components may be performed in the home whenever the policies and procedures required by the American Association of Blood Banks (AABB) can be followed and the procedure itself is cost-effective.

PATIENT SAFETY

The availability of the physician/LIP as well as paramedic services should be determined before the transfusion. Policies should be written for safe administration and compatibility checks, identification checks and verification, transportation of the blood unit or component, emergency measures, registered nurse monitoring (including remaining with the patient for the duration of the procedure and for ~90 minutes after the completion of the transfusion), and signs and symptoms of various types of blood reactions.

VENOUS SAMPLING

Venous sampling for all types of laboratory testing is available in home infusion programs. Peak and trough levels, chemistry panels, CBC, and other tests may be performed depending on the therapy. Venous samples may be drawn through peripheral venipuncture or central line sampling. Procedures should be established for blood draws from central line catheters, including the amount of blood to discard before the sampling, the volume at which to flush the catheter after the draw, and change of any equipment.

HOSPICE

Hospice is a specialized program of care for any person with a limited life expectancy. Hospice seeks to enhance, preserve, and encourage the dignity of life for patients and families by providing medical care, supportive care, and grief educational services. Hospice emphasizes the management of pain and other symptoms, so the patient is comfortable, alert, and able to maintain the highest quality of life possible. One of the major fears of the seriously ill is pain. In a hospice program, medications are prepared for any patient with pain to achieve constant pain control without impairing alertness. A team of physicians/ LIPs, nurses, pharmacists, psychologists, dietitians, social workers, clergy, and volunteers provides 24-hour care. The hospice team develops an individualized plan of care for each patient. Hospice care may be provided in the home with a primary caregiver or in a hospice center when no primary caregiver is available or for short-term acute symptom management that cannot be given at home. Each eligible Medicare patient must decide whether to choose the hospice benefit, which means that the hospice will provide all care related to the terminal illness. Regular Medicare coverage can be used for any services provided by a personal physician/LIP or for illnesses or accidents unrelated to the terminal illness. Hospice care also is provided under other insurances, HMOs, and Medicaid. Currently, many hospice organizations are servicing residents in the long-term care facilities.

SUBACUTE CARE FACILITIES

Ensuring the safe transition of patients from hospitals to SNFs and from SNFs back to the hospital or the community can present significant challenges. Subacute programs are a new level of care for patients in various stages of an acute illness or injury, usually after, but sometimes instead of, hospitalization for an acute episode (Levenson, 2000). **Subacute care** is sometimes called *transitional care*. Two organizations developed the definition: the National Subacute Care Association (NSCA) and The Joint Commission (TJC) (Griffin, 1998). Subacute care facilities respond to the need for the treatment of patients with complex medical conditions and rehabilitation needs and provide for a more cost-effective approach. A description of subacute care is found in Box 23-6.

BOX 23-6   DEFINITION OF SUBACUTE CARE

Subacute care is a comprehensive, cost-effective inpatient level of care for patients who
- Have had an acute event from injury, illness, or exacerbation of a disease process
- Have a determined course of treatment
- Who are stable, yet require diagnostics or invasive procedures

And, the intensity of the patient's condition requires
- Active physician/LIP direction with frequent on-site visits
- Professional nursing care
- Ancillary services
- An outcome-focused interdisciplinary approach utilizing a professional team
- Complex medical and/or rehabilitation care

Adapted from the National Subacute Care Association. (2012). NSCA gives new definition to subacute care: Wound care. http://communityhealthdefinitionhere.blogspot.com/2012/10/nsca-gives-new-definition-to-subacute.html

---

Beginning in the 1980s, the earliest subacute care units were located in SNFs. Later, hospitals began to add subacute units and called them *extended acute care* or *specialty hospitals*. These specialty hospitals typically have 40+ beds or more and usually are located in a separate wing or floor of the host hospital. They have an independent admission and discharge function, are licensed separately as a long-term acute care hospital, and are accredited by TJC. Their costs are 30% to 60% lower than general acute care hospitals.

The extended acute care hospital provides high-quality, cost-effective, long-term care for high-acuity patients. These specialty hospitals manage patients with medically complex conditions who require extended stay, and whose medical condition will resolve sufficiently for transfer to lower levels of care within a few days with an achievable positive outcome for the patient. The types of patients admitted are those who have multiple body system complications with difficult medical and therapeutic needs: patients with challenges of pulmonary care, ventilator dependency, cardiovascular complications, complicated wounds, and major multiple traumas, disease management problems, burns, or other special needs. Infusion therapy treatments include antibiotic or anti-infective therapy, pain management, nutritional support, hydration, and various other infusions, including PICC/midline insertions and central venous catheter care management.

THE INFUSION SUITE OR AMBULATORY INFUSION CENTER

The Infusion Suite or **Ambulatory infusion centers** are another alternative site for delivering infusion therapies. Ideally, the physical layout is self-contained within a hospital setting or adjacent to the facility; it may also be in a medical office building. The standard components are a small laboratory, infusion admixture room, education and training area, medical record station, nourishment area, and individualized patient rooms. The patient is seated in a recliner-type chair, with access to infusion teaching videotapes or other movies during treatment. Laboratory parameters are reviewed, along with the physician/LIP's orders. If needed, additional laboratory studies are obtained and processed. The patient is offered juices and appropriate snacks during the visit. A nurse assigned to and familiar with the patient performs a complete assessment (including vital signs) and initiates treatment, which may take from 30 minutes to more than 4 hours.

AICs may be physician/LIP practice based or hospital based. Some organizations provide a stand-alone infusion center, but this model has faced many reimbursement constraints, limiting its viability and growth. With the introduction of the PPS in long-term care and home care, the need for AICs will be even greater as the pressure to lower costs continues, and the AIC may help patients to avoid rehospitalization.

For infusion therapy provided in AICs, commercial insurers are recognizing the appropriateness of this infusion setting and its cost-competitiveness with other AIC settings. Medicaid coverage varies by state. Medicare's prescription drug plan (Part D) may cover the cost of the infusion drugs, but the costs of AIC services, supplies, equipment, and nursing are not covered. The infusion therapy provider will ascertain coverage for patients and advise on the extent of coverage and patient obligations prior to start of the service.

The patient selection for the AICs depends on reimbursement. The types of patients appropriate for AICs are those who do not have a caregiver in the home or who are unable to learn or perform self-administration. Another appropriate referral is a patient who is not homebound, does not qualify for home care, or does not have insurance coverage for home health care services. Patients can still recover at home and schedule visits for their infusions as prescribed by the physician/LIP.

Other benefits of AICs include teaching, monitoring, follow-up, quality assurance, patient satisfaction, and outcome management. Types of infusion therapy provided at AICs are addressed in Box 23-7. Because this model focuses on positive patient outcomes, other therapies provided may include allergy desensitization injections; diabetes education; hormone therapy; immunizations; protease inhibitors; vaccines for influenza and pneumonia; respiratory therapy (aerosolized pentamidine); and wound care (Bryant-Wimp & Liebert, 1999). Patient care, education, continuity of care, and positive patient outcomes are the keys to patient satisfaction, physician/LIP satisfaction, and the success of AICs.

LONG-TERM CARE

Long-term care (LTC), often provided in SNFs or nursing homes, is part of the continuum of care and an ongoing element of integrated health care. Long-term care services are intended for people of all ages with chronic disabilities and functional deficits to maintain their physical, social, and psychological functioning. The initiation of long-term care services may be preceded by an acute medical illness or the inability to perform activities of daily living (ADL) independently for 90 days or more (Nazarko, 1998). The care ranges from skilled nursing care, to supportive services provided in the home, to informed assistance given by family and friends.

PATIENT SAFETY

The ability to administer infusion drugs in the LTC arena plays a vital role in preventing a patient from having to return to the acute care setting—a top concern for referring hospitals.

BOX 23-7   TYPES OF CARE PROVIDED AT INFUSION SUITES OR AMBULATORY INFUSION CENTERS

Antibiotics/anti-infectives and first dosing
Anticoagulants—heparin therapy
Biologics
Blood transfusion and component therapy
Catheter placement and maintenance (peripheral, peripherally inserted central catheter/midline insertion)
Chemotherapy
Drug monitoring (peak and trough)
Hydration
Intravenous immune globulin
Pain management
Parenteral nutrition
Steroids
Venous sampling

Many residents of long-term care facilities have complex medical problems and receive skilled care for tracheostomies, gastric feeding tubes, ventilators, mobility disabilities, impaired nutrition, IV medications, and deficits in ADL associated with Alzheimer's disease. Acute care and subacute care hospitals, nursing homes, and assisted living centers are the only places that offer 24-hour nursing services with the exception of private duty nursing. Professional nurses are essential to care for the residents by assessing and coordinating patients' needs for care, focusing on rehabilitation and convalescence, providing high-quality care, reducing complications and mortality, and being cost-effective.

Infusion therapy is frequently required for the long-term resident. Commonly used modalities include antibiotic/anti-infective therapy, TPN, pain management, blood products, immune globulin, central venous catheter care and management, and PICC and midline catheter insertion. Credentialed infusion nurse specialists offer educational in-service sessions for the staff to enhance resident care and reduce complications.

As the population ages, chronic illness and disability also will increase, thus creating a growing need for long-term care. The greatest surge in the aging population will occur as the baby boomers reach old age. Estimates are that there will be 86.7 million people over the age of 65 by the year 2050; people in this group would comprise 21% of the total population. Demographic increases also are expected in the segment of the population aged 85 years and older. By 2050, an estimated 27 million people will need some type of long-term care, the majority of which will be delivered in the community (U.S. Census Bureau, 2010).

EVIDENCE FOR PRACTICE

By 2050, there will be 16 million people with dementia; how will that affect practice across the continuum?

FUTURE INFUSION TECHNOLOGY FOR ALTERNATE CARE PROGRAMS

Technology is one of the most important factors affecting infusion therapy for alternate care programs. In the future, patient care will change to accommodate new technologies, new drug therapies, and new equipment. The greatest obstacle will be reimbursement. Many professionals recognize that patients have multiple, medically complex needs that will necessitate more intensive clinical monitoring of the therapy, requiring improvements in staff and caregiver education.

Health care providers are being challenged to become more efficient and cost-conscious about what they do and how they do it. The delivery of antibiotics and anti-infectives is one of the fastest-growing therapies in alternative care programs. Over the years, tremendous changes have occurred in how these therapies are administered. Both high- and low-technology devices and methods are available for these therapies: gravity infusion, stationary infusion pumps, ambulatory electronic pumps, IV push, syringe delivery, and elastomeric devices with rate-restricted IV systems.

Driven by heightened emphasis on cost-effectiveness and cost-containment, and the desire of patients to resume normal lifestyles and work activities while recovering from illness, the alternate-site infusion therapy sector continues to expand. This will only continue to escalate.

However, the overall contribution of home infusion therapy to the health care system is certainly much more significant. The cost of infusion therapy administered in the home or alternate-site care setting is far less than the cost of inpatient treatment. Most infusion therapies can be safely administered in an alternative care environment; the role of the specialty infusion nurse is essential in ensuring positive outcomes.

Review Questions   *Note: Questions below may have more than one right answer.*

1. The fastest-growing alternate clinical setting for infusion is
   A. Home care
   B. Hospice
   C. Ambulatory infusion center
   D. Long-term care

2. The plan of treatment in a home care program is written by the
   A. Pharmacist
   B. Nurse
   C. Physician/LIP
   D. Branch manager

3. A case manager is responsible for which of the following activities?
   A. Initial assessment
   B. Development of a care plan
   C. Appropriate referral and follow-up
   D. All of the above

4. Frequently prescribed home infusion therapies include
   A. Antibiotics
   B. Parenteral nutrition
   C. Antifungals
   D. All of the above

5. The term "competency" refers to which of the following?
   A. Knowledge and skills required to safely practice
   B. Technical skills
   C. Critical thinking
   D. All of the above

6. Home infusion per diem billing codes are commonly referred to as which of the following?
   A. CPT
   B. HIPAA
   C. HCPCS
   D. DRG

7. Types of patients admitted to subacute care facilities include those
   A. With multiple body system complications
   B. Who are ventilator dependent
   C. With complex wounds
   D. With endocarditis

8. Which of the following patients might appropriately receive services at an AIC?
   A. Inadequate insurance coverage
   B. Homebound
   C. Not homebound
   D. Totally independent

9. One type of infusion therapy administered for the long-term patient is
   A. Enteral food supplements
   B. TPN
   C. Transdermal pain patches
   D. Antibiotic intramuscular injections

10. Because of their credentialing and high skill level, the need for infusion nurses in alternate clinical settings will increase in
   A. Subacute hospitals
   B. Ambulatory infusion centers
   C. Long-term care facilities
   D. All of the above

References and Selected Readings   *Asterisks indicate references cited in text.*

*American Medical Association. (2013). CPT—Current procedural terminology. http://www.ama-assn.org/ama/pub/physician-resources/solutions-managing-your-practice/coding-billing-insurance/cpt.page

American Society of Health System Pharmacists (ASHP). (2013). *ASHP Guidelines on Home Infusion Pharmacy Services.* Accessed December 1, 2013. http://www.ashp.org/DocLibrary/BestPractices/SettingsGdlHomeInfusion.aspx

*Baker, G. (2003). Pay for performance incentive programs in healthcare: Market dynamics and business process. *Executive Briefing.* A Research Report sposored by ViPS, Inc. in partnership with Med-Vantage. http://www.leapfroggroup.org/media/file/Leapfrog-Pay_for_Performance_Briefing.pdf

*Barrio, D. (1998). Antibiotic and anti-infective agent use and administration in home care. *Journal of Infusion Nursing, 21,* 50–58.

Benco, L.B. (2000). The exodus escalates: Medicare market pullouts to double in 2001. *Modern Healthcare, 30*(27), 14.

*Billings, D.M., & Halstead, J.A. (2009). *Teaching in nursing: A guide for faculty* (3rd ed.). St. Louis, MO: Saunders Elsevier.

Bowers, M. (1999). *The JCAHO home health mock survey made simple.* New York, NY: Opus Communications.

Bradshaw, M.J., & Lowenstein, A.J. (2007). *Innovative teaching strategies in nursing and related health professions* (4th ed.). Sudbury, MA: Jones and Bartlett.

Bryant-Wimp, J., & Liebert, L. (1999). Partnerships for establishing a hospital-based ambulatory care infusion center. *American Journal of Health System Pharmacy 56*(19), 1974–1977.

Centers for Medicare & Medicaid Services. (2012). *2012 Physician quality reporting system implementation guide.* January 2012, 3.

*Centers for Medicare & Medicaid Services. 2013 *Medicare internet-only-manual publication 100-01.* Washington, DC: Author. http://www.cms.gov/Regulations.

Centers for Medicare & Medicaid Services. (2013, June). *Analysis in support of rebasing and updating medicare home health payment rates.* Retrieved from http://www.cms.gov/Medicare/Medicare-Fee-for-Service-Payment/HomeHealthPPS/Downloads/Analyses-in-Support-of-Rebasing-and-Updating-the-Medicare-Home-Health-Payment-Rates-Technical-Report.pdf

Flores, K. (2004). The nuts and bolts of ambulatory infusion centers: Start up considerations. *Infusion, 10*(6), 15–19.

Government Accounting Office. (2011). *Home infusion therapy: Differences between Medicare and private insurers' coverage.* Washington, DC: GAO.

*Griffin, K. (1998). Evolution of transitional care settings: Past, present, future. *AACN Clinical Issues, 9,* 398–408.

Infusion Nurses Society. (2011a). Infusion nursing standards of practice. *Journal of Infusion Nursing, 34*(Suppl. 1), S1–S92.

Infusion Nurses Society. (2011b). *Policies and procedures for infusion nursing* (4th ed.). Norwood, MA: Infusion Nurses Society.

*Institute of Medicine. (2010). *The future of nursing: Leading change, advancing health—recommendations.* http://www.iom.edu/Reports/2010/The-Future-of-Nursing-Leading-Change-Advancing-Health/Recommendations.aspx?page=4

Joshi, D.K., Bluhm, R.A., Malani, P.N., Fetyko, S., Denton, T., & Blaum, C.S. (2012). The successful development of a subacute care service associated with a large academic health system. *Journal of the American Medical Directors Association, 13*(6), 564–567.

*Levenson, S. (2000). The future of subacute care. *Clinics in Geriatric Medicine, 16*(4), 683–700.

*Martel, D. (2012). Infusion therapy in the home care setting: A clinical competency program at work. *Home Healthcare Nurse, 30*(9), 506–514.

*National Home Infusion Association (NHIA). (2013). *Infusion FAQs.* http://www.nhia.org/faqs.cfm

*National Quality Forum. (2010). National Voluntary Consensus Standards for Home Health Care—Additional performance measures 2008. http://www.qualityforum.org/Publications/2010/10/

National_Voluntary_Consensus_Standards_for_Home_Health_Care_%E2%80%94_Additional_Performance_Measures_2008.aspx

*National Quality Forum. (2013). *National Quality Forum endorsement of measures for home care.* www.qualityforum.org

*Nazarko, L. (1998). Continuing to care. *Nursing Management, 5*(5), 29–33.

*O'Grady, N.P., Alexander, M., Burns, L.A., Dellinger, E.P., Garland, J., Heard, S.O., et al. (2011). Guidelines for the prevention of intravascular catheter-related infections. Centers for Disease Control and Prevention. http://www.cdc.gov/hicpac/pdf/guidelines/bsi-guidelines-2011.pdf

O'Hanlon, S. (2008). Delivering intravenous therapy in the community setting. *Nursing Standards, 22*(31), 44–48.

Pay-for-Performance Research Clearinghouse. (2012). P4P definition—What is P4P? http://www.p4presearch.org/node/36

Poole, S.M., & Nowobilski-Vasilios, A. (1999). To push or not to push. *Infusion, 5*(9), 53–55.

Ross, V.M., & Smith, C.E. (2011). National clinical guidelines and home parenteral nutrition. *Nutrition in Clinical Practice, 26*(6), 656–664.

*The Joint Commission (TJC). (2012). *National patient safety goals.* http://www.jointcommission.org/ltc_2012_npsgs/

*U.S. Census Bureau. (2010). The next four decades: The older population in the United States: 2010 to 2050. http://www.census.gov/prod/2010pubs/p25-1138.pdf

CHAPTER 24

The Future of Infusion Nursing

A Global Approach

Sharon M. Weinstein

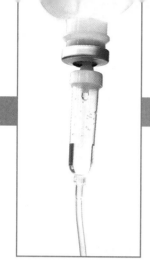

KEY TERMS		
	Brain Drain	Research
	Credentialing	Resilience
	Dual Missions	Shifting Paradigms
	Excellence	Strategic Partnering
	Globalization	Technology
	Interdisciplinary	Workforce
	Education	Workplace
	Leadership	

OVERVIEW

With well over 3 million members, the nursing profession is the largest segment of the nation's health care workforce. Nurses have the opportunity to practice in many settings, including hospitals, schools, homes, long-term care facilities, and community health centers. The educational level of nurses is diverse and extends from the licensed practical nurse to the nurse scientist. Our profession is at a significant time in history. Profound changes in science, technology, patient awareness, advocacy, and our health care environment have led to this change. Nursing, and more importantly, the nurse responsible for infusion therapy, a pivotal health care professional, is highly valued for specialized knowledge, skill, and caring in improving the health status of diverse populations.

The role of nurses in practice, academia, and science will become more critical as an aging population, a challenging environment, and expanded roles define our future. Nurses in clinical practice will continue to enrich nursing education through collaboration and create partnerships between service and academia to enhance education and practice. The role of the infusion specialist has never been more powerful; by partnering with other professionals, institutions, and communities, you make a tremendous difference in achieving quality infusion outcomes.

STRATEGIC PARTNERING

Strategic partnering enables infusion nurses to extend their scope of practice and professional network. Teambuilding, partnering, outreach, and collaboration are terms of the new millennium. Such terms suggest a continuing trend in health care. Partnering and collaboration are the hallmark of many successful models implemented by practice and academic health care settings worldwide. Strategic partnering, within and beyond institutions, provides opportunities for personal and professional growth, outreach, and collaboration (Weinstein, 2004).

Collaboration with like-minded professionals enables each of us to grow as health care professionals. In 2008, the Robert Wood Johnson Foundation (RWJF) and the Institute of Medicine (IOM) launched a 2-year initiative to respond to the need to assess and transform the nursing profession. The IOM appointed the *Committee on the RWJF Initiative on the Future of Nursing*, at the IOM, with the purpose of producing a report that would make recommendations for an action-oriented blueprint for the future of nursing. The committee considered nurses across roles, settings, and education levels in its effort to envision the future of the profession. Through its deliberations, the committee developed four key messages that may be seen in Box 24-1.

NURSING IMAGE

Nurses are often seen as a trusted profession. Yet, nursing sometimes suffers from the contagion of negative perspective that comes from nurses themselves as often as from others. We hear what is wrong with nursing and rarely what is really great about the profession. The general public is aware of the many reasons nursing is considered a hard job, but few could describe why nurses love their work. As nurses, we need to communicate this positive and gratifying part of our experience to balance negative messages. The impression of nursing is improving as a result of programs that celebrate nursing's successes and accomplishments—for example, the Magnet Recognition Program of the American Nurses Credentialing Center.

BOX 24-1 KEY MESSAGES FROM THE IOM REPORT

- Nurses should practice to the full extent of their education and training.
- Nurses should achieve higher levels of education and training through an improved education system that promotes seamless academic progression.
- Nurses should be full partners, with physicians/licensed independent practitioners (LIPs) and other health care professionals, in redesigning health care in the United States.
- Effective workforce planning and policy making require better data collection and an improved information infrastructure.

www.iom.edu/nursing

THE ENVIRONMENT

The environments in which we practice impact how we perceive the profession and our role. Workforce and workplace are critical factors for consideration.

Workforce

Opportunities abound for the nursing profession to intervene and make changes to address current staffing and patient safety problems and the growing nursing shortage. Today's nursing workforce is composed of staff and nursing leaders from four different generational cohorts. Generational diversity, including workforce differences in attitudes, beliefs, work habits, and expectations, has proven challenging for nursing leaders. The nursing workforce will continue to be age diverse for years to come; this is especially true of the infusion nursing workforce. Box 24-2 defines the generational characteristics of these cohorts.

The millennium has become the metaphor for the challenges and opportunities now available to the nursing profession and to those preparing the next generation of nurses. Trends have been driven by forces in demographics, diversity, and more (Table 24-1).

Workplace

Now, more than ever before, we give credence to the term "employer of choice." The American Nurse Credentialing Center's Magnet Recognition Program has made us all aware of the ideal work environment in which nurses are respected for what they bring to the clinical setting. Through clustered components of magnetism, transformational leadership is identified at the organizational level. In the midst of crisis management, leaders may lose sight of the need to care for their employees. And generous compensation and benefits, creative work arrangements, and healthy work environments cannot compete with the forces of our personal lives at times. These forces can make the most capable and motivated worker powerless and ineffective. So, it appears that the pursuit of balance is a delicate act that lies in the hands of the individual.

BOX 24-2 GENERATIONAL CHARACTERISTICS

Veterans (1925–1945)

- Hard working, financially conservative, respectful of authority disciplined

Baby Boomers (1946–1964)

- Strong work ethic, value individualism, empowered in the work setting

Gen X (1963–1980)

- Value self-reliance and work-life balance, less loyal to corporate

Millennials, also known as Generation Y (1980–2000)

- Global generation, accept multiculturalism, technology driven, communicative (via technology), expect more mentoring/coaching

TABLE 24-1 TEN TRENDS TO WATCH THAT IMPACT NURSING	
Demographics and diversity	• Growing life span • Increase in acute and chronic conditions • Disparities in morbidity, mortality, and access • Student demographics
Technology	• The information age • Processing capacity and speed • Affordability • Digital technology • Distance learning
Globalization	• Communication • The "death of distance" • Emerging and re-emerging infections
An educated consumer	• Shared decision making • Public information • Media and Internet • Health promotion and prevention • Wellness • Alternative therapies • Complementary medicine • Palliative and end-of-life advances
Population-based care	• Managed care • Accountable care organizations • Patient care ratios
Cost	• Gross national product • Underinsured and uninsured • Options • Reimbursement challenges • Advanced nurse practitioners • Physicians/LIPs
Policy and regulatory issues	• Increases in regulation at the state and federal levels • Shared responsibility for the Medicaid program
Collaborative practice	• Interdisciplinary teams of health care providers • Leadership and competence
Workforce	• Cyclical shortages • New career opportunities • Care management • Geriatric care managers • Public image • Command of technology
Science and research	• Health behaviors • Symptom management • Disease prevention • Nursing role

*Adapted from Heller, B. R., Oros, M. T., & Durney-Crowley, J. (2011). National league for nursing. http://www.nln.org/nlnjournal/infotrends.htm

Every day, nurses in all clinical settings are faced with the challenges of a changing patient population, a changing work environment, and changing tools with which to do their jobs. Patient and worker safety are key concerns, especially for those who specialize in infusion nursing. On a global level, professional societies have embraced the relationship of healthful practice environments to health outcomes. Based on the conviction, supported by evidence, that quality health care workplaces provide quality patient care, the International Council of Nurses (ICN) launched a global call to address and improve the serious deficiencies currently existing in the health work environment in all regions. The delivery of safe, high-quality, and efficient health services depends on the competence of health workers and a work environment that supports performance excellence. Publication of an information and action toolkit entitled, *"Quality workplaces = quality patient care"* provides data on positive practice environments to all health stakeholders who are interested in improving the delivery of quality services.

Nurses need, and deserve, a positive practice environment consistent with scope of practice, professional licensure, and local culture. Evidence supports the fact that job satisfaction is enhanced when corporate culture supports clinical practice, diversity, leadership, and continuous learning.

Although workplace stress cannot be completely eliminated, the negative stressors can be reduced when nurses make caring for themselves a priority. Self-care can be a barrier to stress-related illness and contribute to your overall well-being. Self-care begins with you! To maintain the delicate balancing act, you must manage your actions and personal/professional life. The universe exists in a state of balance, as should we. We can do anything we wish, but should always do it to moderation, never to excess. Should we do things to excess, they can become addictive, which drains energy and may become negative. Being balanced allows us to act better in situations. If we are sat on the fence, so to speak, we can jump off either way should we desire to.

Goal setting is tantamount to success and well-conceived goals are accompanied by action plans aimed at completion. To get to any goal, break it down into a number of small steps. If you have many small successes, then this will lead to a big success. Remember that a journey towards any destination starts with a single step, and then a second and a third, and as many as required until you reach that destination. Remember to reward and praise yourself for your successes, however small they are. By acknowledging them, you increase your power and will to succeed, strengthening your belief in yourself (Weinstein, 2008).

Safety Implications

Significant pressures are being placed on health care delivery systems to improve patient care outcomes and lower costs in an environment of diminishing resources. The IOM's landmark report attributed medication errors to faulty health care policy/procedure systems as opposed to individual error. Numerous studies have shown that information technology can enhance weak systems. For nursing, information technology plays a key role in protecting patients by eliminating nursing mistakes and protecting nurses by reducing their negative exposure. Information technology is dependent upon user expertise. Nursing is in a unique position to address the challenges of today's health system with respect to outcomes and patient/staff safety.

PATIENT SAFETY

Consider the role that Fatigue plays in your role as a nurse professional. Key considerations are: the role of fatigue in ensuring safe outcomes; operational strategies with a focus on resource allocation and support; and wellness strategies to create and sustain a safe environment.

Changing Technologies

Advances in **technology** continue to affect our practice as well as patient outcomes, regardless of the clinical setting in which care is delivered. Infusion nurses are often the driving force behind innovations that better meet the needs of their patients and those within the medical community. Infusion nurses are credited with the adaptation of vascular access devices from continuous setups to intermittent devices. The term "what if" has led to the creation of multiple technologies such as securement locking devices and taping techniques that have transformed the practice, generated better outcomes, and facilitated the growth of the specialty. This process will continue as a new generation of infusion nurses offers information through surveys, focus groups, market research, and more. As the primary source of patient education, the infusion nurse can contribute greatly to the learning process. As the end user, the infusion nurse's input impacts technology and the quality of products available to us.

Research

This edition of Plumer included references to **research** topics that are currently being explored or that should be developed in an effort to grow the specialty practice. New research ensures sound evidence for practice. Funding may be available through grants and scholarships from professional societies, foundations, and industry. Closing the gap between research and practice requires knowledge, commitment, **resilience**, and confidence that this will further nursing's agenda within the health care arena—especially infusion nursing.

Credentialing

Every day, the delivery of health care becomes more complex as new treatments are discovered and new technologies for diagnosing and treating disease are developed. Today's patients are sicker than ever before. The depth and breadth of knowledge required of the professional are not completely met by the entry-level nursing education available. Today's consumer needs and deserves more.

To better meet the needs of today's patients, nurses often seek additional education and validation of their clinical expertise. Advanced practice requires advanced learning, including baccalaureate and master's degrees, post–master's training, and doctoral degrees. Certification validates one's knowledge, professional skills, and clinical expertise. Requirements for specialty certifications vary, but all include a practice component and an identified body of required knowledge or testing blueprint.

Certification is defined as a process by which a nongovernmental agency validates an individual's knowledge related to a specific area of practice. The National Commission for Certifying Agencies set forth certain basic requirements for all certification examinations, including the requirement that testing reflects current practice in the specialty and measures specified aspects of this practice.

Beyond ensuring basic safety, certification is often thought to promote quality care.

Indicators of quality in health care have drawn consumer interest in recent years. Today, it is not unusual to see hospital morbidity and mortality statistics published in newspapers. In addition, the Centers for Medicare & Medicaid Services (CMS) publish key indicators of hospitals' performance on the Centers' Web site to make this information readily available to the public.

EVIDENCE FOR PRACTICE

Will further confirmation of the link between high quality, safety, and certification drive efforts to support and encourage more nurses and other health professionals to become certified?

Professional societies, such as the Infusion Nurses Society (INS), educate the public to recognize the value of the credentialed nursing professional. Employers increasingly recognize the value of the credential and the enhanced outcomes that result from a certified workforce.

Publications

Today's infusion nurse specialist has the keys to success at his or her fingertips. The plethora of books, journal articles, online training, and more facilitates the process of lifelong learning. Infusion nurses need to continue to share practice through the written word by contributing their knowledge and expertise to journals, newsletters, and more.

Resilience

Resilience is the ability of an individual to positively adjust to adversity and can be applied to building personal strengths in nurses through strategies such as promoting positive and nurturing professional relationships; maintaining positivity; developing emotional insight; achieving life balance and spirituality; and becoming more reflective. Workplace adversity in nursing is associated with excessive workloads, lack of autonomy, bullying and violence, and organizational issues such as restructuring and has been associated with problems retaining nurses in the workforce. However, despite these difficulties, many nurses choose to remain in nursing and survive and even thrive despite a climate of workplace adversity (Jackson, Firtko, & Edenborough, 2007) (Box 24-3).

Leadership

Only when nurses are positioned to have a stronger voice in institutional decision making will they appear at the table in the boardroom. Nurses have what policymakers need—the ability to build the case for change and improve care delivery. Nurses need to become vocal in community forums and public debate. And with care increasingly delivered using team models to promote patient safety and improved outcomes, nurses must be able to lead as well as be an advocate for patients from a holistic nursing perspective (Bleich, 2012).

BOX 24-3   CREATING RESILIENCE

- Personal environment that sustains you
- Bounce back as needed
- Stay in the present and move forward
- Know when to ask for help and where to get it
- Rest, relaxation, quiet time
- Pursuit of passion
- More than avoiding overwork
- Authentic expression
- Personal and professional growth

 PATIENT SAFETY

Think about the multiple ways in which you, as a professional, impact the lives of patients each and every day.

Today's leaders know that nursing is the ideal profession to blend concepts of wellness, balance, and health. As leaders, they should be involved in establishing the evidence base for practice. And, they need balance before they can help others to achieve it. Nurses are key stakeholders and hold important **leadership** roles in health care and education. While their authority and spheres of influence have significantly expanded, more transformational nurse leaders are needed. The transformational nurse leader who understands how to share a vision, how to connect with others, and how to mentor and coach others to exceed expectations and build high-performance teams will be successful in engaging others in the workplace. Transformational leaders are committed to sustainability and recognize the importance of succession planning. They provide mentoring and coaching and understand how to build communities of catalysts for change.

Mentoring and Precepting

The concept of mentoring has gained increasing importance in assisting nurses to reach professional excellence. Beyond role modeling, mentoring implies an experienced individual taking an active role in the professional and personal development of a less experienced person.

Precepting is a term used to describe the relationship between a student clinician and an experienced clinician who supervises and evaluates the student's clinical practicum. In the best of experiences, the preceptor facilitates the student's or novice's clinical learning, acts as a role model, promotes role socialization, encourages independence, and promotes self-confidence leading to clinical competency.

Mentoring is an interaction between an experienced and an inexperienced member of an organization (Figure 24-1). Mentors, as opposed to preceptors, are often self-selected. The story of Mentor comes from Homer's Odyssey. Odysseus, King of Ithaca, fights in the Trojan War and entrusts the care of his household to Mentor, who serves as teacher and overseer of Odysseus' son, Telemachus. After the war, Odysseus is condemned to wander vainly for

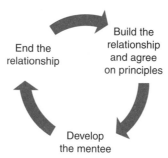

FIGURE 24-1 Components of the mentoring process.

10 years in his attempt to return home. In time, Telemachus, now grown, ventures in search of his father. Athena, Goddess of War and patroness of the arts and industry, assumes the form of Mentor and accompanies Telemachus on his quest. Father and son reunite and cast down would-be usurpers of Odysseus' throne and Telemachus's birthright. The word *mentor* evolved to mean a trusted advisor, friend, teacher, and wise person (Schwiebert, 2000). Table 24-2 lists the qualities of a good mentor.

SHIFTING PARADIGMS

From leadership to first-line management, the rules have changed. The changes ahead for the nursing profession include new rules of engagement based on practice, patient care, outcomes, ethics, and environment. Nursing is at the core of this change process on a global scale. From the hospital to the clinic, from the classroom to the bedside, and from recruitment to retention, nurses are there 24 hours a day, each and every day to advocate for the patient, the profession, and our future.

Across the country and around the world, we hear talk about the Rules of Engagement. Often attributed to migration issues, the rules far surpass the migration concerns and emanate to educating the next generation of nurses, preparing this new cadre of nurse professionals for practice, recruitment and retention, work environment, Magnet status, and more! The rules of engagement are transforming all settings, in all countries of the world. Nurses, nursing, and the health care systems in which we work mandate change. Global

TABLE 24-2	**QUALITIES OF A GOOD MENTOR**

- Demonstrates role expertise and promotes role socialization
- Role models and guides appropriately
- Provides a reflective practice
- Shares values and customs
- Listens actively
- Challenges the protégé by constructing hypotheses
- Sets high-performance standards
- Empowers the protégé to achieve autonomy
- Facilitates essential contacts

nursing impacts healthcare delivery in every corner of the world and will require interventions from all sectors of society (Weinstein, 2007). Infusion nurses can and should share their knowledge, expertise, and passion for the specialty practice with their international colleagues. As the credentialing exam is offered in other countries, the doors to collaboration will open.

INTERNATIONAL MIGRATION

Brain drain, or taking the best health professionals from other countries to compensate for US nursing shortages, is not always the right answer. Organizations such as the International Council of Nurses (ICN) and the World Health Organization (WHO) have stated their concerns publicly. Brain drain deprives developing nations of quality care, whereas global nursing organizations support and advocate on behalf of ethical recruitment of foreign nursing professionals.

A GLOBAL PERSPECTIVE

So, what are the issues nurses and nursing facing today? **Globalization**, the sociopolitical system, the economy, and safety are key concerns. Within our health care system, we worry about economics, the role of government, quality, access to care, patient safety, patient satisfaction, ethics, and bioterrorism. Academic health centers face their own challenges in the form of **dual missions**, health disparities, sick care versus integrative care, an aging population, competition, and succession.

Nurses all face similar problems, regardless of the environment in which they work and the area where they reside. Within their workforce, nurses are concerned with undersupply, knowledge work, fatigue, the work environment, patient/staff safety, and culturally competent care. Models of care delivery that affect outcomes are also a concern, including continuum of care, cost and efficiency, evidence-based outcomes, best practices, sustainability, and wellness incentives. Infusion nursing specialty practice is growing globally; international members have demonstrated their expertise and acumen within the profession.

The professional nurse is a knowledge worker and knowledge manager (Table 24-3). Through continuous learning, the nurse seeks **interdisciplinary education**, technology training, marketing acumen, global mentoring, and emotional intelligence.

This is a great time for nursing. In the future, the public will recognize our vision, our voice, and our vitality. We have the unique opportunity to leverage our talents, skills, and abilities and seek abundant results for ourselves and for our patients.

Professional nursing is at a crossroads, and for those professionals involved in infusion nursing, the future has never been brighter. Value the skills and talents that you have developed as an infusion specialist. Become an active member of the nursing councils within your organization and promote the future of the nursing profession.

EXCELLENCE

The emergence of health systems as a dominant structure for organizing health care has challenged nursing leadership (Arnold et al., 2006). The day-to-day impact of this change places an even greater emphasis on demonstrated outcomes and innovation that may

TABLE 24-3	TERMINOLOGY ASSOCIATED WITH KNOWLEDGE MANAGEMENT

Knowledge Manager

A role with developmental and operational responsibility for promoting and implementing knowledge management principles and practices.

Knowledge Mapping

A process for determining where knowledge assets are within an organization and how knowledge flows. Evaluating relationships between holders of knowledge will then illustrate the sources, flows, limitations, and losses of knowledge that can be expected to occur.

Knowledge Repository

A place to store and retrieve explicit knowledge. A low-tech knowledge repository could be a set of file folders. A high-tech knowledge repository might be a database.

Knowledge Worker

An employee whose role relies on his or her ability to find and use knowledge.

potentially transform nursing practice, quality and safety of care, and the population served. The time for nursing excellence through leadership support and engagement has come.

A SOLID PAST AND A SECURE FUTURE

When the late Ada Plumer became the first "official IV nurse" in the country at Massachusetts General Hospital in 1940, she was a pioneer. It is that "pioneer" spirit that led to the creation of the Infusion Nurses Society (INS), formerly the National Intravenous Therapy Association (NITA). Ms. Plumer, with her colleagues, chartered a path that has developed exponentially into the thriving practice that it is today. Although the responsibilities of the IV nurse and team were quite different at that time, the intention was the same—that of providing quality, safe care to those receiving infusion therapies. It is that proud past that helped to secure our future.

Nursing and health care face many challenges in today's world and in the future. Society expects—and rightfully should demand—safe, high-quality care. The public and health care–accrediting bodies want to find the best indicators of quality so that care can be evaluated more comprehensively. The future of infusion therapy is in the hands of those who deliver care each and every day.

Our professional organizations promote quality, credentialing, and more. To attain success, an interdisciplinary team of health care professionals must work cohesively to ensure positive outcomes. Infusion nurses are in unique position to drive change, to enhance outcomes, to work as members of the interdisciplinary team to ensure safety, and the growth of the profession. An innate belief in the practice model, the process, and the profession contribute to a future without limits. We are challenged to shape the future of infusion nursing. We share a common passion for the profession and for the practice. We must think critically about solutions that benefit the society, the profession, our patients, and our practice.

Review Questions   *Note: Questions below may have more than one right answer.*

1. Which of the following is true of strategic partnering as it relates to infusion nursing?
   A. Allows one to extend scope of practice
   B. Facilitates professional networking
   C. Limits implementation of advanced practice
   D. A and B only

2. All of the following statements are true concerning preceptorship except
   A. A preceptor supervises and evaluates the student's clinical practicum
   B. A preceptor facilitates the student's or novice's clinical learning
   C. A preceptor discourages role socialization
   D. A preceptor acts as a role model

3. Which of the following terms has become the metaphor for the challenges and opportunities now available to the nursing profession and to those preparing the next generation of nurses?
   A. Gen Z
   B. Millennium
   C. Gen X
   D. Baby boomers

4. Terminology associated with knowledge management includes all of the following except
   A. Manager
   B. Mapping
   C. Depository
   D. Worker

5. Key issues facing professional nursing today include
   A. Globalization
   B. Dual missions

C. Economics
D. All of the above

6. Changes ahead for the nursing profession include which of the following?
   A. New rules of engagement
   B. Global warming
   C. A only
   D. A and B

7. Mentoring has its roots in which of the following?
   A. The Bible
   B. Homer's Odyssey
   C. The Iliad
   D. Homeric Hymns

8. Professional organizations promote which of the following?
   A. Quality
   B. Credentialing
   C. A and B
   D. B only

9. Which of the following factors is affected by advances in technology?
   A. Practice
   B. Certification
   C. Outcomes
   D. A and C

10. Closing the gap between research and practice requires
    A. Knowledge
    B. Commitment
    C. Resilience
    D. All of the above

References and Selected Readings   *Asterisks indicate references cited in text.*

Aiken, L.H., & Poghosyan, L. (2009). Evaluation of "magnet journey to nursing excellence program" in Russia and Armenia. *Journal of Nursing Scholarship, 41*(2), 166–174.

Alexander, M., Corrigan, A., & Hankins, J. (2009). *Infusion nursing: An evidence-based approach.* St. Louis, MO: WB Saunders Company.

American Board of Nursing Specialties. (2006). Promoting excellence in nursing certification. http://www.nursingcertification.org/index.html

American Nurses Association. (2002). Nursing's agenda for the future: A call to the nation. www.nursingworld.org/naf

Arnold, L., Bakhtina, I., Brooks, A.M., Coulter, S., Hurt, L., Lewis, C., et al. (1998). Nursing in the newly independent states of the former Soviet Union: An international partnership for nursing development. *Journal of Obstetric and Gynecologic Neonatal Nurseries, 27*(2), 203–208.

*Arnold, L., Drenkard, K., Ela, S., Goedken, J., Hamilton, C., Harris, C., et al. (2006). Strategic positioning for nursing excellence in health systems: Insights from chief nursing executives. *Nursing Administration Quarterly, 30*(1), 11–20.

Auerbach, D.I., Buerhaus, P.I., & Staiger, D.O. (2007). Better late than never: Workforce supply implications of later entry into nursing. *Health Affairs, 26*(1), 178–185.

*Bleich, M.R. (2012). The future of nursing report and direct care nurses. *American Journal of Nursing, 112*(2), 11.

Briggs, L.A., Brown, H., Kesten, K., & Heath, J. (2006). Certification a benchmark for critical care nursing excellence. *Critical Care Nurse, 26*(6), 47–53.

Brown, C.E., Wickline, M.A., Ecoff, L., & Glaser, D. (2009). Nursing practice, knowledge, attitudes and perceived barriers to evidence-based practice at an academic medical center. *Journal of Advanced Nursing, 65*(2), 371–381.

Byrne, M.W., & Keefe, M.R. (2004). Building research competence in nursing through mentoring. *Journal of Nursing Scholarship, 34*(4), 391–396.

Coulon, L., Mok, M., Krause, K. L., & Anderson, M. (2008). The pursuit of excellence in nursing care: What does it mean? *Journal of Advanced Nursing, 24*(4), 817–826.

Goss, L., & Carrico, R. (2002). Get a grip on patient safety: Outcomes in the palm of your hand. *Journal of Infusion Nursing, 25*(4), 274–279.

Hadaway, L. (2012). Infusion teams: The future is now. *Newsline, 34*(3), 1.

Halbesleben, J.R., Wakefield, B.J., Wakefield, D.S., & Cooper, L.B. (2008). Nurse burnout and patient safety outcomes nurse safety perception versus reporting behavior. *Western Journal of Nursing Research, 30*(5), 560–577.

Haley-Andrews, S., & Winch, A. (2001). Mentoring, membership in professional organizations, and the pursuit of excellence in nursing. *Journal for Specialists in Pediatric Nursing, 6*(3), 147–148.

Harrison, M., Henriksen, K., & Hughes, R. (2007). Improving the healthcare work environment: Implications for research, practice, and policy. *The Joint Commission Journal on Quality and Patient Safety, 33*(11), 81–84.

*Heller, B.R., Oros, M.T., & Durney-Crowley, J. (2011). The future of nursing education: Ten trends to watch. *Robert Wood Johnson Foundation and the Institute of Medicine Consensus Report.* The National Academy of Sciences. http://www.nln.org/nlnjournal/infotrends.htm

Infusion Nurses Society. (2012). INS mission statement. *INS Web site.* http://www.ins1.org

*Jackson, D., Firtko, A., & Edenborough, M. (2007). Personal resilience as a strategy for surviving and thriving in the face of workplace adversity: A literature review. *Journal of Advanced Nursing, 60*(1), 1–9.

Jasovsky, D.A., Grant, V.A., Lang, M., Devereux, B.F., Altier, M.E., Bird, S.R., et al. (2010). How do you define nursing excellence? *Nursing Management, 41*(10), 19–24.

Kimball, B., & O'Neil, E. (2002). *Health care's human crisis: The American nursing shortage.* Princeton, NJ: The Robert Wood-Johnson Foundation. http://www.rwjf.org/research/researchdetail.jsp?id=1108&ia=137

Kowalski, K., Horner, M., Carroll, K., Center, D., Foss, K., Jarrett, S., et al. (2007). Nursing clinical faculty revisited: The benefits of developing staff nurses as clinical scholars. *The Journal of Continuing Education in Nursing, 38*(3), 69.

Laschinger, H.K.S., & Leiter, M.P. (2006). The impact of nursing work environments on patient safety outcomes: The mediating role of burnout engagement. *Journal of Nursing Administration, 36*(5), 259–267.

Malloch, K., & Porter-O'Grady, T. (2010). *Introduction to evidence-based practice in nursing and health care.* Sudbury, MA: Jones & Bartlett Learning.

Mattox, E.A. (2012). Strategies for improving patient safety: Linking task type to error type. *Critical Care Nurse, 32*(1), 52–60.

McMahon, D.D. (2002). Evaluating new technology to improve patient outcomes: A quality improvement approach. *Journal of Infusion Nursing, 25*(4), 250–255.

Meredith, E.K., Cohen, E., & Raia, L.V. (2010). Transformational leadership: Application of magnet's new empiric outcomes. *The Nursing Clinics of North America, 45*(1), 49.

Milton, C.L. (2008). Accountability in nursing reflecting on ethical codes and professional standards of nursing practice from a global perspective. *Nursing Science Quarterly, 21*(4), 300–303.

Morgan, S.H. (2009). The Magnet (TM) model as a framework for excellence. *Journal of Nursing Care Quality, 24*(2), 105–108.

Moureau, N. (2006). Vascular safety: It's all about PICCs. *Nursing management, 37*(5), 22.

Page, A. (Ed.). (2003). *Keeping patients safe: Transforming the work environment of nurses.* Committee on the Work Environment for Nurses and Patient Safety. Washington, DC: Institute of Medicine. http://books.nap.edu/catalog/10851

Peate, I. (2008). Coding the path for practice accountability. *British Journal of Nursing, 17*(6), 353.

Phaneuf, M. (2003). Resilience and nursing. *Infiressources, clinical crossroad, section mental health and communication.* http://www.infiressources.ca/fer/Depotdocument_anglais/Resilience_and_nursing.pdf

Polit, D.F., & Beck, C.T. (2007). *Nursing research: Generating and assessing evidence for nursing practice.* Philadelphia, PA: Lippincott Williams & Wilkins.

Puglise, K. (2012). We lead a message from the president. *INS Newsline.* http://www.ins1.org/i4a/pages/index.cfm?pageid=3482

Ravert, P., & Merrill, K.C. (2008). Hospital nursing research program: Partnership of service and academia. *Journal of Professional Nursing, 24*(1), 54–58.

Robertson, K. (2005). Active listening—More than just paying attention. *Australian Family Physician, 34*(12), 1053–1055.

Rothschild, J.M., Landrigan, C.P., Cronin, J.W., Kaushal, R., Lockley, S.W., Burdick, E., et al. (2005). The Critical Care Safety Study: The incidence and nature of adverse events and serious medical errors in intensive care. *Critical Care Medicine, 33*(8), 1694–1700.

*Schwiebert, V.L. (2000). *Mentoring: Creating connected, empowered relationships.* Alexandria, VA: American Counseling Association.

Scott, L.D., Hofmeister, N., Rogness, N., & Rogers, A.E. (2010). An interventional approach for patient and nurse safety: A fatigue countermeasures feasibility study. *Nursing Research, 59*(4), 250–258.

Simpson, R.L. (2005). Patient and nurse safety: How information technology makes a difference. *Nursing Administration Quarterly, 29*(1), 97–101.

Smolenski, M.C. (2005). Credentialing, certification, and competence: Issues for new and seasoned nurse practitioners. *Journal of the American Academy of Nurse Practitioners, 17*(6), 201–204.

Stanley, J.M., Gannon, J., Gabuat, J., Hartranft, S., Adams, N., Mayes, C., et al. (2008). The clinical nurse leader: A catalyst for improving quality and patient safety. *Journal of Nursing Management, 16*(5), 614–622.

Stone, P.W., Mooney-Kane, C., Larson, E.L., Horan, T., Glance, L.G., Zwanziger, J., et al. (2007). Nurse working conditions and patient safety outcomes. *Medical Care, 45*(6), 571–578.

Strout, K. (2012). Wellness promotion and the Institute of Medicine's Future of Nursing Report: Are nurses ready? *Holistic Nursing Practice, 26*(3), 129–136.

Swanson, K.M. (2007). Nursing as informed caring for the well-being of others. *Journal of Nursing Scholarship, 25*(4), 352–357.

Wachter, R.M. (2010). Patient safety at ten: Unmistakable progress, troubling gaps. *Health Affairs, 29*(1), 165–173.

Watson, R. (2006). Is there a role for higher education in preparing nurses? *Nurse Education in Practice, 6*(6), 314–318.

Weinstein, S. (2000). Certification and credentialing to define competency-based practice. *Journal of Intravenous Nursing, 23*(1), 21–28.

Weinstein, S. (2002). A nursing portfolio: Documenting your professional journey. *Journal of Infusion Nursing, 25*(6), 357–364.

*Weinstein, S.M. (2004). Strategic partnering. *Journal of Infusion Nursing, 26*(5). www.hospitalconnect.com/ahanews/jsp/display.jsp?

Weinstein, S.M. (2008). *B is for balance: a nurse's guide for enjoying life at work and at home* (pp. 19, 68). Indianapolis, IN: Nursing Knowledge International.

Weinstein, S.M. & Brooks, A.M. (2007). *Nursing without borders: values, wisdom, success markers* (pp. 45, 46). Indianapolis, IN: Nursing Knowledge International.

Zrelak, P., Utter, G., Sadeghi, B., Cuny, J., Baron, R., & Romano, P. (2012). Using the agency for health-care research and quality patient safety indicators for targeting nursing quality improvement. *Journal of Nursing Care Quality, 27*(2), 99–108.

ANSWERS TO REVIEW QUESTIONS

CHAPTER 1
1. C
2. A, B, C, D
3. A
4. B
5. B, C

CHAPTER 2
1. B
2. C
3. C
4. A
5. C
6. C
7. B
8. D
9. D
10. D

CHAPTER 3
1. D
2. D
3. A
4. A, B
5. B
6. A
7. D
8. D
9. D
10. C

CHAPTER 4
1. D
2. A
3. B
4. C
5. D
6. B
7. B
8. D
9. B
10. D

CHAPTER 5
1. D
2. D
3. D
4. D
5. D
6. C

7. B
8. C
9. C
10. D

CHAPTER 6
1. B
2. A, B, C, D
3. C
4. A
5. D
6. A, B, C
7. C
8. D
9. D
10. A

CHAPTER 7
1. A, B, C, D
2. D
3. D
4. A, B, C
5. A
6. D
7. D
8. D
9. C
10. C

CHAPTER 8
1. A
2. D
3. A
4. A
5. A, B
6. A
7. A, B, C, D
8. A, B, C
9. A
10. B

CHAPTER 9
1. B
2. A
3. A
4. B, C
5. A
6. A
7. D
8. B

9. A, B
10. D

CHAPTER 10
1. A
2. A
3. C
4. B
5. D
6. D
7. D
8. D
9. D
10. B

CHAPTER 11
1. C
2. A
3. A
4. D
5. D
6. A
7. A
8. B
9. A, B, D
10. B, D

CHAPTER 12
1. D
2. A
3. D
4. B
5. A, C
6. D
7. D
8. A
9. D
10. B

CHAPTER 13
1. D
2. B
3. C
4. B
5. D
6. C
7. A
8. B, D
9. B
10. A

CHAPTER 14
1. D
2. C
3. B
4. D
5. A, B, D
6. D
7. B, D
8. A
9. D
10. A

CHAPTER 15
1. A
2. A
3. B, C
4. D
5. D
6. D
7. C
8. B
9. B
10. D

CHAPTER 16
1. C
2. B
3. D
4. A
5. A
6. D
7. B
8. D
9. A
10. D

CHAPTER 17
1. A
2. A, B, D
3. D
4. A
5. B
6. C
7. C
8. B
9. D
10. B

CHAPTER 18
1. D
2. C
3. A, B, C, D
4. B
5. A, B, C
6. D
7. D
8. C
9. D
10. D

CHAPTER 19
1. B
2. D
3. A
4. A
5. C
6. D
7. C
8. B

9. C
10. A

CHAPTER 20
1. C
2. A, B
3. A, D
4. B
5. A, B
6. D
7. D
8. A
9. A, B, C, D
10. A, C, D

CHAPTER 21
1. C
2. B
3. D
4. B
5. D

6. A
7. C
8. B
9. C
10. B

CHAPTER 22
1. D
2. C
3. A, B
4. C
5. B
6. C
7. D
8. C
9. B
10. A

CHAPTER 23
1. A
2. C

3. D
4. D
5. D
6. C
7. A, B, C
8. C
9. B
10. D

CHAPTER 24
1. D
2. C
3. B
4. C
5. D
6. C
7. B
8. C
9. D
10. D

ABO system—a basic hereditary blood group system used to classify a person's blood group

Absorption—process by which medication moves from drug administration sites to vasculature

Acidosis—blood pH below normal (<7.35)

Active transport—the passage of a substance across a cell membrane by an energy-consuming process, permitting diffusion to occur

Adjuvant chemotherapy—the addition of drug therapy to surgery and/or radiation therapy to eradicate metastatic disease

Admixture—combination of two or more medications

Adsorption—attachment of one substance to the surface of another

Advocate—informing patients of their rights, ensuring information exchange, and supporting patients in decisions they make

Agglutination—clumping of red blood cells when incompatible bloods are mixed

Agglutinin—an antibody causing agglutination with its corresponding antigen

Alarm fatigue—a national patient safety hazard associated with ignoring alarm systems

Alkalosis—blood pH above normal (>7.45)

Alkylating agents—agents that kill cells by cross-linking DNA strands (i.e., disturbing the normal structure) in the DNA molecule

Alopecia—the loss of hair from the body and/or the scalp

Alpha (α)—(a) the level of statistical significance designating the probability of committing a type I error. Also known as the P value; (b) a reliability coefficient, such

as Cronbach's alpha, to estimate internal consistency

Alternate site care—care that is delivered beyond the confines of an inpatient facility

Ambulatory infusion device—electronic infusion device specifically designed to be worn on the body to promote patient mobility and independence in the home or work environment

Analgesia—freedom from nociceptive stimuli; absence of pain

Analogue—a compound that resembles another in structure (e.g., fluorouracil is an analogue of uracil)

Anorexia—absence or loss of appetite for food

Antibody—a substance present in the plasma that incites immunity and that can react with the specific antigen that caused its production

Antidiuretic hormone (ADH)—hormone secreted from a pituitary mechanism that causes the kidneys to conserve water

Anti–free-flow administration set—an IV administration device that stops when removed from the electronic infusion device, yet allows gravity flow when the user takes action

Antigen—an immunizing agent capable of inducing the body to form antibodies

Antimetabolites—anticancer drugs that substitute for or block the use of an essential metabolite

Antimicrobial—an agent that destroys or prevents development of microorganisms

Antimicrobial ointment—a semisolid preparation used to prevent the pathogenic action of microbes

Antineoplastic agent—a medication or treatment for cancer

Antitumor antibiotics—anticancer drugs that interfere with cellular production of DNA and/or RNA

Arterial pressure monitoring—monitoring of arterial pressure through an indwelling arterial catheter connected to an electronic monitor

Arteriovenous (AV) fistula—the surgical anastomosis of an artery and a vein

Arteriovenous (AV) grafts—the insertion of a synthetic device connecting a vein and an artery

Aseptic technique—mechanism used to reduce potential contamination

Assay determination—decision based on an analysis and/or examination

Auscultation—process of listening to or for sounds in the body

Autologous—products or components of the same individual

Bacteria—microorganisms that may potentiate disease and infection

Benchmarking—comparing one's systems to others

Beta (β)—(a) statistical testing term referring to the probability of making a type II error; (b) the standardized regression coefficient in the regression equation indicating the relative weights of the independent variables

Biotherapy—therapeutic use of biological materials or biological response modifiers

Biotransformation–metabolism—the enzymatic alteration of a drug molecule

Blood grouping—the testing of red blood cells to determine antigens present and absent

Body surface area—surface area of the body determined through use of a nomogram; important when calculating drug dosages

Bone marrow—the inner spongy tissue of a bone in which red blood cells, white blood cells, and platelets are formed

BSPECLD—method of determining levels of pain in the pediatric patient

Cancer—the general name for more than 100 diseases in which abnormal cells grow out of control; a malignant tumor

Cannula—a hollow tube made of plastic or metal used for accessing the vascular system

Catheter—a hollow tube made of plastic used for accessing the vascular system

Cell kill—the number of cancer cells killed at a given dose by an antineoplastic drug

Cellular kinetics—study of mechanisms and rates of cellular changes

Central venous bundle—the process of grouping key actions to prevent CRBSIs and CLABSIs

Certification—recognition of a specialized body of knowledge, experience, and/or skills demonstrated by the achievement of standards; sponsored by a professional organization

Competency—expected level of performance integrating knowledge, skill, and clinical reasoning

Chemical incompatibility—a change in the molecular structure or pharmacologic properties of a substance, which may or may not be visually observed

Chemotherapy—the chemical treatment for cancer patients with agents designed to kill cancer cells

CLABSI—central line–associated bloodstream infection

Cognitive—behaviors that place primary emphasis on mental or intellectual processes

Cold agglutinin—a red blood cell agglutinin that acts at a relatively low temperature; part of a disease process caused by a transient infectious disease; may be idiopathic

Color coding—system developed by manufacturers that identifies products/medications by color. These color code systems are not standardized and may vary with manufacturer.

Compartment syndrome—compression of circulation evidenced by impaired pulses, compromised circulation, and pain

Compatibility—capacity for being mixed and administered without undergoing undesirable chemical and/or physical changes or loss of therapeutic action

Compatibility test—all tests performed on donors and recipients to determine compatibility of blood; also known as *cross-matching*

Complement—a group of proteins in normal blood serum and plasma that, in combination with antibodies, cause the destruction of particular antigens

Complex Regional Pain Syndrome—see RSD

Contamination—introduction of pathogens or infectious material from one source to another

Corrective action—a defined plan to eliminate deficiencies

CRBSI—catheter-related bloodstream infections

CRNI®—the nursing credential awarded to qualified candidates by the Infusion Nurses Credentialing Corporation (INCC)

Cross-contamination—movement of pathogens from one source to another

Curative—healing or corrective

Cutdown—surgical procedure for exposure and catheterization of a vein

Cytoprotectant—drug to minimize toxicities of chemotherapy without compromising the cytotoxic effects of drugs on cancer cells

Delayed reaction—in relation to blood transfusions, adverse effect occurring after 48 hours and up to 180 days after the transfusion

Delivery system—product that facilitates administration of drug(s);

can be integral or have component parts. Delivery systems encompass all products used, from the solution container down to the cannula.

Dermatomes—segmental distribution of the spinal nerves. Dermatomes are labeled according to their exit point on the spinal cord. The spinal canal has 31 dermatomes. Dermatome pathways are not defined or determined through dissection but by observation of patients with spinal cord injuries for the resultant neurologic effects.

Diffusion—passage of molecules of one substance between the molecules of another to form a mixture of the two

Disinfectant—an agent that eliminates all microorganisms except spores; generally used on inanimate objects

Distal—farthest from the heart; farthest from point of attachment; below previous site of catheterization

Distention—expansion owing to pressure within

Document—a written or printed record that contains original, official, or legal information

Documentation—a recording in written or printed form containing original, official, or legal information

Dome—a plastic component used in hemodynamic monitoring

Dose-limiting toxicity—the degree of toxicity that dictates the maximum amount of drug that safely can be administered

Drug–nutrient interaction—an event that occurs (a) when nutrient availability is altered by a medication or (b) when a drug effect is altered or an adverse reaction is caused by the intake of nutrients

Ecchymoses—bruising resulting from escape of blood from injured vessels into subcutaneous tissue

Electronic infusion device (EID)—an electronic instrument that regulates the flow rate of the prescribed therapy

Embolus—a blood clot or other foreign substance that is carried in the bloodstream and has the potential to impede and/or obstruct circulation

Enteral nutrition—nutrition provided via the gastrointestinal tract

Epidemiology—the division of medical science concerned with defining and explaining the interrelationships of the host, agent, and environment in causing disease

Epidural—a potential space that is part of the spinal canal outside the dura mater. This space contains a network of large and thin-walled veins as well as fat that is proportional in volume to a person's body fat.

Epithelialization—the growth of epithelial cells over a wound or over and around a catheter site

Erythema—redness

Evidence-Based Practice—incorporates the best available evidence with the expertise of the nurse and the patient preferences in the context of care delivery

Extravasation—inadvertent escape of a solution or medication (usually a vesicant) into surrounding tissue

Factor V Leiden—the most common hereditary blood coagulation disorder in the United States; causes blood to have an increased tendency to clot (also called factor V Leiden)

Filter—a porous device used to prevent the passage of undesired substances

Filtration—process of passing fluid through a filter using pressure

Free flow—referring to nonregulated, inadvertent administration of fluid

Fungi—vegetable cellular organisms that subsist on organic matter

Gram-negative bacteria—organisms that remain unstained by Gram method, including *Klebsiella*, *Escherichia coli*, *Pseudomonas*, *Serratia*, etc.; associated with infusate contamination and arterial catheters

Gram-positive bacteria—organisms holding the dye after being stained by Gram method, including *Staphylococcus aureus*, *S. epidermidis*, and others; associated with venous catheter contamination

Grounded theory—theory that is constructed from theoretical propositions based on data obtained in the real world

Health literacy—an individual's ability to access, read, interpret, and comprehend health information

High fidelity—as close to a live patient situation as possible, placing the learner in a realistic environment

Hematocrit—an expression of the volume of red cells per unit of circulating blood

Hematogenous—produced by or derived from the blood; disseminated through the bloodstream or via circulation

Hematoma—usually refers to uncontrolled bleeding at a venipuncture site, generally creating a hard, painful lump

Hemodynamic pressure monitoring—the measurement of pulmonary artery pressure, arterial pressure, cardiac output, and so forth, via an electronic monitor and internally placed catheter

Hemoglobin—the iron-containing pigment of red blood cells; functions primarily in transporting oxygen from the lungs to the body tissues

Hemolysis—rupture of the red blood cell membrane causing the release of hemoglobin

Hemorrhage—abnormal discharge of blood, either external or internal

Hemostasis—cessation of the flow of blood through a port or vessel

HLA system—human leukocyte antigens; a complex array of genes that are involved in immune system regulation and cell differentiation

Homeostasis—ability to restore equilibrium under stress

Human patient simulators—fully automatic mannequins with comprehensive clinical functioning and react to the learner's actions or inactions.

Hypercalcemia—serum calcium concentrations above normal levels

Hyperkalemia—excess of potassium in the blood

Hypertonic—solution more concentrated than that with which it is compared; a fluid having a concentration greater than the normal tonicity of plasma

Hyperuricemia—uric acid blood concentrations above normal levels

Hypodermoclysis—use of the subcutaneous route as a vehicle for absorption of IV isotonic

Hypokalemia—low potassium concentration in the blood

Hypotonic—solution less concentrated than that with which it is compared; a fluid having a concentration less than the normal tonicity of plasma

IgA—immunoglobulin A; a class of immunoglobulins in body secretions

IgG—immunoglobulin G; a class of immunoglobulins or circulating antibodies in the blood that frequently causes sensitization

IgM—immunoglobulin M; a class of immunoglobulins or circulating antibodies in the blood that is capable of binding complement

Immediate reaction—in blood transfusions, an adverse effect occurring immediately or up to 48 hours after the transfusion

Immunocompromised—having decreased resistance to disease

Immunoglobulin—a protein with antibody activity

Immunohematology—the study of blood and blood reactions

Implanted port or pump—vascular access device placed totally beneath the skin surface by surgical procedure

Incident—an unusual occurrence that requires documentation and action because of potential or implied consequences

Incompatible—incapable of being mixed or used simultaneously without undergoing chemical or physical changes or producing undesirable effects

Infection—invasion of the body by living microorganisms

Infiltration—the inadvertent administration of a nonvesicant solution or medication into surrounding tissues

Infusate—parenteral solution administered into the vascular system

Integumentary—cutaneous; dermal

Interferons (IFNs)—cytokines that initiate immune responses that are antiviral, antitumor, and immunomodulatory

Interleukins—cytokines that stimulate the migration of active immune cells to the tumor

Intermittent intravenous therapy—IV therapy administered at prescribed intervals with periods of infusion cessation

International normalized ratio (INR)—the PT (prothrombin time) ratio that would have been obtained using the World Health Organization reference PT reagent

Interval variables—an ordered set of categories if categories form a set of intervals that are all exactly the same

Intraosseous—within the cavity of a bone that is filled with marrow

Intrathecal—a space that contains cerebral spinal fluid and bathes the spinal cord. The intrathecal space runs parallel to the epidural space. The two spaces are separated by the dura mater.

Intrinsic contamination—contamination during product manufacture

Isolation—the separation of potentially infectious persons and/or materials

Isotonic—solution having the same concentration as that with which it is compared (i.e., plasma)

Laminar flow hood—a contained work area in which the air flow within the area moves with uniform velocity along parallel flow lines with a minimum of eddies

Latex injection port—a resealable rubber cap over any opening, designed to accommodate needles; for administration of solutions into the vascular system or for access to a vial

Leukopenia—total number of leukocytes in the circulating blood less than normal, the lower limit of which generally is regarded as 5,000/μL

Low fidelity—a teaching environment that is not realistic but with a focus on skill development

Lumen—the interior space of a tubular structure, such as a blood vessel or cannula

Lymphedema—swelling of an extremity caused by obstruction of the lymphatic vessel(s)

Magnet recognition—recognizes health care organizations for quality patient care, nursing excellence, and innovations in professional nursing practice

Malignancy—uncontrolled growth and dissemination of a neoplasm

Malnutrition—any disorder of nutritional status including those resulting from a deficient intake of nutrients, impaired nutrient metabolism, or overnutrition

Medical act—procedure performed by a physician/licensed independent practitioner

mEq— milliequivalent; the measure of the chemical-combining power of an ion with hydrogen

Metastasis—the spread of cancer to sites distant from the site of origin

Microabrasion—break in skin integrity, which may predispose the patient to infection

Microaggregate—microscopic collection of particles, such as platelets, leukocytes, and fibrin, that occurs in stored blood

Microaggregate blood filter—device that removes potentially harmful microaggregates and reduces nonhemolytic febrile reactions

Microorganisms—extremely minute living matter that can be seen only with the aid of a microscope

Midline—peripherally inserted catheter with tip terminating in the proximal portion of the extremity, usually 6 inches long

Monoclonal antibody—antibody produced by a clone of cells derived from a single cell in large quantities for use against a specific antigen

Morbidity—number of infected persons or cases of infection in relation to a specific population

Mortality—ratio of number of deaths in a population to number of individuals in that population

Multiple-dose vial—medication bottle that is hermetically sealed with a rubber stopper and designed to be entered more than one time

Nadir—the lowest level; in chemotherapy, the nadir is the lowest level to which the blood count drops in response to an antineoplastic agent.

Needle—a slender, pointed, hollow metal device

Neoadjuvant—the use of chemotherapy prior to treatment for localized cancer when the local therapy is less than completely effective

Neoplasm—a new growth or tumor, either benign or malignant

Nitrosoureas—anticancer drugs that produce metabolites that attack DNA in a manner analogous to alkylating agents

Nominal variables—names of categories

Nonpermeable—able to maintain integrity

Nonvesicant—intravenous medications, including, but not limited to, medications administered for cancer; these medications generally do not cause damage or sloughing of tissue

Nutrients—proteins, carbohydrates, lipids, vitamins, minerals, trace elements, and water

Nutritional assessment—a comprehensive evaluation to define nutritional status; includes medical history, dietary history, physical examination, anthropometric measurements, and laboratory data

Nutritional screening—the process of identifying characteristics known to be associated with nutrition problems, particularly in individuals who are at risk for malnutrition or who are malnourished

Nutritional support—provision of specially formulated and/or delivered parenteral or enteral nutrients to maintain or restore optimal nutrition status

Occlusion—a blockage, which may result from precipitation or clot formation

Oncology—the study of tumors

Oncotic—within the tissue; relating to tissue pressure

Opiate receptor sites—cells that receive only one particular kind of drug. These are located in the dorsal horn of the spinal cord and the periaqueductal gray region of the brain. The discovery of spinal opiate receptors in 1973 led to the development of selective spinal opiate analgesia.

Opioids—narcotics that stimulate the opiate receptor site to produce analgesia

Ordinal variables—sets of ordered categories

Osmolarity—number of solutes contained in solution measured in milliosmoles per liter

Outcome—the interpretation of documented results; educational goal

Palliative—treatment that may be provided for comfort and/or temporary relief of symptoms but that does not cure

Palpable cord—a vein that is rigid and hard to the touch

Palpation—examination by touch

Parenteral—denoting any route other than the alimentary canal, such as intravenous

Parenteral nutrition—nutrients that are administered intravenously, comprising carbohydrates, proteins, and/or fats, and additives, such as electrolytes, vitamins, and trace elements

Paresthesia—abnormal spontaneous sensations (e.g., burning, prickling, tingling, or tickling without physical stimulus)

Particulate matter—relating to or composed of fine particles

Pathogens—disease-producing microorganisms

PCA—patient-controlled analgesia

Peak level—time of highest drug concentration

Percutaneous puncture—puncture performed through the skin

Peripheral—pertaining to veins of the extremities, scalp, and external jugular; not central

Peripheral neuropathy—dysfunction of postganglionic nerves, ranging from paresthesia to paralysis

Peristalsis—progressive wave-like movement that occurs involuntarily

Phlebitis—inflammation of a vein; may be accompanied by pain, erythema, edema, streak formation, and/or palpable cord; rated by a standard scale (see "Phlebitis" topic); a possible precursor to sepsis

Phlebotomy—withdrawal of blood from a vein

Physical incompatibility—an undesirable change that is visually observed

Plant alkaloids—anticancer drugs derived from plants, such as the periwinkle (vincristine and vinblastine) in the *Vinca* family

Point of care testing—medical testing at or near the site of patient care

Port—usually refers to device implanted into subcutaneous tissue. See Implanted Port. May refer to hub of catheter tubing for infusion access

Positive pressure—maintaining a constant, even force within a lumen to prevent reflux of blood; achieved while injecting by clamping or withdrawing needle from cannula

Postinfusion phlebitis—inflammation of a vein occurring after cannula removal and often due to a specific drug

Pounds per square inch (psi)—a measurement of pressure; 1 psi equals 50 mm Hg or 68 cm H_2O

Preservative free—containing no added substance capable of inhibiting bacterial contamination

Priming—initial filling of the administration set with infusate

Process—actual performance and observation of performance based on compliance with policies, procedures, and professional standards

Product integrity—state of product that is intact and uncompromised; condition suitable for intended use

Professional development—lifelong process of continuing education to remain current in one's career or occupation

Proximal—nearest to the heart; closest to point of attachment; above previous site of cannulation

Pruritus—itching

Psychomotor—referring to behaviors that place primary emphasis on the various degrees of physical skills and dexterity as they relate to the thought process

Purpura—condition in which spontaneous bleeding occurs in subcutaneous tissue resulting in purple patches visible on the skin

Purulent—containing or producing pus

Push—direct injection of a medication into a vein or access device

Quality indicator—a systematic process for monitoring, evaluating, and problem solving

Radiopaque—able to be detected by radiography

Ratio variables—interval variables with an absolute zero point, indicating absence of a point being measured

Reference range—the parameter or context in which to interpret results; it is established by testing a large number of healthy people and observing what appears to be normal for this group. This term is preferred over *normal range* because the reference population can be clearly defined.

Reflective practice—a planned and organized method of making sense of one's experiences, situations, or activities

Reflex sympathetic dystrophy (RSD)—a condition of burning pain, stiffness, swelling, and discoloration occurring in an area of injury, such as intravenous access

Research—systematic inquiry using an orderly method to answer a question and designed to contribute to generalizable knowledge

Rh system—a blood group system denoting the presence or absence of the D (Rh) red blood cell antigen

Risk management—process that centers on identification, analysis, treatment, and evaluation of real and potential hazards

Roller bandage—a roll of gauze or other material used for protecting an injured part, for immobilizing a limb, for keeping dressings in place, and so on

Sclerotic—referring to fibrous thickening of the wall of the vein resulting in decreased lumen size; on palpation, usually feels hard to the touch

Semiquantitative culture technique—a laboratory protocol used for isolating and identifying microorganisms

Sensitization—the initial exposure of an individual to a specific antigen that results in an immune response

Sentinel event—an unexpected occurrence involving death or serious physical or psychological injury, or the risk thereof

Sepsis—infectious microorganisms or their toxins in the bloodstream

Septum—a wall dividing two or more cavities

Simulation—a technique to mimic a situation or experience with the goal of allowing individuals to practice, learn, and understand a skill or more complex system of human interactions

Single-use vial—medication bottle intended for one-time use that is hermetically sealed with a rubber stopper

Skin–cannula junction—point at which the cannula enters the skin

Spike—insertion of the administration set into the solution container

Statistics—the science of collecting, classifying, and interpreting information based on the numbers of things

Stomatitis—sores on the inside of the mouth

Structure—describes the elements on which a program is based. Elements may include resources such as federal and state laws, professional standards, position descriptions, patient rights, policies and procedures, documentation forms, quality controls, corrective action programs, and so on.

Stylet—a rigid metal object within a catheter designed to facilitate insertion

Surfactant—material whose properties reduce the surface tension of fluid

Surveillance—the active, systematic, ongoing observation of the occurrence and distribution of disease within a population and of the events or conditions that increase or decrease the risk of such disease occurrence

Sympathetic—referring to the part of the autonomic nervous system responsible for the fight-or-flight response. The sympathetic system is dominant when a person experiences pain. The effects on the body are from a release of norepinephrine in the body, resulting in increased heart rate, blood pressure, and respiration.

Systemic—pertaining to the whole body rather than one of its parts

Tamper-proof—impossible to alter

Task trainer—a life-like model of a body part or organ, or a nonanatomical device to teach a skill, such as a specialized stethoscope to learn heart sounds.

Thrombocytopenia—decrease in thrombocyte or platelet count

Thrombolytic agent—a pharmacologic agent capable of dissolving blood clots

Thrombophlebitis—inflammation of the vein with clot formation

Thrombosis—formation of a blood clot within a blood vessel

Total nutrient admixture—parenteral nutrition formulation containing carbohydrates, amino acids, lipid, vitamins, minerals, trace elements, water, and other additives in a single container

Trace elements—minute amounts of essential elements present in the body

Transfusion reaction—any adverse effect to the transfusion of whole blood or its components or derivatives

Transitional feeding—progression from one mode of feeding to another, while continuously administering estimated nutrient requirements

Transparent semipermeable membrane (TSM)—a sterile dressing that allows visualization, repels water, and allows air to permeate it

Trendelenburg—a position in which the head is lower than the feet, used to increase venous distention

Trough level—time of lowest drug concentration

Tunneled catheter—a central catheter designed to have a portion lie within a subcutaneous passage before exiting the body

Valsalva maneuver—the process of making a forceful attempt at expiration with the mouth, nostrils, and glottis closed

Vascular access—means of approaching or entering the vascular system

Vascular access devices—catheters placed directly into the venous system for infusion therapy and/or phlebotomy

Venipuncture—puncture of a vein for any purpose

Ventricular reservoir—a device that, once implanted, provides direct access to the cerebrospinal fluid (CSF) without the need to perform a spinal tap

Vesicant—intravenous medication that causes tissue injury when it escapes into the surrounding tissue(s)

Volumetric—relating to measurement of a substance by its volume

INDEX